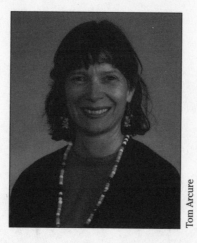

Tom Arcure

## *About the Author*

KATHI J. KEMPER, M.D., M.P.H., is a pediatrician on the faculty of Children's Hospital, Harvard Medical School, and the Mind-Body Medical Institute in Boston, Massachusetts. She has an international reputation as a pediatric researcher and educator and is director of the first center for holistic pediatric education and research in the United States, as well as a member of the prestigious American Pediatric Society. Dr. Kemper is former president of the Ambulatory Pediatric Association, as well as the first chair of its Special Interest Group on Holistic Medicine.

# THE HOLISTIC PEDIATRICIAN

# THE HOLISTIC PEDIATRICIAN

SECOND EDITION

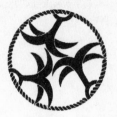

A Pediatrician's Comprehensive Guide to Safe and Effective Therapies for the 25 Most Common Ailments of Infants, Children, and Adolescents

✳

## Kathi J. Kemper, M.D., M.P.H.

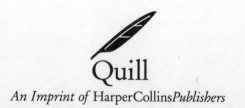

Quill

*An Imprint of HarperCollinsPublishers*

*This book is intended to educate parents about a variety of approaches to children's health care needs. This book should not be a substitute for the personal care and treatment of a qualified physician, but, rather, should be used in conjunction with a physician's care in order to consider the full range of health care options available to your child. The author and publisher expressly disclaim responsibility for any adverse effects resulting from the information contained herein. Before giving your child any of the herbal treatments recommended in this book, consult a physician or pharmacist for possible drug interactions.*

First Perennial edition published 1996.

First Quill edition published 2002.

*Designed by Nancy Singer Olaguera*

Library of Congress Cataloging-in-Publication Data

Kemper, Kathi.
   The holistic pediatrician: a pediatrician's comprehensive guide to safe and effective therapies for the 25 most common ailments of infants, children, and adolescents / Kathi J. Kemper.
      p. cm.
   First ed. published with subtitle: A parent's comprehensive guide to safe and effective therapies for the 25 most common childhood ailments.
   Includes bibliographical references and index.
   ISBN 0-06-008427-8
   1. Pediatrics—Popular works. 2. Holistic medicine. 3. Children—Diseases—Alternative treatment. I. Title.

RJ61 .K325 2002
618.92—dc21

2001039856

02 03 04 05 06 ❖/RRD 10 9 8 7 6 5 4 3 2 1

To Daniel Alexander Kemper

# CONTENTS

Contents

# FOREWORD TO THE SECOND EDITION

I am delighted to write the foreword to this outstanding reference work by my friend and colleague at Harvard Medical School, Dr. Kathi Kemper. I have known Dr. Kemper since she was recruited to the Boston Children's Hospital and Harvard Medical School in 1998.

This is an exciting time for medicine, but it is also a time that calls for caution and common sense. There is excitement as we begin to understand the basic mechanisms for ancient healing techniques such as meditation and the placebo effect. New diagnostic methods, medications, and procedures are developing rapidly, and the dissemination of health information is at an all-time high. The explosive growth in knowledge about genetics and immunology will soon render our current knowledge obsolete. On the other hand, hucksterism and quackery are alive and well. Con men manipulate millions via mass media and the Internet, and it takes a physician experienced in both traditional and alternative medicines to keep perspective in the face of sales tactics appealing to nature, forgotten mysteries, and forbidden fruits.

Modern medicine must be founded first of all on compassion for individual suffering and on a commitment to alleviating that suffering whenever possible. It must also be based on sound scientific principles and a basic understanding of human physiology, psychology, culture, and spirituality. Modern healers must maintain the dedication to their calling that defines professionalism. And we must be adept at evoking in our patients the fundamental experience of remembered wellness, of calling on the wondrous healing capacity, derived through evolution, that is present in every individual.

*The Holistic Pediatrician* reflects these values in abundance. Shortly after her arrival at Children's Hospital, Dr. Kemper's photogenic face graced the cover of *Boston Magazine,* in its feature on the "Best Doctors in Boston." The cover story was a wake-up call to physicians to remember that doctoring must encompass the *whole* patient—body, mind, emotions, and spirit—in the context of each patient's family, culture, and community. Dr. Kemper is widely known as *the* holistic pediatrician, and with good reason.

She has published more than sixty articles in peer-reviewed scientific and medical journals, including *The New England Journal of Medicine* and *The Journal of the American Medical Association.* She has lectured extensively, urging her audiences to become attuned to all of the factors affecting children's health—from social factors such as poverty and racism, to environmental factors such as organic foods, to psychological factors such as maternal depression. In the process, she has opened up new ways of providing health care to individuals and groups of children.

*The Holistic Pediatrician* provides a balanced, thoughtful approach to the common conditions affecting children and adolescents. Although I'm not an advocate of alternative medicine, I respect sound scientific researchers who critically examine the evidence for a variety of healing techniques and then synthesize this information to benefit others. This book achieves those goals admirably. I highly recommend *The Holistic Pediatrician* to all who have questions about their children's health, and desire a balanced, safe, and responsible guide.

*Herbert Benson, M.D.*
*President, Mind-Body Medical Institute*
*Associate Professor of Medicine,*
*Harvard Medical School*

# ACKNOWLEDGMENTS AND THANKS

No great work is accomplished in isolation. This was as true during the revision process as it was in writing the very first draft of *The Holistic Pediatrician*. I am deeply grateful to many people who supported me during this process of writing, talking, teaching, and practicing. Direct contributions that vastly improved the quality of this effort were made by:

The librarians in Boston and Seattle who performed amazing feats in locating all of the references: Alison Clapp at the Children's Hospital and Julia Whelan at the Massachusetts College of Pharmacy;

Research assistants, organizational and secretarial support: Elizabeth Hopfinger, Thomas Delaney, and Beth Allee;

Pediatric collaborators at Children's Hospital—holistic pediatricians one and all—Lisa Albers, Chuck Berde, Hank Bernstein, Danny Coles, Jack Maypole, Shari Nethersole, Wanessa Risko, Cassandra Walcott, Wendy Wornham, and the many residents, fellows, students, and attending staff at the Children's Hospital and the Dana Farber Cancer Institute. Special thanks to Dr. Allan Crocker and the members of the Children's Hospital Task Force on Holistic Pediatrics;

Help with herbs: Dr. Paula Gardiner, Lana Dvorkin, and June Riedlinger at Massachusetts College of Pharmacy; Andey Amata-Kynvi, who provided the organizational energy and skill to keep the Longwood Herbal Task Force and the Interent Herbal Education Project on track;

Help with mind-body therapies: Dr. Herbert Benson at the Mind-Body Medical Institute; MaryJane Ott, A.R.N.P., M.N.; the entire staff of the University of Massachusetts Medical Center Mindfulness Based Stress Reduction program, especially Saki Santorelli, Jon Kabat-Zinn, and Florence Meyer;

Help with acupuncture: Ellen Silver Highfield and Ted Kaptchuk;

Help with massage: Mary McLellan;

Help with homeopathy: Ted Chapman, Christine Luthra, Richard Moskowitz, and Janet Levatin in Boston and Jennifer Jacobs in Seattle;

The students who kept me energized and humble, especially Anne (CC) Lee and Catherine Chu;

Reiki Masters and guides: Roy Bauer, Larraine Bossi, and Dora Kunz;

The many friends, parents, and health care professionals who reviewed early drafts and continued to support and inspire me, especially Dr. Nancy Rudner (friend, nurse practitioner, public health advocate, and mother); Dr. Cora Breuner; Dr. Dedra Buchwald; Toni Weschler, M.P.H., Mary Gardiner; Melissa Ross; James, Juan, and Julia Cofield; Linda Barnes, Becky Sarah; and Frank Ackerman;

Colleagues and leaders in holistic medicine: Andy Weil, Herb Benson, David Eisenberg, Jim Gordon, Rick Leskowitz, Michael Lerner, James Dillard, Rachel Remen, Marilyn Schlitz, John Astin, Wayne Jonas, Tim Culbert, Greg Plotnikoff, Tracy Gaudet, Jim Overall, Fayez Ghishan, and all the wonderful folks in Arizona, Boston, and around the world who light the candles, dispelling darkness.

# INTRODUCTION

"We heard you were open to holistic medicine, and we wanted you to see our daughter, Shelly," Lisa and Larry Bradshaw began. "She's had asthma since she was nine months old, and she just isn't getting over it. We don't like the idea of giving her drugs every day, but we don't want her to be sick, either. We've treated ourselves with Chinese herbs and homeopathic remedies, but we aren't sure what's safe for a two-year-old like Shelly. Can you help?"

Lisa and Larry are typical of the growing number of parents who have sought and used alternative therapies for themselves and who want to provide the safest, most effective care for their children. There has been a veritable explosion in the number of books on holistic medicine over the last twenty years, but few of these books are aimed at providing pediatric care.

This book was written to educate and empower you to exercise your options in taking care of your child's health care needs. Parents are the primary providers of their children's health care. Parents manage their children's home environment, diet, and medical care. Mothers characteristically cope with most minor illnesses using home or folk remedies, and ask for advice from relatives and friends before seeking help from a health care professional. Parents are generally very competent in caring for their children's illnesses. With government, professional organization, and university-grade information available over the Internet, parents have become well-educated consumers of a variety of goods and services. In my practice, I see parents as the primary providers of health care and myself as their coach.

Many books written by physicians and psychologists discuss child development, behavior, health, and illness. However, none integrates the best of modern medical science with proven therapies from herbal medicine, homeopathy, and other healing techniques in a truly holistic approach to common childhood illnesses. This book does just that.

*Who needs another book on holistic medicine?* Parents do! A 1993 study in the *New England Journal of Medicine* reported that nearly one out of every three American adults used alternative medical therapies in 1990; by 1997, this percentage rose to over 40%. Many parents also seek alternative therapies for their children. When given an option between a non-drug home remedy and a drug, nearly 85% of parents prefer the home remedy. The families most likely to seek complementary and alternative care have children who suffer from a serious, chronic disease, such as rheumatoid arthritis, or children for whom traditional medical care has not been of much help, such as children suffering from recurrent ear infections or allergies. However, parents of healthy kids often use echinacea or vitamin C when their child has a cold, or try a back rub when the baby can't sleep.

Parents want the best for their children—safe, effective, personal care that is low in cost and side effects. Practitioners of "natural" therapies are often seen as providing more personalized care, listening to parents' concerns and preferences better than the average general practitioner. Most parents who seek alternative care are intelligent and well educated, and most take their children to regular medical doctors in addition to other types of health care providers.

*What is holistic medicine?* Holistic medicine has as many definitions as there are people. At times it seems that the term is used more as a marketing tool than as a description of a distinct approach to health care. Here's my definition:

Holistic medicine is the foundation of good medicine. It promotes the well-being and optimal functioning of the child in the context of family, culture, and community. Holistic practitioners see the whole child—body, mind, emotions, spirit, and relationships with others. From a variety of potential treatments, holistic practitioners choose those that are best suited to the individual child and family and integrate those therapies into a unique plan for each child and family.

One of the most holistic doctors I've ever met is Dr. David Heimbach, a burn surgeon at Harborview Medical Center in Seattle. You might wonder if a surgeon could really be holistic. Dr. Heimbach has assembled a team of plastic surgeons, nurses, physical and occupational therapists, pediatricians, nutritionists, social workers, and psychologists to help meet the needs of children who have suffered severe burns. When he takes care of a burned child, he looks not only at the burn, but at the whole child and the child's family. He makes sure that out-of-state families have a place to stay while their child is being treated and has implemented a fund to help pay for their housing. He asks about the child's school, friends, and church. On one occasion, he even made arrangements for a seriously burned child to be visited in the hospital by his puppy. (Yes, hygiene was maintained, and the visit was a rousing success for both boy and puppy.) The psychologists on the team use hypnosis to help children cope with the pain of the initial burn and the subsequent surgeries. Nutritionists help ensure that children are not only getting enough calories, but also additional vitamins and minerals to hasten healing. For children whose families are far away, Dr. Heimbach asks for volunteers from the community to play with, read to, and hold injured children. Yes, even surgeons in major academic medical centers can be holistic physicians.

On the other hand, practitioners who believe that all ailments can be traced to allergies, yeast infections, or vitamin deficiencies are no more holistic than those who believe that all illness is due to germs. Some worrisome providers refuse to refer a sick feverish child to a medical doctor because they think the problem can be fixed with an alternative therapy alone. These practitioners may call themselves holistic, but in fact they are ideologues with good marketing skills. Not all unconventional therapies are holistic, nor is mainstream medical practice necessarily NOT holistic. A single therapy, be it medication, surgery, nutrition, supplements, herbs, exercise, or massage is not holistic unless it is done in the context of the whole child.

I try to avoid the terms "alternative" and "unconventional" medicine, despite their widespread use, because they are very difficult to define. One's definition of "alternative" depends very much on what one considers mainstream. For many Americans, Chinese medicine is an alternative. But for Chinese-Americans, it is mainstream. Other so-called alternatives, such as chiropractic, are as American as apple pie. Hypnosis and acupuncture used to be considered unconventional, but they are now used in major medical centers across America. Rather than try to define mainstream, alternative, and unconventional medicine, we'll look at the therapies themselves (Chapter 1) and how they can complement each other.

*Illness versus disease.* Disease is an abnormal condition in the body. Illness is one's experience of abnormal or suboptimal functioning. You can have a disease such as cancer for weeks or months before symptoms develop and you feel ill. In general we *cure* disease and *heal* illness.

*Healing versus curing.* In this book, curing means the elimination of symptoms or signs of a disease. For example, a child is cured of pneumonia when the fever and the cough are gone, and signs of infection are gone from the X ray. There are no cures yet for many illnesses that affect children. The symptoms of cystic fibrosis may be minimized, but the underlying disease will not be eradicated until we come up with genetic therapies. Yet, even children with chronic or genetic diseases such as cystic fibrosis can be considered healed if they feel happy and loved and function as well as they'd like. Being healed is a state of mind and spirit. Being cured is a physical phenomenon. We can compare the cure rates of different therapies, but we cannot yet scientifically measure healing. When I describe the effectiveness of different therapies, I am talking about the effectiveness of those therapies in curing, not healing.

## About the Author

I am a pediatrician, a medical doctor specializing in the care of children. My medical training has spanned many years at several institutions—the University of North Carolina (M.D. and master's degree in Public Health, specializing in maternal and child health), the University of Wisconsin (internship and residency in pediatrics), and Yale University (fellowship training in pediatric research). In 1988, I joined the faculty of the University of Washington, where I taught medical students and pediatric residents how to be good pediatricians. In 1994, I joined the staff of Swedish Medical Center in Seattle, helping to train family doctors in pediatrics. Shortly after the first edition of *The Holistic Pediatrician* was published, I was elected president of the Ambulatory Pediatric Association—an international academic organization of some of the top pediatricians in the world. That was also the year I became a mom, and I can assure you that being a doctor is far easier than being a mother! In 1998, I was recruited by Harvard Medical School to become the first director of the new Center for Holistic Pediatric Education and Research at Children's Hospital in Boston—the first such center in the country. I have had over sixty scientific articles and chapters published in medical journals such as the *New England Journal of Medicine* and the *Journal of the American Medical Association*. I have also been a consultant and writer for popular magazines and Internet sites.

Throughout my training and professional experience, I have learned and been stimulated to do research the most by my patients and their families. And now, of course, by my son, who is the best teacher in the world. My colleagues in Seattle and Boston and now throughout the United States have taught me an enormous amount about healing, about teaching, about writing grants and proposals, about starting and maintaining a new enterprise, and mostly about myself. To all of these teachers and mentors, I am thankful.

## About the Book

This book is organized for you to read selectively. You do not need to read it from cover to cover. I suggest that you read the first and second chapters, and then skip to the chapters that are pertinent for your particular child. By reading the first chapter first, you will be better able to understand all of the rest of the chapters. Chapter 1, "The Therapeutic Mountain," describes a paradigm for integrative medicine which I developed in 1994 and have taught to thousands of pediatricians and parents to help us understand the relationship between different types of therapies. This chapter covers the therapies, the professionals who recommend them, and how to select a practitioner for your child. Chapter 2, "Trust Me, I'm a Doctor," is a short description of how you can evaluate claims for different treatments and decide which are effective for your child.

*Note on organization:* To maintain a consistent, systematic, comprehensive approach, all of the chapters on a particular illness and conditions are organized the same way, outlined in Chapter 1. If you want a quick summary of how to treat a particular condition, see the last section in each chapter, "What I Recommend."

*Note on gender:* To avoid using cumbersome phrases such as he/she and him/her, I have alternated males and females by chapter throughout the book. All of the case stories are composite descriptions of patient encounters; to preserve patient confidentiality, fictitious names, gender, and ethnicity are used.

# THE HOLISTIC PEDIATRICIAN

# 1

# THE THERAPEUTIC
# MOUNTAIN

"I've taken my child to so many doctors, I've lost count," Helen began. "The pediatrician put him on antibiotics to prevent any more ear infections, but the medicines gave him diarrhea and a yeast infection. The chiropractor said that adjusting his neck would help, but I didn't think it helped much and I didn't like all the X rays. The naturopath recommended some herbs and vitamins, but my insurance wouldn't pay for them. None of these doctors thought the other ones did any good; they all seemed more interested promoting their own particular therapy than in working with each other to help my child. I'm frustrated and confused. How can the best, the safest, and most effective of all available treatments be combined for my child?"

Helen's story epitomizes many families' complaints about the health care system. In the 1990s, my colleague at Harvard, Dr. David Eisenberg, published two landmark scientific surveys in the *New England Journal of Medicine* and the *Journal of the American Medical Association;* his research showed that the percentage of Americans using complementary and alternative medical (CAM) therapies increased from about 30% to over 40% in less than ten years. Dr. John Astin followed this work with extensive interviews to find out why CAM was so popular in an era in which mainstream medicine and public health had achieved unprecedented success; he found that many people felt that CAM therapies and therapists relied on values and worldviews that were more consistent with their personal beliefs than the very objective, technology-rich world of modern medicine.

Different kinds of practitioners have different theories, rely on different treatments, and often compete rather than cooperate with one another. It doesn't have to be this way. Rather than being polarized and competitive, healing can be family-centered, integrated, cooperative, and holistic. In her bestselling books, *Kitchen Table Wisdom* and *My Grandfather's Blessings*, pediatrician Dr. Rachel Remen has shared story after beautiful story about the heart of healing.

The bedrock underlying all true healing is the clear intention to express and embody *compassion*. Whether the health care provider is a physician, nurse, acupuncturist, herbalist, or parent, concern for the patient's well-being is the first prerequisite for healing. Healers also need to be deeply mindful of the most peaceful, harmonious aspects of themselves and bring that awareness to the fore when working with infants, children, adolescents, and their families. I believe that the best healers are incredibly *mindful*, and I encourage my students, residents, and colleagues to commit to a daily meditation practice (such as the ones described by Jon Kabat-Zinn in *Full Catastrophe Living* and by Saki Santorelli in *Heal Thy Self*) to strengthen this nonjudgmental awareness in themselves.

Ideally, both professionals and parents lay aside their personal concerns when faced with an ill child. The focus should be on the child's and family's goals for wellness and healing.

## GOALS OF HEALING

- Cure disease
- Manage or mitigate symptoms
- Prevent disease or disability
- Promote health and vitality; rehabilitation
- Eliminate toxins and minimize stress
- Enhance harmony, connections to family and community; be present
- Promote inner peace

My patients and colleagues have taught me that many different goals can be valid and held simultaneously. Most doctors immediately think of the goal of *curing disease;* this is appropriate and achievable when the problem is pneumococcal pneumonia, but it is not feasible for all patients with all conditions. Mainstream medicine is also pretty good at another goal, *managing* or *mitigating symptoms;* we can use eyeglasses to manage near-sightedness, insulin to manage diabetes, and ibuprofen or massage to relieve pain. Pediatricians promote immunizations as a cost-effective way to *prevent* serious infectious diseases such as whooping cough, tetanus, and rubella; in fact, modern public health has effectively eradicated the scourge of smallpox and is on its way toward eliminating polio, too. Most primary care physicians are also interested in broader issues of *health promotion,* such as avoiding tobacco smoke, encouraging exercise, and counseling about healthy diets and sleep; many alternative and complementary therapies such as massage, homeopathy, and naturopathy are also geared toward health promotion. The *elimination of toxins* is an old idea in medicine; however, aside from environmental medicine, it doesn't hold much appeal for doctors. On the other hand, psychologists and many complementary therapists are keenly interested in ridding stress, pesticides, genetically modified foods, hormones, antibiotics, and chemicals from our environments and bodies. Ideas of *harmony* and being present or connected with each other are well described in Native American and Asian medical systems, and are incorporated to at least some extent in Western mainstream medicine in terms of the importance of the "doctor-patient relationship." Goals such as *serenity* and *inner peace* are often thought of as spiritual goals, but certainly for those at the end of life, these become the primary objectives of care. Obviously, a person and a family can hold several

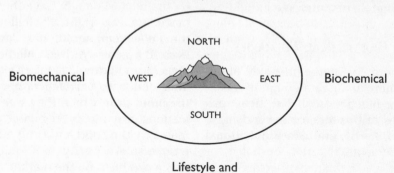

Therapeutic Mountain

Bioenergetic

NORTH

WEST        EAST

Biomechanical                                    Biochemical

SOUTH

Lifestyle and
Mind-body

goals simultaneously, and it is important to clarify which goals are being sought with particular therapies or therapists.

In addition to the traditional models of Eastern and Western medicine, there are many other healing traditions. Massage, herbal medicine, ritual, and prayer have been used around the world since ancient times. Chiropractic and osteopathy are nineteenth-century American inventions. The use of vitamins and nutritional supplements to prevent and cure illness is largely a twentieth-century phenomenon. Nowadays, dietary supplements are the fastest growing market in health care.

I have spent many years thinking about the different kinds of healing techniques, trying to find ways to bridge the gulf that exists between different kinds of health practitioners. I wanted to put the patient back in the center of the picture, and to create a paradigm or model in which all therapies could be seen as related and complementary to one another, on common ground in their pursuit of the highest and best for their patients. The image that emerged has gone through many iterations—a wheel, a cross, a four-leaf clover, and finally the Therapeutic Mountain. Over the many years I have now used this model, it has held

up well and been adopted by thousands of healers and researchers across the United States and around the world.

The mountain is an archetypal symbol of a high goal, achieved with dedication, preparation, persistence, and hard work. Such is the nature of healing. The goal is the well-being of the patient in the context of the family and greater community. Regardless of background, the healer must be dedicated to this goal, undergo months and years of training, and continue to learn from and listen to each patient, refining and enhancing his or her skills.

There are many sides to a mountain and many ways to reach the top. For the sake of simplicity, we will picture all of the primary healing modalities as occurring on one of four sides of the Therapeutic Mountain.

## THERAPEUTIC MOUNTAIN

1. East Side:     Biochemical Therapies
2. South Side:    Lifestyle and Mind-Body Therapies
3. West Side:     Biomechanical Therapies
4. North Side:    Bioenergetic Therapies

Therapies on each side of the mountain are grouped together because of their functional similarities. Let's look at each side of the Therapeutic Mountain in more detail.

## SIDE 1 (EAST): BIOCHEMICAL THERAPIES

All of the therapies on the east side of the Therapeutic Mountain share a common mechanism of action: biochemistry. The three primary techniques of this side of the mountain are medications, herbs, and other nutritional or dietary supplements.

### BIOCHEMICAL THERAPIES

- Medications
- Herbal Remedies
- Nutritional or Dietary Supplements

Each molecule of a therapeutic compound—whether it is a medication, an herb, or a vitamin—interacts with tiny molecules far smaller than even a single cell.

### Medications

When most of us think of medical therapy, the first thing that comes to mind is taking *medication*. Medication is any compound that is taken into or applied to the body with the intent of healing. Medications have very specific meanings legally that have implications for the standards by which they are manufactured and marketed. Today, most medicines are chemically synthesized, but originally many were derived from plants.

Amoxicillin is a good example. The most common medicine used to treat children with ear infections, amoxicillin is a modern version of penicillin. In 1928, a Scottish microbiologist, Alexander Fleming, noticed that a blue *Penicillium* mold growing on his laboratory cultures of *Staphylococcus* was killing the bacteria. Just as he was about to throw the ruined cultures away, he realized that the mold's deadly effect on the bacteria might have therapeutic importance. He was right. Penicillin, derived from the *Penicillium* mold, has saved millions of lives. By using synthetic medications such as penicillin, children can take a simple pill, syrup, or injection to get well rather than ingesting the mold from which they were derived. Medications are highly regulated in the United States by the Food and Drug Administration to ensure safety, purity, uniformity, and potency of the products on the market.

Medications are lifesaving when it comes to acute, severe illnesses such as shock, meningitis, and septicemia. They are also highly effective in managing certain chronic illnesses such as diabetes and asthma and in curing previously fatal diseases such as childhood leukemia. However, medications are practically useless in curing many common childhood illnesses such as colds and coughs. Even used properly, medications have side effects. Antibiotics, for example, commonly cause stomachaches, diarrhea, and diaper rashes; for 1 in 10,000 children they cause a severe allergic reaction that can lead to death.

Though many medications can be purchased by parents over the counter, prescription medication is available only with a physician's order. M.D.'s (Doctors of Medicine), D.O.'s (Doctors of Osteopathy), and dentists are fully licensed to prescribe medications. Nurse Practitioners have master's degrees, and they are licensed to prescribe many common medications. Physician's Assistants (P.A.'s) prescribe only under physician supervision. Only a handful of states license Naturopathic doctors (N.D.'s); most allow naturopaths to prescribe from a small list of certain medications, but do not allow them to prescribe other kinds of medication. Other health care providers are not licensed to prescribe regulated medications.

Always ask about the risks, benefits, side effects, and alternatives to prescription medications. Many pharmacies carry drug information sheets that describe specific medications and their effects in detail. Internet sites for large pharmacy chains also often provide this kind of information. In this book, each chapter on a particular illness will give you information on nonprescription and prescription medications used in treating that particular condition. A number of academic, governmental, and commercial sites on the Internet provide information about medications, and even the old standard, the *Physicians Desk Reference* (PDR) is available online.

## Herbs

Herbal, botanical, or phyto-therapeutic medicines have been used around the world since ancient times to prevent and cure disease. Herbal medicines contain a complex mixture of chemicals. Some people feel Nature combined the ingredients in plants for good reason, more wisely than a chemist distilling out a single active ingredient. For many herbal remedies, the active ingredient has not yet been identified, extracted, or synthesized in a laboratory. For example, chamomile tea (prescribed by Peter Rabbit's mother) is used around the world to soothe distressed babies and children. Its therapeutic effect does not depend on a single ingredient, but on a complex mixture of different chemicals that has not been duplicated in any lab.

Regardless of whether you take the chemically isolated, active ingredient (medication) or an herbal compound, herbs and medicines work basically the same way. That is, the active ingredient interacts with particular molecules in the body or bacteria to achieve their beneficial effect. Medication is more highly purified and herbs contain more of the original natural ingredients, but their effectiveness is due to the same principles of organic chemistry.

Herbs tend to be both more subtle and more variable in their effects than medications. Because herbs are natural products, their potency and purity vary. As recent studies commissioned by the *New York Times, Los Angeles Times, Boston Globe,* and other publications have pointed out, the concentration of active ingredients can vary ten- to a hundred-fold in products made by the same manufacturer. This is particularly scary for products such as ephedra, in which the margin between help and harm is narrow. Many herbal products contain none of the active ingredients listed in the label. This makes the potential for being ripped off when buying herbal products high. Mercury, arsenic, and lead contaminate many herbal remedies imported from developing countries. About one-third of Asian patent medicine (herbs compounded and sold in pill form) are intentionally "spiked" with medications such as steroids and antibiotics to enhance their effectiveness; the labels typically do not provide this information in English. At Children's Hospital we cared for a boy whose seizures were being treated with both mainstream medications and a Chinese patent medicine; he became sleepier and sleepier, and when he ended up in the intensive care unit, the toxicologist determined that the "herbs" he was taking actually contained high concentrations of phenobarbital and bromides, potent anticonvulsants that could cause a fatal interaction with his other medicines. Fortunately, the mystery was solved and he recovered, but it was a powerful lesson for all of us of the dangers of using Asian patent medicines.

Currently, herbal products are not regulated by the FDA the same way as medications, so standardization and quality control are quite variable. Safety is only addressed after a product is on the market and the FDA begins to receive reports of serious side effects. This lack of regulation doesn't matter very much if you're treating a stomachache with home-grown peppermint tea, but it could cause problems if you are using more potent herbs or use adult-sized doses for a child. The use of adult-sized doses of Chinese herbal medicine, Jin Bu Huan, resulted in the near-fatal poisoning of three children in 1993, and since then there have been numerous reports of serious toxicity associated with using herbal products. *You cannot assume that a product is safe simply because it is natural.* Nor can you assume that government regulations provide consumer protection for herbs the same way they do for medications.

Family members, friends, folk healers, shamans, medicine men, chiropractors, naturopaths, Ayurvedic physicians, practitioners of traditional Chinese medicine, and even some medical doctors recommend herbal remedies. No one has to have a degree in botany or biochemistry to prescribe herbs. Herbs are not a panacea. Practitioners should be aware of when a child's illness is amenable to herbal therapies and when another type of therapy (medication, vitamins, massage, etc.) would be more effective. Beware of anyone who claims that herbs can cure anything that ails your child. That is no more holistic than claiming that medications cure everything. I do not recommend you use an herb unless you or someone you trust can recognize the herb and has overseen the preparation of the product you use for your child. For scientific information about herbs, see the website we developed for the Longwood Herbal Task Force in conjunction with the Massachusetts College of Pharmacy: http://www.mcp.edu/herbal/. For objective information about the different commercially available products, check the website for ConsumerLabs: http://www.consumerlabs.com.

## Nutritional or Dietary Supplements

Vitamins and minerals are essential for maintaining health. A deficiency of any of the essential vitamins or minerals causes illness. British sailors recognized and effectively prevented scurvy by bringing along a supply of vitamin C–rich limes, hence their nickname Limeys. Normally, the body's needs for vitamins and minerals can be met adequately with a healthy diet emphasizing fruits, vegetables, and whole grains.

Nutritional supplements, including foods such as garlic extracts, are also recommended as treatments for a variety of ailments. Vitamin C can reduce the duration of common cold symptoms in adults. Extra vitamins A, D, E, and K are required by children with the genetic disease cystic fibrosis. Magnesium given intravenously can help children hospitalized with asthma. Children who require daily seizure medicine may need nutritional supplements to counteract some of the medication's effects. Toddlers who drink more than three or four glasses of cow's milk a day often need extra iron. Supplements may also be useful for children who do not eat a balanced, healthy diet. It turns out that only about 1% of American children meet their required dietary allowance (RDA) of nutrients through their diet. I typically recommend a good daily multivitamin/multimineral to just about everybody. Because brands and formulations change so often, you may want to check with the Center for Science in the Public Interest (CSPI) publication, Nutrition Action Newsletter (http://www.cspinet.org/nah/index.htm) or Consumer Reports on Health (http://www.consumerreports.org/services/health.html). These groups regularly compare vitamin products.

As with medicine, high doses of certain vitamins and minerals can have dangerous side effects. Although vitamin A is important for normal vision, too much can cause problems in the brain, liver, bones, and skin. Excessive vitamin C causes diarrhea. Iron overdoses can be fatal. Garlic poultices cause burns if left too long on delicate skin. Nature designed us to be in balance. When we take super-high doses of any one substance, we run the risk of upsetting the balance. That which has the power to cure also has the power to harm.

As with herbal remedies, no particular license is required to recommend nutritional supplements, and there are a lot deceptive claims (pro and con) about the need for supplementation. Unfortunately, there is little standardization in nutrition education and far too little research on optimal use of supplements in children. Medical doctors and osteopaths receive more training than in the past, but most rely on trained nutritionists (registered dietitians, R.D.'s) to help children who have complex nutritional needs. I have found dietitians to be among the most knowledgeable health professionals when it comes to dietary supplements. Naturopaths and chiropractors also receive nutrition education, but it may not be specifically geared to children's needs. Be sure to ask your health care practitioner about his or her training in pediatric nutrition, because it is a specialized field.

## SIDE 2 (SOUTH): LIFESTYLE THERAPIES

All of the therapies on the south side of the Therapeutic Mountain have such common-sense benefits that we sometimes forget how potent they are. The techniques of this side of the mountain are integral to healing traditions worldwide.

### LIFESTYLE THERAPIES

- Nutrition
- Exercise
- Environment
- Mind-Body Therapies

All of these factors are primarily regulated by the child and family with occasional profes-sional advice. Nutrition, exercise, environment, and mind-body interactions are a habitual part of daily life. As components of lifestyle, they are under our control, but paradoxically take more effort to change than using a pill or syrup. It's harder to transform a fast-food diet into a healthy whole foods regimen than to take vitamins. It's more challenging to develop and maintain an exercise program than to take high blood pressure medicine. Despite the challenges involved in changing lifestyle and habits, parents who are interested in their child's lifelong health make the effort to learn about and use these therapies.

### Nutrition

"You are what you eat." Proper nutrition is the backbone of a healthy lifestyle. A child's nutritional needs change as he develops. Appropriate nutrition for the child begins with the mother's diet at the time of conception. It includes not only what she eats and drinks, but just as importantly, what she avoids, e.g., alcohol, tobacco, and drugs. After delivery, newborn babies need mother's milk, not fruits and vegetables. Young children increase their food vocabulary one food at a time and gradually adopt their families' eating habits. By the time children reach adolescence, the nutritional patterns for a lifetime have been established.

Nutritional therapy is especially important for children suffering from chronic conditions (such as cystic fibrosis and cancer) and for children recovering from major trauma (such as injuries and burns). For everyday problems (such as constipation), you can easily treat your child with extra servings of fruit and bran muffins. Children with special health care needs or suspected food allergies need the help of a trained dietitian.

Anyone, regardless of training, can offer nutritional advice. Registered Dietitians (R.D.'s) have advanced training in nutrition. Be a smart consumer of nutritional advice. When someone recommends a particular diet (macrobiotic, low fat, etc.), ask to see the data showing that it has proven helpful in a child like yours. Children can grow perfectly well on vegetarian diets, but I have seen several young children who were growing and developing poorly because their parents had been erroneously advised to put them on a low-fat diet before they'd completed their infant growth spurt. (See Chapter 2 for more advice on evaluating health claims.) Check your sources before making radical changes in your child's diet. *What is helpful for adults may not be helpful for children.*

You can help your child heal and prevent future problems by modifying your own lifestyle. Avoiding cigarette smoke is a crucial element of therapy for childhood asthma, allergies, colds, and ear infections. Smoking, excessive drinking, and drug use have obvious adverse effects. These habits almost always start during adolescence, and are often learned from the child's primary role models—parents. Save your child the later struggle of overcoming an addiction by quitting these habits yourself *now*. Demonstrate your commitment to your child's healthy nutrition and the future health of the planet we share by planting an organic garden. Your child will be delighted to learn where real food comes from, have a better appreciation of the work involved in obtaining it, and perhaps develop a healthy hobby for the rest of his life!

## Exercise

A proper balance of exercise and rest is basic to maintaining health and is an important element of healing when we become ill. Exercise releases the body's own antidepressants and painkillers. Exercise improves circulation, lung function, and brain function. Whether it is organized soccer or a backyard game, exercise is good for children. Other habits, such as excessive time in front of the television, pro-

mote a sedentary lifestyle and compete with more active pursuits. Developing a routine of regular physical activity during childhood is an antidote to the frightening national epidemics of obesity and "couch potatoitis."

Exercise therapy includes everything from strengthening muscles and joints after an injury to yoga breathing exercises to help with asthma. Exercise can help children deal with stress, lift layers of depression, and build self-esteem.

Outside the specialized area of sports medicine, professional training in exercise therapy for children is limited. A therapeutic exercise program should be tailor-made for each individual child.

Most children suffering from a short-term illness such as a cold, flu, ear infection, or diarrhea will rest more and exercise less. Rest is as important as exercise in allowing the body's energy to be redirected to healing. Do not push your child to romp and play when he's acutely ill.

## Environment

Children are extraordinarily sensitive to their physical and emotional environments. Unhealthy environments, burdened with pollution, noise, violence, poverty, sexism, and racism are leading causes of illness in children. When trying to help heal a child, paying attention to the environment pays off. Environmental activism is simply health care on a larger scale. Specific examples of environmental therapies for children are:

- Air filters to remove airborne allergens
- Tepid baths to reduce the itching of chicken pox or eczema
- Phototherapy (special waves of sunlight) to reduce newborn jaundice
- White noise to soothe a colicky baby

- Ice packs to minimize swelling of a sprained ankle
- Mist tents for croup

Never underestimate the therapeutic value of the smell of home cooking or the presence of the child's favorite blanket or stuffed animal. Like herbal and nutritional therapies, no formal degrees or licenses are required to make recommendations about environmental therapy. Much of the wisdom about environmental therapies is simply based on experience or common sense. If you want to play a more active role, check out the Environmental Health Coalition (http://www.environmentalhealth.org/links.html) or Toxic Environments Affect Children's Health, TEACH (http://www.tr-teach.org/index.html). The Environmental Protection Agency's website also contains a wealth of free information that is relevant for families (http://www.epa.gov/ow/citizen/health.html).

## Mind-Body Therapies

Mind-body therapies encompass a range of techniques from behavior management to self-hypnosis and professional psychological counseling. Perhaps the most well-known technique for relaxing the mind is the Relaxation Response, described by my warm, wise colleague at Harvard, Dr. Herbert Benson. Around the world, the Relaxation Response and other meditative techniques are used to calm the mind and emotions of patients with high blood pressure, cancer, and other chronic illnesses.

Even infants learn to calm themselves by sucking on their hands or a pacifier. Older children learn more complex techniques to calm themselves. Relaxation therapies have beneficial effects on conditions ranging from asthma to chronic diarrhea. They can also improve concentration for tests and sports.

Despite its popular image as a theatrical technique used to get hapless victims to embarrass themselves in public, *hypnosis* is a safe, effective therapy used with thousands of children. It has been endorsed by the American Psychiatric Association, American Psychological Association, and American Dental Association. It is widely used by pediatricians, pediatric psychologists, and behavioral therapists to assist children confronted by pain, chronic headaches, and behavioral problems such as bedwetting. Hypnosis is simply a state of focused, concentrated attention. Lamaze breathing to reduce the pain of childbirth is one type of hypnosis. Parents and children can learn to use hypnotic techniques to improve health and to manage the discomfort of medical procedures such as injections and sutures. These techniques can be as simple as focusing on breathing, becoming absorbed in a story or fantasy, or counting sheep.

Remember mood rings? By turning a deep blue when your hands were relaxed and warm, they gave you *biofeedback* that blood flow was increased to your fingers. Every moment, your child regulates his temperature, heart rate, breathing, muscle tone, and millions of other functions that are not part of his conscious awareness. If he receives help in focusing on one of these processes and gets feedback about it, he can begin consciously to regulate that function. For example, children can learn to increase and decrease the temperature in their fingers if they are given feedback by a machine in the form of sound or lights. This technique has been helpful in reducing the frequency and severity of migraine headaches. Biofeedback is also helpful in severe, chronic constipation in which bowel function has been abnormal for so long that the child needs to learn again how to sense and respond to the body's signals.

Biofeedback is generally taught by psychologists, but formal training and licensure are not required. Before taking your child to a therapist for biofeedback, ask for and check references to other parents whose children were treated. Also ask about fees and how much of the cost your insurance might be expected to cover.

*Meditative* practices such as focusing on the breath or a word can result in profound states of relaxation. Meditation is simply a way of paying attention on purpose. Many scientific studies have shown that meditation can help lower blood pressure and reduce ulcer symptoms and many types of pain. More and more centers across the United States are starting programs to teach meditation to children, who can learn and practice it readily.

There are no particular licensure requirements for teaching meditation techniques. Almost every town has one or more centers that teach meditation. And some clinics and medical centers offer classes, too. Many of these are modeled after Dr. Benson's program at Harvard and Dr. Kabat-Zinn's program at the University of Massachusetts. There is no evidence that one form is more effective than another, so you can choose whatever kind fits with your personal beliefs and is convenient and covered by insurance.

Many types of therapists provide *counseling* and *psychotherapy* to parents and their children. Treatment by counselors, support groups, behavioral therapists, psychologists, and psychiatrists can be helpful in addressing the thoughts and emotions that affect children's health. Like adults, children experience stress and negative emotions. Children whose parents are going through a divorce, for example, are prone to behavior problems, school problems, sleep problems, stomachaches, and headaches. Children who suffer from chronic illnesses such as cancer or asthma or who depend on wheelchairs to get around can benefit from support groups of similarly affected peers. Such groups offer kids the opportunity to share strategies for managing their common problems. Many such groups have formed Internet sites that make it easier for geographically isolated families to feel connected.

If you seek professional assistance because of a serious behavioral or psychological problem, please ask about the therapist's training in pediatrics and family issues; ask for and check references. Licensing requirements for psychologists vary from state to state.

## SIDE 3 (WEST): BIOMECHANICAL THERAPIES

All of the therapies on the west side of the Therapeutic Mountain work biomechanically. Whereas the therapies on the east side work biochemically, the therapies on the west side affect larger tissues and organs by stimulating, realigning, moving, or removing, them.

### BIOMECHANICAL THERAPIES

- Massage and Physical Therapy
- Spinal Manipulation (Chiropractic and Osteopathic Adjustments)
- Surgery

### Massage and Physical Therapy

*Massage* is an ancient healing technique used in every culture around the world. Parents practice informal massage when they encourage burps by rubbing or patting babies' backs. Formal massage techniques range from Swedish massage to Rolfing, deep tissue massage, and physical therapy to rehabilitate muscles and joints after an injury. The various massage techniques all contribute to relaxation and well-being by stimulating blood flow, calming nervous impulses, and stretching and relaxing the tendons and ligaments that hold the bones and joints together. Massaging one part of the body can help draw attention away from another painful part of the body, reducing discomfort. The close personal interaction during massage also enhances the bond between parents and children.

Many massage therapists use oils or lotions to help reduce friction between the therapist's hands and the patient's body. Oil lubricates the skin and makes massage more comfortable. By adding aromatic oils (such as eucalyptus) to the base oil (usually some sort of vegetable oil), the massage can have even more benefit. In my family, our parents massaged Vicks VapoRub or Mentholatum into our necks and chests when we had colds. The camphor and eucalyptus oil helped unclog our noses while the massage itself comforted and reassured us that we were loved and cared for, no matter how miserable we felt.

Massage oils can be stimulating (such as bergamot, grapefruit, lavender, geranium, and cardamom); calming (such as sandalwood, sage, chamomile, and rose); and even sedating (such as vanilla, hyacinth, jasmine, and valerian). Some massage oils have natural antibacterial effects. Tea tree oil, for example, was used by Australian medics during World War II to prevent wound infections. Today it is a common ingredient in natural dandruff shampoos. Massage therapists must be licensed, but licensing requirements vary by state. The first complementary clinician hired by our Center for Holistic Pediatric Education and Research at the Children's Hospital in Boston was Mary McLellan, a nurse and licensed massage therapist. She has been in high demand since the day she started, and her primary role is to teach parents how to provide massage for children.

If you learn to give a good massage to your child, the cost of care goes way down. Daily massage has proven helpful for low birth weight babies, depressed teenagers, kids with asthma, children with painful arthritis, and a variety of other conditions. It is about the most under-utilized therapy with proven effectiveness. I recommend massage for just about every patient I see.

## Spinal Manipulation

*Chiropractic* therapy was invented by an Iowa grocer, Daniel Palmer, in 1895. Palmer believed that all human ailments were due to misalignment (subluxation) of the spine, and that therefore all ailments could be cured by manually realigning the spine. Today there are two main types of chiropractors—those who still believe that manipulating the spine can cure all ills, and those who make more limited claims about treating neck, back, and injury-related pain. Many chiropractors also recommend nutritional and herbal therapies as well as spinal manipulation. Chiropractic treatment is used by about 10% of American adults and 5% of children.

Scientific studies have documented the effectiveness of chiropractic treatment in helping adults with back and neck pain. However, few studies have evaluated effectiveness of chiropractic manipulation for children. Children rarely experience back pain; when they do, serious diseases such as spinal infections and cancer must be considered. The studies done so far have not shown that chiropractic is effective for treating asthma or colic. Reliance on repeated X rays to document spinal changes puts children at risk from exposure to excessive radiation.

Chiropractors are licensed to practice in all fifty states. Most insurance covers chiropractic treatments. Chiropractors are not specially trained to recognize or treat serious childhood illnesses, and they are not licensed to prescribe medications or to perform surgery. They may be helpful if your child has a wrenched back or stiff neck from an injury, but be wary about claims to cure serious problems such as diabetes or infections.

*Osteopathic* manipulation was invented by

the American Dr. Andrew Taylor Still in the late 1800s. Still believed that manipulating the spine and other joints would improve the circulation and lead to more balanced functioning of the nervous system. Although Still rejected the use of all drugs (including homeopathic remedies), his descendants have adopted a more holistic approach. Some osteopaths do not perform spinal or joint manipulation, while others have expanded the scope of therapy to include manipulation of the cranium (head) and sacrum (pelvis). Studies evaluating the effectiveness of this type of treatment for children are under way at the University of Arizona. Osteopathic physicians (D.O.'s—Doctors of Osteopathy) are licensed in all fifty states and have the same prescriptive and practice privileges as medical doctors (M.D.'s). My son's pediatrician, Dr. Henry Bernstein, is an osteopathic physician.

## Surgery

*Surgery* has been practiced since ancient times. Lancing a boil is a surgical procedure as is repairing a hernia or removing an inflamed appendix. Surgeons set fractures, remove brain tumors, perform skin grafts, and deliver babies. Modern techniques have made surgery far safer than it was fifty years ago. Simple surgical procedures (such as the placement of ear tubes in children with recurrent ear infections) can be done on an outpatient basis. Surgeons undergo at least five years of training after completing medical (or osteopathic) school. Becoming board-certified in pediatric surgery requires at least two years of additional training. Before you agree to a nonemergency surgical procedure for you child, ask for a second opinion. Some insurance companies now require a second opinion anyway. Ask the surgeon about his or her credentials, alternatives to surgical treatment, and references to parents of children who have undergone the procedure recommended for your child.

## SIDE 4 (NORTH): BIOENERGETIC THERAPIES

All of the therapies on the north side of the Therapeutic Mountain are based on the principle of an invisible, vital energy or spirit that animates, flows through, and surrounds the body. The aim of all of these techniques is to restore a harmonious balance of energy which, in turn, improves the functioning of molecules, cells, tissues, and organs.

### BIOENERGETIC THERAPIES

- Acupuncture
- Therapeutic Touch, Reiki, Healing Touch, *Qi Gong*
- Prayer and Ritual
- Homeopathy

Some people think that the therapies on the north side of the Therapeutic Mountain are nonsense because they are not based on the known laws of chemistry and physics that govern everyday life. Despite their enigmatic nature, these therapies have proven effective in diverse circumstances. Acupuncture, for example, is effective in reducing pain in racehorses. Prayer effectively enhances plant growth. Homeopathy reduces diarrhea among infants too young to understand the power of suggestion. These therapies work—at least for some children, some of the time. We just don't know how they work or the best way to elicit their effects on a consistent basis (yet).

## Acupuncture

*Acupuncture* has been practiced in China for over 2,000 years. It is based on the theory that illness is caused by an imbalance in the body's flow of energy, called *Qi* or *Chi*. Treatment is aimed at restoring balance of the yin and yang (negative and positive aspects of *Qi*) along the twelve meridians or vessels that carry *Qi* throughout the body. In classical acupuncture, the points along the meridians are stimulated by needles or heat (moxibustion), but they can also be stimulated with vigorous massage (*shiatsu*), tiny hammers, lasers, or electrical currents. *The Web That Has No Weaver*, by Ted Kaptchuk, O.M.D. is the best book about acupuncture and Chinese medicine. Ted is one of my best friends and colleagues at Harvard, and I often turn to him with questions about the theory and practice of Oriental medicine.

Like surgeons' knives, acupuncture needles actually penetrate the body. But, unlike surgery, in which healing is effected through rearranging tissues, in acupuncture treatment the needles' purpose is to restore proper energy flow.

Most of the scientific studies of acupuncture's effectiveness have been performed on adults, but more and more studies are being done on children as well. In 1997, the National Institutes of Health (NIH) convened an expert panel on acupuncture; this panel concluded that acupuncture is effective for a number of painful conditions and for treating certain kinds of nausea. More than one-third of the pain treatment programs at pediatric teaching hospitals in North America now offer acupuncture. In a survey we performed of pediatric patients at Boston Children's Hospital, of those who had undergone acupuncture therapy for severe pain only 1 in 50 reported it was uncomfortable, and most actually thought it helped, even when other therapies didn't. The second complementary clinician we hired at the Boston Center for Holistic Pediatric Education and Research was Ellen Highfield, a licensed acupuncturist. Within a few months of her hire there, the nearby Dana Farber Cancer Institute hired an acupuncturist, too. Our New England patients had quickly discovered what the Chinese have known for thousands of years—acupuncture works.

Acupuncture treatment is complex. Proper training is extensive. The Chinese, Japanese, and Koreans all have somewhat different styles of acupuncture, but there are no studies suggesting substantial differences in their effects. Choose a therapist who has a title, Lic.Ac. or L.Ac. (Licensed Acupuncturist) or Dipl.Ac. (a Diplomate of Acupuncture from the National Commission for the Certification of Acupuncturists). If your child's physician practices acupuncture, ask whether he or she belongs to the American Academy of Medical Acupuncture. Traditional Chinese doctors carry the title O.M.D. (Oriental Medical Doctor), indicating additional training in herbal medicine. These initials *do not* indicate that the practitioner has any training as an M.D. Be sure that your acupuncture therapist uses disposable needles to reduce your child's risk of acquiring AIDS or hepatitis. Insurance reimbursement and licensing requirements for acupuncture therapy vary from state to state and are changing rapidly. Check with your state's medical licensing board and with your insurance carrier.

## Therapeutic Touch, Reiki, Healing Touch, Laying on of Hands

The practice of healing by transmitting energy from the therapist's hands to the patient's body has been around since the beginning of time. The formal technique, *Therapeutic Touch,* was developed by Dr. Dolores Krieger, a professor at the New York University School of Nursing, in conjunction with my teacher, Dora Kunz in the 1970s. This technique develops intuition, enabling practitioners to sense blockages in the energy flow in and around the patient and to help correct the energy flow. Therapeutic Touch is akin to massage, but its practitioners do not need to actually touch the body; rather, they work just on the surface or in the energy fields surrounding it. Laying on of hands, the Chinese technique known as *Qi Gong,* Reiki, and Healing Touch are all variations on this same theme. Therapeutic Touch has undergone scientific study and has proven useful in the treatment of pain, high blood pressure, anxiety, headache, and wound healing. Therapeutic Touch is practiced primarily by nurses. It has been taught and is practiced in over eighty countries around the world. Although formal training is available, certification and licensure are not required to practice Therapeutic Touch. Spend some time asking your prospective practitioner about his or her philosophy of healing, references, and experiences in working with children.

Many children's hospitals have nurses on staff who are trained in Therapeutic Touch or Reiki. The hospitals have developed policies about who can provide these services and the circumstances in which they may be used. In recent years, my colleagues MaryJane Ott and Larraine Bossi (both advanced nurses at Boston Children's Hospital and the Dana Farber Cancer Institute) and I have trained over a dozen nurses, social workers, and physicians in Boston to provide Therapeutic Touch. Since I received the Reiki Master initiation from Roy Bauer in October 2000, I have incorporated Reiki into my practice as well. In 2001 the most frequent reason I was consulted in the hospital was to provide Reiki and Therapeutic Touch for children in the intensive care unit, those recovering from major surgery, or those with cystic fibrosis or cancer. The pediatric residents who train at Children's Hospital were so intrigued with the benefits their patients reported from receiving these treatments, they asked MaryJane, Larraine, and I to provide a workshop for them. We provided the first such training in April 2001, and it was attended by more than forty pediatricians in training. I predict that over the next ten years you will see a huge increase in the number of doctors and nurses who talk openly about the value of Therapeutic Touch, Reiki, *Qi Gong,* and other forms of energy healing.

## Prayer

Intercessory *prayer* asks the Unseen Power (God, Spirit, Great Absolute) to heal the patient. Prayer forms an invisible connection between the patient and the Universal Energy or Spirit, thus restoring balance, wholeness, and health. Prayer and spiritual rituals are as old as the human race. Effective prayer does not require formal training or licensure. One does not need to practice a particular religion. Prayer has proven effective for numerous conditions in numerous studies. *Healing Words,* by Dr. Larry Dossey (editor of *Alternative Therapies in Health and Medicine*), is the best book summarizing the numerous scientific studies demonstrating that prayer works. Another wonderful book summarizing years of research and common sense is *The Healing Power of Faith* by a physician from Duke, Dr. Harold Koenig. Although prayer does not *cure* in every case, sincere prayer often brings a sense of peace and genuine *healing* to both the person praying and the patient. I recommend prayer as a therapy for all kinds of conditions in children whose family beliefs include this spiritual tradition.

## Homeopathy

*Homeopathy* was founded by a German physicist and chemist, Samuel Hahnemann, at the end of the eighteenth century. This was an era when the other main type of medical practice (called allopathy by Hahnemann) had little to offer patients except bleeding, sweating, and purging. Given the allopathic alternatives at the time, homeopathy was definitely a safer treatment! In the intervening years, homeopathy has remained largely unchanged, whereas allopathic medicine has developed advanced diagnostic and surgical techniques, antibiotics, and effective treatments for cancer and other killer diseases. Although homeopathy is disparaged by most American physicians, it is widely used in India and Europe.

Homeopathy is based on two principles. The first principle is: *Like cures like.* Hahnemann said that a substance that produces symptoms in a healthy person cures those same symptoms in a sick person. For example, Belladonna causes flushing, fever, and a rapid heart rate. Thus, it would be the remedy of choice for a child with a sudden onset of fever, flushing, and a fast heartbeat. The theory behind this principle is that the body will tend to react to the remedy, fighting the symptoms it provokes, and thereby fighting the symptoms the body is experiencing. By paying careful attention to the whole range of the child's experience, the homeopathic practitioner matches the remedy that comes closest to causing those symptoms, and therefore cures them. Homeopathic practitioners are very interested in the entire constellation of symptoms the child experiences; they ask a lot of questions and don't rely much on laboratory tests.

The second principle has to do with the bioenergetic or spiritual aspects of homeopathic remedies. It is: *The more the remedy is diluted, the more potent it is.* Homeopathic remedies are diluted anywhere from 1:10 to 1 in billions. The theory states that the 1:10 remedies are not as powerful as the 1:1,000,000 remedies. During each dilution, the compound is vigorously shaken or succussed, which is thought to further increase its potency. Of course, this principle violates our current concepts of chemistry and physics, which is why homeopathy is disparaged by most medical doctors. Nevertheless, several scientific studies have demonstrated homeopathy's effectiveness in treating hayfever, childhood diarrhea, and even ear infections. One of the early

directors of the NIH Center for Complementary Therapies was Dr. Wayne Jonas, a family physician, medical researcher, and homeopath. Some of the most prominent researchers in modern homeopathy are also physicians—Dr. Jennifer Jacobs, who is a family doctor in Washington state, Dr. Edward (Ted) Chapman in Massachusetts, and Dr. David Reilly from Scotland.

Bach flower remedies, invented in the 1930s by Dr. Edward Bach, are an offshoot of homeopathy. Dr. Bach was a British homeopathic physician who used his intuition to select trees, flowers, and other plants used in dilute doses to heal the negative emotions underlying physical illness. Perhaps the most famous of the thirty-eight remedies is Rescue Remedy, a combination of cherry, plum, clematis, impatiens, rock rose, and star of Bethlehem. Rescue Remedy is said to be useful in treating the shock resulting from a startling experience or acute injury. The remedies contain water and brandy in addition to the flower essences. They are available without prescription, and are sold at many health food stores and by mail order from British distributors. There are no scientific studies demonstrating the effectiveness of Bach flower remedies in treating children.

Legally, homeopathy can only be practiced by health professionals who are licensed to prescribe medications. In most states this means that homeopathic practice is legally limited to M.D.'s, D.O.'s, dentists, nurse practitioners, naturopaths, and chiropractors. Despite these regulations, many people without formal pediatric training prescribe homeopathic remedies, and remedies can be purchased through mail order catalogs and at many grocery stores and even convenience stores. Be aware that there is no uniformity in the training standards for homeopathic practice. Although the remedies themselves are probably safe, the danger is that an untrained practitioner may not recognize that your child is seriously ill and in need of other types of therapy.

## SUMMARY

The four sides of the Therapeutic Mountain cover the gamut of healing techniques. No one technique—no matter how organic or high tech, ancient or modern—is a panacea. Do you know the story of the carpenter whose only tool was a hammer? Using his hammer when he needed to replace a light, the bulb shattered. Some problems are best treated with therapies from one side of the mountain and some respond better to others. The challenge for parents is to figure out what kind of therapy and practitioner will be most helpful for their child's problem. Although practitioners often draw upon an array of therapies, they are usually best trained in and most familiar with only a few.

## PRACTITIONERS

*Medical doctors* (M.D.'s) and *osteopathic doctors* (D.O.'s) prescribe medicine; give advice about lifestyle; do counseling about child behavior, growth, development, nutrition; and safety; and may perform surgery. Osteopaths are also trained in performing spinal manipulation. An increasing number of regular physicians (more than 50% and less than 70% as of 2001) recommend herbal medicines, vitamins, meditation, hypnosis, acupuncture, or some other complementary therapy. The old image of the closed-minded doctor who hates complementary medicine is just plain out of date. You might be surprised to learn that your family doctor or pediatrician has attended a continuing medical education course or studied complementary medicine through the Internet or during residency. Things are changing fast.

To become an M.D. or D.O., physicians must complete a college degree, medical school, and one to five years of additional residency training. After completing years of training at approved institutions, a physician is eligible to take a grueling set of examinations to become board-certified. Pediatricians are required to recertify every seven years to ensure up-to-date knowledge and practice. If you want to be sure your doctor has met these standards of training, ask if he or she is board-certified in Family Medicine or Pediatrics. If your child's physician practices a specialty (e.g., cardiology or allergy medicine), ask if he or she is board-certified in that subspecialty.

Most important, you need to be able to trust your child's physician. Get a recommendation from someone you trust, such as a coworker, relative, or friend. Even if someone is highly trained and competent, you may not "click" or be on the same communication wavelength of values and style. Ask questions. Don't be afraid to let a physician know that you are interviewing a number of physicians to find the best one for your family. You probably spent at least a few weekends shopping for your last automobile; the choice of your child's physician is at least as important as your choice of cars. The American Holistic Medical Association is a voluntary medical association that maintains an extensive list of physicians who describe themselves as holistic.

*Naturopathy* as a separate healing tradition was born in Germany in the early twentieth century, though its roots in the health spa movement go back considerably further. Early naturopaths emphasized the importance of mineral baths, steam baths, and fasts. The founder of the modern movement, Benedict Lust, strongly believed in the body's own regenerative powers, and decried the use of coffee, white flour, sugar, tobacco, and alcohol. Naturopathic physicians complete a four-year curriculum covering a wide range of therapies: herbal and homeopathic remedies, nutrition, exercise, and environment, massage and spinal manipulation. Not all naturopaths use all of these therapies. They reject the use of surgery and medications except as a last resort. Fewer than fifteen states currently license naturopaths.

*Traditional Chinese Medicine* is one of the most ancient and holistic of all healing systems. The theory on which it is based—the flow and balance of *Qi* or energy in the body—is not intuitively obvious to most Westerners. Yet, numerous studies have shown the effectiveness of Chinese herbs and acupuncture treatments. Other traditional Chinese therapies include diet, exercise (such as *Tai Chi*), meditation, massage, spinal manipulation, *Qi Gong* (transfer of healing energy from the practitioner to the patient), and bone setting.

*Ayurvedic medicine* is an ancient system of medicine from India that has been recently popularized by Dr. Deepak Chopra. The theory behind Ayurvedic medicine is similar to traditional Chinese medicine: balancing the flow of the body's life force or life energy—*prana,* as it is known in the Ayurvedic tradition. Ayurvedic therapies include herbs, proper nutrition, meditation, environmental changes (aromatherapy and sound therapy), and massage.

## PAYING FOR HOLISTIC HEALTH CARE

The payment systems for financing health care are changing rapidly. Many more therapies are covered by insurance today than they were five years ago, but the situation is far from optimal. This means you could end up paying "out of pocket" for the therapy of your choice. Be sure to talk with your child's health care provider about payment and insurance coverage right up front. Ask not only about professional fees, but also about the cost and coverage for treatments and devices that the provider might recommend (such as vitamins, herbs, psychotherapy, or biofeedback devices). It's also a good idea to check your insurance policy and call your agent about coverage for specific services or treatments before you start a course of therapy for your child. Get the agent's statement about coverage in writing in case there are any questions later.

## GENERAL ADVICE

Practitioners work best when they know the whole story about your child. If you seek care from more than one practitioner, let everyone know what kind of care your child is receiving and from whom. Ask the different practitioners if they are willing to cooperate with each other and send each other copies of their records, recommendations, phone numbers, and Internet addresses. You can contact your state department of licensing regarding regulations for the various kinds of health professionals in your state. Ask questions. Ask for references. Doubt claims about panaceas. If something sounds too good to be true, it probably is. How do you know what to believe? That's what Chapter 2 is all about.

# 2

# "Trust Me, I'm a Doctor"

"Dr. Kemper, I'm so glad you're here. I really wanted to talk with a doctor about natural therapies for cancer. I read somewhere that there was this boy in California who had cancer, and he was cured with cat's claw. My cousin's son was just diagnosed with cancer. Do you think he should take cat's claw, too?" So began a recent conversation with friend, Toni Lozano.

When a child is ill, we all want to help. In general, we prefer remedies that are natural, safe, good for the environment, and in harmony with our beliefs about ourselves and the world. Stories about dramatic cures are inspiring and give us hope that we, too, can overcome the painful challenges of a child's illness.

*"I know that I can't trust everything I read,"* Toni continued. *"There are so many claims out there about certain foods or whatever being bad for you and other foods or vitamins being good for you. It's everywhere—magazines, billboards, TV, radio talk shows, the Internet, friends, and neighbors. And they're all saying different things. Sometimes I feel overwhelmed, and I don't know who to trust. How do I know what really works and what is safe for my family?"*

Several years ago, a colleague gave me an aphorism I adore. I immediately put it on my office door, and it has hung there ever since:

*In God we trust; everyone else must have data.*

This is the era of the skeptic. Given political scandals and the graceless falls of athletic heroes, many of us have lost faith in traditional authority figures. Before trusting their child to a surgeon's knife, many well-informed parents ask for a list of potential alternative treatments, possible side effects, evidence of effectiveness from recent studies and a second opinion. When it comes to your child's health, skepticism is your right as a loving and prudent parent.

## "In God We Trust . . ."

Most of us do have faith in something or someone. Many have complete faith in their own doctor, though they distrust others. Some believe in the power of prayer. If you have complete faith in something, you don't need any evidence to know what to do. You follow your faith. Faith alone can be one of the most healing powers on earth. I have seen miraculous healings based on faith.

More and more hospitals now allow and encourage various types of spiritual healers (such as Native American medicine men) to visit patients and perform healing rituals. On my very first day at Boston Children's Hospital back in 1998, I was asked by a dying teenager and his family to find a spiritual healer. We successfully found a wonderful shaman who visited the boy, performed a ceremony in his hospital room, and brought great comfort and peace to everyone involved. Numerous scientific studies have demonstrated the healing power of prayer. Prayer is effective whether the seeker is Christian, Jewish, Muslim, Buddhist, or Hindu—the words and the form don't matter. It is the faith and the intent that count.

On the other hand, I have also witnessed the suffering of children whose parents slavishly adhered to religious doctrines—a child who died of meningitis because the parents saw the illness as a test of their faith rather than seeking "worldly" antibiotics. Another child suffered for days from a low blood count following a serious injury because the parents refused a transfusion. Children have been bruised and battered, permanently scarred and brain damaged because parents felt they needed to "beat the devil" out of them. These parents put their rigid interpretation of religious doctrine before the community's common sense.

Our cultural beliefs, our sense of who we are, our connectedness to family and community, and the meaning of health and illness are vital to the healing process. In many Eastern and Native American cultures, illness is seen as a lack of balance within a person or between a person and their environment. Western culture looks at disease in terms of cause and effect (e.g., germs cause illness). It is impossible for science to prove whether Eastern or Western philosophies are more "true." But science can compare the effectiveness of different kinds of therapies in healing and curing children with different kinds of diseases.

We all have values that guide our judgments about what is best for our children. Some believe that natural methods are better than chemicals. Some believe that purified chemicals are safer than unregulated herbal mixtures. Some believe in vitamin C and others believe in chicken soup.

*Toni believed in natural remedies, but she wasn't sure if an herb was powerful enough for a disease like cancer. She wondered if natural methods are always better.*

Given equal effectiveness and safety, we'd all choose natural therapies over artificial ones. But keep in mind that many modern conveniences such as central heating, hot running water, and jet airplanes are not natural. The lowest infant mortality rates in the world are found in the technologically advanced nations. There are some lifesaving advantages to modern medicine. On the other hand, many times physicians and families take the easy way out and choose a drug when a change in nutrition, exercise, or environment would do more good in the long run. We all have to balance our values, priorities, and resources when choosing therapies.

## THE OLD PARADIGM: THEORY, TRADITION, AND PERSONAL EXPERIENCE

Prior to this century, medicine was largely unscientific. Medical practice was based on tradition and theory. Unfortunately, practices based on *theory* alone, while they may be well intentioned, can be disastrous for the patient. For example, the practice of bloodletting using leeches was based on the reasonable-sounding theory that it would rid the body of evil humors. It is now believed that excessive bloodletting is what ultimately killed the first U.S. President, George Washington. Many therapies that sound good in theory turn out to be at best ineffective and at worst deadly in actual practice.

Despite spectacular advances in medicine, much of health care continues to be based on *tradition*. Health care practitioners, like all human beings, tend to do things the way we were taught. But traditions change. My early professors taught me to follow up children diagnosed with an ear infection two weeks after their diagnosis to ensure that the fluid had cleared; by the time I became a fellow at Yale, the tradition had changed to three weeks. We now know that only 50% of children clear that fluid within four weeks of a diagnosis, and many pediatricians do not recommend ear recheck visits at all unless the child is still having a problem. Is it wrong to recommend things based on tradition and experience? Not necessarily. Some traditions are simple common sense, and experience can be our greatest teacher.

On the other hand, some traditions based on short-term successes turn out to be hazardous or costly. Though it is a traditional herbal remedy for coughs, coltsfoot has recently been shown to be a cancer-causing liver toxin, and it is no longer regarded as safe. Even ten years after scientific evaluations indicated that aggressively treating healthy jaundiced babies was probably unnecessary, physicians continued to order phototherapy. Why? In part because of tradition, and in part because we doctors feared that if we broke with tradition and anything bad happened, we would be held liable. Stepping outside of our traditions can be scary.

Our own *experience* shapes our attitudes and recommendations. Recently a prominent pediatrician related the story of his teenage patient who had very smelly feet. The pediatrician had counseled him extensively about hygiene to no avail. One day the boy showed up for a routine physical exam, and the physician braced himself for the overwhelming aroma before entering the exam room. To his surprise, the foot odor was completely gone. He began to congratulate the boy on his hygiene, but the boy told him it had nothing to do with washing his socks. "Zinc," he said. "I started taking some of my mom's zinc supplements and the smell went away." The pediatrician was dubious. The boy said he, too, thought it was just a fluke, so he stopped the zinc. Within a few days the odor returned, so he resumed the zinc. On the basis of this experience, this physician now recommends zinc supplements to his patients with smelly feet. While zinc is probably safe in low doses, there are no studies demonstrating its effectiveness in treating foot odor. It may not affect other boys the same way. The boy may have adopted other healthy habits, diet or exercise changes at the same time. Even impressive experiences such as that of the boy with smelly feet are not necessarily a solid scientific foundation for making treatment suggestions to others.

If we can't trust authorities, theories, tradition, and our own experience, what can we trust?

## THE NEW PARADIGM: EVIDENCE-BASED MEDICINE

If you're like most people, you care less about theory and tradition than about how well a treatment actually works. *Evidence-based medicine* means that you look at the scientific evidence that a treatment is effective rather than relying on tradition, theory, or anecdotal experience when making a medical decision. Evidence-based medicine relies on several *levels of evidence* to evaluate the effectiveness of therapies. Let's look at these different levels of evidence.

## The Lowest Form of Evidence: The Anecdote or Case Report

*Child with fatal cancer, cured with coffee enema!*

*Ancient Amazon ointment reverses ravages of acne!*

These stories usually begin, "I had a patient (friend, cousin, etc.) once who . . ." This is the kind of claim that caught Toni's eye and impressed my colleague with the power of zinc. We're intrigued by the possibility of instant or miraculous cures. The more exotic, mysterious, or organic the treatment, the greater the appeal. Those who market "the cure" may cite impressive and rational-sounding philosophical theories to support their claims.

These stories are called *anecdotes* in the popular press and *case reports* in scientific journals. They usually take the form of a hopelessly ill child who is cured with a wondrous or unexpected therapy. Anecdotes grab our attention, pique our curiosity, and give us hope. In the typical anecdote there is insufficient information to tell if the child in the story is similar to your child or if the illness is really like your child's illness. It is also difficult to tell what other therapies the child may have been receiving and exactly what is in the miracle cure.

Be very wary of people marketing miracle cures by phone, Internet, or direct mail. Many of these "cures" are available only with a substantial outlay of cash up front. Or they promise you untold, easy riches if you, too, join the marketing pyramid. Although case reports may be intriguing, they do *not* provide a sufficient basis for recommending a certain therapy for any but the most desperate parents who have exhausted all proven remedies.

## The Case Series: A Collection of Anecdotes

*We treated one hundred feverish children with Brand X, and they all felt better within hours.*

*Colicky babies, treated with chiropractic, dramatically improve within six weeks.*

*I have used vitamin C with my patients for years, and they've all done very well.*

A *case series* is simply a collection of anecdotes. Although the numbers make the claim sound scientific, a case series is also weak evidence that a treatment works. Consider the first claim—children treated with Brand X felt better within hours. Why did they have a fever? What other therapies were they given? Would they have gotten better regardless of what kind of therapy they received, or if they didn't receive any therapy? Case series provide promising leads for scientists to test. But a collection of hopeful anecdotes is not sufficient grounds for saying that a therapy has proven effectiveness. Colicky babies treated with chiropractic do improve over six weeks, but so do colicky babies who never visit a chiropractor.

## Variations on the Theme of Case Series: The Twenty-first Doctor

*"I took my child to twenty doctors, and none of them could figure out what was the matter with him. Nothing they recommended worked, and they pronounced him incurable. Just when I was about to give up, I took him to Dr. Jones. He put my baby on these food supplements, and now he's like a different child. Now he's active and full of life. I'm sure glad we took him to Dr. Jones. Maybe you should take your son to him, too. Or maybe you just want to try these supplements. . . ."*

This scenario is the prototype for *"the twenty-first doctor syndrome."* It is really just a variation on the anecdote or case report. The story starts off with a difficult illness, resistant to the ministrations of numerous healers. The parent is frustrated and about to give up, but tries one last doctor or therapy. The story is usually told by someone who is genuinely convinced that the final treatment caused the cure.

In some cases, it does take one unique healer or one unique treatment to cure a child. However, in many more cases, the marvelous cure is the result of the parents' own strong hope and faith or the illness having finally run its course (such as an infant who outgrows colic). Was the child about to get better anyway? Perhaps. Does this make the cure less remarkable or less true? Of course not. These stories remind us that the human mind and spirit are among the most powerful healing tools available. But bear in mind that the visible trigger (the doctor or the diet) for this particular cure may not be the key to healing for your child.

*"Well, this is all very disappointing,"* Toni complained, *"If I can't trust friends' stories, and if I can't trust doctors' theories, how do I know who to trust? My husband says that all this holistic stuff is nothing but a placebo anyway. Just what is a placebo?"*

## THE PLACEBO EFFECT: A PSYCHO-NEUROIMMUNOLOGIC MODULATOR?

Anecdotes about miraculous cures, stories about spontaneous remission, and the twenty-first doctor syndrome all raise the issue of the *placebo effect*. A placebo is an inert or inactive substance, such as water or sugar pills. The word *placebo* comes from the Latin *placere,* "to please." Placebos were originally devised to satisfy demanding patients who did not need

or would not benefit from real medicine. A placebo can be anything—a word, pill, diet, exercise, or operation. For example, a patient takes the inert sugar pill, believing it will help him, and he is healed. Dr. Herbert Benson refers to placebos as "remembered wellness."

You might think that placebos work only for the weak-minded and suggestible, but you would be wrong. The placebo effect occurs in about 20 to 30 percent of *all* patients with every imaginable disease. It benefits the gifted as well as the gullible. It can reverse real disease as well as overcome imaginary symptoms. It illustrates the amazing capacity of the power of the mind to bring about healing.

Recently I have begun telling my medical students and residents that we should replace the word placebo with the phrase *Psycho-Neuroimmunologic Modulator (PNIM)*. Why should we use such a cumbersome phrase? Because many people associate the word placebo with something that is worthless. But placebos are often very valuable. After many years of research, we know that there are direct connections between the mind (psycho), the nervous system (neuro), and the immune system (immuno). In themselves placebos may be nothing, but by modulating psycho-neuroimmunologic interactions, they release a powerful healing force that can effectively cure real diseases.

Although placebos are effective in helping some children sometimes, they do not always cure everyone. Another active ingredient in addition to the PNIM is sometimes necessary to kill the bacteria or restore balance to the system. The difficulty in scientific research is in figuring out how much better the proposed therapy is than a placebo.

*"Well,"* Toni said, *"as good as placebos may be, I want something better for my family. What kinds of studies prove a treatment is better than a placebo?"*

## Comparative Studies

*American children who are not immunized have the same rate of polio as those who are immunized.*

*Children who are breast-fed are smarter than those who are fed formula.*

These kinds of claims compare one group of patients to another. Such studies look very scientific, and they are a big improvement over case studies, but they can also be misleading. What would you think of the first example if I told you that the rate of polio was nearly zero for both groups? The risk of polio for any child in the United States is nearly zero because of the success of the polio vaccine. What about breast-feeding and IQ? IQ scores are generally a few points higher among infants who are breast-fed than among formula-fed infants. However, American babies who are breast-fed generally also have parents with higher IQs and better education. Is the higher IQ due to the breast milk, the intelligence genes of their parents, or the environment?

Sometimes this type of *comparative study* is the best that can be done in the situation. A scientist can't tell 100 new mothers: "Now you fifty are going to breast-feed for at least four months, and you other fifty are going to feed your baby nothing but formula for the first four months. At the end of that time, we'll measure your babies and see how smart they are." You just can't force people to have certain health habits (what they eat or how much they exercise or whether or not they smoke or meditate or pray). It's likely that the people who practice one healthy habit are healthier in other ways, too. All of this makes it challenging to figure out exactly what's making children healthy (or sick). Many factors must be taken into account before you can conclude that the one thing you're interested in is the thing that matters.

"Well," Toni continued, "what do you think about using remedies that have been proven to work in adults?"

## Children Are Not Sophisticated Rodents or Small Adults

*Rats who are fed only 80% of their needed calories live twice as long.*

*Herbal remedy kills bacteria in test tubes.*

*Cold medicines reduce symptoms in adults.*

What's good for other animals isn't necessarily what's best for human beings. Calves thrive on cow's milk while human infants do best with their own mother's milk. What happens in isolation in a test tube bears little resemblance to what happens inside a complex human being. Therapies that work in adults don't necessarily work in babies and young children. Cold medicines do reduce adults' symptoms, but are useless in infants. Unless a therapy has been proven useful in humans, I don't recommend it. If it has been proven useful in adults, it's worth testing in children, and may be worth trying if it is safe and you've run out of other options.

"Aren't there any *studies I can really trust?*" Toni pleaded.

## The Gold Standard: The Randomized, Controlled, Double-Blind Clinical Trial

Although all studies have shortcomings, the gold standard of scientific evidence is the *randomized, controlled, double-blind clinical trial.* Randomization means that each child in the study has a 50–50 chance of getting the study treatment or the comparison treatment. The treatment decision is determined by the luck of the draw. That way the group of children who receive the experimental treatment are nearly certain to be similar to the group of children who receive the comparison treatment. This is important because without randomization, certain families would be more likely to believe in and choose one treatment over another. The differences between the families who choose different treatments might very well outweigh the differences in the therapies themselves.

Good studies have a control or comparison group. If you give aspirin to children with fever, the fever will go down. But the fever would go down eventually anyway. A comparison group is needed to see if the fever goes down faster with aspirin than without it. (Yes, aspirin is an effective fever fighter.) The strongest evidence for an effective therapy is one that has been tested in children (not adults, animals, or test tubes), randomizing them into active treatment and placebo groups and assessing the results when no one knows exactly who got which treatment.

*Double-blinding* is when neither researcher nor parent nor child knows whether the child received the study treatment or the comparison treatment until after the study is over. If the child and family don't know what treatment is being given, but the researcher does know, that's *single-blinding*. In a study of the effectiveness of acupuncture, the patient and parent may not know whether the needles are being placed in real points, but the acupuncturist must know whether the needle is going in a real point or not. If the family knew the child was getting the "better" study treatment, their expectation about its benefit would modify the psycho-neuroimmunologic response. This would give the new treatment an unfair advantage or a bias toward appearing to be more effective. Keeping everybody in the dark until the study is over helps minimize the bias that might arise if everyone knew which treatment the child was getting.

*"Well that randomized, placebo-controlled, double-blind trial sounds just about perfect—that is, if it was easier to pronounce!"*

It does sound perfect, but remember, if something sounds too good to be true, it probably is. Randomized controlled trials aren't perfect either. Because they are so costly and difficult to perform, they are usually limited to just one patient group (in terms of age, race, gender, geographic area, or stage of illness), which may not be all that similar to your particular child. Also, the folks who enroll in studies are a pretty special breed. How desperate do you have to be to agree to be randomized and perhaps endure extra doctor visits, blood draws, questions, phone calls, etc., especially when there's a chance you aren't going to get the "new, improved" treatment? The people who actually complete the study are only a subset of those who start, and your family might be more like those who stop participating than those who stick it out to the bitter end. And that's just the logistics of the study itself. We haven't even begun to talk about who funds these studies (which determines which therapies and conditions get studied in the first place) or about the possibilities of the patients somehow learning what treatment they receive.

## SUMMARY

*"Whew! Let me see if I've got this straight,"* Toni said. *"The lowest level of evidence is the case report and the case series. Stories about eventual success with a certain doctor or therapy are really just the same thing. Studies of success in adult patients may not apply to children. Studies in children are good if there is a comparison group to make sure the therapy is better than a placebo. And the strongest evidence is from a randomized, double-blind, controlled trial in children. But even those aren't perfect and have to be taken with a grain of salt, right?"*

Exactly. If the only evidence for a therapy is based on tradition, a case series, or case report, I consider it an interesting possibility, but unproven. If the evidence is from a comparative trial in adults or children, I'll tell you it's worth trying, but not recommended until better studies are done in children. The therapies I'm most likely to recommend in this book are those that have been tested with a controlled clinical trial in children. I also like to see them used for at least a few years so we know something about the safety and long-term effects of the therapy.

Do people combine faith with evidence? Of course we do. If you generally believe in herbal medicine, you may just hear one neighbor's story about how echinacea conquered her daughter's cold before you try it for your own child. On the other hand, if you're skeptical about antibiotics, you may doubt your doctor even when she cites randomized controlled trials. In all cases, you will end up judging my recommendations by your own faith, values, and experiences. We all have our own biases. Be open-minded and remember the levels of evidence when you hear or read about possible therapies for your child.

Ask yourself:

- Have clinical studies in children demonstrated that the therapy is more effective than a placebo treatment?
- How will the therapy affect your family's lifestyle and pocketbook?
- What are the risks and alternatives?
- Who is recommending the therapy, what are their qualifications, and do they have a vested interest in you choice?

*New truths commonly begin as heresies, but all too often end as superstitions.*
                                —T. Huxley, 1885

# 3

# ACNE

Gerald Taylor came to see me last spring about his acne. He was an industrious seventeen-year-old who worked part-time at a fast-food restaurant to earn money for college. Gerald was upset about his skin; the senior prom was coming up in two months, and he wanted to wipe out his acne by then. I asked him what he'd tried so far. "Oh, the usual stuff," he replied. "I tried some of that benzoyl something or other, but it didn't work and it just made my face red. My mom says I should stop eating french fries, but it's hard because I get them for free where I work. My friend Marco got this prescription from his doctor for some kind of antibiotic, and his face looks real good. I'd really like something natural, but if that doesn't work, I guess I'd use antibiotics." Before writing a prescription to clear up Gerald's face, I wanted to clear up some of his ideas about acne, where it comes from, what causes it, and what he needed to do to make it better.

The principle players in the acne story are *sebum, hormones, bacteria*, and the *immune system*. Most of the action occurs deep beneath the skin surface in the tiny hair shafts on the face, the chest, and the back. The hair shafts are lined with sebaceous glands that produce a complex oily lubricant called *sebum*. Sebum normally moves smoothly up the hair shaft to the skin surface. Just before adolescence begins visibly, increasing levels of *androgen hormones* stimulate sebum production. Sebum builds up, forming a plug under the skin surface. Dead skin cells mix with sebum in the hair shaft, stick together, and worsen plugging.

Plugged pores are perfect breeding grounds for the bacteria, *P. acnes*. When *P. acnes* proliferate, they break down sebum into irritating *fatty acids*. The bacteria also attract infection-fighting *white blood cells*, starting a cascade of inflammation—redness, swelling, warmth, and pain.

### Acne

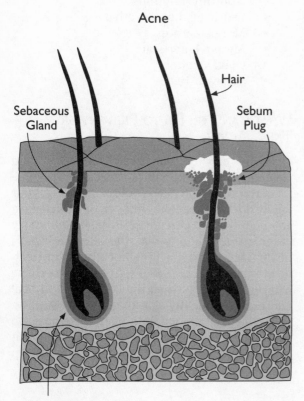

Hair

Sebaceous Gland

Sebum Plug

Hair Bulb

Together the dead cells, sebum, bacteria, and fatty acids form a plug deep within the skin. As the plug pushes to the surface, it is visible as a *blackhead*. Contrary to popular belief, the black color does *not* come from dirt on the skin, but from pigment in the dead skin cells. Albinos (people who lack skin pigment) can get acne, but they do not get blackheads.

Although blackheads are unsightly, they are eventually extruded without a problem.

If a plug gets so big that it blocks its own exit, it makes trouble. The expanding plug eventually bursts the walls of the hair shaft, spilling irritating fatty acids into the skin tissues. White blood cells rush to the site and release even more irritating chemicals. On the surface, this process initially appears as a white-head (plugged hair shaft), eventually becoming a raised red pimple, and then a pustule (a pimple that has come to a head), or, in the worst cases, a scarring nodule or cyst. It takes four to eight weeks for the plugs beneath the skin surface to become visible as acne. This is why THERE ARE NO OVERNIGHT ACNE CURES; it takes several weeks for changes beneath the surface to become visible at the skin surface.

### ACNE AGGRAVATORS

- Higher hormone levels (puberty, males)
- Higher sebum production (stress)
- More irritating fatty acids
- More rapid cell death and sloughing
- Skin irritation
- Certain medications
- Oily air or oily cosmetics
- More *P. acnes* bacteria
- More aggressive immune system

Most American teenagers (over 80 percent) face acne and a third of them worry that their acne is the first thing other people see about them. About 10 percent of adults continue to deal with acne into their thirties and forties. Most people treat their acne on their own; only about a third ask their doctor for a prescription medicine.

Boys tend to have more severe acne because they have more *androgen* hormones. Many women experience acne flares just before menstrual periods when *progesterone* hormones (chemically similar to male androgen hormones) are highest. Athletes who bulk up on *androgen steroids* also tend to get worse acne, among many other more severe side effects. *Stress* from lack of sleep, major exams, or emotional tension also increases sebum production and free fatty acids, exacerbating acne. Acne-causing medications include the seizure medicine *dilantin;* a drug for bipolar disorder, *lithium;* an anti-tuberculosis drug, *isoniazid;* and *iodine.*

*Oily air* can block pores, contributing to acne. Fast-food restaurants (filled with deep fat fryers), refineries, garages, and some chemical plants have high oil levels in the air. Airborne oil settles on the skin and blocks pores.

*I advised Gerald that his job might contribute to his acne, because of the oily air. If he continued to work there, he would need to wash his face with a gentle soap after every shift to help minimize blocked pores.*

Common "treatments" can actually worsen acne. Despite the popular idea that *sun* dries up acne, increased *sweating* from summertime sunbathing on humid days can also block pores, aggravating rather than improving acne. *Overzealous facial scrubbing*, friction, frequent rubbing, picking, and pinching increase the breakdown of sebum into irritating fatty acids and further provoke the immune system. *Friction* from clothing, football pads, hair, headbands, and resting the face on the hand can also aggravate acne. *Oily cosmetic coverups* can block pores, preventing the normal outflow of sebum and dead skin cells. Whenever possible, use water-based rather than oil-based cosmetics. All makeup should be thoroughly removed before bed. Avoid skin lotions or cosmetics containing acne-aggravating ingredients. Read labels carefully.

## COSMETIC INGREDIENTS TO AVOID

- Acetylated PEG 15, PEG 75, or plain lanolin
- Butyl stearate
- Cocoa butter or coconut butter
- Glyceryl-3-diisostearate
- Hydrogenated vegetable oil
- Isopropyl anything
- Lauric acid or laureth 4
- Monostearate
- Myristyl myristate
- Oleyl alcohol
- Stearath 10

## WHAT CAN YOU DO TO PREVENT OR TREAT ACNE?

Acne can be effectively prevented and treated. Many treatments are available without a prescription. If you need professional help, your family doctor, nurse practitioner, or pediatrician can help with 95 percent of all acne. Refractory cases usually end up at the dermatologist's office. There are no overnight cures. Most treatments take *at least eight weeks to work* because it takes that long for all the old lesions to heal and the new healthy skin to get to the surface. Let's consider the whole range of therapies to learn what works and what doesn't. If you want to skip to my bottom-line recommendations, flip to the end of this chapter.

## BIOCHEMICAL THERAPIES: MEDICATIONS, HERBS, NUTRITIONAL SUPPLEMENTS

### Medications

The medications used to treat acne fall into three categories: those that prevent or destroy sebum plugs, those that affect hormone levels, and those that kill bacteria. The most effective treatment regimens combine these three strategies.

## ACNE MEDICATIONS

### PRESCRIPTION AND NONPRESCRIPTION AVAILABLE

- Plug busters: benzoyl peroxide or salicylic acid

### PRESCRIPTION MEDICATIONS

- Hormonal treatments
- Antibiotic lotions
- Antibiotics taken by mouth
- Accutane (only from a dermatologist)

### Plug Busters

Some of the most effective treatments for preventing and destroying sebum plugs are inexpensive and available without a prescription. Some also have antibacterial effects. Most of them irritate the skin. Your face may actually look worse the first three days you try them; don't give up the first week. To minimize initial irritation, start with low concentrations and nighttime applications.

*Benzoyl peroxide* is one of the most effective and widely used nonprescription acne treatments. Numerous brands are available (Acne-10, Benoxyl, Clearasil Maximum Strength Acne Treatment, Cuticura Acne, Fostex 10%, Oxy 5, Theroxide, Vanoxide, and others); you can save money by buying generic brands. Benzoyl peroxide generates free oxygen radicals deep in the hair follicles; it breaks down sebum plugs and kills acne-causing bacteria. Strengths range from 2.5% to 10%. Start with the lower strengths (2.5% or 5%) once a day at night until your skin gets used to it. Then advance to twice daily. If you haven't noticed any improvement after six weeks and your skin tolerates it, you can advance the strength.

Side effects of benzoyl peroxide include irritation, stinging, drying, itching, redness, and peeling. Benzoyl peroxide inactivates topical vitamin A preparations (see below), so the two should not be applied simultaneously. Nonprescription benzoyl peroxide is available in either alcohol-based or water-based formulas. Alcohol is more drying and irritating than water-based forms. Prescription-strength benzoyl peroxide comes as a gel; the gel penetrates the skin more deeply and is more effective, but it also causes more redness and irritation. Benzoyl peroxide is more irritating when applied to wet skin, so wait 20 minutes after washing and drying your face to apply it.

About 1 to 2 percent of adolescents become allergic to benzoyl peroxide. Benzoyl peroxide is a bleach; be careful around colored fabrics, especially silk shirts! It can also bleach skin; darkly pigmented teens may prefer nonprescription salicylic acid remedies.

For over one hundred years, *salicylic acid* has been used to treat acne. It breaks apart sebum plugs by "ungluing" the sticky webs between dead skin cells. Salicylic acid is as effective as benzoyl peroxide for most acne. It is the active ingredient in many of the over-the-counter acne remedies, such as Stri-Dex, Clearasil Medicated Cleanser, and Therapads Plus. Strengths vary from 0.5% to 2%. Start with the lowest strength; as your skin tolerates it, try higher ones. As with other topically applied acne medicines, the main side effect is redness and irritation. This is usually mild and doesn't mean that you have to stop treatment; just reduce the strength or frequency of use. A new prescription acne product, *azelaic acid* (Azelex), busts plugs, fights bacteria, and reduces inflammation and skin discoloration, but its expense and side effects (irritation, redness, and dryness) have made it less popular than other acne remedies.

### Prescription Hormonal Treatments

*Birth control pills* containing estrogen (female hormones) suppress acne-causing hormones. Most birth control pills contain a combination of estrogen and progesterone. Low-progesterone pills are the most effective for reducing acne, especially if there are other signs of hormonal imbalance, such as facial hair. It takes several months for benefits to become apparent, and therapy may last one to two years. Birth control pills obviously are *not* recommended for male acne sufferers. Nevertheless, they are among the best treatments for women afflicted with acne.

Another hormone, *spironolactone*, also has anti-androgenic effects.[1] Although it is used mainly to lower blood pressure, it can also improve acne. Patients who take spironolactone need to have their blood pressure and blood chemistry levels checked regularly; some women who take it develop irregular menstrual periods and breast pain. I rarely recommend it.

Although high doses of anti-inflammatory *steroids* (such as *prednisone* for asthmatic teenagers) can make acne worse, low doses seem to improve the picture. Because of the severe side effects of long-term prednisone, it is not a first-line acne remedy. Steroids can be injected directly into large, cystic acne lesions. This is done only for severe acne, and usually only by dermatologists.

## Antibacterial Agents

Antibiotics kill off *P. acnes* bacteria that cause acne. They do *not* clear up pimples that already exist. To stop pimples before they reach the surface, antibiotics should be applied to *all* acne-prone areas, not just those that have already broken out. Antibacterial agents can be applied topically or taken by mouth (orally). Both topical and oral antibiotics take several weeks to have visible effects. Because of the overuse of antibiotics and the emergence of bacteria resistant to commonly used antibiotics, many patients and physicians opt for alternative remedies.

### BACTERIA KILLERS

- Soap: Chlorhexidine (Hibiclens)—nonprescription
- Antibiotics (topical)— prescription
- Antibiotics (oral)—prescription

Do *not* use abrasive cleansers and scrubs; they cause too much friction and irritation, worsening acne. Most soaps don't penetrate deeply enough or stay on the skin long enough to kill acne-causing bacteria. *Chlorhexidine* (Hibiclens) skin cleanser is widely used in hospitals because it does such a good job of killing skin bacteria. When used twice daily, it has proven effective as an acne fighter in a randomized, placebo-controlled trial. It is as effective as 5% benzoyl peroxide and is less drying and irritating. Washing with it more than twice daily confers no additional benefits.

The four most widely used prescription antibiotic lotions are: clindamycin (Cleocin), tetracycline, erythromycin, and meclocycline (Meclan). A fifth option is sulfacetamide-sulfur (Sulface-RT, Novacet); sulfur is an ancient acne remedy, but it smells so bad that newer formulations of this product (omitting the sulfur) are being developed and tested. Combinations of antibiotics and zinc or antibiotics and benzoyl peroxide are also available; the combinations are more effective (and expensive) than single remedies.[2]

Topical antibiotics work, but because all people are different, some folks do better with one than another. If you decide to use antibiotics, start with a prescription for the least expensive type for three months. If it is too irritating or doesn't work very well, try another. Antibiotic lotions are often alternated with benzoyl peroxide or salicylic acid—one type of medicine applied in the morning and the other used in the evening.

Do *not* apply plug busters and antibiotics at the same time (such as both benzoyl peroxide *and* erythromycin lotion in the morning). Combinations can aggravate side effects and reduce effectiveness, but they do *not* improve acne. By alternating medications—antibiotic lotion in the morning, benzoyl peroxide or salicylic acid in the evening—you can reduce side effects and get better results than with either one alone. Antibiotic lotions are nearly as effective as taking antibiotics by mouth.[3] Very little of the antibiotic lotion is absorbed into the system, so there are fewer side effects than with oral antibiotics. Antibiotic lotions are also less irritating than benzoyl peroxide and salicylic acid. Be careful with tetracycline creams; they glow under ultraviolet light. Your face may attract unwanted attention if you apply tetracycline to it before visiting a nightclub featuring "black" lights!

*Oral antibiotics* kill bacteria on the entire skin surface, in the intestines, and everywhere else. Acne-fighting antibiotics include tetracycline, erythromycin, and minocycline. Oral antibiotics are more effective than antibiotic lotions in treating severe, widespread acne, but it takes about four months before the benefits are really noticeable. Because so many people have been using tetracycline to treat their acne, bacteria have become more resistant to it, and your doctor may prescribe a different antibiotic or urge you to avoid antibiotics altogether. Frankly, I think avoiding antibiotics is a good idea except in cases of severe infections like pneumonia or meningitis.

One of the main side effects of oral antibiotics for teenage girls is the risk of developing vaginal yeast infections. Other side effects include upset stomach, allergies, increased sun sensitivity, and changes in skin color. Antibiotics kill normal intestinal bacteria and can cause diarrhea. If you take an antibiotic daily, make sure you eat yogurt (with active cultures) daily, too, to replace the healthy bacteria in your system. *Tetracycline should not be taken by children under eight years of age or by pregnant women* because it turns developing teeth an ugly brown. Erythromycin is usually the least expensive of all the acne antibiotics. Minocycline (Minocin) is taken twice daily and can be taken with meals; however, it has recently been shown to have severe side effects such as arthritis, hepatitis, and systemic lupus erythematosis (SLE). Although these terrible side effects are rare, they have led many doctors to avoid minocylcine.

Isotretinoin (Accutane) is the most powerful prescription acne medication. It reduces sebum production by 90% and helps kill acne-causing bacteria. Along with power comes the potential for *serious side effects*. It is reserved for patients with severe, deep, widespread acne. Women should not use it unless they abstain from sex or use a reliable form of contraception, because isotretinoin can cause serious birth defects if taken during pregnancy. It can also cause dry eyes, headaches, nosebleeds, and changes in blood lipids. It is available only with a prescription. If your child's acne is bad enough that you are considering this medication, see a dermatologist.

### Herbs

Tea tree oil (from the Australian *Melaleuca alternifolia* tree) has proven benefits for acne. It kills bacteria. An Australian study on 124 acne patients showed that a 5% tea tree oil *gel* was as effective as 5% benzoyl peroxide.[4] It has not been compared to stronger acne treatments. Do *not* use straight, undiluted tea tree oil because the oil can block pores, aggravating acne. Be sure tea tree oil is packaged in a child-proof container; swallowing as little as 1 to 2 teaspoons can put a toddler in a coma.

Many other herbs have been used as traditional acne remedies, but none has been tested against standard therapies in scientific studies. Teas made of catnip, chamomile, comfrey, lavender, thyme, or yarrow root are used as facial rinses. Calendula is thought to soothe irritated skin. Folk remedies for acne include poultices of grated carrot, cucumber, aloe vera, and lemon juice. An Ayurvedic remedy is a paste made with turmeric and sandalwood powder mixed with water. Herbal masks containing equal parts of green clay and corn flour, with one or two drops of the essential oils of chamomile, lavender, juniper, and patchouli have also been used. Native American herbal cures include burdock root, echinacea, Oregon grape, and goldenseal. Test-tube studies evaluating the bacteria-killing power of several natural products—cashews, apples, green tea—have had promising results, but have not been thoroughly tested in actual acne sufferers. Until studies document the effectiveness of these herbal remedies, I do *not* recommend them. Too many other effective treatments are available to waste your time and money on unproven remedies. On the other hand, if you've tried one and your skin is better, keep using it.

## Nutritional Supplements

### VITAMINS AND MINERALS FOR ACNE

#### PROVEN HELPFUL

- Vitamin A (Retin-A) cream or gel—prescription only

#### UNCERTAIN BENEFIT

- Vitamin B6
- Vitamin A (oral supplements)—nonprescription
- Zinc
- Selenium
- Chromium

#### PROVEN HARMFUL

- Vitamin B12
- Iodine

### Proven Helpful for Acne

*Tretinoin or topical Vitamin A acid (Retin-A).* The topically applied form of vitamin A is very effective against acne. Tretinoin normalizes skin sloughing, breaks down sebum plugs, and creates an unwelcome environment for *P. acnes*. It works synergistically with plug busters (benzoyl peroxide or salicylic acid) and antibiotic lotions because it makes the skin more receptive to other medications. It should *not* be applied at the same time as other medications, but it can be alternated; for example, tretinoin in the morning and either benzoyl peroxide or an antibiotic lotion in the evening. This is actually my favorite combination because it works so well.

Tretinoin comes in several strengths (0.025%, 0.05%, and 0.1%) and in both a cream and gel; all require a prescription, and all are fairly expensive ($20 to $30 per month). The gel formations and the higher concentrations are more potent and have more side effects (red skin and peeling); side effects can be reduced by starting with lower concentrations. Start by using it at night once every other day, gradually to every night as tolerated. Topical vitamin A also makes skin more sun sensitive, so *be sure to use a good sunscreen if you're using tretinoin*. Treatment usually lasts six to eight months. Tretinoin does not cause birth defects or any of the problems associated with overdoses of oral vitamin A supplements.

Recently, two new forms of topical retinoids have come on the market. Adapalene (brand name Differin) comes as a 0.1% alcohol-free gel or solution; it is less irritating that tretinoin (Retin-A) and is more effective at decreasing inflammation. Tazarotene (brand name Tazorac) is another prescription type of retinoid; it was originally developed to treat psoriasis, but it's also an effective acne remedy. However, it is more expensive and more irritating than tretinoin, so it is rarely prescribed.

*Retin-A is usually one of the first medications I prescribe for teenagers with acne who have already tried benzoyl peroxide. For Gerald, I wrote a prescription for Retin-A (0.025% cream) to be used at night after his evening wash with chlorhexidine soap. I suggested that he continue his morning treatment with nonprescription benzoyl peroxide, explaining that he should see some improvements by prom time, but that he might have some redness and irritation for the first week or so. We took a picture in the office to compare to his later appearance because the improvement is sometimes so gradual that teenagers aren't aware of it until they compare before and after pictures.*

### Uncertain Benefit for Acne

Anecdotally, some women who have acne flare-ups with their periods benefit from taking 50 milligrams per day of *vitamin B6, pyridoxine*.[5] However, there are no comparison studies proving its effectiveness. It may be worth a trial of vitamin B6, but to reduce the risk of side effects, start with lower doses such as 10 milligrams twice daily, increasing as tolerated to 25 milligrams twice daily.

*Vitamin A* supplements were previously recommended for acne based on reports of improved skin with vitamin A therapy.[6] However, there was no comparison group in this study, and the high doses used (300,000 to 500,000 International Units daily) can result in severe headaches, dry skin, cracked lips, and blurred vision.[7] I do not recommend vitamin A supplements in higher doses than are found in nonprescription multivitamins (10,000 International Units daily). *The best plan is to eat a diet rich in vitamin A containing fruits and vegetables—at least seven servings daily.*

Interestingly, zinc levels are lower than normal in many male acne sufferers. Higher zinc levels inhibit sebum production and make sloughed skin cells less sticky. Studies about the effectiveness of zinc supplements are conflicting: a Swedish study showed that 45 milligrams taken three times daily was more helpful than placebo in reducing acne;[8] other studies have not duplicated these results.[9] The body tries to maintain a balance between zinc and copper. Too much zinc can suppress immune function. Do not overdose on zinc. If you take zinc supplements, take it as part of a balanced multivitamin/multimineral supplement. If you aren't getting enough zinc in your diet, you may not be getting enough of several other nutrients either. *I'm less in favor of supplements than of a healthy, balanced diet, especially during the teenage years of rapid growth and development.*

A Swedish study indicates that *selenium* supplementation (0.2 milligrams taken twice daily) may be helpful in treating acne for people who live in areas that have low soil levels of selenium and eat crops grown in these areas.[10] This study did not include a comparison group and has not been duplicated in the United States where soil levels of selenium are higher. If you take a multivitamin supplement that includes selenium, you probably don't need any additional selenium.

Theoretically, supplemental *chromium* may improve the skin's sugar metabolism, thereby reducing the food supply for acne-causing bacteria. However, there are no studies indicating that chromium supplements are actually beneficial for acne sufferers.

### Proven Harmful for Acne

Beware of *vitamin B12* supplements. High doses can promote an acnelike rash.[11]

Excessive *iodine* may worsen acne in some sensitive teenagers. Fast foods often contain extraordinary amounts of iodine. Sushi wrapped in *seaweed* and *kelp* supplements are other potential sources of excessive iodine. Regular iodized table salt is OK if used sparingly.

## LIFESTYLE THERAPIES: NUTRITION, EXERCISE, ENVIRONMENT, MIND-BODY

### Nutrition

Does a bad diet cause acne? Despite the nearly universal fears of fried foods, chocolate, and sweets, there are few scientific studies evaluating their effects on acne. One randomized, controlled study from 1969 showed that eating chocolate did *not* make acne worse.[12] However, the comparison group was eating a very fatty diet. Though frequently cited, this study has not been replicated, it did not focus on patients who felt that chocolate made their acne worse, and did not control for dietary fat.

Studies of acne in different countries suggest that people who eat a diet low in animal fat, low in saturated fats, and higher in olive oil have a lower risk of acne (especially Mediterranean diets low in red meat, butter, and milk).[13] There have not been any good scientific studies evaluating the effectiveness of a low fat (less than 30% of calories from fat) diet, or of the effectiveness of switching from saturated animal fats to unsaturated vegetable fats for acne. Nevertheless, the Mediterranean diet has a lot going for it in terms of preventing heart disease and reflecting a generally healthier lifestyle. I recommend this diet to adolescents interested in lifelong nutritional health, whether or not they have acne.

Nor have there been any good studies on the effectiveness of cutting down on refined sugar in reducing acne. Several older studies suggested that poor sugar metabolism in the skin made acne worse. A 1937 report from Bellevue Psychiatric Hospital in New York noted that six psychotic teenagers treated with insulin shock therapy (which dramatically drops blood sugar and was standard therapy at that time for schizophrenia) had a marked improvement in their acne.[14] Based on this observation, two British physicians began to give insulin injections to nondiabetics in the late 1930s to improve their acne. Similarly, when oral medications became available to reduce blood sugar, they were given to London patients in the 1950s. Although these treatments were reported to be effective, these studies did not contain comparison groups, and the patients ran the risk of going into shock from low blood sugar. Possible problems with sugar metabolism form the basis for recommending *yeast supplements* for acne sufferers;[15] yeast contains high amounts of *chromium*, which plays an essential role in helping tissues metabolize sugar. However, there are no studies proving that chromium supplements are effective in treating acne. I do not recommend chromium supplements as an acne treatment. On the other hand, I think we can all reduce our sugar intake to reduce our risks of obesity and tooth decay, and a sugar-free diet may have other benefits as well.

In a relatively small number of people, acne is exacerbated by a particular food, but even in these patients the effect is inconsistent.[16] For those who are convinced that chocolate, peanut butter, french fries, or some other food makes their acne worse, eliminating the suspected offender is worth a try. Even if your skin is sensitive to a particular food, prepare to endure six to eight weeks of continued symptoms. It takes that long for just about any treatment to start to make a difference.

### Exercise

There is no exercise that has been proven to improve acne. Serious sweating can block pores, so be sure to shower after exercising to clear the skin. Fear of acne is not a good reason to become a couch potato. If you easily overheat or sweat a lot, consider swimming.

### Environment

Acne is *not* caused by dirt. Washing twice a day is plenty to prevent blocked pores. However, teenagers who work in fast-food restaurants, like Gerald, or in a garage with lots of airborne grease, may find that washing after work helps reduce the oil on their skin.

Some people feel that acne improves during the summertime with increased exposure to the sun. However, there is a condition called tropical acne, in which acne is induced by the high temperatures and humidity in the tropics. With all of the concerns about excessive exposure to sunlight increasing risks of skin cancer, I cannot recommend sunbathing as a treatment for acne.

## Mind-Body

No doubt about it—*stress* makes acne worse. Acne itself is a major stress for most teenagers. In fact, it's usually rated among the top health concerns of adolescents.[17] When British teenagers suffering from severe acne were offered a choice of $1,000 or a cure for their acne, 87% chose the acne cure![18] Failure to get enough rest contributes to overall stress levels. Teenagers need a lot of sleep to get through growth spurts and rapid developmental changes.

Acne sufferers should find a relaxation technique that works for them—listening to music, meditation, self-hypnosis, breathing exercises—and stick with it. *Relaxation techniques are most useful if practiced daily, not just when major stress occurs.* Parents can help by offering emotional support. For severely stressed teens, hypnotherapy and psychotherapy may be helpful in reducing stress and stopping behaviors that worsen acne such as picking at the sore spots.

## BIOMECHANICAL THERAPIES: MASSAGE, SPINAL MANIPULATION, SURGERY

### Massage

Massage oils can block pores, making acne worse. Though massage may be wonderfully relaxing and helpful in stress reduction, there are no studies yet documenting its effectiveness in treating acne. If massage is used to decrease stress, use water-based lotions rather than oils. If oils are used, use light ones that are easily absorbed such as jojoba oil, rather than heavier sesame or avocado oils. Aromatherapists favor bergamot, chamomile, cedarwood, eucalyptus, juniper, lavender, lemongrass, and sandalwood as essential oils to add to the basic massage lotion.

### Spinal Manipulation

There are no scientific studies documenting the effectiveness of spinal manipulation such as chiropractic adjustments, osteopathic adjustments, or craniosacral therapy in treating acne.

### Surgery

Some dermatologists use a long-handled thin extractor to remove blackheads. The extractor has a round end that fits around blackheads. By pressing down on the round loop, the plug is forced up and out. Extraction is a less irritating technique than pinching or pushing. It does *not* prevent pimples, but can help reduce the number of cosmetically disturbing blackheads.

A variety of plastic surgery treatments are available to treat acne scars. With cryosurgery acne scars are sprayed with a freezing-cold liquid; the frozen surface layers eventually peel away, leaving smoother skin. Chemical peels work the same way. Dermabrasion, in which the skin is scraped with a wire brush, is reserved for more severe scarring. For deep scars, the individual areas are cut out, then grafted or stitched. Collagen or silicon can be injected under the skin to push up broad, flat, scarred areas. These procedures should only be undertaken by a plastic surgeon and only when the acne is no longer active.

## BIOENERGETIC THERAPIES: ACUPUNCTURE, THERAPEUTIC TOUCH/PRAYER, HOMEOPATHY

### Acupuncture

Several case series report that acupuncture is a helpful treatment for acne.[19] Before you get your hopes up, you should know that there was no comparison group in these studies, so it is impossible to tell how many patients would have improved without acupuncture. There was also no mention of concurrent treatments that may have played a role. It took an average of sixteen treatments for improvements to appear. If you are paying out of your own pocket, acupuncture becomes a very expensive therapy with very uncertain benefits. I do not typically recommend it as an acne cure.

### Therapeutic Touch/Prayer

There are no studies specifically evaluating the effectiveness of prayer or Therapeutic Touch or any other distant or local healing treatment for acne, but if these practices are consistent with your beliefs, I encourage you to consider them. Let me know how they work for you.

### Homeopathy

Homeopathic remedies taken internally for acne include *Antimonium crudum, Carbo animalis, Hepar sulfur, Kali bromatum*, and *sulfur*. There are no scientific studies documenting the effectiveness of homeopathic remedies for treating acne. They are safe, but until more studies are done evaluating effectiveness, I do not recommend that you spend money on them.

✳

# WHAT I RECOMMEND FOR ACNE

*Remember, it will take 8 to 12 weeks to see the effect of almost any therapy. Treatment must be persistent and you must be patient!*

1. *Lifestyle—nutrition.* Eat a healthy diet with at least seven servings of fruits and vegetables daily. Eat less red meat, whole milk, cream, butter, and other sources of animal fat. Consider taking a multivitamin containing vitamin B6 and zinc.

2. *Lifestyle—environment.* Avoid prolonged exposure to oily environments such as fast-food restaurants and car repair shops. Avoid sunbathing, especially on hot, humid days. Minimize friction to your face and other acne-prone areas. Don't try to cover the acne with long hair. Avoid abrasive soaps and scrubs. Do *not* pick at your pimples. Wash acne-prone areas twice a day with chlorhexidine or a gentle, mild antibacterial soap.

3. *Lifestyle—mind-body.* Practice stress-reduction techniques such as meditation, yoga, self-hypnosis, or progressive muscle relaxation every day to lower your stress levels.

4. *Lifestyle—cosmetics.* If you use cosmetics, use only water-based kinds. Avoid the following ingredients: acetylated lanolin, PEG 15, PEG 75 or plain lanolin, butyl stearate, cocoa butter or coconut butter, glyceryl-3-diisostearate, hydrogenated vegetable oil, isopropyl anything, lauric acid or laureth 4, monostearate, myristyl myristate, oleyl alcohol, oils of avocado, mink, or sesame, propylene glycol, red dyes, stearath 10.

5. *Biochemical—nutritional supplements.* For women who note an increase in acne with menstrual periods, consider supplemental vitamin B6 (25 milligrams twice daily) and asking your health care professional about birth control pills.

6. *Biochemical—nutritional topical medications.* If you want to try nonprescription treatments, consider:
- tea tree oil gel, applied twice daily
- salicylic acid, applied twice daily
- benzoyl peroxide, applied twice daily; start with a daily application of the 2.5% strength before bedtime. As tolerated, increase to twice daily; then increase to higher strengths.

*See your health care professional if these measures haven't helped within two months. You may benefit from topical treatments with:*

- *Vitamin A cream, retinoic acid.* Retinoic acid can make skin sun-sensitive, so avoid sun exposure and use a good sunscreen—at least SPF 15.

- *Antibiotic lotions* such as tetracycline, clindamycin, erythromycin, or meclocycline. Do not use at the same time as other skin creams. If you're using another treatment such as benzoyl peroxide, use one in the morning and the other in the evening.

For severe acne that has not responded adequately to the other therapies, talk with your doctor about *antibiotics.* For women, talk to your doctor about starting birth control pills. If you take antibiotics daily, increase the amount of yogurt (with active cultures) that you eat to reduce the side effects of the antibiotics.

For severe acne that does not get better even with oral antibiotics, it is time to consult a dermatologist for a thorough evaluation and consideration of even stronger medication (such as isotretinoin—Accutane). Remember, the stronger the medicine, the stronger the side effects.

## RESOURCES

### Internet

American Academy of Dermatology
http://www.aad.org

National Institute of Health
http://www.nih.gov/niams/healthinfo/
acne/acne.htm

Stop Spots (an international acne support group)
http://www.stopspots.org

# 4
# ALLERGIES

Every spring Yvonne sneezes and gets itchy, watery eyes and a runny nose.

Every time Cory eats strawberries, he breaks out in hives.

Aaron has chronic diarrhea, eczema, and asthma. He also has dark circles under his eyes and is not growing as well as his brothers.

Every time Anne wears inexpensive earrings, her earlobes swell painfully.

Twelve-year-old Joannie has spina bifida and severe reactions to latex balloons.

These are all examples of allergies. Allergies cause many different symptoms in different people at different ages and are triggered by different things. Symptoms can range anywhere from fussiness to fatal shock. Allergies affect more than 30 million Americans, account for 2 million days lost from school, and cost approximately $1 billion annually in doctor visits and medications. Food allergies affect about 2 to 5 percent of children, skin allergies affect 3 to 10 percent, and nasal allergies such as hay fever affect as many as 30 percent. The number of children and adolescents who suffer from various allergies is climbing, and no one is exactly sure why.

Allergies are confusing to most parents and many physicians because the body reacts to what it perceives as allergies in different ways; many allergic symptoms mimic other illnesses. On the other hand, many symptoms blamed on allergies on not true allergies. Despite their complaints to the contrary, most kids are not allergic to homework, algebra, or Latin. The vast majority of people who can't tolerate milk aren't allergic to it, but lack the enzyme needed to digest milk sugar. About 1 to 2 percent of people of Northern European ancestry have celiac disease, which is sensitivity to gluten (a component of wheat and other grains); this can cause upset stomach and diarrhea, problems with nerves and balance, and poor growth. Kids who have an upset stomach after eating a chili dog slathered with onions may have poor judgment, but probably don't have allergies to chili or onions. Belching and passing gas after eating raw vegetables or beans are not due to allergies, either. "Chinese restaurant syndrome" is a direct chemical effect of the flavor enhancer MSG, monosodium glutamate, not an allergy to bean sprouts. Red eyes after swimming are due to irritation, not allergies.

## COMMON ALLERGY SYMPTOMS

*Skin:* hives, eczema, swelling, itching

*Nervous system:* headache, fatigue, confusion, difficulty concentrating, decreased attention span,[1] depression, insomnia and other sleep problems[2]

*Eyes:* red, itchy, watery eyes; dark circles under the eyes; swollen eyelids

*Nose:* watery, itchy nose; sneezing, congestion; horizontal wrinkle across tip of nose

*Mouth:* itchy roof of the mouth, swollen tongue, lips; sore, scratchy throat

*Lungs:* asthma, wheezing, coughing, feeling of tightness in the chest

*Heart:* rapid heart rate, irregular heartbeats

*Muscles and joints:* muscle pain, joint pain, arthritis

*Intestines:* colic, diarrhea, nausea, vomiting, constipation, abdominal pain, itchy anus, bloody diarrhea

*Urinary system:* sense of urgency or frequent need to urinate

Kids who suffer from allergies are truly miserable. Troublesome daytime symptoms seem worse at night, keeping restful sleep at bay. A tired, itchy, sneezing child is apt to have a hard time paying attention in class and being well-behaved. As if that's not enough, the medications that are often used to control the symptoms (such as antihistamines) tend to make kids drowsy and dopey-feeling. All of this can interfere with school performance and contribute to underlying anxiety, depression, and low self-esteem. Treating the allergies (without sedating antihistamines) can clear up a host of problems.

*What causes allergies?*

Allergies are symptoms of an *oversensitive immune system*. They occur when the immune system decides that something that has come in contact with the body is dangerous and needs to be fought. Fights on one front may lead to symptoms in another system; for example, food allergies trigger breathing problems in about 10% of kids with asthma.

*My child is allergic to pollen, cat dander, mold, and dust mites. How many different kinds of allergies are there?*

Even though a person could be allergic to hundreds of different things, there are just four main types of allergic reactions, sensibly called Type 1, Type 2, Type 3, and Type 4. Type 1 and Type 4 are most common, but we'll cover all the bases, just to be complete.

*Type 1 allergic reactions* are immediate; they are usually due to reactions of the immune molecule, immunoglobulin E (IgE). IgE molecules trigger the mast cells in the immune system to release histamine—the chemical that causes swelling, itching, and watering. Type 1 reactions cause watery eyes, sneezing, hives, itching, swelling, and in the most extreme cases, shock. People who are allergic to latex rubber (such as Joannie, who had several operations in which the operating team used latex gloves) can become so sensitive that they develop symptoms if they even enter a room in which latex was used.[3] Fortunately, severe Type 1 reactions are treatable with medication.

*Just as we were about to close the clinic one warm summer evening, Bill Aylers rushed in the door carrying his pregnant wife, Judy. She was weak to the point of collapse, wheezing and dotted with hives. Bill told me that he and Judy had been visiting relatives in the country. As they got in the car, Judy was stung by a bee. She felt weak and started wheezing almost immediately. As he frantically drove down the road, he saw our clinic lights on and pulled in. Within minutes after a shot of adrenaline (epinephrine) and a dose of Benadryl (diphenhydramine), Judy roused, the hives faded, and the wheezing lessened. Bill's quick action and our clinic's readiness for this kind of emergency saved his wife's (and unborn baby's) life.*

This kind of immediate, life-threatening Type 1 allergic reaction is called *anaphylaxis*. In sensitive people, insect stings, certain medications, or even common foods, such as eggs, nuts, strawberries, or shellfish, can trigger anaphylaxis. Parents whose children have had an anaphylactic reaction to common foods such as eggs or wheat must be vigilant about the ingredients in prepared or processed foods such as breads, cakes, snacks, and candy because they may contain the fatal allergen. Type 1 allergic reactions to food cause about one hundred deaths in the United States each year—about twice the number of deaths due to allergic reactions to insect stings.

Most of the time, the IgE molecule causes Type 1 immediate reactions that are less serious. The reactions most people get to ragweed pollen or cats happen within an hour or two of exposure—watery, itchy eyes, sneezing, wheezing, coughing, and hives. This less serious variety of Type I reaction is far more common than

anaphylaxis. It is the main reason for the booming industry in antihistamines. Many food allergies are also caused by IgE molecules. These allergies trigger asthma symptoms and eczema for many children; in fact, among children who suffer from both severe, chronic eczema and asthma, eggs induce symptoms in 50% and wheat causes reactions in 20%.[4]

*Type 2 allergic reactions* are those in which antibodies attack not just a molecule but a whole cell. This is the kind of reaction that destroys red blood cells if the wrong type of blood is given during a transfusion. Type 2 reactions are uncommon.

*Type 3 allergic reactions* occur when antibodies bind to foreign proteins, forming big clusters that deposit in various tissues such as the kidneys and the joints. Wherever they settle, these clusters cause problems such as allergic arthritis. It usually takes several days after the initial clusters form to develop symptoms. This may be the mechanism by which allergies to certain foods and food additives trigger joint pain and arthritis.[5]

*Type 4 allergic reactions* are typified by the common responses to poison ivy, perfumes, and to nickel jewelry (contact dermatitis). They usually take twelve to twenty-four hours after contact to become visible. Type 4 reactions cause intense itching and a blistering rash, but are rarely life-threatening. Just about everyone is allergic to poison ivy. About 25% of children are allergic to other contact allergens such as nickel.[6]

### How much allergen does it take to trigger symptoms?

Some allergies don't depend on the dose of allergen—one bee sting or one bite of eggs may be enough to trigger a severe reaction. Other allergic responses do depend on the dose. A child who is allergic to cow's milk may tolerate a half cup of milk on his cereal in the morning, but experience severe bloody diarrhea if he drinks a quart of milk in a day. Some allergies (such as that to animal dander) are perennial (all year round) and some only occur during certain seasons (such as ragweed season in the fall or tree pollen allergies in the spring). Some allergies are lifelong, and others are outgrown; for example, about 5% of children less than three years old have food allergies, but this decreases to 1 to 2 percent in adults.[7] Hay fever becomes more common with age, peaking between twenty and forty years old.

### Why do some kids develop allergies and others don't?

No one knows for sure exactly why some people develop allergies and others don't. Allergies run in families, but the number of people with allergies is rising much faster than our genetic heritage changes.[8] Although being an only child of wealthy, older parents is good for preventing most health conditions, it is actually associated with an increased risk of hay fever and grass allergies; when it comes to allergies, you're much better off being the youngest child in a large family or starting day care in the first six months of life.[9] Current theories about the increase in allergies focus on recent changes in the environment—from what we eat to what we breathe, to how many people we live with, to what infections we get. There is a huge concern about the potential effects of processed foods, pesticides, hormones, genetically modified foods, and antibiotics given to livestock. Others believe that the problem is due to decreases in breast-feeding rates, increases in air pollution, decreases in exercise, increases in urbanization (decreased exposure to pets and farm animals), or something else entirely.[10] One of the weirder and most intriguing ideas about what's causing the increase in allergies is that we've been too successful in eliminating parasitic worms (called *helminths* in medical lingo) from our intestinal tract. This theory says that our immune systems evolved over millions of years to combat these critters, and when we eliminate them, our bored immune systems started picking on other things.[11] Another theory blames the *H. pylori* bacteria. This bacteria causes ulcers and is found in more adults than children (just the reverse of food allergies, which are much more common in children than adults), but in one study of unfortunate adults who had both ulcers *and* allergies, treating the ulcer with antibiotics resulted in dramatic improvement in allergy symptoms. This certainly isn't the first thing I'd think of when seeing a new child with allergies, but if the child also has an ulcer or has a history of *H. pylori*, I'd certainly try to get rid of that darned bacteria!

## COMMON ALLERGY TRIGGERS

### OUTDOORS

- Plants and their pollens: such as poison ivy and poison oak, ragweed, grass
- Chemicals: such as insecticides, pesticides, fertilizers, fumigants
- Air pollution: sulfur dioxide and particulates
- Insect venom, such as bee stings

### INDOORS

- Animal dander, saliva, or urine
- Dust and dust mites
- Foods: such as nuts and peanuts, cow's milk, soy, fish, eggs, wheat, oranges, strawberries, chocolate, tomatoes, corn
- Herbs: such as feverfew, chamomile, parrow, tansy
- Irritants: such as wool, fabric finishes, dry-cleaning solvents

- Chemicals: such as perfumes, soaps, detergents, cosmetics. cleaning products, disinfectants, solvents, turpentine, paint, formaldehyde
- Food colorings, additives, preservatives, hormones, antibiotics
- Medications: such as aspirin, antibiotics, morphine, X-ray contrast material

In addition to not feeling well, children who suffer from allergies frequently suffer from other problems. For example, they tend to grow poorly. So much of their energy is consumed with the allergy, there just isn't enough left over to grow. Chronic nasal allergies lead to nasal obstruction, mouth-breathing, and can eventually lead to deformities of the face, necessitating later orthodontic intervention. Children with hay fever–type allergies can have more frequent ear infections, sinus infections, and delayed language development.

When children eat foods to which they are allergic, the normal intestinal barrier is breached, promoting sensitivity to even more foods.[12] Fortunately, many children outgrow food allergies over one to three years.[13] Those whose symptoms come on immediately or within a few hours are more likely to outgrow their allergies than those children whose symptoms occur several hours or days after eating the allergenic food.[14]

## Could It Be Something Else?

Yes. It is often difficult to diagnose allergies in babies because allergic symptoms can easily be attributed to other problems: colds, diarrhea, eczema, and sleeping problems. Sometimes it's hard to tell the difference between a cold and an allergy, both cause runny or stuffy noses and sneezing. Children who have diarrhea and gas after drinking milk due to lactase deficiency have similar symptoms to children suffering from true milk allergies. If you are not sure whether your child's symptoms are due to allergies or something else, take him to be evaluated by a professional who is experienced in treating allergies.

## Diagnosing Allergies

The basis of all allergy diagnosis is the relationship of the child's symptoms to his exposure to allergens. Physical examination is also useful. Keep a careful symptom diary, noting what kinds of symptoms your child develops, the timing, previous exposures, etc. This will be the most helpful tool in figuring out what's causing allergic symptoms. Some triggers work immediately—the child develops hives within minutes of exposure to the trigger—whereas others are more delayed, with symptoms not appearing for 6 to 12 hours. Be alert for hidden exposures; one woman who was allergic to numerous foods and pollens, and who made every effort to eliminate them, continued to have symptoms until she realized that her shampoo contained apricot—to which she was allergic. Changing shampoos dramatically improved her symptoms.

A variety of allergenic foods are hidden in common foods and ingredients.[15] Sometimes food manufacturers use the same equipment to make different products. One product may call for eggs, and even if the next recipe doesn't require eggs, tiny amounts of egg may remain on the equipment and contaminate the next product. All manufactured, processed foods must be suspect for highly allergic children. Kids may have severe reactions the very first time they knowingly eat an allergenic food; or they might not have any problems the first few times and then develop a severe reaction.

| INGREDIENTS AND FOODS THAT MAY CONTAIN EGGS | |
|---|---|
| *Ingredients* | *Foods* |
| albumin, binder, coagulants, egg white, egg yolk, emulsifier, globulin, lecithin, ovalbumin, powdered egg, vitellin, whole egg | baked goods, baking mixes, batters, Bearnaise sauce, breakfast cereals, cake flours, cookies, custard, egg noodles, French toast, hollandaise sauce, ice cream, lemon curd, macaroni, malted drinks, mayonnaise, meringues, muffins, noodles, omelettes, pancakes, puddings, sherbets, souffles, spaghetti, tartar sauce, waffles |

Milk protein also shows up in a lot of prepared foods:

| INGREDIENTS AND FOODS CONTAINING MILK PROTEIN | |
|---|---|
| *Ingredients* | *Foods* |
| butter flavor, butter fat, buttermilk solids, caramel color, casein, caseinate, cheese, cream, curds, dried milk, dry milk solids, high-protein flavor, lactalbumin, lactose, milk protein, milk solids, natural flavoring, rennet, casein, skim milk powder solids, whey, whey powder, whey protein concentrate, yogurt | batter-fried foods, biscuits, bread, breakfast cereals, cakes, chocolate, cookies, cream sauces or soups, custard, gravy and gravy mixes, ice cream, sour cream, imitation sour cream, instant potatoes, margarine, muesli, muffins, canned soups, packaged soups, pies, puddings, sherbet |

Soy protein is called by several different names on ingredient lists. It's hard to avoid in processed foods.

## SOY PROTEIN

- Gum arabic
- Bulking agent
- Emulsifier
- Guar gum
- Hydrolyzed vegetable protein
- Protein or protein extender
- Soy protein, soy protein isolate, soy sauce, soybean oil
- Stabilizer, starch
- Textured vegetable protein, thickener
- Tofu
- Vegetable broth, vegetable gum, vegetable starch

Peanut allergies affect about 1% of all children;[16] these allergies can be quite severe and are seldom outgrown.[17] Many products contain peanuts or peanut oil—a significant hidden hazard for those who are allergic to it. Be particularly careful of Chinese, African, and Thai cuisines, which often include frying in peanut oil or using peanut butter in sauces.

A variety of diagnostic tests have been developed to test for allergies.

## DIAGNOSTIC TESTS FOR ALLERGIES

- Symptom diary
- Skin prick, intradermal, scratch or patch tests; DMSO patch test
- Double-blind, placebo-controlled food challenges
- Blood tests: RAST, FICA, cytokins, CAP FEIA, levels of IgE, IgG, and histamine

Health professionals rely on a variety of tests to diagnose allergies.[18] *Skin prick, intradermal, patch or skin scratch tests* are the most widely available and widely used allergy tests. The intradermal (or intracutaneous) progressive dilution test is endorsed by mainstream medical groups as the most reliable type of test for food allergies (other than the double-blind, placebo-controlled food challenge described below).[19] In a skin test, the child's skin is scratched and a liquid containing the suspected allergen is dropped on the scratched or pricked area. The test is considered positive if the skin develops hives at the scratch site. The prick or scratch tests have a fair number of false positive results. This means that your child could have a positive test and not really have an allergy. These tests can also have false negatives; this means that it looks like the substance is not a problem for your child when it actually is a trigger. If you strongly suspect a substance is allergic for your child, but the skin test is negative, ask the physician to repeat the test using *freshly* prepared extracts to avoid missing the diagnosis.

DMSO is a chemical that makes the skin very permeable to other compounds. It is used in some skin tests as a replacement for a scratch or prick. The DMSO is mixed with the suspected food and applied to the skin as a patch. Positive reactions include anything from mild redness to severe blistering. Because the skin is not actually punctured, the DMSO test seems to cause fewer systemic reactions than the prick or scratch or injection tests, making it one of the safest skin tests around.

For diagnosing food allergies, the most common and reliable test is a *double-blind, placebo-controlled food challenge*. In this test, all potentially allergic foods are withheld for several days; then the child is given a capsule containing either a suspected allergen or an inert substance (placebo). Neither the child, the parents, nor the physician know whether the capsule contains the allergen or the placebo. After taking the capsule, the child is carefully watched for any type of reaction. A more extreme permutation of this test requires hospitalization in a special low-allergy unit and going on a fast or severely restricted diet, gradually reintroducing substances and assessing the child's reactions as each thing is added—a food, a pollen, dust, etc. This kind of evaluation is expensive, time-consuming, and stressful for the family and child, so it is not often done. In severe cases, it may be the best alternative.

A number of blood tests have been developed to try to spare kids the discomfort of having large areas of skin exposed to potential allergens in the various scratch, prick, and injection tests. On the other hand, sometimes you get what you pay for. Blood tests are easier and less costly than doing a double-blind food challenge. However, most of them are not very reliable. The *RAST (radioallergosorbent test)* is one of the most commonly used tests for allergies because it is convenient and pretty good for inhaled allergens such as pollen and dander, but it can be inaccurate for food allergies. The *FICA (food immune complex assay)* is another blood test. *Cytotoxic blood tests* for allergies are fairly controversial. In this test, the child's white blood cells are mixed with the suspected allergen; if the white cells react, the child is thought to be allergic to that substance. The problem is that white cells in a test tube don't necessarily react the same way they do in the body surrounded by other cells and molecules. The test is also very dependent on the skill of the person looking at the white blood cell reaction; there is a lot of variability in interpreting the test results. A new lab test is the *FEIA (fluorescent enzyme immunoassay)*, which may eventually replace the gold standard for food allergies, the double-blind placebo-controlled food challenge test. Work is ongoing.

Kids who have allergies typically have higher than normal levels of several immunoglobulins (immune proteins) in their blood; these include IgE and IgG. They can also have higher than normal levels of certain immune cells such as basophils and other immune chemicals such as histamine. This just means that your child has a revved-up immune system, which you probably already knew; it does not tell you what is triggering the allergy or what the best treatment is.[20] Though practitioners who use them come up with theories that sound convincing, there is no known scientific basis for fads such as urine autoinjection, kinesiology testing, Vega testing, or electrodermal diagnostic techniques.[21]

Remember, the best test for allergies is *careful observation*. Keep a diary of your child's symptoms and exposures. You may be able to figure it out yourself with some careful detective work. The son of one of my colleagues was allergic to corn (among other things). She noticed that he developed a severe diaper rash every time she gave him a common pain relieving medication. Finally she checked the label—sure enough, it contained corn syrup. When she switched to a product free of corn syrup—no more diaper rashes. Another child seemed to be allergic to a number of medications, but it turned out that all three contained red dye no. 40; it was the dye, not the active ingredients themselves that caused the problems. If you suspect an additive, and the label doesn't list *all* the ingredients, contact the manufacturer.

## WHAT'S THE BEST WAY TO PREVENT AND TREAT ALLERGIES?

The best preventive strategy is to avoid the allergen (Lifestyle—environment). When children are inundated with allergens, their immune systems get revved up, and it takes very little of another allergen to trigger a big reaction. On the other hand, if your child is allergic to three things—cats, dust, and pollen, for example—and you markedly reduce her exposure to two of those things (say cats and dust), she will be much less likely to react to the third (pollen). If you can eliminate most of your child's allergy triggers by changing things you can control (dust and pets), you may also reduce her sensitivity to other triggers over which you have less control (pollen). Let's tour the Therapeutic Mountain to find out what treatments have proven effectiveness. If you want to skip to my bottom-line recommendations, flip to the end of the chapter.

## BIOCHEMICAL THERAPIES: MEDICATIONS, HERBS, NUTRITIONAL SUPPLEMENTS

### Medications

The overwhelming variety of allergy medications can be confusing. There are several classes of effective medications that work different ways.

### ALLERGY MEDICATIONS

- Antihistamines
- Leukotriene inhibitors
- Mast cell stabilizers
- Steroids
- Desensitization therapy
- Epinephrine
- Decongestants
- Saline
- Others

*Antihistamines* are the mainstay of medical allergy treatments. They work by blocking the histamine released from mast cells. There are many types, varieties, and brands of antihistamines. It's impossible to tell which antihistamine is most effective for your child unless you try different kinds. Most people start with the least expensive nonprescription remedy. If these don't help or have unacceptable side effects, see your physician about other (more expensive) prescription medications. More expensive antihistamines are not necessarily more effective, but they may be less sedating.

### ANTIHISTAMINES

- *Nonprescription:* triprolidine (Actidil), diphenhydramine (Benadryl), chlorpheniramine, maleate (Chlortrimeton), brompheniramine (Dimetane), clemastine fumarate (Tavist)
- *Prescription:* hydroxyzine (Atarax), cyproheptadine (Periactin), promethazine (Phenergan)
- *Prescription (nonsedating):* astemizole (Hismanal), loratadine (Claritin), fexofenadine (Allegra), cetirizine (Zyrtec), azelastine (Astelin nasal spray)

Many antihistamines are available without a prescription. Nearly all of them require doses every few hours and have side effects such as a dry mouth, difficulty concentrating, and drowsiness; a few children also have problems with urination and constipation. Some children become irritable and hyperactive from antihistamines. Antihistamines do a good job with runny noses, but they don't help much with congestion. That's why many allergy preparations contain a *decongestant* as well as an antihistamine. Decongestants have additional side effects: increased blood pressure, irritability, insomnia, nervousness, increased heart rate, and decreased appetite.

Because most people don't want to spend the entire hay fever season sleeping, they often ask physicians for prescription antihistamines that are less sedating, such as Claritin, Zyrtec, or Allegra. These medications only require dosing once or twice daily. They are, however, extremely expensive compared to nonprescription antihistamines; astemizole (Hismanal) is approved for children six years and older and loratidine and cetirizine are approved for those two years and older. These should *not* be taken at the same time your child is on erythromycin-type antibiotics or antifungal medications such as ketoconazole because of the risk of liver toxicity. Some patients have had serious and even fatal irregular heart rhythms while taking astemizole ; cetirizine has caused fewer heart problems and doesn't seem to interact with as many other medications as terfenadine or astemizole, but it is more sedating.[22] Be sure to ask both the physician and your pharmacist about potential interactions before starting any new medication. Because they are so much less sedating than other antihistamine medications, they may be the safest option if your child needs to drive or operate heavy machinery during peak allergy season.[23] On the other hand, steroid nasal sprays (see below) don't cause any sedation and may be more effective than antihistamines, particularly for kids with severe allergies and asthma; more and more physicians are turning to nasal steroid sprays instead of antihistamines for first-line treatment.[24]

If your child's allergy symptoms are mostly related to the nose (runny nose, itching, sneezing), you may want to consider azelastine (Astelin) nasal spray. In comparison trials, using Astelin nasal spray twice a day was as effective as the nonsedating antihistamines that are taken by mouth. Also, because it's sprayed in the nose, Astelin is less likely to cause systemic side effects and less likely to interact with other medications. It may sting for a minute right after administration and some kids complain that it tastes bad, but I think it's a good option because it's less likely to interact with other medications.

When using an antihistamine, give it to your child *before* symptoms occur rather than after your child is miserable. Remember, antihistamines work by inhibiting the reaction to allergens. If your child's symptoms are worse when he goes to visit his cat-loving friend, giving him an antihistamine 30 to 60 minutes before he gets to the friend's house is more effective than delaying treatment until he's coughing and sneezing.

You can also increase your child's tolerance to the sedating effect of antihistamines by starting him on doses before he goes to bed, when it doesn't matter if he's sleepy. Then add low daytime doses and gradually increase the dose as his body gets used to it.

Although antihistamines help relieve allergic symptoms, they do not address the underlying sensitivity that causes allergies. Go ahead and use them if your child has mild or occasional symptoms and to help your child feel more comfortable while you take other measures to address the underlying problem.

A new class of prescription medications that were developed to treat asthma are also finding their way into the allergists' toolkit. These medications affect the production and attachment of leukotriene chemicals, which are inflammation-causing compounds produced throughout the body. These medications include zafirlukast (Accolate), which is approved in children seven years and older, montelukast (Singulair), which is approved for children six years and older, and zileuton (Zyflo), which is approved for teenagers and adults; all of these medications can interact with other medications.

*Mast cell stabilizers* are medications that calm the mast cells that release histamine. These medications require a prescription. They are also best given *before* symptoms start. Unlike antihistamines, they have very few side effects, and I recommend them for children who have year-round or predictable allergies, such as to dust mites or ragweed. Cromolyn is effective in preventing food allergy symptoms as well as allergic asthma.[25]

## MAST CELL STABILIZERS (ALL REQUIRE PRESCRIPTION)

- Loxamide (Alomide) eye drops
- Olopatadine (Patanol) eye drops
- Cromolyn (Nasalcrom) nasal spray
- Nedocromil (Tilade) inhaler and eye drops

Mast cell stabilizers have fewer side effects than other allergy preparations because they target just one area. For example, Alomide and Patanol eye drops are just put in the eye, Nasalcrom is sprayed in the nose, and Tilade is inhaled into the lungs. They prevent the release of histamine from the mast cells where they're applied but do not affect other tissues such as the brain or heart. They have specific rather than general effects. They are safe to use in combination with other more general treatments such as antihistamines or steroids. They also tend to be less expensive than oral, nonsedating antihistamines or orally administered steroids.

*Steroid medications* are available in several forms to treat different kinds of allergic reactions. Steroid medications are very similar to the body's own anti-inflammatory messengers. They help reduce swelling, pain, and irritation.

## STEROID PREPARATIONS FOR ALLERGIES

- *Creams or ointments:* such as Cortaid—prescription and nonprescription hydrocortisone
- *Nasal sprays:* such as Vancenase and Beconase (beclomethasone), Flonase (fluticasone), Nasalide (flunisolide), Nasonex (mometasone), Nasacort (triamcinolone), Rhinocort (budesonide)—all prescription only
- *Metered dose inhalers* for allergic asthma: such as Aerobid, Azmacort, Beclovent, Decadron, Vanceril—prescription only
- *Oral steroids* for systemic symptoms: such as cortisone, Decadron, Medrol, Pedi-pred, Prelone, Prednisone—prescription only

The mildest kind of *steroid creams* (0.5% and 1% hydrocortisone, Cortaid) are available without a prescription. They are helpful for allergic rashes such as poison ivy. Prescription-strength steroids are available as *nasal sprays* to treat runny nose and congestion due to allergies. Some (such as mometasone, fluticasone, and budesonide) are effective even with once-a-day dosing;[26] steroid nasal sprays are best used as a preventive therapy before symptoms start.[27] It takes several days to a week for improvements to be noticeable. Steroids are available in *inhaled form* (metered dose inhalers, MDIs) to treat children with allergic asthma. For children with more severe, system-wide symptoms, *steroid pills or liquid* may be needed to get symptoms under control. When taken by mouth, steroids can have powerful side effects—suppressing the immune system, raising blood sugar, increasing blood pressure; they should be used for as little time as possible. When steroids are applied directly to the affected area (such as creams to rashes and sprays to the nose), they have few side effects and are safe even for young children.

*Allergy shots (desensitization therapy)* are a series of injections of minute amounts of whatever is causing the allergy. By giving extremely small doses, the immune system is stimulated to produce the "good" kind of immune globulin, IgG. IgG blocks the allergy-causing immune globulin, IgE. Allergy shots are most effective for allergies to bee stings,[28] pollen, dust mites, and animals;[29] they are less effective for mold and food allergies.[30] Desensitization therapy usually lasts three to five years and, interestingly, may help protect against developing new allergies.[31] A few children suffer relapsing symptoms when the shots stop, but most (especially those getting shots for allergies to insect stings) continue to be protected.[32] A few allergists, particularly in Europe, are trying *noninjection desensitization;* this involves giving drops of tiny doses of the allergen under the tongue; it may work better than placebo, but it can still result in serious allergic reactions and should only be tried with an experienced allergy doctor.[33] Desensitization therapy can be dangerous because if the dose is advanced faster than IgG builds up, the child can have a severe allergic reaction. That's why allergy shots should only be given in the office of a physician who has emergency equipment on hand.

If your child ever has a major allergic reaction (anaphylaxis) to a food, bee sting, or anything else, please have him wear a *Medic-Alert bracelet* and ask your physician for a prescription for *epinephrine* for emergency use. Keep one at home and one with the child wherever he may come in contact with the allergen. Epinephrine can be lifesaving if your child has an anaphylactic reaction. The only drawback is that epinephrine has to be given by a shot. An inhaled epinephrine treatment does not work very well, partly because it requires a lot of "puffs" to get the same amount of medicine delivered by an injection, and also because the stuff tastes so bad, kids don't want to inhale it.[34]

If your child's main symptom is a stuffy nose, you may be tempted to use a nonprescription *nasal decongestant spray*. Don't. Although these products (such as Afrin) are effective in reducing congestion, they do so at a price. Because the blood vessels swell when allergies strike, shrinking them helps open up the nasal passages and results in symptomatic relief. However, the blood vessels quickly become dependent on the medication, requiring higher and more frequent doses to achieve

the same effect. It only takes a few days to become dependent on (or addicted to) decongestant nasal sprays. If your child suddenly quits taking them, he could have rebound swelling and worse congestion than ever.

For those children who have become dependent on their nasal spray, don't make them quit cold turkey. The rebound swelling will just make them miserable and tempted to return to the spray for relief. Instead, spray only one nostril for three days. The unsprayed nostril will initially swell up and feel stuffy, but your child can still breathe through the sprayed side. When the unsprayed side returns to normal in two to three days, stop spraying the other side. It will be congested for a day or two, but your child can breathe through the now normal side. Within a week, both sides will have returned to normal and your child will have overcome the dependence on nasal sprays nearly painlessly.

If you want to help keep nasal secretions loose, give your child simple *saline nose drops* (¼ teaspoon of salt in 8 ounces of water—or buy premixed saline drops, Na-Sal). One or two drops on each side can be given as often as you like to help with congestion. In fact, some parents find that frequent nose washes help rinse out the allergy-causing pollen.

You may be hearing about a new medical treatment for children with allergies. *Atrovent (ipratropium bromide)* has been used for several years to treat adults with nasal allergies and asthma. There is preliminary evidence that it may be useful for children, too.[35]

## Herbs

### HERBAL REMEDIES

- *Scientifically proven useful:* ephedra
- *Scientifically unproven but widely used:* angelica, skullcap, coleus root, eyebright, goldenrod tea,

goldenseal, licorice root, magnolia, nettle leaves, plantain, green clay, and calendula
- *Herbs that may cause allergic reactions*: chamomile, echinacea, others

*Ephedra tea (Ma Huang)* has long been used by the Chinese as a treatment for allergies, asthma, hay fever, and the common cold. It is the original source of *ephedrine* which has been chemically synthesized and is an ingredient in many cold and allergy medications. Ephedra is a decongestant, and it has some anti-inflammatory effects.[36] It is contraindicated for long-term use because with frequent, repeated use, higher and higher doses are required to achieve the same results. Ephedra also has side effects such as high blood pressure and rapid heart rate, so it should not be used by children who have weak hearts or who already have high blood pressure. Due to the many reports of severe and even fatal reactions to it, the federal government and many states have greatly restricted the availability and dosing recommendations for ephedra. Products that remain on the market contain quite variable concentrations of the active ingredients. I do not recommend ephedra; safer alternatives are available.

In addition to having a beautiful ornamental flower, the *angelica (Dong Quai)* plant has been used by Chinese herbalists since ancient times to treat allergies, eczema, and hay fever.[37] *Chinese skullcap tea* decreases inflammation and inhibits the immune system's allergic response. One of the chemical constituents of *coleus root* demonstrated antihistamine properties in animal studies. However, there are no studies that demonstrate the effectiveness of angelica root, Chinese skullcap, or coleus root in treating children with allergies. I do not typically recommend them.

*Eyebright tinctures* have long been used to treat the burning watery eyes and runny nose associated with hay fever–type allergies. You can find tincture of eyebright in natural food stores. *Euphrasia* is also one of the most commonly recommended homeopathic remedies for allergies (see the Homeopathy section below), but its sap can be very irritating. The anti-inflammatory properties of *goldenseal* have made it a favorite herbal remedy, but natural supplies of wild herb have been overharvested and it is no longer commonly recommended. Scientific studies have not evaluated the effectiveness of any of these herbs in treating childhood allergies. I do not recommend them.

*Goldenrod tea or tinctures* are controversial allergy remedies because goldenrod actually causes allergies when it is inhaled. Some physicians believe that drinking goldenrod tea may cause a severe allergic reaction; others who believe in the healing principle of "like cures like" believe that goldenrod tea or tinctures make the perfect preventive medication and antidote to inhaled allergens. Although both sides of the argument can be quite vocal, there are no studies showing either marked benefits or severe risks of goldenrod tea in treating childhood allergies.

*Licorice root* has anti-allergy and anti-inflammatory effects because it blocks the breakdown of cortisol, which is a naturally produced hormone that decreases inflammation.[38] However, due to the other effects of this hormone (which affects the kidneys as well as the immune system), large doses or chronic use of licorice can result in fluid retention, high blood pressure, headache, and significant potassium loss.

*Magnolia* flower buds reduce histamine release in test tube studies, but have not yet been evaluated in children.[39] *Nettles* are common remedies for allergic reactions, particularly for runny nose and watery eyes. In a randomized controlled trial of 98 adult allergy sufferers, those given freeze-dried nettle were more likely to report dramatic or marked improvement in their symptoms over the next week than those patients given placebo pills; however, the differences were not significant statistically.[40] Because brushing up against a nettle plant usually causes stinging and hives, it is also a commonly recommended homeopathic remedy for allergies. Again, there is no scientific evidence that it is useful. It needs more study.

For those suffering from allergic skin rashes, *plantain* poultices are said to be soothing. Others recommend an application of a paste made of *green clay* and water to the affected area. Many people find *calendula* creams and ointments soothing for allergic skin irritation. However, there are no scientific studies documenting the effectiveness of any of these remedies in treating allergic rashes.

Many herbs can actually cause allergic reactions. The most famous culprits are members of the daisy family—echinacea, chamomile, feverfew, and others. These reactions can be life-threatening.[41] Fortunately, they are pretty rare.

## Nutritional Supplements

### NUTRITIONAL SUPPLEMENTS FOR ALLERGIES

- Vitamin C
- Essential fatty acids: fish, flax, and evening primrose oils
- Other vitamins and minerals
- Red peppers (capsaicin)

Large doses of *vitamin C* (2 grams per day) alleviate allergy symptoms in adults with allergic asthma and hay fever.[42] No studies have yet evaluated the benefits of vitamin C for allergic children, but it is so safe, I often recommend it for children with allergies and asthma. If you'd like to try vitamin C, give about 250 milligrams twice daily for children between three and six years old and 500 to 1,000 milligrams twice daily to older children. Vitamin C is excreted very rapidly, so look for extended release formulations. If your child develops diarrhea (an early symptom of vitamin C overdose) reduce the dose.

Other supplements, such as *vitamins A, B6, E, beta-carotene, selenium,* and *zinc* have been recommended as allergy remedies, but there is little research to support their use in treating children with allergies, and I do not typically recommend them.

Supplemental *essential fatty acids (EFA)* are sometimes given to children with allergies and eczema. Two main types of EFA are recommended—omega-3 fatty acids (found in fatty fish, fish oils, cod liver oil, and flax seed oil) and omega-6 fatty acids (found in evening primrose, black currant, and borage oils). Some allergic families have a blockage in fatty acid metabolism, which makes the immune system more prone to allergies and inflammation. For example, children who are prone to allergies and eczema have lower than normal levels of EFA in their blood and their moms seem to produce less omega-3 fatty acids in their breast milk.[43] By giving large doses of EFA, the immune system may become more stable. In scientific studies, doses of two capsules (1,000 milligrams) three times daily of evening primrose oil were helpful in treating children suffering from eczema (see Chapter 18, Eczema); it takes about eight weeks for any benefits to become noticeable. The data are not strong enough to suggest that all allergic children have to take cod liver oil or evening primrose oil, but unless they're allergic to fish, I think that all kids who are prone to allergies should eat fatty fish (such as salmon or mackerel) at least twice a week, and try to include flaxseed oil in their salad dressings.

*Capsaicin*, the spicy, pungent molecule in red peppers, decreases airway sensitivity to irritants such as tobacco smoke. Spicy foods such as peppers, horseradish, and hot mustard have long been part of folk remedies for respiratory allergies. In animal studies, capsaicin decreases a variety of airway allergic responses.[44] There are no studies yet evaluating the effects of hot peppers in allergic children, but see if your child's symptoms improve following a spicy meal.

One theory holds that food allergies are due to the passage of small molecules of undigested food across a leaky gut wall into the bloodstream. Those who hold to this theory believe that *digestive enzymes* such as *papaya enzyme tablets* and *bromelain* may be helpful in preventing allergies. Others believe that allergic reactions are causes, not consequences, of leaky intestines.[45] Although papaya is one of my favorite foods, it has not been scientifically evaluated for its effectiveness in treating childhood allergies.

*Bee pollen supplements* are another favorite allergy remedy, which have not been scientifically studied in children.

## LIFESTYLE THERAPIES: NUTRITION, EXERCISE, ENVIRONMENT, MIND-BODY

### Nutrition

Food allergies, remember, are much more common in children than in adults. About 5 to 8 percent of kids have food allergies, but most kids outgrow them so that only about 1 percent of adults have food allergies;[46] the most common food triggers are cow's milk, eggs, wheat, soy, fish, citrus, strawberries, peanuts, and tree nuts (such as Brazil nuts, almonds, and hazelnuts)—some of the most frequently eaten foods in childhood! Allergies to rice have been reported, but are rare.[47] Food allergies often run in families; for example, kids whose parents are allergic to peanuts are more likely to have peanut allergies than kids whose par-

ents have no allergies.[48] (It pays to pick your parents wisely!) Fortunately there's good evidence that avoiding allergy triggers early in life can help reduce sensitivity later on by 30 to 60 percent.

By now you've probably noticed that I recommend breast-feeding as a preventive therapy for just about every condition. What about allergies? Yes, breast-feeding helps prevent allergies, especially for kids whose families are prone to allergies and eczema and especially when parents are able to stop smoking and mothers minimize their intake of allergenic foods such as peanuts.[49] One study even found that breast-feeding for more than six months helped protect kids against developing allergies, eczema, and asthma for the next seventeen years![50] Moms need to be extra careful about what they eat and drink while they're nursing because the foods they eat are often concentrated in breast milk; for example, the protein from cow's milk is concentrated in breast milk, so if a mom drinks cow's milk, her nursing child is exposed to cow's milk protein.[51] For breast-feeding moms who've battled allergies triggered by cow's milk, avoiding cow's milk during pregnancy and while breast-feeding protects the baby against exposure to cow's milk proteins and reduces the risk of becoming allergic to cow's milk by about 60%.[52] If for some reason you need to feed formula, choose a hypoallergenic formula, preferably a hydrolyzed formula.[53] Moms who are allergic to peanuts, fish, eggs, wheat, corn, or other common allergens should avoid eating them during their last trimester of pregnancy and the whole time they are nursing the baby.[54]

*Mare's milk,* anyone? I know it sounds weird, but milk from horses is actually closer to human milk than milk from cows. And it seems to cause far fewer allergies than cow's milk.[55] It's pretty hard to find unless you raise your own horses, though.

You may have also recognized that I'm a big fan of yogurt and other cultured or fermented dairy drinks that contain pro-biotics or healthy bacteria. If your child can tolerate cow's milk–based products, it may be worth boosting his intake of yogurt, kefir, and other foods rich in *Lactobacillus, Bifidobacterium,* and *Strep thermophilus.* These healthy bacteria suppress the growth of bad bacteria in the intestines and also seem to stimulate healthy immune responses. Eating yogurt regularly can decrease the production of IgE, the immune compound responsible for a good many allergic reactions.[56] There are few contraindications or side effects. And you don't need a doctor's prescription.

Children who are fed a variety of solids before six months of age are more susceptible to developing allergic skin rashes than children who solely breast-feed for six months.[57] Do not feed your child anything besides mother's milk or formula in the first four to six months of life. Feeding beef before the baby is six months old also increases the risk of allergies. Even future cowboys don't need to start eating beef before six months of age!

Omitting an allergenic food from the diet may be your only practical alternative if your child has a serious Type I anaphylactic reaction to certain foods. Some clinicians recommend that a severely suffering patient go on a total fast for four to five days to clean all potential allergens out of the system before reintroducing possible offenders (one every few days). I do *not* recommend fasts for children under six years old; nor should they be undertaken in older children without the supervision of a dietitian or nutritionist. Eliminating major dietary staples such as milk or wheat runs the risk of developing serious nutritional deficiencies.[58] Most children who consume milk-free diets get too little calcium unless they receive supplements.

Be aware of potential cross-reactions between inhaled allergens and foods. For example, many who suffer from ragweed allergies (worse in the fall) are also allergic to melon (cantaloupe, honeydew, or watermelon). Those who are allergic to birch tree pollen may react to apples, carrots, cherries, pears, peaches, or potatoes. Keep a diary of your child's exposures to foods and pollens and their allergic symptoms to help sort out these associations.

I do not recommend that most children eat much red meat because of its high fat and cholesterol content, the widespread use of hormones and antibiotics in the meat industry, and the tremendous drain on the ecosystem involved in producing meat compared with other sources of protein. However, lamb is one of the least allergic foods available, and you can include it as a source of protein in a "few foods" diet for your allergic child. Try to buy meats labeled as "organic" or free of hormones and antibiotics or use wild game to reduce your child's exposure to these chemicals.

Sugar has been blamed for a variety of childhood problems from acne to tooth decay to hyperactivity to allergies. Sugar comes in a variety of forms including table sugar (sucrose), the milk sugar found in human, cow, and goat milk (lactose), and fruit sugar (fructose). There are no studies showing that children have fewer allergy symptoms when they avoid sugar. However, kids don't need candy or soft drinks to grow well. They can get plenty of calories to grow and be healthy from whole foods without adding sugar. I recommend that most parents keep a lid on their child's sugar consumption, but you don't necessarily need to take extra precautions if your child has allergies.

Despite widespread recommendations to avoid "mucus-producing foods" such as dairy products, there have not been any scientific studies showing that dairy products produce more mucus than any other kind of food. True milk allergies typically cause diarrhea, upset stomach, anemia, chronic lung problems, and eczema.[59] On the other hand, yogurt may be a helpful preventive therapy for children suffering from allergies. Yogurt containing live cultures increases the level of gamma interferon, one of the body's own infection and allergy-fighting chemicals. Start feeding your child yogurt several months before allergy season starts to build up gamma interferon levels. Better yet, eat yogurt all year round!

Remember, many children outgrow their food allergies.[60] It's most common to outgrow allergies to cow's milk, eggs, and soy protein. It's easiest to outgrow these allergies if the triggers are completely avoided for six to twelve months. Some food allergies are *not* outgrown. Kids who are allergic to peanuts, nuts, and fish tend to stay allergic to them, even if they're not exposed for years. Peanuts are especially hazardous because peanut oil is used in a lot of prepared foods and can trigger a life-threatening reaction in an unsuspecting youngster. If your child is allergic to peanuts, you *must* read food labels carefully, let the school, camp, and coach know about the allergy, and be prepared with epinephrine and an antihistamine. And if you decide to try to reintroduce an allergic food to see if your child still reacts, *please* do it in a physician's office, just in case your child has a severe reaction.[61]

## Exercise

Vigorous exercise can make allergy symptoms worse. Not only does outdoor exercise expose children to pollens and air pollution, but some children actually get hives just from getting overheated. Some children have worse food allergy symptoms if they exercise immediately after eating.[62] For example, they might have no symptoms if they eat wheat (to which they are allergic) and didn't exercise, but they might have a severe reaction if they eat wheat and then exercise. One adult had repeated life-threatening allergic reactions when exercising

after eating hazelnuts. No one knows exactly why this happens, but perhaps it's another reason for the conventional wisdom to rest for half an hour after eating before engaging in vigorous exercise. Some sensitive kids may have to wait eight to twelve hours after eating certain foods to avoid having an allergic reaction to them;[63] I say, avoid the foods and get the exercise!

## Environment

The primary treatment for allergies is environmental: avoid the allergen! The three most common non-food allergens are: pollen, dust mites, and pet dander. The majority of people who are allergic to one thing are sensitive to other triggers as well. The bigger the burden of allergens, the more likely your child is to react to something. If you reduce your child's exposure to common allergens, it may reduce his reaction not only to those, but to other allergens over which you have less control. Minimizing your child's exposure to house dust mites early in life can also help prevent a variety of later allergic reactions.[64]

If your child is allergic to pollens, take a few minutes each day to check on the daily pollen count. Radio and television stations and local Internet weather sites usually have this information, or call your local weather service. Pollen counts are generally highest in the morning, so you may want to limit your child's outdoor activities until the afternoon and keep the windows closed in the morning.

Between 5 and 10 percent of Americans are allergic to cats or dogs. About twice as many children are allergic to cats as are allergic to dogs. Interestingly, children who live with cats as infants often develop tolerance to cats and are less likely to be allergic later on than children initially raised without them.[65] Children can also be allergic to guinea pigs, mice, hamsters, and rats. Even if the animal is removed from the home and you start an aggressive cleaning campaign, it can take four to six months for animal allergen levels to clear. Washing the cat makes for an unhappy cat (and a pretty scratched-up cat owner) and needs to be done every five to six days to really reduce shedding of allergenic cat dander;[66] still, it may be better than getting rid of a beloved pet. Same for dogs, though in my experience they don't put up as much of a fuss at bath time as cats do.

## TIPS FOR REDUCING ALLERGENS IN THE HOME

1. Thoroughly dust (using a damp cloth or mop) and vacuum the house every week. Change the vacuum's dust bag frequently. Keep your child out of the vacuumed room for an hour after you've finished to allow the dust to settle.
2. Avoid using chemical cleaners that leave a lingering smell. Cleaning with bleach helps eliminate molds from damp areas. Bleach (5% in water) eliminates other allergens, too.
3. Remove all dust-catchers from your child's room. This means carpeting, stuffed animals, ruffled bedclothes, and draperies. Avoid wool blankets and synthetic pillows in your child's room. Wash all of your child's bedding in hot water (at least 130 degrees Fahrenheit) weekly to destroy dust mites. To avoid additional pollen, do not dry the bedding outdoors. Dry cleaning does not reduce allergens as much as cleaning in very hot water.[67]
4. Encase your child's mattress and pillow (favorite homes of the dust mite) in allergy-proof nylon or vinyl casings. This makes a big difference.

5. Install a high-efficiency particulate arresting (HEPA) air filter in your child's room. Keep the windows closed between 5 and 10 A.M. when pollen counts are highest. Install an electrostatic air filter on your furnace or air conditioner.[68]
6. Add air-cleaning house plants (such as philodendrons and spider plants) in your child's room. They help remove indoor air pollutants.
7. Do not allow furred or feathered pets in your child's room. Preferably, pets should be kept outside. If your pets are as much a loved and integral part of your family as mine are, you can keep them in the house if you bathe them weekly.
8. Keep the humidity in your house below 50% to discourage molds and dust mites.
9. Kill dust mites by spraying an acaricide-dust mite killer (such as Acarosan) or tannic acid (Allersearch-Ads) on all your carpeting, upholstery, and draperies at least twice yearly; thoroughly vacuum a day later to clean up the residue of dead dust mites. You can obtain Acarosan by calling (800) 882-4110, (800) 621-5545, or (800) 422-3878.
10. DO NOT SMOKE AND DO NOT ALLOW OTHERS TO SMOKE IN YOUR HOME.

Housecleaning is a key therapy to reduce allergy symptoms due to dust mites, dust, and danders. (Unfortunately, I don't know of any health insurance companies that will pay to have someone come clean your home!) The biggest exposure to dust mites is in bed, where children typically spend eight to ten hours a day. Washing bedding, even in cold water, reduces dust mites by one hundred–fold, but it doesn't kill them all, and they reaccumulate within two weeks. If your child is sensitive to mites, you need to wash all his bedding weekly. Adding eucalyptus oil to the laundry detergent (3 ounces of eucalyptus oil to 1 ounce of detergent for a single load of bedding in a top-loading machine) kills significantly more mites than washing in detergent alone.[69] Keep the mattress enclosed with a finely woven polyester fabric to keep the mites in the bed away from your child. Dust mites actually seem to prefer growing on synthetic pillows to down pillows; keep the feathers and down unless your child is specifically allergic to ducks or geese.[70]

High-efficiency particulate arresting filters (HEPA) will not eliminate dust mites, but they can help lower the amount of dander in the air. If you have a pet and your child is allergic to it, keep the pet out of the child's bedroom and run a HEPA air filter in the bedroom 24 hours a day; the filter will also help reduce the amount of mold in the air.[71] If you make the wrenching decision to find another home for your dog or cat, recognize that it may take six to twelve months for the levels of animal dander in your home to fall enough to make a dent in your child's allergy symptoms.

Keep the relative humidity below 50% in your home to discourage the growth of dust mites and molds. Molds thrive in damp basements, so if your basement gets wet every time it rains, you could be harboring some serious allergens. If your child's allergies or asthma flare up at school, talk with the school about the humidity there as well. Allergies to molds typically affect kids year round and can trigger sinus infections when molds are at their worst in the damp winter months. Watch out for volatile organic chemicals (VOCs), which trigger allergy symptoms in many children; these chemicals are given off by vinyl flooring and many types of carpeting; check with the salespeople before you buy new flooring. Try to stick to hardwood floors that don't accumulate molds and can be damp-mopped to remove dust and danders.

Environmental therapies can also help treat many allergic reactions. For example, to treat reactions to insect stings, immediately apply ice. Ice numbs the pain and reduces swelling. Remove the stinger by scraping it off; pulling it can release more venom into the skin. Children whose reaction consists of hives and swelling at the sting site are not at increased risk of a life-threatening reaction in the future.

On the other hand, some people break out in hives wherever an ice cube is rubbed on their skin. The runny nose caused by going in and out of the cold is called "skier's nose."

## HOME REMEDIES FOR POISON IVY AND OTHER ALLERGIC RASHES

1. Rub them with ice. Ice helps numb the area, reducing itch.
2. Make a paste of baking soda and water, and rub it in. Baking soda seems to be most helpful for blistering rashes, not plain old hives.
3. Some patients have tried applying milk of magnesia (MOM)—usually used for upset stomachs—when they were desperate and there was nothing else in the house. They reported that it was useful. I've recently learned that some of my colleagues actually recommend MOM as a soothing lotion for itchy rashes. It's readily available and free of side effects, but I don't think anyone has actually studied its effectiveness as an allergy remedy in scientific studies.
4. Other parents report that zinc-oxide (the active ingredient in the strongest sun blocks and diaper rash preparations) is also an effective anti-itch treatment.

Heat typically makes itching worse—whether the itching is due to eczema, chicken pox, or poison ivy. However, allergy sufferers can achieve four to six hours of relief from inhaling hot steam.[72] Again, I don't know of any insurance companies that will pay for your gym membership so that your child can sit in the steam room several times a week, but if you can afford it (and your child doesn't have any other medical problems that contraindicate heat), you might try it.

Running the air conditioner may also help reduce the pollen count in your home. I know many parents hate air conditioning, but it can make allergy sufferers much more comfortable because it filters allergens out of the air. For maximal benefits, keep the windows and doors closed (even when the temperature isn't high) and keep the pollen out. If you don't need the cold air, just run the fan; this will circulate air through the filter. Clean the filter at least twice yearly with a bleach or vinegar solution or use disposable filters.

Tepid water may be soothing for a child suffering from irritating allergies. Try putting a cup of plain, dry oatmeal in an old stocking and toss it in the bathwater. Oatmeal is very soothing to irritated skin, no matter whether the underlying problem is allergies, eczema, or chicken pox.

Bathing and shampooing at night will help wash out all the pollens and other allergens that have clung to your child's skin over the day. Rinsing off in the evening ensures that your child doesn't have to deal with allergens when he's asleep.

### Mind-Body

Several startling experiments have proven that the mind indeed affects allergic reactions.[73] In one experiment, hypnotized subjects were told that a leaf was poison ivy. After the leaf touched their skin, all of the subjects broke out in a typical poison ivy rash, even though the leaf was actually from a maple tree. In another experiment, subjects who were tested with varying strengths of allergen reacted differently depending on what mood they were in when the test was placed; they had much smaller reactions when they felt happy or lively than when they felt down or listless.

Anecdotes from psychiatry also lend credence to the power of the mind in mediating allergic reactions. Some patients suffering from multiple personality disorders display an interesting allergic phenomenon: one of their personalities can be severely allergic to a food, such as oranges, while another personality has no reaction to that food at all. So if the person eats an orange in personality A, she may break out in hives, but if she eats oranges while she is personality B, she can eat as many as she wants without any reaction.

Stories such as these tell us that the connection between the mind and the immune system is far more complex than we currently understand. Clearly hypnotized subjects and patients with multiple personalities have only one body and one immune system, but their allergic reactions vary depending on their mental state. We don't need to fully understand the mechanism of this interaction to use it. Hypnosis and even conscious suggestion can markedly reduced symptoms of food and inhaled allergies in children.[74]

If your child suffers from chronic annoying allergies, consider taking him to a hypnotherapist. Hypnotherapy can help uncover the source of the problem (if it is emotional), provide powerful suggestions to prevent reactions, and give you and your child useful techniques to help deal with symptoms such as shortness of breath.[75] The image need not be elaborate. As you apply whatever treatment you use for your child's allergy, remind him that this is a healing treatment and that it will make him better. Hypnosis is not for everyone; in some studies, few people were able to affect their immune reactions to allergic triggers using hypnosis.[76] On the other hand, it's very safe and may be empowering, and I often recommend it if kids and families can make the commitment to regular practice.

*Anne was able to cool off the itchy reaction to her earrings by imagining herself skiing down a snowy mountain on a clear, cold day with her cap off.*

It has been said that allergic reactions are a manifestation of unexpressed emotions, particularly anger. Although it is difficult to imagine that a six-month-old's anger results in an allergy to cow's milk, it is easy to imagine how the stress of pent-up emotions in the family can trigger a variety of physical symptoms. Infants and children are particularly sensitive to the emotions of other family members. Emotional stress affects the immune system (the key factor in allergies) in profound and as yet unexplained ways. Whether or not your child's allergy symptoms are directly due to family emotional issues, it makes sense to put such issues on the table and resolve them quickly. Professional counseling may help.

## BIOMECHANICAL THERAPIES

### Spinal Manipulation

*Osteopathic manipulation* was the most commonly recommended treatment by the American psychic Edgar Cayce during his trance readings for children suffering from allergies. Cayce recommended relaxing adjustments of the upper neck and back areas and stimulating adjustments for the lower back. Although these recommendations are fascinating and the patients reported remarkable improvements, neither chiropractic nor osteopathic treatment for allergies have undergone scientific evaluation and I do not routinely recommend them.

## BIOENERGETIC THERAPIES: ACUPUNCTURE, PRAYER/REIKI/ THERAPEUTIC TOUCH, HOMEOPATHY

### Acupuncture

Acupuncture has been a mainstay of allergy treatment in China for hundreds of years. Acupuncture is best when used as *preventive* therapy, *before* symptoms occur. For example, acupuncture treatment 15 minutes prior to exposure to an itch-inducing allergen can markedly reduce symptoms. It is less effective after symptoms have already appeared. Allergic patients who receive acupuncture three times a week for four weeks have gradual changes in their white blood cells that are associated with being less allergic.[77] Recently, acupuncture treatment was compared to antihistamine treatment in 45 adults with nasal allergies. Antihistamines were taken three times daily for seven weeks and acupuncture treatment was given for 15 minutes every other day. Both treatments resulted in significant improvement.[78] In another study acupuncture treatment was compared with traditional desensitization injections in 143 adults. The desensitization group was treated for a year; the acupuncture group was treated every one to three days for a total of five to ten treatments (less than a month). Significantly more patients treated with acupuncture had major improvements in their symptoms than patients who were treated with desensitization therapy. This was true whether their primary symptoms were asthma, nasal allergies, or hives.[79] These results are impressive. If you are tired of the side effects of chronic allergy medication and are considering taking your child to an allergist for desensitization shots, you may want to try acupuncture first. Please seek an acupuncturist who has extensive experience in dealing with children and their fears of needles.

## Prayer/Reiki/Therapeutic Touch

Although the power of prayer to help heal is acknowledged by just about every culture on earth, there are no studies specifically evaluating its benefits in treating allergies. Similarly, I use Reiki and Therapeutic Touch in my daily medical practice and would not hesitate to offer them to a patient suffering from allergies, but neither has been systematically studied for this problem.

## Homeopathy

Homeopathy is more closely related to allergy desensitization treatments than it is to any other conventional medicinal therapy. Based on the principle of "like cures like," the primary homeopathic remedy for hay fever is *Ambrosia* (ragweed). Like all homeopathic remedies it is given in extremely minute doses. *Allium cepa* (spring onion) is a common homeopathic remedy for burning, watery eyes. Apis homeopathic remedy is an extract of crushed bees—rather like a crude form of the allergists' injections for bee sting allergies. Euphrasia (eyebright) is used for the allergic symptoms in which the eyes are primarily affected (redness, watering, burning, feeling rough or gritty). *Urtica urens* (stinging nettle) is the homeopathic remedy for treating hives. Homeopathic remedies for hay fever–like allergies (usually to inhaled allergens such as pollen) include *Arsenicum, Kali bic, Natrum mur, Nux vomica* (poison nut), *Pulsatilla* (windflower), *Sabadilla* (cevadilla seed), Sulfur, and *Wyethia* (poison weed). Many of these remedies are poisonous undiluted. However, homeopathic remedies are extremely dilute and there is no danger of poisoning. Homeopathic remedies for skin allergies (contact dermatitis) include *Bryonia* (wild hops—said to be good for food allergies as well), *Rhus,* and Sulfur.

Europeans commonly rely on homeopathic remedies to treat allergies. In a 1990 survey of nearly 300 Dutch general practitioners, almost half reported that they believed homeopathic remedies are effective in treating hay fever.[80] Several European studies have demonstrated that homeopathic remedies are superior to placebos in treating hay fever; however, some patients notice a brief worsening of their symptoms when they start homeopathy.[81] A review of the world's scientific studies on homeopathic remedies concluded that the trials on treating hay fever showed an overall positive result;[82] the strength of the homeopathic remedies used as the standard in these studies was 30 C (remedy diluted 1:100 thirty times). If you choose homeopathic remedies, please take your child to a homeopathic physician who has extensive experience in treating children with allergic disease. *Do not rely* on homeopathy alone for severe, life-threatening allergic reactions.

✳

# WHAT I RECOMMEND FOR ALLERGIES

## PREVENTING ALLERGIES

1. *Lifestyle—environment.* Clean up. No matter whether your child's allergies are from pollen, poison ivy, or peaches, the best prevention is to reduce your child's exposure to the allergen. Also reduce exposure to pollution and irritants. Do not smoke and do not allow others to smoke around your child.

2. *Lifestyle—nutrition.* Breast-feed for at least the first year of life. If your family is prone to allergies and eczema, try avoiding cow's milk during pregnancy and while nursing. When you start cow's milk, consider making it in the form of yogurt or kefir with live cultures. Do not feed your child solids before she is at least four months old. When you introduce solids, try no more than one new food a week; don't try several new foods within a day. Don't start beef until the child is at least six months old. If your child has allergies at predictable times of year (spring or fall pollen season), try giving him a half to one cup of yogurt daily for two months preceding allergy season.

## TREATING ALLERGIES

1. *Biochemical—medication. For severe, life-threatening allergic reactions such as ana- phylaxis from a bee sting, seek emergency care immediately.* If your child has a severe reaction, ask for a prescription for an epinephrine. Get your child a medic-alert bracelet.

For symptomatic relief of minor symptoms, try nonprescription antihista- mines. Follow package directions on doses and be aware of potential side effects.

For moderately severe respiratory allergies (affecting the eyes, nose, sinuses, and lungs), consider safe prescription medications such as cromolyn (Intal), nedocromil (Tilade), or steroid nasal sprays. Or ask your doctor about antihista- mine nasal sprays or nonsedating antihistamine medications. Or ask your doctor about the newer anti-leukotriene medications.

For respiratory allergies to pollens and pets, consider desensitization therapy (after cleaning up the environment to prevent symptoms and *after* trying non- prescription antihistamines and prescription mast cell blockers.)

2. *Biochemical—nutritional supplements.* For respiratory allergies, try vitamin C supplements; start with 250 to 500 milligrams twice daily. Back off if diarrhea develops. For children whose food allergies appear as skin rashes, consider fish oil,

flaxseed oil, or evening primrose oil supplements, 500 milligrams to one gram three times daily.

3. *Lifestyle—nutrition.* If you suspect that your child has moderate or severe food allergies, seek the help of a health professional, nutritionist, or dietitian in developing an elimination or few foods diet. Consider making fatty fish such as salmon a regular part of your diet. Watch your child's weight; obese children have higher levels of inflammatory chemicals in their blood stream and are more likely to have allergic problems such as asthma.[83]

4. *Lifestyle—environment.* Wash thoroughly and immediately after contact with poison ivy or other skin sensitizers. Use ice compresses to reduce swelling and itching. Try tepid baths with or without oatmeal to relieve itching. Keep pets away from kids who are allergic to them and consider running an air filter in the child's bedroom. Wash the child's bedding at least weekly.

5. *Lifestyle—mind-body.* For any type of allergy, consider taking your child for hypnotherapy or biofeedback therapy with a therapist trained in treating children.

6. *Bioenergetic—homeopathy.* For hay fever symptoms, consider seeing a homeopathic physician who is experienced in treating children.

7. *Bioenergetic—acupuncture.* If your child is comfortable with the idea of needle therapy, consult an acupuncturist who is trained in treating children.

## RESOURCES

Food Allergy Network
4744 Holly Avenue
Fairfax, VA 22030-5647
(703) 691-3179
(800) 929-40401

Enviracaire HEPA Air Filters
Honeywell Environmental Air Control
747 Bowman Avenue
Hagerstown, MD 21740
(800) 332-1110

American Academy of Allergy, Asthma, and Immunology
611 East Wells St.
Milwaukee, WI 53202
(800) 822-2762
http://www.aaaai.org/

National Allergy Supply, Inc
4400 Georgia Hwy 120
PO Box 1658
Duluth, GA 30136
(800) 522-1448
http://www.natallergy.com/

Allergy Control Products, Inc.
96 Danbury Rd.
Ridgefield, CT 06877
(800) 422-DUST
http://www.allergycontrol.com

*Internet*

Food Allergy and Anaphylaxis Network
(also known as Food Allergy Network)
http://www.foodallergy.org

National Institutes of Health (food allergy
information)
http://www.nlm.nih.gov/medlineplus/
foodallergy.html

Peanut Allergies
http://www.peanutallergy.com/

# 5

# ASTHMA

Yolanda Jefferson awoke suddenly in the middle of the night, hearing her youngest son, Devante, cough again. Neither of them was getting any sleep. Yolanda was exhausted from the lack of sleep, caring for three children and two cats, getting the kids to day care while she worked, making meals, and trying to keep the house clean. Devante seemed to cough more than other kids when he caught a cold. His cough was worse at night; sometimes he coughed even when he didn't have a cold. Yolanda was beginning to wonder if he had asthma. His grandmother, who lived with them, continued to smoke though she had asthma, and Devante's two older brothers had asthma, too. Yolanda couldn't believe Devante was starting to get sick already; he was only eighteen months old. She wanted to know what she could do to ease his symptoms and if there was anything she could do to stop it from getting worse.

If your child suffers from asthma, you are not alone. About 5 to 15 percent of American children suffer from asthma, making it the most common chronic condition of childhood. Asthma accounts for 10 million missed days of school each year. Over the last thirty years, asthma has become even more common and more severe. Between 1980 and 1995 pediatric asthma rates climbed over 70% and asthma deaths jumped a whopping 40%.[1] Asthma rates have also increased dramatically in other countries, such as England, Ireland, Scotland, and New Zealand.[2] These countries have the highest asthma rates in the world; much lower rates are found in India, China, and Greece.

Asthma is epidemic in America, and it is particularly problematic in our inner cities.[3] It is more common among children who are born prematurely (especially those who had lung problems as newborns), those living in crowded conditions and in poverty, those who have had pneumonia or other lung infections, and those living with a smoker.[4] Although asthma is more common in American Indian, Alaska Native, Puerto Rican, and African American children, the fastest increase in asthma has been among middle-class Caucasian children.[5] Asthma and obesity often go hand in hand. No one knows exactly why.[6] Perhaps kids with asthma exercise less and perhaps fat cells make more inflammatory chemicals that tend to make asthma worse. Asthma is more common among boys before puberty and more common in girls after puberty starts. Asthma tends to be milder right after ovulation (about days 19 to 25 of the cycle) when estrogen levels are at a sustained peak, and more severe in the peri-menstrual period (days 26 to 4 of the cycle) when estrogen levels fall and stay low for several days.[7] Like allergies, asthma runs in families. Symptoms improve for many children when they reach adolescence. On the other hand, some children first experience asthma as teenagers.

Children with asthma can do just as well in school, sports, and social situations as their peers without asthma. In the 1984 Olympics, 67 of 597 U.S. athletes had exercise-induced asthma. They brought home fifteen gold, twenty-one silver, and five bronze medals.

Asthma is one disease with several symptoms.

## ASTHMA SYMPTOMS

- Dry cough (especially at night)
- Wheezing (high-pitched whistling sounds) during exhalation
- A feeling of tightness in the chest
- Having difficulty breathing; can't catch breath

Sometimes children will have only one of these symptoms—usually the cough. Many children have symptoms just once or twice and never have them again. Coughing and wheezing can be caused by other health problems, too.

## OTHER CAUSES OF COUGH AND WHEEZING

- Viral infections
- Aspirating food or other objects into lungs
- Genetic lung diseases
- Airway abnormalities

Viral infections such as colds and bronchitis, aspiration (when food or a small object is inhaled into the airways), and genetic diseases such as cystic fibrosis are all marked by coughing and wheezing. Abnormal airways—such as floppy tracheas or having a blood vessel mistakenly wrap around a breathing tube—can lead to wheezy breathing, too. X rays, blood tests, and lung function tests may be necessary to make the correct diagnosis. A child is called asthmatic only if his symptoms occur at least three times, several family members have asthma, or there is some other reason to suspect that symptoms will recur.

*Devante had classic asthma symptoms. His diagnosis was confirmed by his physical examination and response to treatment. Yolanda wanted to know what was happening in his lungs to cause Devante's symptoms. She also wanted to know what might trigger his asthma so she could prevent flare-ups.*

Three changes in the small airways *(bronchioles)* cause asthma symptoms.

## LUNG CHANGES IN ASTHMA

- Inflammation and swelling of the walls of the bronchioles
- Increased mucus production, blocking the bronchioles
- Bronchospasm, muscle tightening around the bronchioles

When the airways become inflamed during an infection or allergy, the walls of the bronchioles become swollen and irritated, blocking airflow to the tiny air sacs (alveoli) at the end of the bronchioles. The irritation also triggers coughing. Normally, mucus helps clear the airways, but when there is too much mucus, it clogs air passages. Irritation also stimulates the muscles around the bronchioles to tighten or constrict, further cutting off airflow. These changes lead to coughing, wheezing (the sound the air makes as it tries to flow through narrowed tubes), and feelings of tightness and an inability to catch one's breath.

Very few children have asthma symptoms all the time; most just have symptoms triggered occasionally. The National Heart Lung and Blood Institute (NHLBI) of the National Institutes of Health (NIH) has sponsored a lot of asthma research and has published guidelines for diagnosing and treating asthma. It categorizes asthma in four levels of severity. The severity depends on the frequency and intensity of symptoms and the lungs' maximal function (also known as peak flow rate).

| ASTHMA SEVERITY | |
| --- | --- |
| Mild, intermittent | • Daytime symptoms twice or fewer times weekly<br>• Nighttime symptoms twice or fewer times monthly<br>• No school absence; no need for emergency room<br>• Peak flow rates more than 80% of predicted |
| Mild, persistent | • Daytime symptoms more than twice weekly<br>• Nighttime symptoms more than twice monthly<br>• Peak flow rates more than 80% of predicted<br>• Symptoms may affect activities |
| Moderate, persistent | • Daily symptoms<br>• Nighttime symptoms more than once a week<br>• Peak flow rates between 60% to 80% of predicted<br>• Symptoms regularly affect activities |
| Severe, persistent | • Continuous symptoms unless treated<br>• Peak flow less than 60% of predicted<br>• Symptoms often limit physical activities |

The goals of asthma education and treatment are to restore normal lung function and minimize symptoms.[8] The different degrees of asthma severity mean different kinds of treatments are needed. Regardless of the severity of asthma symptoms, every child who suffers from asthma needs an Asthma Action Plan.[9] This means that you work out goals, strategies, and contingencies to minimize the chance that your child will end up in the emergency room or hospital. You should write this plan down and review it regularly to keep it updated; it should be posted on the refrigerator at home so everyone can easily refer to it. Give a copy to the school nurse, coaches, and camp counselors, too.

*What triggers asthma and how do you keep track?*

Sometimes an asthma trigger works immediately—the child starts wheezing as soon as he walks outside on a pollen-filled spring day. Sometimes triggers have delayed effects; a child is exposed to a cat in the afternoon and does not have symptoms until he goes to bed. Keeping a diary of your child's asthma symptoms can help you figure out what triggers the flare-ups.

## COMMON ASTHMA TRIGGERS

- Airway irritants: cigarettes, air pollution, wood smoke, gas heat/stove
- Allergies, including food sensitivity
- Exercise
- Cold air
- Infections: colds, sinus infections, bronchitis
- Medications: aspirin, angiotensin converting enzyme (ACE) inhibitors
- Stress
- Acid reflux

*Cigarette smoke* is the number-one preventable trigger of asthma. Even if your child doesn't smoke, being around smokers will almost certainly make your child's asthma worse. Maternal smoking during pregnancy affects a child's lung development and increases his risk of having asthma later.[10] *Do not smoke and do* not *allow other people to smoke around your child!*

*Air pollution* also aggravates asthma. Today's energy-efficient houses trap indoor mold, dust mites, and animal danders in the house, aggravating asthma symptoms. Children who live near busy roads, factories, power stations, and other sources of pollution are barraged by bad air. City emergency rooms log more asthma visits when pollution levels are higher. In general, city dwellers have much higher asthma rates and more severe asthma than their country cousins.[11] Children who live in rural areas have their own sources of pollution: wood smoke from stoves and fireplaces, dust, animal dander, and agricultural chemicals.

Ragweed and pollen provoke *seasonal allergies* in some children and asthma in others. Other asthma-inducing allergens are molds, grasses, dust, dust mites, fleas, and cat and dog dander. *Food allergies* (such as to peanuts, eggs, and wheat) can also trigger asthma symptoms in some sensitive children. Kids who are extremely sensitive may even develop asthma flares-ups just smelling the offending food, which makes cooking for the whole family a little tricky. Cow's milk is a well-known but rare trigger for asthma symptoms; children who are truly allergic to milk almost always have other symptoms as well, such as hives, diarrhea, or eczema. *Food additives*, such as yellow dyes, sodium benzoate, and sulfites, also trigger asthma in some children.[12] If you think your child might be allergic to foods or food additives, please have him tested by an allergist before you make radical changes in his diet. Many children outgrow their food allergies, though no one knows why (see Chapter 4, Allergies).

*Exercise, especially in cold, dry air,* triggers symptoms in nearly 90% of asthmatics. Frequent, vigorous exercise in cold, dry air may actually induce chronic asthma. More than half of Swedish elite cross-country skiers have asthma, and about 30% of figure skaters also wheeze after a performance.[13] Fortunately, exercise-induced asthma can be effectively prevented and treated. *There is no reason for your child to avoid exercise just because he has been diagnosed with asthma.*

Cold and sinus *infections* are among the most common triggers for asthma. Cold viruses trigger wheezing in 80 to 85 percent of asthmatic children. They can even provoke wheezing and coughing in people who don't have asthma. Sinus infections in children can be subtle and difficult to diagnose. If your child has frequent bouts of asthma, is troubled by nighttime coughing, or has had a cold that lasts more than ten days in a row, talk with your health care provider about the possibility of a sinus infection. Treating the infection can dramatically improve asthma symptoms.

The most common *medication* causing asthma flare-ups is aspirin. Steer clear of aspirin, and other non-steroidal anti-inflammatory drugs (NSAIDS) such as ibuprofen. Acetaminophen (e.g., Tylenol) does *not* trigger asthma attacks. Prescription medications known as beta-blockers (such as propanolol), used to prevent migraine headaches and treat high blood pressure, can also trigger asthma symptoms. The high blood pressure medicines known as ACE inhibitors frequently cause coughing that may either trigger or mimic asthma. Some of the contrast dyes used in fancy X rays can also trigger asthma symptoms. Whenever your child sees a new doctor for any reason, be sure to mention that your child has asthma to minimize the chances of an inappropriate prescription.

Emotional *stress* can cause a tight chest and labored breathing in almost anyone. It's not surprising that children with asthma are more prone to having symptoms at stressful times such as the first day of school or during a divorce. Previously it was believed that dysfunctional parents contributed to childhood asthma, and children were sent away to boarding schools to get away from their "toxic" families. A recent study demonstrates that, on the contrary, children's illnesses contribute to parental stress and dysfunction. The more serious the child's illness, the more disruptive for the family.[14]

Does *dirt* make asthma worse? There's little doubt that air pollution, cat and dog hair, dust mites, and cockroaches can make asthma worse. But interestingly, kids growing up in the dusty countryside tend to have less asthma than urban kids. It might be that certain microbes and parasites actually offer some protection against asthma and eczema.[15] While I don't recommend that you intentionally expose your child to dirt or worms, I think an extra bit of the healthy bacteria found in yogurt and kefir might help promote healthy immune responses.

Heartburn not only feels bad, it can trigger asthma symptoms. *Acid reflux* (also known as heartburn or gastro-esophageal reflux disease, GERD) triggers asthma symptoms for many people. Medications that minimize stomach acid reduce asthma symptoms in over 70% of adults who suffer from acid reflux–triggered asthma.[16] Treating the heartburn actually improves the asthma. Two for the price of one—a welcome but uncommon bargain in medicine.

Asthma can be deadly. If your child has any of the following symptoms, take him for professional care.

**SEEK IMMEDIATE PROFESSIONAL CARE IF YOUR CHILD IS:**

- Having a hard time breathing
- Breathing much more rapidly than usual
- Making a grunting noise when he breathes out
- Getting tired or agitated with his shortness of breath
- Getting blue in the lips or fingertips
- Sucking in the spaces between his ribs with each breath

**MAKE AN APPOINTMENT IF:**

- Symptoms interfere with sleep or other activities
- The child has a high fever
- The child has a poor appetite

## Diagnosing and Monitoring Asthma

Observations of coughing, wheezing, and breathing patterns have long been the mainstays of monitoring asthma symptoms.

### MONITORING ASTHMA SYMPTOMS

- Daily diary: symptoms, triggers, treatments
- Peak flow meter
- Visits to health care professional four times yearly

Today you can measure your child's lung function at home using a peak flow meter. Peak flow meters cost less than $30 and may be covered by your insurance. A peak flow meter measures how forcefully your child can exhale (blow air out). A low reading on the peak flow meter is an early warning sign that symptoms will soon slide downhill. Children as young as six years old can learn to use a peak flow meter reliably. Those with frequent symptoms should measure their peak flow at least twice daily (morning and evening) and record it in an asthma diary along with symptoms and triggers. Such information will be very helpful in mapping out the best treatment plan for your child. See your doctor four times yearly to monitor your child's growth and response to therapy and to receive support and information about new treatment strategies.

## Preventing and Treating Asthma

There are no cures for asthma yet, but many treatments can help control its symptoms. Optimal treatment is based on careful observation, and relies on a combination of therapies. Let's tour the Therapeutic Mountain to find out what works; if you want to skip to my bottom-line recommendations, flip to the end of the chapter.

## Biochemical Therapies: Medications, Herbs, Nutritional Supplements

### Medications

Modern medications are lifesaving for acute asthma attacks. Do not rely on nonprescription medications for asthma. They are not strong enough or enduring enough to help, and you may be giving yourself false assurance that you are doing something useful.

Inhaled cromolyn (Intal) and nedocromil (Tilade) help *prevent* asthma symptoms by blocking histamine release. When lungs are irritated (by tobacco smoke, vigorous exercise, or cold viruses, for example, they release small amounts of histamine. Histamine causes inflammation, and thus, asthma symptoms.

## MEDICATIONS (ALL ARE PRESCRIPTION ONLY)

- *Preventive:* cromolyn or nedocromil, influenza vaccine, allergy shots
- *Maintenance and treatment:* steroids (sprays and oral forms)
- *Prevention and treatment:* beta-agonists (albuterol, bitolterol, pirbuterol, and terbutaline)
- *Prevention and maintenance:* leukotriene inhibitors
- *Other:* theophylline, ipratropium, adrenalin, heliox

These medications only work when taken *before* the lungs get irritated; they are useless in treating acute attacks. These are my first choice for preventing symptoms in children who have symptoms three or more days a week, particularly for exercise-induced asthma. For maximal effectiveness, cromolyn and nedocromil must be taken several times daily for at least two to four weeks before improvements are detectable. Few side effects have been reported from either medication, but they are not of much use in an acute attack.

Inhaled asthma medications, such as cromolyn and nedocromil, steroids and beta agonists, are delivered directly to the lungs by either a nebulizer (a device that turns the medication into a fine mist) or a metered dose inhaler (MDI or "puffer"). MDIs are the most widespread and convenient way to take inhaled asthma medications. A canister containing the medication inserts in a plastic dispenser. Pressing the canister releases a premeasured amount of medication from the dispenser. The child inhales the medication, delivering it right to the lungs. Some of the newer MDIs only deliver the medication when the child takes a breath, enhancing efficiency. Metered dose inhalers are as effective as nebulizers if they are used correctly.[17] Even infants can use *MDIs if they use a spacer and mask.*[18]

## HOW TO USE AN MDI

1. Shake canister while taking deep breath in and out.
2. Hold can one inch from mouth (or preferably, use a spacer).
3. Release medication at the beginning of the next breath in (inhalation).
4. Breathe the medication mist in deeply.
5. Hold breath to count of 10; exhale.
6. Wait one minute; repeat.

Although these directions sound simple, it takes a fair amount of coordination to get the timing right to dispense the medication just as the child breathes in. If the child has finished inhaling by the time the medicine is dispensed, the medicine just evaporates into the surrounding air rather than reaching the lungs. A *spacer* is a device that holds the medicine in a confined space after its release from an MDI. The medication remains suspended, waiting for the child to take the next breath. Some fold up so they can be carried in a purse or backpack; some make sounds to let the child know when the medication has been inhaled properly. Some spacers come with face masks that cover the nose and mouth, so even infants can receive MDI medication without a nebulizer. Many spacers and masks are covered by insurance; they usually cost between $15 and $35. I always write a prescription for a spacer at the same time I write the initial prescription for metered dose medications. And I always make sure the child and family can demonstrate proper MDI technique before they leave the office. It's one of the things we recheck at our quarterly visits.

Children with asthma can have especially severe symptoms with *influenza*. If your child has asthma, please *get the influenza vaccine every fall;* it definitely helps prevent asthma flare-ups.[19] I get the flu vaccine myself every year to reduce my chances of getting influenza and passing it on to others. The vaccine is especially worthwhile for kids who require medications daily, even steroid medications.[20] If your child has moderate or severe asthma, I'd consider having everyone in the household vaccinated against influenza, just to protect the child from a heavy exposure from someone at home.

More physicians are prescribing *inhaled steroids* (such as Aerobid, Azmacort, Beclovent, Decadron, and Vanceril) nowadays to both prevent and treat moderate or severe asthma. Inhaled steroids get the needed medicine right to the lungs;[21] they should almost always be used if your child has moderate to severe persistent asthma.

## INHALED STEROIDS FOR ASTHMA

- Beclomethasone (Beclovent, Vanceril)
- Budesonide (Pulmicort)
- Flunisolide (Aerobid)
- Fluticasone (Flovent)
- Triamcinolone (Azmacort)

Steroids effectively decrease airway inflammation and swelling; they both prevent and treat asthma symptoms. Given when peak flow meter readings start to fall, steroids can prevent asthma flare-ups and are among the most cost-effective treatments for children with chronic asthma.[22] When used for an acute attack, steroids can prevent emergency room visits and hospitalization. Inhaling these steroid medications in an emergency works even faster and better than taking them by mouth.[23] Most only need to be taken once or twice daily to keep symptoms under control.[24] Giving inhaled steroids only once a day is less likely to limit your child's growth than giving them twice daily.[25]

These are *not* the kind of steroids that athletes use to bulk up. Also, when steroids are given by MDI they go directly to the lungs; very little is absorbed into the bloodstream, resulting in very few side effects.[26] A recent analysis of over 800 children showed that inhaled steroids do *not* usually impair growth; however, several studies have shown that a few kids who take very potent inhaled steroids several times daily may lose an inch or two in eventual height, so if your child requires inhaled steroids, he needs to have his growth monitored three to four times yearly.[27] You can reduce the impact on growth either by decreasing the daily dose or by giving a larger dose once a day as opposed to smaller doses twice daily.[28] Inhaled steroids can cause sore throat, hoarseness, and yeast infections in the mouth. You can prevent these side effects by using a spacer (so more of the medicine goes to the lungs and less stays in the mouth) and gargling with plain water after "puffing" to rinse it out of the mouth. Even though most of us are scared by steroids' potential side effects, children who have moderate or severe asthma end up spending less time in the hospital and less time in the emergency room if they use inhaled steroids daily rather than relying solely on beta-agonist medication.[29]

Children with severe asthma may need to take *steroids by mouth*. Because of their potential side effects (e.g., decreased growth, unstable blood sugar levels, cataracts, easy bruising, impaired immunity), oral steroids should be taken for as short a time as possible. Generally, three to five days of oral steroids are sufficient for most children with a severe asthma attack and may help prevent a hospitalization;[30] taking steroids for less than a week does not increase the risk of serious infections or other side effects associated with long-term use of steroid medicines.[31] For children who are coughing too hard to take medicine by mouth, a single steroid injection is as effective as three to five days of oral therapy.[32] This is a good thing because most steroid syrups taste awful, and many parents would rather give their child a shot than struggle with them several times a day to take a vile-tasting medicine.

*Beta-agonists* (such as albuterol, bitolterol, pirbuterol, and terbutaline) are the most commonly prescribed asthma medications. They relax airway muscles, and allow the air passages to expand. Beta-agonists effectively prevent exercise-induced asthma; inhaled twenty to thirty minutes prior to vigorous exercise, they reduce breathing problems. You may have seen athletes using them before practices and competition. Beta-agonists are also useful for the quick relief of flare-ups caused by an allergy or a cold. They start to work in about twenty minutes; benefits last for four to six hours. A longer-acting (twelve-hour) beta-agonist medication, salmeterol (Serevent) is a preventive medication for children and teenagers who need beta-agonist medication every day.[33] Using it regularly may decrease the need for steroid medications.[34] Another new beta-agonist medication is formoterol (Foradil), which is approved for children five years and older. Do *not* overuse beta-agonist inhalers; if your child thinks he needs his inhaler more than twice a day, you need to see your physician to consider other medicines. Overuse results in dependence, needing higher and higher doses to achieve the same benefit; this is a very dangerous situation that is best avoided before your child gets into serious trouble.[35]

As with cromolyn, nedocromil, and inhaled steroids, beta-agonist medications are best given by MDIs and spacers; nebulizers offer no real advantage over the hand-held "puffers."[36] For infants and toddlers, beta-agonists can also be given by mouth, but this is not as effective as inhaled treatments, because not as much medicine goes directly to the lungs, and there are more side effects.

The main side effects from beta-agonists are like the side effects from drinking too many cups of coffee: racing heart, high blood pressure, high blood sugar, reduced appetite, or feeling a little "hyper." If your child requires more than two doses in a day or more than three times a week, see your doctor about additional or alternative preventive therapies so you can cut down on the beta-agonist treatments.

Could your child's medicine be making him sick? Some of the antibacterial agents added to medications to ensure that they don't become contaminated with bacteria or fungi may actually trigger asthma symptoms. The latest culprit is BAC (benzalkonium chloride). BAC is added to nebulized medicines to keep them fresh, but it can trigger asthma. It is *not* part of MDIs. However, the CFCs (chlorofluorocarbons) used to power MDIs cause problems with the earth's protective ozone layer and are being banned. A whole new breed of MDIs have been developed to replace CFCs; they may take some getting used to, but eventually your child should do just fine, and the environment will do much better!

In the 1970s and early 1980s, *theophylline* and its cousin, *aminophylline,* were the treatments of choice for children with asthma. Both are chemically related to caffeine; they expand airways and decrease inflammation.[37] Blood levels need to be monitored closely to minimize side effects. They fell out of favor because of many reported side effects: hyperactivity, decreased attention span, decreased appetite, and increased risk of seizures. This bad reputation may not be entirely deserved.[38] Low doses of theophylline may decrease the doses of steroids needed to control symptoms for patients with moderate or severe asthma.[39]

Aminophylline may also be useful if your child's symptoms are severe enough to land him in the hospital.[40] Using theophylline is a complicated decision you'll need to make with your child's physician.

Inhaled *ipratropium bromide* (Atrovent) is a relatively new but cost-effective treatment for asthmatics suffering from severe attacks who need emergency treatment.[41] It is chemically related to the older, plant-derived drug, atropine. Some adults use it daily, but only for severe symptoms that are not well controlled with inhaled steroids. It works best when used with beta-agonist medications.[42] One product (Combivent) combines ipratropium with albuterol; it is mostly used by elderly asthmatics and has not caught on as a pediatric remedy. Perhaps it should.[43]

A new class of asthma medications helps prevent inflammation and allergic-type reactions: *anti-leukotriene medications*.[44] These medications are taken by mouth to *prevent* symptoms. They are especially helpful for children whose asthma is triggered by aspirin because they block the enzyme involved in this reaction. Asthma specialists are currently debating whether anti-leukotriene medications should be used in place of inhaled steroids for children with mild to moderate asthma. In general, they are quite safe and have fewer side effects than steroids.[45] Check with your doctor to learn the very latest recommendations; this is a rapidly changing area of treatment.

## ANTI-LEUKOTRIENE MEDICATIONS

- Montelukast (Singulair)
- Zafirlukast (Accolate)
- Zileuton (Zyflo)

Even though it is effective, *zileuton* is probably not a good choice for most kids because it must be taken four times a day; it can also interfere with blood levels of other medicines.[46] Similarly, *zafirlukast* is moderately effective for mild to moderate asthma in children, including exercise-triggered asthma, but it has to be taken twice daily on an empty stomach and it can interfere with other medications.[47] *Montelukast* is fairly effective for moderate, persistent asthma or asthma triggered by exercise and it only has to be taken once daily;[48] it is approved for use in children and can reduce reliance on steroid medications.[49] Not surprisingly, kids who are old enough to take pills generally prefer to take pills than to use puffers; nearly everyone prefers taking a medicine once or twice daily to one that requires dosing every four to six hours, and every parent I know would prefer just about anything to steroids.

One of the quickest treatments for children with an acute attack of severe asthma is a shot of *epinephrine* (Adrenalin). Adrenaline works well, but it wears off quickly. In the 1970s clinicians started using *terbutaline* instead of adrenaline because it lasts longer. Because adrenaline and terbutaline require injections, they were replaced in the 1980s by inhaled medications. For children with severe asthma who are hospitalized in intensive care units, terbutaline shots are still sometimes given to help open up the airways when inhaled medications just can't get through blocked air passages.

*Allergy shots* are useful for children whose asthma symptoms are triggered by a few specific airborne allergens such as pollen, but they offer limited benefits of uncertain duration for other kids with multiple allergies such as food and dust mites and cats.[50] In an emergency, for severe asthma being treated in the hospital, your physician may call on the old remedy *heliox* to treat your child's asthma.[51] Heliox is a combination of helium and oxygen. The helium replaces the air's nitrogen; helium is lighter than nitrogen, and it's easier to breathe heliox than room air, so your child doesn't have to work as hard to get the oxygen into his system. He may talk like Mickey Mouse, but it may spare him from needing a breathing tube.

## Herbs

Herbs have been used to treat asthma by traditional healers around the world. However, there are few scientific studies evaluating their effectiveness compared with other treatments. They are *not* as effective as medications and are not tightly regulated by the FDA, so you cannot be sure you are getting what you're paying for. Do not abandon your current medications in favor of herbs. You need to discuss *all* treatments with your doctor before making major changes. Even if you're just using herbs as supplements, you need to tell your doctor and pharmacist so they can help you avoid adverse interactions.

Perhaps the most well known herbal asthma remedy is *ephedra*, the original source of the old asthma medication ephedrine and the modern decongestant pseudoephedrine. The Chinese have used ephedra *(Ma Huang)* for nearly 5,000 years to treat asthma. It is chemically related to epinephrine and it has similar side effects: high blood pressure, rapid heartbeat, decreased appetite, and feeling overstimulated, eventually resulting in severe fatigue. Sadly, ephedra gained notoriety in the 1990s as adolescents tried using it to get high. The U.S. Food and Drug Administration received over 600 complaints of adverse effects, including 22 deaths, related to ephedrine. This led to tighter state regulations governing the availability and strength of ephedra-containing products. Independent testing of commercially available ephedra products show huge discrepancies between what the label says and what's actually in the bottle; some contain none, some contain too much, and the difference even between lots of the same

brand can vary ten-fold. I do not recommend it—at least until the herbal products industry is better regulated and we can count on pure products of known potency.

Other mainstays of Chinese herbal therapy are *Chinese skullcap (Huang Qin)* and *ligusticum* which have anti-inflammatory properties similar to cromolyn, and *Angelica sinensis (Dong Quai),* which relaxes bronchospasm and reduces reactivity to allergens. *Cordyceps* is a fungus which is a common ingredient in Chinese herbal asthma remedies; it affects immune reactions in test tubes, but there are no studies yet comparing it to standard asthma medicines in real live human beings.[52]

*Licorice root (Glycyrrhiza glabra radix)* has been used in folk medicines around the world to treat coughs. Licorice root's active compounds, glycyrrhetinic acid and carbenoxolone, block the breakdown of steroids, which means it offers both the benefits and side effects of steroids.[53] As recently as the 1960s licorice was used successfully by American physicians to treat Addison's disease (a serious steroid deficiency). On the other hand, licorice can cause fluid retention, swelling in the feet and ankles, hypertension, headaches, blood chemistry imbalances, lethargy, and muscle weakness.[54] No studies have yet evaluated the risks and benefits of including licorice root as a standard pediatric treatment regimen for asthma. Patients using licorice should be closely monitored for steroidlike side effects.

*Minor Blue Dragon* is a combination of several herbs, including licorice, ginger, ephedra, and cinnamon.

Like the new leukotriene-inhibitor medications, the ancient Asian herbal combination remedies, *Shinpi-To* and *Saiboku-To*, inhibit the body's chemical pathway that leads to inflammation in the lung.[55] Saiboku-To contains five herbs that slow steroid breakdown, possibly increasing the risk of side effects in patients who need to take steroid medications, but it reduces the need for anti-inflammatory medications in adult asthmatics who take it for several months.[56] Shinpi-To contains seven herbs, including ephedra, licorice, apricot, and magnolia.

Other healing traditions also rely on herbal remedies for asthma.[57]

## TRADITIONAL HERBAL REMEDIES FOR ASTHMA

* *China and Japan:* Ephedra *(Ma Huang):* Chinese skullcap, angelica *(Dong Quai),* licorice root; Minor Blue Dragon; Saiboku-To, Shinpi-To, Moku-Boi-To, Sho-Saiko-To, Sho-Seiryu-To, and others
* *Europe and America:* Coffee and tea, coltsfoot, ginkgo, onions, bee pollen
* *Hawaii: Sophora chrysophylla* (mamane), *Piper methysticum* (kava kava), nightshade
* *India: Adhatoda vasica* (malabar nut), *Coleus forskholii, Verbascum thapsus* (mullein*), Tylophora indica*, and others
* *Latin America:* Aloe vera, *Galphimia glauca*, red onions, *Siete jarabes, Agua maravilla, Jarabe maguey*

In the 1800s *coffee* was the treatment of choice for asthma. In general, folks who drink more coffee tend to have fewer respiratory symptoms than those who don't. Xanthine, coffee's chemical cousin to theophylline, helps relax lung spasms and reduces inflammation. In a large Italian study, adults who drank two to three cups of coffee daily had about 25% less asthma than adults who abstained.[58] There are no recent randomized controlled trials evaluating the effects of caffeine on childhood asthma symptoms, nor on the interaction between coffee, tea, colas, and modern asthma medications. Still, everybody knows what the side effects of coffee are, and it may be worth trying as long as you don't overdo it.

*Onions (Allium cepa)* are a common folk remedy for asthma. Nine different compounds in onions inhibit the synthesis of inflammatory chemicals.[59] Onion extracts reduce asthma in guinea pigs.[60] Onions are extremely safe in normal diets. Allergies are rare. Additional research is needed to determine the best dose and frequency and the optimal variety of onion supplements for asthmatic children. In the meantime, I often advise patients to eat more onions.

*Bee pollen* is widely touted as a natural remedy for asthma, allergies, and eczema. There are no clinical trials evaluating the effectiveness of bee pollen in treating childhood asthma. Serious allergic reactions and even fatalities have been reported.[61] Bee pollen is *not* a safe adjunctive therapy for your child.

*Ginkgo biloba* is one of the most ancient trees in the world. It was used in Chinese medicine long before becoming one of the biggest selling herbal remedies in Europe. Standardized Extract of Ginkgo biloba (EGb), is sold under several different brand names: Ginkgobil, Rokan, Tanakan, Tebonin, and Kaveri. Ginkgo's active ingredient, ginkgolide, decreases inflammation in the lungs.[62] Ginkgo is also a powerful antioxidant.[63] Despite its long historical use and biochemical rationale, only one small pilot study has evaluated ginkgo's effectiveness as an asthma remedy, finding it protective against both allergic and exercise-induced asthma.[64] Ginkgo can cause bleeding problems. It has not been extensively tested in children. If you decide to try it for your child, please let your doctor know, and discontinue use two weeks before any planned surgery.

*Coleus forskholii* is an herb used in Indian Ayurvedic medicine to treat asthma. It contains chemicals that work like theophylline and beta-agonist medications, and helps relax lung muscles.[65] Another Ayurvedic herbal remedy, *Tylophora indica*, has proven beneficial in controlled, double-blind crossover studies of patients with both allergies and asthma, but optimal dosages and long-term effects on children are unknown; tylophora leaves cause nausea.[66] *Boswellia serrata* is another Ayurvedic asthma remedy; it blocks inflammatory chemicals (5-lipoxygenase) in animals, and it looked promising in a pilot study of asthmatic adults.[67] One dose of *Solanum xanthocarpum* and *S. trilobatum* improved lung function for six to eight hours in a small study of asthmatic adults, but these herbs were not as powerful as standard medications.[68] I am not very familiar with Ayurvedic herbs, and I do not typically recommend them.

Other traditional remedies for asthma include: coltsfoot, yerba santa, wild cherry bark, ginger root, peppermint, red clover, comfrey, lobelia, marsh mallow root, nettle, parsley, and thyme. Adding a strong solution of thyme tea to bathwater is believed to help all kinds of coughing illnesses and is very safe. Thyme is also added to home steam inhalation treatments to soothe irritated airways. Slippery elm bark and wild cherry bark are both helpful for scratchy throats from dry, hacking coughs. Kava kava is a Polynesian herb that eases anxiety, but it can cause serious liver problems.

Many home remedies contain multiple herbal ingredients. For example, the Puerto Rican remedy, *Siete jarabes,* is a honeyed syrup containing almond oil, castor oil, wild cherry, licorice, and cocillana.[69] Similarly, Asian herbal remedies, such as Saiboku-To, typically contain twelve or more ingredients.

Herbs are not necessarily safe just because they are natural. Unfortunately, herbal remedies are poorly regulated by the FDA. About one-third of Chinese patent medicines are intentionally spiked with medications such as steroids, resulting in significant side effects.

During harvesting, sometimes the wrong plants, pesticides, herbicides, animal residues, etc., get into the material. During processing, products may become contaminated with heavy metals such as lead and arsenic; strengths and dosing are not standardized, and significant variation in purity and potency have been reported. This means that you might be paying for herbs you are not really getting; or you may be unknowingly giving your child an overdose. Until there is better research on their safety and effectiveness and better government regulation protecting consumers, I do *not* typically recommend herbal remedies for asthmatic children.

## Nutritional Supplements

The most commonly recommended dietary supplements for asthma include vitamin B6, vitamin C, magnesium, and fish or flaxseed oils.

### NUTRITIONAL SUPPLEMENTS FOR ASTHMA

- Vitamin B6 (pyridoxine)
- Vitamin C
- Magnesium
- Avoiding salt
- Fish oils/flaxseed oil

Supplemental *Vitamin B6 (pyridoxine)* has proved helpful in both adults and children suffering from asthma. For example, among adult asthmatics who had low blood levels of pyridoxine, supplementation reduced the severity and number of wheezing episodes.[70] For steroid-dependent adult asthmatics, 300 milligrams daily of Vitamin B6 supplements improved airflow significantly better than placebo pills.[71] Vitamin B6 supplements in doses of 50 to 200 milligrams daily over several weeks helped reduce the number of asthma attacks, the severity of symptoms, and the need for medications in asthmatic children.[72] Pyridoxine may be particularly helpful for children who take theophylline because theophylline can deplete body stores of this vitamin. Like a few other nutritionally minded pediatricians, I routinely recommend pyridoxine supplements to asthmatic children.

Adults and children who consume the most foods rich in *vitamin C* (such as citrus fruits, strawberries, and kiwi) have the least wheezing and asthma;[73] those who eat the least vitamin C have a five times greater risk of having twitchy lungs.[74] In ancient days, the relationship between scurvy (severe vitamin C deficiency) and asthma was well known. However, in modern days since few folks suffer from scurvy, giving megadoses of vitamin C supplements to treat asthma is controversial. Vitamin C reduces reactivity to histamine, the lung chemical that causes bronchospasm; vitamin C and other antioxidants also help protect the airways against asthma triggers, including ozone.[75] Ozone triggers a lot of asthma attacks,[76] and giving extra vitamin C (500 to 1000 milligrams daily for adults) protects against those attacks.[77] This does *not* mean that we should ignore air pollution, but while we're cleaning up the air, it may be worthwhile to give asthmatic kids foods that are rich in vitamin C, and consider vitamin C supplements as well. For some children, 500 milligrams daily of vitamin C protects against exercise-induced asthma.[78] In a double-blind comparison study, taking 1 gram of vitamin C daily significantly improved symptoms in adult asthmatics.[79] Giving your child 500 to 1,000 milligrams (½ to 1 gram) per day is safe; I recommend sustained-release vitamin C supplements to all of my asthmatic patients. Other antioxidants that may prove helpful include selenium, vitamin E, and beta carotene, but these have not been as well studied as vitamin C, so I do not routinely recommend them.

People who eat fewer foods containing *magnesium* tend to have more wheezing illnesses than those who consume more magnesium-rich diets. Higher dietary and blood levels of magnesium are associated with fewer and less severe breathing problems such as asthma and bron-

| MAGNESIUM-RICH FOODS | |
|---|---|
| Banana | 35 mg per 1 banana |
| Beans (pinto, northern, black, navy) | 100 mg per 1 cup of cooked beans |
| Beans (garbanzo or lima) | 80 mg per 1 cup of cooked beans |
| Cereal (all-bran) | 120 mg per ½ cup |
| Cereal (raisin bran) | 80 mg per 1 cup |
| Lentils | 70 mg per 1 cup of cooked lentils |
| Nuts (almonds, cashews) | 80 mg per 3 tablespoons |
| Peanut butter | 50 mg per 2 tablespoons |
| Rice, brown | 85 mg per 1 cup of cooked rice |
| Spinach | 75 mg per ½ cup of cooked spinach |

chitis.[80] In serious emergency asthma attacks, magnesium (300 milligrams to 2 grams depending on the child's weight) is now given by vein as a standard treatment in many emergency rooms.[81] In a randomized, controlled study, daily magnesium supplements (400 milligrams) significantly improved asthma symptoms and reduced the need for some medications in adults.[82] Too much magnesium (e.g., patients taking a lot of magnesium-containing antacids) can cause diarrhea. I haven't found any studies evaluating magnesium supplements for childhood asthma. Magnesium supplements are not part of mainstream medical care for asthma yet, but I always recommend that the asthmatic child's daily multivitamin contains magnesium and that she eats magnesium-rich foods.

Salt seems to make airways more twitchy, but large studies have *not* found an association between dietary salt and asthma.[83] On the other hand, there's no data showing that extra salt is good for asthma, and it's certainly not helpful for those with high blood pressure.

Omega-3 fatty acids, such as those found in *flaxseed oil* and *fatty fish* may reduce levels of inflammatory chemicals and reduce the risk of asthma.[84] People who regularly eat fresh oily fish have significantly better lung function and reduced risk of asthma compared with those who avoid eating fish.[85]

In one study, 29 children with chronic asthma were given daily fish oil supplements; over ten months their symptoms gradually improved, but they also underwent a major cleanup in their environment.[86] In another study, adults who took *omega-3 fatty acid* (docosahexanoic acid, DHA—the active ingredient in fish oil) supplements for one year had fewer asthma symptoms than others who took placebo pills.[87] Another study also supports taking omega-3 fatty acid supplements to improve lung function.[88] However, a similar study in asthmatic children did not show any change in symptoms over six months.[89] It may

| OMEGA-3 FATTY ACIDS IN FISH | |
| --- | --- |
| Bass, freshwater | 0.9 gm |
| Halibut | 0.6 gm |
| Herring, Atlantic | 1.9 gm |
| Mussels, steamed | 0.7 gm |
| Perch, ocean | 0.4 gm |
| Salmon, Atlantic | 1.9 gm |
| Salmon, smoked | 0.4 gm |
| Salmon, sockeye | 1.2 gm |
| Sardines, in oil | 1.3 gm |
| Trout, rainbow | 1.0 gm |

take nine months to a year for supplemental omega-3 fatty acids to make a difference in asthma symptoms—that's a long time to wait for an uncertain benefit.

Canned tuna as well as fresh mushrooms, shrimp, dried fruits, guacamole, and salad bar ingredients may contain sulfites that trigger asthma in some children. However, fresh fish are generally well tolerated. It's too early to tell if you should be forcing your child to take cod liver oil every day, but a moderate intake of fish is part of a healthy diet.

## LIFESTYLE THERAPIES: NUTRITION, EXERCISE, ENVIRONMENT, MIND-BODY

### Nutrition

Modern America has an obesity epidemic; Evidence is growing that obese children are more prone to developing asthma than children who have an optimal weight.[90] There are *no* studies suggesting that restricting your child's calories and making her super-thin is helpful, but bulking up is bad for asthma as well as diabetes, arthritis, self-esteem, etc.

Many children with asthma, especially those who also have allergies or eczema, notice that certain foods seem to trigger symptoms, and that carefully avoiding these foods improves asthma control.[91] A Swedish study of asthmatic adults showed an improvement on a diet low in tryptophan, an amino acid found in milk, cheese, turkey, and bananas.[92] Asian children who eat a typical Asian diet have a lower risk of asthma than Asian children who eat a more American type of diet.[93] Some physicians routinely advise asthmatics to follow an elimination diet (restricting major allergenic foods), a minimal diet (allowing only a restricted number of foods), vegan diets, or diets excluding certain foods such as dairy products.[94] These physicians and their patients are often impressed with the improvement in asthma symptoms. For example, in a study of adult asthmatics, 79% of those who had tried a restricted diet reported an improvement in their asthma symptoms.[95] In a Danish study, the symptoms of hospitalized adult asthmatics improved when they were placed on a hypoallergenic, elemental diet.[96] Many parents believe that milk increases mucus and worsens asthma symptoms.[97] This idea was tested in a randomized, controlled trial in asthmatic adults. Milk did not cause coughing, wheezing, or impair lung function.[98] Milk does *not* make asthma worse, not unless you know that your child is allergic to milk. Calcium is a particularly important nutrient for children with steroid-dependent asthma because of its protective effects on bones.[99] While restricted diets may be helpful in a minority of asthma patients, they must be done only under the strict supervision of a nutritionist and for brief trials to avoid developing deficiencies of calcium, protein, iron, and other critical nutrients.

On the other hand, some interesting studies suggest that certain foods may protect against asthma.

## NUTRITIONAL THERAPIES FOR ASTHMA

DO:

- Breast-feed
- Give plenty of water
- Try onions and spicy foods
- Try coffee


DON'T:

- Ingest sulfites, preservatives, yellow dyes

Start your child's life right by *breast-feeding*. Breast-feeding reduces wheezing in the first month of life, and the benefits in reducing the risk of asthma persist throughout the first seventeen *years* of life.[100] Make sure that your child gets plenty of *water*. Water helps keep secretions thin and loose, preventing mucus in the lungs from getting dry, sticky, and difficult to clear.

Certain compounds in *onions* and *spicy foods* such as red peppers can reduce the release of histamine and other inflammatory chemicals responsible for asthma's symptoms.[101] I have no idea how many onions a child needs to eat to improve asthma symptoms nor which species or variety, cooked or raw, is most effective. Some parents believe that hot spices such as horseradish, mustard, and chili peppers are also helpful in preventing asthma symptoms. Since onion and hot spices are common cooking ingredients, you may want to experiment yourself: note onion and spice intake and asthma symptoms in your child's asthma journal to see how much better (or worse) he is on the days he eats (or doesn't eat) these foods.

*Coffee* for asthma? In the 1800s it was the treatment of choice. Caffeine is chemically related to the asthma medication theophylline. (See above section on supplements.) There is no benefit to drinking more than three cups daily. There are *no* recent studies evaluating the effects of caffeine on childhood asthma. Don't try to substitute caffeine-containing colas; colas can actually trigger asthma symptoms in some children. Coffee is relatively inexpensive and widely available. If you want to try it for your child, remember that less coffee would be needed for smaller children than for adults and that coffee can have significant side effects.

*Sulfite preservatives, benzoic acid, MSG,* and *yellow dyes* can trigger asthma. Sulfites (chemically related to the sulfur dioxide in smog, which clearly makes asthma worse) are commonly sprayed on fresh fruits and vegetables (beware of restaurant salad bars!), added to certain snacks, orange drinks, beer, and wine. It may be that the real culprit for food-triggered coughs is either allergies to additives or sensitivity to the temperature or acidity of the food being eaten. If you are not sure if your child is sensitive to preservatives or dyes, read labels for all prepared food and wash all fresh fruits and vegetables thoroughly before serving them. Given all the uncertainties in today's food supply, I think the best option is to buy and serve only foods that are organically grown.

## Exercise

*Exercise,* especially in cold, dry air triggers symptoms in nearly 90% of asthmatics. However, children with asthma should still be encouraged to exercise. The overall health benefits of cardiovascular fitness are well known. Asthma is easier to control in patients who are physically well conditioned, and exercise-induced asthmatic symptoms can be readily controlled. Many Olympic athletes have asthma and have set world records for athletic performance. Don't let your asthmatic youngster become a couch potato.

*Yoga exercises*, particularly yogic breathing exercises *(pranayama),* improve lung capacity and reduce the number of asthma attacks in young adults.[102] The physical exercises *(asanas)* alone are helpful, but they're even better when combined with breathing exercises.[103] These exercises emphasize slow, regular breaths in which the ratio of time for inhalation (breathing in) to exhalation (breathing out) is 1:2. For example, have your child breathe in for a count of 5 and breathe out to a count of 10. The benefits can be enhanced by breathing hot, moist air.[104] Regular yoga practice can even reduce the need for steroid medications and frequent inhalers.[105] Yoga has long-term benefits; follow-up studies in India show improvements for at least two years when young adult asthmatics keep practicing yoga, and doing yoga helped them participate in other sports as well.[106] Yoga is straightforward, inexpensive, and free of side effects. I recommend yoga for all of my asthmatic patients. Classes are taught in nearly every community, and at least a dozen books about yoga for children are available at big booksellers and on the Internet.

Another good breathing exercise for asthmatic children is called *pursed lips breathing.*[107] In this technique, children purse their lips and blow out as if blowing a kiss. Adults with severe chronic lung disease who practice this technique are able to increase their blood oxygen levels during pursed lips breathing alone without any other therapy.

Other types of *breathing exercises* frequently suggested as complementary therapies for asthma combine aspects of physical training and mind-body interventions. Training sessions may include voice training, relaxation, postural changes, and breathing exercises.[108] In a randomized, controlled trial of German adults with mild asthma, breathing exercises significantly improved pulmonary function—long-term improvements that were comparable to the short-term benefits of inhaled beta-agonist medications.[109]

A recent fad hitting the Internet is Buteyko breathing. This technique is named after a Russian physician, Konstantin Buteyko, who believed that deep breaths or "over-breathing" causes asthma, and that to reduce asthma symptoms, patients should be trained to "breathe less." In one Australian study, teenagers and adults who received training in Buteyko's breathing techniques showed some improvement in their asthma symptoms over four months compared with a control group who received standard asthma education;[110] they needed fewer treatments with beta-agonist medications and reported better quality of life.[111] Nevertheless, I remain pretty skeptical about this technique. It may help simply by helping asthmatics focus on breathing while remaining calm so that when problems do arise, they can react more objectively and with less panic.[112] I prefer yogic breathing exercises, but you should be aware of the scientific data about all the therapies out there.

*Swimming* is a great exercise for youngsters with asthma. Swimming may not be significantly better than other aerobic conditioning programs, but swimming programs do improve overall fitness, swimming ability, and self-esteem.[113] Spa treatments (swimming in hot spring/mineral water) may be even better. In a study of adults with severe, steroid-dependent asthma, 69% given spa treatments reported significant improvement; rates of improvement were even higher among those with more severe disease.[114] Similar studies have not been done in children, nor are insurance companies likely to race to reimburse you for spa memberships. Remember that some kids are sensitive to the high chlorine levels in public pools, and that the most important thing to do is to keep your child exercising.

## PREVENTION STRATEGIES FOR EXERCISE-INDUCED ASTHMA

- A fifteen- to thirty-minute warm-up period before vigorous exercise
- Breathing in through the nose—not the mouth—to warm and filter outside air before it hits the lungs
- Covering the nose and mouth with a loose-fitting scarf or bandanna when exercising outdoors on especially cold days

## Environment

*Avoiding environmental triggers* is the best way to prevent your child from having asthma flare-ups. It has been estimated that if typical environmental triggers at home (such as tobacco smoke, furry pets, and gas ovens or stoves) were eliminated, there would be about a 39% reduction in the amount of asthma in the United States.[115]

## REDUCING AIRBORNE ASTHMA TRIGGERS

- *No smoking* anywhere near the child
- Changing from gas to electric furnaces and stoves
- HEPA air filters; furnace and air-conditioner filters
- Houseplants: philodendrons, spider plants
- Windows closed 5 A.M. to 10 A.M. when pollen counts are high
- Get rid of cockroaches
- Reduce air pollution: ride a bike or take a bus

Avoiding cigarette smoke reduces the risk of many heart and lung diseases, including childhood asthma. Secondhand cigarette smoke may be responsible for up to 50% of asthma episodes in children. Don't smoke and don't let anyone else smoke around your child.

Free-standing HEPA electronic air filters efficiently remove airborne asthma triggers inside the home, but filters alone don't remove dander and dust lying on the floor or furniture.[116] Potting soil and common houseplants (such as spider plants, philodendron, bamboo palm, and English ivy) also absorb some indoor air pollutants.[117] Change or replace your furnace filter and air-conditioning filter regularly. Consider installing an electrostatic air filter on your furnace; such filters can effectively remove over 90% of airborne irritants and allergens. Check *Consumer Reports* for the best buys. Keep your child indoors when air quality is bad. Pollen counts are usually highest between 5 and 10 A.M., so keep the windows closed during early morning hours. To reduce outdoor air pollution, think of carpooling, using buses or bicycles, and working for tougher anti-pollution laws as ways of helping your child stay healthy throughout life. Electric cars, anyone?

Many children who suffer from chronic asthma are sensitive to *dust* and microscopic *dust mites.* By reducing the levels of household dust and dust mites, you can help your child reduce asthma and allergy symptoms. Eliminate dust-catchers such as old carpeting and dust ruffles. Dust mites love to live in mattresses and pillows. Keep them away from your child by encasing the mattress and pillow in a plastic or vinyl fitted sheet.[118] Wash your child's sheets, pillow cases, and blankets weekly in hot water to kill dust mites. Engage in a weekly cleanup campaign to fight dust and mold in the child's room; damp mopping helps remove dust without stirring it up.[119] Consider spraying carpets and upholstery with a dust mite killer. Use a 3% tannic acid solution or benzylbenzoate (chemicals that kill the dust

mite) every two to three months.[120] Clean thoroughly after spraying to remove all of the dead dust mite particles.

Furry pets should not sleep in your child's bedroom. Furry pets should be confined either to the outdoors or to a non-carpeted room that is easily cleaned and in which the child does not spend a lot of time. If your child is visiting a home with furry pets, pretreat the child with anti-inflammatory asthma medication prior to the visit.

*Mold*, a common asthma trigger, is a problem in humid climates and in households that cook a lot of pasta or rice, because of all the water vapor in the air. Try to keep household humidity less than 50% with a dehumidifier, and clean any visible mold or mildew with a 10% bleach solution.

Negative *ion generators* have *no* proven benefits for asthmatic adults or children.[121] I do *not* recommend them. While mist and steam from vaporizers are often soothing for children with colds, sinus infections, and bronchitis, they are not very helpful for children with asthma.

*Infections* are common triggers for asthma symptoms. This is particularly true for the common cold viruses that run rampant in the fall when kids return to school. There's not much you can do about this except to try to keep your child in less crowded classrooms. Interestingly, there are some new studies showing that a few patients with severe, chronic asthma are actually suffering from a form of walking pneumonia (caused by Mycoplasma or Chlamydia bacteria), and that when they receive several weeks of antibiotic treatment (with erythromycin or clarithromycin), their symptoms improve dramatically.[122] Sinus infections are also major asthma triggers. If your child has cold symptoms that are not getting better within ten days, take her to the pediatrician to make sure she doesn't have a sinus infection.

Rid your home of cockroaches. New studies indicate that more than one-third of children are allergic to cockroaches, and those who are often exposed (such as urban apartment dwellers) have a much higher risk of asthma.[123]

## Mind-Body

Stress is a major trigger for asthma symptoms.[124] Depression and stress combined with inadequate social support play a major role in making asthma worse and increasing the risk of emergency care and hospitalization.[125] Stress management can take a variety of forms and be helpful for both parents and children. Mind-body therapies for asthma include hypnosis, autogenic training, biofeedback, meditation, music therapy, and several relaxation therapy hybrids. These therapies can be helpful, even with a relatively short training period. For example, in one study of asthmatic children, just three sessions of systematic relaxation training improved lung function.[126]

*Hypnosis* and guided imagery have proven useful in improving symptoms and lung function, enhancing parental confidence in managing their children's asthma, and reducing the amount of medication and number of physician visits for asthma, even among preschoolers.[127] Physicians experienced in using clinical hypnosis may help patients reduce allergic reactions, the need for steroid medications and even hospitalization rates. Additional studies are needed to assess optimal training frequency and duration of hypnotic training and the patients for whom it is likely to be most helpful.

*Relaxation* and *guided imagery* are extremely safe. A trained therapist should be able to get you started on a home program of your own, and your child can practice by listening to cassette tapes of the therapist's voice, leading her through the relaxation exercises. In the meantime, it is important for you to remain calm and confident when your child has an asthma attack. Plan your strategy in advance. When parents stay calm and relaxed, children have an easier time relaxing, addressing the problem, and reducing symptoms.

Like self-hypnosis, *autogenic training* has proven effective in reducing chronic asthma symptoms.[128] Daily practice is essential for maximal effectiveness of mind-body therapies. *Transcendental meditation* has also proven helpful for adult asthmatics who practice it regularly.[129]

*Biofeedback* can also be a useful therapy for asthmatics.[130] In a fifteen-month follow-up of seventeen adult asthmatics who were trained with biofeedback devices to improve their breathing, there were fewer and less severe asthma attacks, requiring less medication and resulting in fewer visits to the emergency room for over a year following training.[131] Other studies have also reported success in children and adolescents; if your child has persistent, recurrent symptoms, biofeedback may be worth trying.[132] Give it five to ten sessions, and if there's no improvement by then, it's probably not going to work at this point in your child's life.

A novel mind-body therapy for asthma and other chronic diseases is "journaling." Adult asthmatics who were assigned to write about their stressful experiences three times a week for twenty minutes at a time had a marked reduction in asthma symptoms and had improved lung function over the next four months.[133] Interestingly, these journals were not discussed with a therapist, and no particular therapy was initiated on the basis of writing. It looks as though just getting those stressful thoughts out on paper helps reduce stress which in turn can improve lung function. This is very simple and straightforward, and I recommend you try it.

Seek *support* from other families who have asthmatic children. Sharing stories and strategies helps decrease isolation and makes stress more manageable.

## BIOMECHANICAL THERAPIES: PHYSICAL THERAPY, MASSAGE, SPINAL MANIPULATION

### Physical Therapy

Physical therapy treatments (pounding on the chest to help clear mucus) have been proved *not* to benefit asthmatic children.[134]

### Massage

Massage not only feels good, it helps reduce stress and anxiety which may contribute to asthma. In a study of 32 asthmatic children, massage was compared with relaxation therapy; parents were instructed in either technique and provided the therapy to their child each night before bed for one month. The youngest children had the biggest gains with massage—less anxiety, lower stress hormone levels, better attitudes and better lung function—but even the older children with more chronic asthma had an improvement in some lung functions.[135] Once parents are trained, they can provide the therapy, and if the therapy is provided by parents, the cost is low and the side effects, if any, are minimal. This is one therapy that I regularly recommend for families try to assist their children with asthma.

### Spinal Manipulation

Spinal manipulation or spinal adjustments are provided by chiropractors, naturopaths, and osteopaths to treat asthma. Randomized clinical trials have found no real benefit of chiropractic adjustments in treating asthma in adults or children.[136] Chiropractic not only offers no proven clinical benefit, but its costs in terms of frequent visits, X rays, and encour-

aging reliance on costly visits several times a week may actually increase dependence on health professionals and overall health care costs. I do not regularly recommend chiropractic therapy for asthmatic children.

## BIOENERGETIC THERAPIES: ACUPUNCTURE, THERAPEUTIC TOUCH, PRAYER, HOMEOPATHY

### Acupuncture

Chinese medical practitioners claim that asthma readily responds to acupuncture, but data from controlled trials are not yet conclusive.[137] Twelve acupuncture treatments given over four weeks (that's three sessions a week!) can calm down an overactive immune system and many clinical studies support a modest role for acupuncture for adult asthmatics.[138] Asthmatic children treated with acupuncture twenty minutes before exercise have milder symptoms than untreated children.[139] Even in China, however, acupuncture is not usually the only remedy for people with asthma but is used in combination with herbs or Western medications. Additional studies are needed to determine the cost-effectiveness of acupuncture and optimal treatment regimens for asthmatic children. Acupuncture should not be relied upon to replace conventional asthma medication, but it can be a reasonable adjunct therapy to try if your child is willing to try it; actually, although many kids are initially a bit fearful, they find acupuncture pleasant rather than some kind of needle torture.[140]

### Therapeutic Touch

There have not been any studies of the effectiveness of Therapeutic Touch in treating asthma symptoms. However, in my own practice I have watched children's oxygen levels climb and their breathing relax during Therapeutic

Touch treatments. I incorporate Therapeutic Touch and Reiki into my therapy for children during acute asthma attacks and for children with all kinds of breathing problems, especially those hospitalized in the intensive care unit. A group of German asthmatics reported great improvement in their asthma symptoms and a decrease in their need for medications when they received treatments from a "hands on" healer;[141] it's not clear from this study exactly what kind of healing or how many sessions might be helpful for children with asthma. Hands on healing, Therapeutic Touch, and Reiki are all very safe. Clearly, more research is needed to determine the optimal strategy for using these different techniques for children.

### Prayer

Many of my patients tell me that they feel more relaxed and peaceful when they pray; they also feel that prayer helps them manage their asthma better.[142] This makes sense to me. I recommend prayer if it is consistent with your family's values and beliefs.

### Homeopathy

Homeopathy shows some promise in treating allergic asthma in adults, but the quality of the research studies is not very good, and treatment is highly individualized.[143] Common asthma remedies include Arsenica, Antimonia, Chamomilla, Ipecac, Lobelia, *Nux vomica,* and Pulsatilla. However, there are *no* published studies of homeopathy in preventing or treating asthmatic children. Homeopaths themselves advise parents not to treat symptoms of acute asthma with homeopathic remedies alone. If your child has allergies as well as asthma, I think homeopathy might be a reasonable route to explore, but only as an adjunct, not a replacement for asthma medications and lifestyle changes.

## WHAT I RECOMMEND FOR ASTHMA

### PREVENTING ASTHMA

1. *Lifestyle—nutrition.* Start your child off right by breast-feeding. Give plenty of fluids, especially when your child has a cold.

2. *Lifestyle—environment.* Do *not* smoke and do not allow others to smoke around your child. Avoid allergy triggers. Drive less. Work for clean air in your community. Try to avoid crowds where your child will catch another respiratory virus. Keep your house clean and wash your child's bedding in hot water at least twice a month to minimize dust mite exposures.

3. *Biochemical—medications.* Get your child immunized.

*See your health care professional if your child is:*

- Having a hard time breathing

- Breathing much more rapidly than usual

- Making a grunting noise when breathing out

- Getting tired or agitated with his shortness of breath

- Getting blue in the lips or fingertips

- Sucking in the spaces between his ribs with each breath

- Having symptoms that interfere with sleep or other activities or has a high fever or poor appetite

- Or get help if you have *any* concerns about your child's breathing or he is not improving with home therapies

## TREATING ASTHMA

*Work with your doctor to develop a written asthma plan. Help children monitor their symptoms; obtain and use a peak flow meter and keep a record of symptoms, triggers, treatments, and peak flow meter readings. Treat all symptoms promptly.*

1. *Biochemical—medications.* Work with your physician or other health care professional to develop the best plan for using medications to prevent and treat asthma. In general, cromolyn and nedocromil help prevent symptoms and have few side effects; steroids can help prevent or treat symptoms, and beta-agonists are used when your child has symptoms. Make sure your clinician demonstrates and your child understands how to use a metered dose inhaler (and a spacer). Have your child immunized against influenza every fall. Do *not* rely on nonprescription medications.

2. *Biochemical—nutritional supplements.* Consider supplemental B6 (pyridoxine), magnesium, fish oil, vitamin C.

3. *Lifestyle—environment.* Don't smoke and don't let anyone else smoke around your child. Avoid triggers such as allergens, dust and mold, and foods that trigger your child's asthma. Don't let furry pets sleep in your child's room. Drive less. Work for cleaner air in your home and in your environment. Thoroughly clean your child's room weekly. Wash your child's bedding in the hottest possible water twice a month. Consider using an electronic air filter and adding houseplants such as philodendron to your child's room.

4. *Lifestyle—exercise.* Keep your child moving. Asthma symptoms can be controlled even during vigorous exercise. Have your child try yoga (especially yogic breathing), pursed-lips breathing exercises, or swimming. Have your child warm up before exercise; breathe through the nose, not the mouth; and cover nose and mouth with a scarf when exercising in very cold weather.

5. *Lifestyle—mind-body.* Consider training in self-hypnosis, meditation, or biofeedback training. Get support. Communicate with other adults who care for your child about your child's asthma. Teachers, day care workers, baby-sitters, and relatives need to know what symptoms to look for, what your care plan is, and how to reach your child's health care professional in case of an emergency. Remind yourself and your child to have fun! Asthma can be serious, but with an appropriate treatment plan, your child should be able to have a happy, normal childhood.

6. *Lifestyle—nutrition.* Consider supplemental onions and spicy foods. Give your child foods rich in vitamin C, vitamin B6, magnesium, and include fish in his diet. Avoid sulfite preservatives.

7. *Biomechanical—massage.* Get a book, a video, or a massage therapist to teach you how to give a massage to your child every day.

8. *Bioenergetic—acupuncture.* Acupuncture may be a helpful adjunctive treatment, but more research is needed before it becomes routine. Although there is little research on hands-on healing techniques or prayer, I recommend both if they are provided free or at low cost and are consistent with your family's beliefs.

## RESOURCES

American Lung Association
1740 Broadway
New York, NY 10019–4374
(800) LUNG-USA or (212) 315-8700
http://www.lungusa.org/asthma/

American Academy of Allergy Asthma and
    Immunology
http://www.aaaai.org/

American Academy of Pediatrics
    http://www.aap.org

Asthma and Allergy Foundation of
    America
1717 Massachusetts Avenue
Washington, D.C. 20036
(800) 727-8462
http://www.aafa.org/

Allergy and Asthma Network Mothers of
    Asthmatics, Inc.
2751 Prosperity Avenue, Suite 150
Fairfax, VA 22031
(800) 878-4403 or (703) 641-9595
http://www.aanma.org/

National Heart Lung and Blood Institute,
National Asthma Education Program
(301) 251-1222
http://www.nhlbi.nih.gov/guidelines/
asthma/asthgdln.htm

## Asthma Diaries

Asthma Peak Flow Diary
http://www.pedipress.com/products/
DiaryADPF.html
http://thriveonline.oxygen.com/medical/
asthma/tools/worksheet.peakdiary.
html

## Air Cleaners and Other Allergy Products

Allergy Control Products (800) 422-DUST

Allergy Resources (800) USE-FLAX

Gazoontite.com
http://www.gazoontite.com

## Peak Flow Meters

Clement Clarke (Mini-Wright's peak flow
meter)
(800) 848-8923
http://www.clement-clarke.com/
respiratory/index.htm

## Books

Bock, Steven J.; Bock, Kenneth; Bruning,
Nancy P. *Natural Relief for Your Child's
Asthma*. New York: HarperCollins, 1999.
Plaut, Thomas F. *Children with Asthma: A
Manual for Parents*. 2nd ed. Amherst,
Mass.: Pedipress, 1988.
Rogers, A. *Luke Has Asthma Too*. Burlington,
Vt.: Waterfront Books, 1987.

# 6
# BED-WETTING (ENURESIS)

Maggie Murphy brought her seven-year-old son Matthew in to see me several months ago for his annual checkup. When I asked what concerns they had about Matt's health, they looked at each other sheepishly. "Well," Maggie began, "Matt wants to join the Scouts this year, but they have overnight camping trips, and he can't always make it through the night without an accident." Matt looked down at the floor. I looked directly at him. "There's no need to be embarrassed about this, Matt. Lots of boys your age have the same problem. Let me ask you a few more questions and then we'll do some tests on your urine, and I can suggest a few ideas for things to try at home." Matt looked cautious but hopeful. "OK, but am I going to have to take drugs or have a blood test?" "No. You definitely don't need a blood test today, and most boys learn to manage this problem just fine without any medication."

Bed-wetting (or *enuresis* as it's known in medical circles) is the most common bladder problem affecting children. Everyone starts life without control over their bladder. We don't expect babies or toddlers to stay dry by themselves. Bladder control is usually learned after bowel control. Most children are dry during the daytime many weeks or even months before they are dry at night (usually by three to four years old). Many children don't develop full control of their bladders until about school age, and some take a bit longer.

Bed-wetting was noted as a medical problem in papyrus writings dating back to 1550 B.C. In more modern times, we know that between 5 and 15 percent of seven-year-old boys occasionally wet the bed, and about two-thirds of their parents go to a doctor for help.

There are two kinds of enuresis: *primary* (never has been dry at night) and *secondary* (was dry at night at one point and is now wetting again). Primary enuresis is the most common kind of bed-wetting. It is more common in *boys* and tends to run in families.

*Matt had never been completely dry at night, though he had been fine during the daytime for two years. He didn't wet every night, but there was a problem at least three nights a week. His mother told me that Matt's father had had the same problem when he was a boy, and hadn't outgrown it until he was ten. Both parents wanted Matt to be spared the embarrassment of having an accident while he was out camping or spending the night with friends. It sounded to me as if Matt had a classic case of primary enuresis, but I wanted to check his urine, just to make sure he didn't have a secondary reason for bed-wetting.*

*Secondary enuresis* can be a sign of an underlying medical problem (such as a bladder infection, constipation, or diabetes) or a sudden emotional stress (such as birth of a new sibling), causing the child's behavior to regress. Unfortunately, another cause of bed-wetting in girls who have been dry in the past is sexual abuse or molestation. If your child has been dry at night for a while and suddenly starts wetting again, it's a good idea to have him checked by your health care professional.

*Constipation* is a common cause of secondary enuresis and bladder infections. When the colon is stretched full, it rubs against the bladder, irritating it, putting pressure on it and making the child feel as if he has to urinate even though his bladder isn't full. If your child is constipated and wets the bed, treat the constipation first (see Chapter 12). Once the constipation has resolved, the bed-wetting may no longer be a problem.

Children suffering from enuresis also frequently suffer from *allergies* such as hay fever, hives, and eczema. This has led many people to believe that enuresis is just another manifestation of food allergies. Rather than causing a skin rash or wheezing, these allergic reactions are thought to irritate the bladder, sending it into spasms. Commonly blamed food allergens are milk, chocolate, eggs, wheat, and citrus fruit. *Caffeine* is a known bladder irritant. Like coffee and tea, *chocolate* contains caffeine and should be avoided by children suffering from enuresis.

Many parents think that bed-wetting is a sleep problem. It's not. Extensive studies have shown that children who wet the bed are *not* necessarily deep sleepers. Children who wet the bed sleep normally. Bed-wetting doesn't just occur during deep sleep or dreaming sleep; it occurs when the child's bladder is full.

Enuresis is also *not* necessarily a sign of psychological or emotional problems. It is not a sign of bad parenting or that the child is bad, willful, or lazy. On the contrary, enuresis can *cause* humiliation and lower self-esteem. Punishing a child who suffers from enuresis just adds to the burden of guilt and makes it less likely that the child will be able to summon up the inner resources to overcome the problem. Successfully resolving the problem boosts a child's self-esteem and improves performance in school and social situations as well.

*Matt's urine test showed no sign of infection or diabetes. Neither he nor his mother could identify any recent stresses, except the stress of bed-wetting. His parents were divided about how to handle it. Maggie just wanted to use a plastic mattress cover, change the sheets when they needed it, and wait until Matt outgrew it. His father thought Matt should lose TV privileges for his wet nights and not be allowed to go on overnight trips until he learned better. It sounded like both parents needed to learn more about enuresis.*

At school age, about 10% of children still wet the bed regularly; this means that three children in a class of thirty first graders have a problem with nighttime wetting. By fifteen years of age, 2% of children still suffer from occasional bed-wetting. Remember, unless there is an anatomic problem or underlying illness, everybody eventually "outgrows" enuresis.

## CAUSES OF ENURESIS

- Genetic—runs in families
- Small bladder
- Slow hormonal maturation

Like many problems, enuresis tends to *run in families*. A child whose father was a bed-wetter has a 40 to 50 percent chance of being one, too. If both parents suffered from enuresis, the child has a 70 to 80 percent chance of being a bed-wetter. For unknown reasons, enuresis is more common in boys than girls. Enuresis is more common in crowded living conditions and families in which one or both parents smoke.

Children with enuresis tend to have *smaller bladders* than other children. Children with small bladders have to make frequent trips to the bathroom. You can check your child's bladder capacity by having him hold his urine as long as he can after he feels he has to go (in the daytime), and then have him void into a container. A normal child should be able to hold (and void) his age in years plus two in ounces. For example, a seven-year-old should be able to void: 7 + 2 = 9 ounces.

The adult bladder capacity is reached between ten and fourteen years of age.

| NORMAL BLADDER CAPACITY | |
| --- | --- |
| *AGE IN YEARS* | *VOLUME IN OUNCES* |
| 6 | 8 |
| 8 | 10 |
| 10 | 12 |
| 12 | 14 |

The brain monitors the balance of salt and water throughout the body. It sends hormonal messages to the kidneys about how much salt and water to save and how much to release. The brain's hormonal messenger antidiuretic hormone (ADH) tells the kidneys how much urine to make. Lower ADH levels tell the kidneys to make more urine, and to make the urine more dilute (watery). Higher ADH levels tell the kidneys to make less urine and to make the urine more concentrated.

As a child grows and develops, the brain gradually makes more ADH during the nighttime and less ADH during the day. More ADH at night means less urine is produced, so the bladder doesn't fill as quickly. This is what saves us from having to urinate every three to four hours at night. Low daytime ADH levels tell the kidney to make more urine when it is easy to empty a full bladder.

Many children suffering from enuresis secrete the same amount of ADH around the clock. They don't develop the difference in daytime vs. nighttime ADH secretion at the same age as other children. This means their kidneys keep producing urine as fast at night as during the day, filling their (relatively small) bladders every few hours. Some enuretic children have such low levels of nighttime ADH they produce enough urine to fill four normal bladders at night. A full bladder needs to be emptied. If the child doesn't wake up when the bladder is full, it empties while he's asleep, and the bed is wet. Most children eventually develop the day-night differences in ADH secretion that allow them to go through the night without urinating. In the meantime, they need to be trained to wake up when their bladder is full so they can empty it in the toilet rather than in the bed.

## HOW TO TREAT ENURESIS

No matter how you decide to help your child with enuresis, make at least one visit to your health care professional to make sure your child doesn't have a bladder infection, early diabetes, or some other reason for excessive urination. These problems account for less than 5% of enuresis, but they are the kinds of things you wouldn't want to overlook. Let's tour the Therapeutic Mountain to find out what works for treating enuresis. If you want to skip to my bottom-line recommendations, flip to the end of the chapter.

## BIOCHEMICAL THERAPIES: MEDICATIONS, HERBS, AND OTHER DIETARY SUPPLEMENTS

Medications and herbs are not the first choices for treating enuresis. The primary treatment for enuresis is changing the lifestyle: diet, exercise, environment, and behavior (mind-body). Nevertheless, if changes in lifestyle alone do not cure the problem, biochemical therapy may be helpful for some children.

### Medications

Nonprescription medications are not useful in treating enuresis. If you want to try a medication, you'll need a prescription.

#### PRESCRIPTION MEDICATIONS FOR ENURESIS

- Imipramine (Tofranil)
- DDAVP pills or nasal spray (Minirin)
- Oxybutynin (Ditropan)

Several types of powerful medication have been used to treat enuresis. For several years, the most commonly prescribed medication was *imipramine (Tofranil)*. Imipramine is an antidepressant, but it helps enuresis by increasing bladder capacity and decreasing

spontaneous bladder contractions. It is taken just before bedtime. It is effective for many children while they are taking it, but then many children relapse after they stop the medication. *Overdoses of imipramine can be fatal.* I do not prescribe imipramine because of the obvious hazards of having a potentially fatal drug around a child who has low self-esteem or depression secondary to his enuresis.

The new favorite medication for enuresis is *DDAVP*, a synthetic form of antidiuretic hormone (ADH), which tells kidneys to make less urine. DDAVP is one of only a few drugs that is as effective when given as a nasal spray as it is when taken by mouth. It reduces the number of wet nights from an average of four or five per week to an average of two or three. It is especially effective when used in combination with behavioral and environmental therapies such as sticker charts (rewards for dry nights) and alarms.

Unfortunately, bed-wetting frequently reoccurs when the medication is stopped because DDAVP doesn't really change hormonal maturation or bladder capacity. DDAVP is also pretty expensive ($50 to $100 per month). About 4% of children have significant side effects with DDAVP. Their kidneys overconcentrate the urine, resulting in water-salt imbalances throughout the body and even seizures in some children. This risk can be minimized if the child does not drink anything after dinner. Nevertheless, DDAVP is safer than imipramine; it has become the medication of choice (when medications are needed) for treating children who wet the bed. Over the long term, DDAVP is less effective than lifestyle approaches. I do not recommend it unless other treatments have failed or the child needs it occasionally to avoid embarrassment on an important overnight trip. Even then, DDAVP is far from 100% effective.

A third drug, *oxybutynin (Ditropan)*, decreases bladder contractions, but in a controlled trial, was not found to be helpful in treating children with enuresis.[1]

## Herbs

Although herbal teas have historically been recommended to treat enuresis, there are no scientific studies evaluating the effectiveness of any herbal remedy in treating bed-wetting. Children who suffer from enuresis should *avoid* hops, kava kava, valerian, skullcap, and passionflower. These herbs promote deep sleep, potentially impairing the ability to awaken when the bladder is full. Horsetail and juniper are weak diuretics, which means they tend to increase urination. Juniper irritates the kidneys. *Uva ursi* (bearberry leaves) decreases bladder inflammation; it is a common ingredient in kidney and bladder teas sold in Europe where it is used to prevent bladder infections in adult women. Cranberry helps prevent bladder infections in women prone to recurrent urinary tract infections; there are no studies evaluating its effectiveness in treating normal childhood bed-wetting. Until studies are performed comparing herbal remedies to other effective treatments, I do not recommend them for bed-wetting.

Similarly, no vitamins or minerals or other dietary supplements have proven safe and effective in treating bed-wetting.

## LIFESTYLE THERAPIES: NUTRITION, EXERCISE, ENVIRONMENT, MIND-BODY

### Nutrition

*Do not let your child drink any fluids for at least one or two hours before going to bed.* This helps reduce the strain on a small bladder capacity to make it through the night without being emptied.

Some have suggested that enuresis can be caused by *intolerance or allergy* to cow's milk or other foods (chocolate, eggs, grain, citrus fruit). Although some investigators have reported success with elimination diets (which drastically limit the kinds of foods eaten), their studies did not include control groups and there was probably a strong placebo effect at work.[2] One study that compared dietary restriction to imipramine (medication) showed that the medication was far more effective.[3] I do not recommend that you embark on an elimination diet for your child unless:

- He has other allergy symptoms (eczema, hay fever, wheezing, diarrhea)
- Other treatments for the enuresis have failed
- You seek professional guidance from a nutritionist to make sure your child maintains a balanced diet

There are a small group of children who have persistent enuresis whose problem is partially due to having too much calcium in their urine.[4] Urine tests can show the ratio of calcium to other substances in the urine (such as creatinine—a normal excretion product) to find out if this is the problem. Appropriate dietary restrictions combined with special medicine can help correct this problem and resolve the enuresis. This is a rare condition, and dietary restrictions should not be undertaken without a thorough medical examination, urine tests to confirm the condition, and ongoing expert advice from a pediatric nutritionist and pediatrician.

### Exercise

If your child has a small bladder, try *bladder-stretching exercises* during the day. Bladder-stretching exercises have proven effectiveness in treating enuresis:

## BLADDER-STRETCHING EXERCISE I

1. Agree in advance on some small reward (stickers or vouchers that can be redeemed for a larger reward such as a trip to a ball game) for successfully delaying voiding.

2. Ask your child to notice when he has to urinate and ask him to hold his urine.

3. Set a portable timer for 5 minutes and have him try to wait until the timer goes off until he actually voids.

4. Gradually increase the time on the timer to 10 minutes during the second week of practice, then 15 minutes the third week.

This exercise gets him in the habit of overcoming the initial bladder spasms.

## BLADDER STRETCHING EXERCISE 2

1. Have your child drink 8 to 12 ounces of water.

2. Have him note his initial urge to urinate.

3. Have him count as high as he can while he holds his urine until it becomes uncomfortable.

4. Measure and record the amount voided and the number reached during counting.

5. Give rewards for being able to hold the urine longer and counting higher until he has to void. Make a game to see how high he can count before he has to void.

A third exercise helps children gain a sense of control over the urination process.

## BLADDER STRETCHING EXERCISE 3

While the child is voiding, have him practice:

1. Stopping (interrupting the stream)

2. Holding it a second

3. And restarting the stream

Practice at least once a day until the child gains a sense of mastery in being able to start and stop at will.

Bladder-stretching exercises work best if you are calm about both success and failure and do them as interesting games or challenges rather than do or die situations. Progress is gradual, as it is with all types of exercise. Relapses are common when a child is overexcited, overtired, afraid, or anxious. Don't emphasize your child's misses; instead, reward his successes. Remeasure his bladder capacity once a week to see how well the bladder is stretching. Celebrate successes!

## Environment

If your child is still potty training and is having a hard time making it to the bathroom in the middle of the night, consider putting the potty chair in his bedroom so he doesn't have as far to go. Obviously, you should not run a tabletop fountain or waterfall within earshot of the sleeping child.

## Mind-Body

Bed-wetting is not a sign of parental or child failure. It is simply a sign of a small bladder and a possible delay in developing hormonal rhythms for antidiuretic hormone. While the bladder is stretching and the hormones are coming into balance, a number of mind-body remedies have proven effectiveness in helping a child learn to awaken when his bladder is full.

### MIND-BODY THERAPIES FOR ENURESIS

- Tracking on a calendar
- Rewards
- Alarms
- Hypnotherapy
- Biofeedback

Some parents believe that punishment will stop enuresis. This is misguided. It is not helpful to yell at, humiliate, allow siblings to tease, or physically punish the child. These punishments just make the child feel more ashamed and lower the child's sense of self-esteem. It is helpful to be calm and to give the child responsibility for cleaning up his clothing and bedding (changing clothes and putting the wet things in the washing machine or laundry basket). It is helpful to *track* dry nights on a calendar. It is also helpful to give praise and other *rewards* for dry nights.

One of the most effective treatments for enuresis is the *bed-wetting alarm*. Bed-wetting alarms have a cure rate of 70 to 90 percent, which is higher and longer lasting than any medication. Alarms also raise a child's self-esteem because they actually train him to wake up rather than simply create a dependency on a drug. They are especially useful to train children with small bladders to awaken when the bladder is full. Most alarms are lightweight and are easily attached to the child's pajama bottoms. The devices are sensitive to just a few drops of urine. When urine is sensed, the alarm rings, awakening the child, and alerting him to finish voiding in the bathroom.

Several different brands of alarms are available. Many are available for less than $50—about the price of one visit to the doctor. Some doctors and clinics have inexpensive rental programs for bed-wetting alarms. Some insurance policies will cover an enuresis alarm if the health professional writes a prescription for it as a medical device.

Make sure you tell your child that this is *his* alarm, and he is responsible for hooking it up, testing it out, and responding to it. Success with this treatment is directly tied to the child's motivation and the family's support. Help your child by making sure he wakes up the first few times the alarm goes off; encourage him to get to the bathroom, change pajamas, reattach the alarm, and put a towel over the wet spot on the bed or change the sheets. It usually takes a couple of months to achieve consistent dryness. Continue using the alarm for a few weeks after dryness has been achieved, just to be sure he has learned to wake up on his own. Alarms are especially effective in combination with bladder-stretching exercises (described on page 94). Nearly 100% effectiveness can be achieved by combining alarms with rewards for following the instructions.

### ALARM INSTRUCTIONS

1. Turn off the alarm
2. Get out of bed
3. Go to the bathroom to finish voiding
4. Cover the wet area or change the sheet
5. Reset the alarm
6. Go back to bed

If you want to try something even simpler and less expensive than special bed-wetting alarms, set a regular *alarm clock* for three hours after the child goes to sleep. When the alarm goes off, wake him up and have him empty his bladder in the toilet. Do this several nights in a row. Do not set the alarm for more than two awakenings at night or you could interfere with his sleep so much that he has trouble functioning during the day. Gradually reduce the time to two hours, then one hour, then have the child wake himself. One study showed a 92% success rate within one month of using the alarm-clock treatment. I think this is one of the most sensible and low-cost treatment options, and I almost always recommend this as a first step in treating bed-wetting.

*Hypnotherapy* is another technique that has helped thousands of children. It is my treatment of choice during an initial visit for enuresis. Actually, I combine hypnosis with 1) keeping a calendar, 2) rewarding dry nights, 3) bladder-stretching exercises, and 4) an alarm clock. Hyp-

nosis or *imagining therapy* has proven as effective as medication and the results are more long-lasting.[5] You do not need to be a professional therapist to use these techniques yourself at home.

The technique I use involves using the child's imagination to visualize the connections between his brain, his bladder, and the muscles that allow the urine to flow out or keep it in. Help the child visualize these parts by drawing a picture.

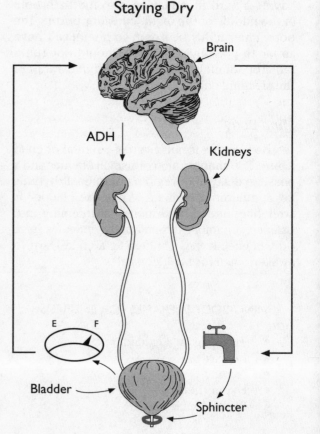

## Staying Dry

He can imagine or pretend what it feels like to have a full bladder, see the nerves telling the brain the bladder is full and the brain deciding whether to tell the nerves and muscles to keep the urine in or let it out. If the brain decides to let the urine out, it can wake up the rest of the body so the child can urinate in the bathroom rather than in bed. The brain can tell the nerves and muscles to keep the urine in until he gets out of bed and goes to the bathroom. Remind your child that the bladder, nerves, brain, and muscles are already doing this job very well during the day. Assure your child that you are confident that they can do this job at night, too. You can help your child practice imagining this picture during the day and right before he goes to sleep. Reward your child for success in making it to the bathroom before he urinates.

*Biofeedback* therapy can effectively treat enuresis in those rare children who have an incoordination between the bladder and sphincter contractions. Biofeedback for these particular muscles is tricky and requires professional guidance.[6] Newer equipment is available that makes biofeedback more feasible that it was ten years ago; still, it is mostly reserved for children who have not responded well to simple alarm systems or to guided imagery/hypnosis or medication.

## BIOMECHANICAL THERAPIES: SPINAL MANIPULATION, SURGERY

### Spinal Manipulation

One study found an insignificant benefit for real compared to sham chiropractic treatment for enuresis. Another showed no benefit of chiropractic treatment compared with just keeping track of the number of dry nights.[7] The chiropractors who did this study concluded that chiropractic was not a useful therapy in the treatment of enuresis. I agree.

### Surgery

Surgery is unnecessary for treating ordinary enuresis. If your child continuously dribbles urine throughout the day or has frequent bladder infections, have him evaluated for an anatomic problem underlying his enuresis. Surgery can often correct these problems.

## BIOENERGETIC THERAPIES: ACUPUNCTURE, HOMEOPATHY

### Acupuncture

Several studies report good success using acupuncture to treat enuresis.[8] Most treatments require repeated needle treatments over several weeks.[9] An Italian study showed that acupuncture decreases bladder spasms.[10] A study comparing acupuncture to DDAVP indicated that the combination of both treatments was most effective and that acupuncture alone was comparable to DDAVP.[11] If acupuncture needles are acceptable for you and your child, it may be worth a try if other treatments (rewards for dry nights, bladder-stretching exercises, alarms, and imagery techniques/ hypnosis) have failed.

### Homeopathy

Homeopathic remedies traditionally used to treat bed-wetting include: Belladonna, Causticum, Equisetum, Kreosotum, Phosphorus, Pulsatilla, Sepia, and Sulfur. There are no studies evaluating the effectiveness of homeopathic remedies in treating children with enuresis. I do not recommend them.

# WHAT I RECOMMEND FOR ENURESIS

*See a health care professional to make sure the child doesn't have bladder infection, diabetes, or some other treatable condition.*

---

*Also consult a professional if:*

- Home treatments don't seem to help after two or three months

- Your child has burning or pain with urination

- Your child starts wetting during the day

- Your child's stream of urine seems abnormal to you

- You have any questions or concerns

---

A combination approach using sticker charts (positive rewards for dry nights), education, bladder-stretching exercises, decreased fluid intake before bedtime, decreased caffeine intake, using an alarm, and helping the child change his own sheets resulted in significant improvement in a majority of children and is far less expensive than any medication.

1. *Lifestyle—mind-body.* Keep a calendar marked with dry nights. Focus on the positive, desired outcome. Give your child positive rewards (such as stickers or vouchers) for dry nights. Do not punish your child for wet nights.

   Put your child in charge of changing pajamas, changing the wet sheets, and putting the wet bedding in the laundry basket. He is responsible but not guilty or being punished.

   Have your child imagine the nerves going from the bladder to his brain, telling his brain that the bladder is full and needs to be emptied. Have him visualize the nerves from the brain to the bladder muscle, telling him to hold the urine a little longer. The brain then sounds the alarm so he can wake up and go to the bathroom before the brain tells his bladder it's OK to go. Help him practice this imagination exercise twice a day, especially before he goes to sleep.

   Set an alarm and awaken your child three hours after he goes to bed so he can get up and void again. If this is not successful within six weeks, try an enuresis alarm.

2. *Lifestyle—nutrition.* Do not give your child anything to drink in the two hours before bed. Have him avoid caffeine and chocolate. If he has other symptoms, consider having him evaluated for food allergies.

3. *Lifestyle—exercise.* Have your child try one or more bladder-stretching exercises described in this chapter. Remeasure bladder capacity every week.

4. *Biochemical—medication.* If the child is still wet at night, see your health care professional about the possibility of medication, especially if your child needs short-term help (e.g., going to camp or slumber parties).

5. *Bioenergetic—acupuncture.* Alternatively, consider acupuncture therapy if lifestyle remedies haven't worked.

RESOURCES

Center to Assist Regulation of Enuresis
Division of Urology
Children's Memorial Hospital
2300 Children's Plaza
Chicago, IL 60614
(312) 880-4000

*Enuresis Alarms*

*Nite Train'r Alarm*
Koregon Enterprises
735 SW Sunshine Ct.
Baverton, OR 97005
(800) 544-4240
http://www.nitetrain-r.com

*Nytone Alarm*
Nytone Medical Products
2424 S. 900 West
Salt Lake City, UT 84119
(801) 973-4090
http://www.w2.com/docs2/n/nytone.html

*Wet Stop Alarm*
Palco Laboratories
8030 Soquel Ave
Santa Cruz, CA 95062
(408) 476-3151 or (800) 346-4488
http://www.palcolabs.com/pediatrics/

*Books*

Allison Mack. *Dry All Night: The Picture Book Technique That Stops Bed-Wetting.* Boston: Little, Brown, 1990.

*Internet*

American Academy of Family Practice
http://www.aafp.org/afp/990301ap/1205.html

Cochrane collaboration and McMaster University
http://hiru.mcmaster.ca/cochrane/cochrane/revabstr/ab002112.htm

Virginia Urology Center
http://www.uro.com/enuresis.htm

# 7
# BURNS

Brian West brought his two-year-old daughter, Cora, into the clinic to be treated for a scald burn first thing one morning before dropping her off at day care. Heavy hearted, he told me he'd had a cup of coffee and a bran muffin sitting on the sink, so he could eat breakfast while getting ready for work. Before he knew it, Cora came in and pulled his cup off the sink, splashing hot coffee on her left shoulder, arm, and chest. The coffee had been sitting out for a few minutes, so he didn't think it was very hot, but Cora had cried immediately and loudly. He'd put cold water on the burn, which was pink and had a few small blisters. He'd also given her some Tylenol. Brian's wife was out of town on a business trip, and he wasn't sure what else to do. He'd called his mother, who said to put butter on it. Brian wanted to know if there was anything else he could put on the burn to prevent complications. Because Cora was screaming, he also wanted something stronger to help with her pain.

Each year over 23,000 American children are hospitalized and nearly 1,500 die from burn injuries. Burns can be caused by heat, caustic chemicals, electricity, or radiation. The most common burns in children are sunburns and scald burns. The most deadly burns are due to fires and electricity.

It may take a day or two after a burn before you can really tell how deep it is. Have you ever spent the day at the beach and returned home thinking you had escaped a sunburn only to awaken the next day to red, painful skin? Many burns appear to be less serious initially than they are. It sometimes takes forty-eight hours after the burn before even a physician can accurately determine how deep it is.

| DEGREE OF BURN | HOW DEEP | APPEARANCE |
| --- | --- | --- |
| First degree | Superficial | Pink, no blisters; dry; painful |
| Second degree | Partial thickness | Pink or red with blisters, moist, very painful |
| Third degree | Full thickness | Red, white, or charred; not painful in center |

Sunburn typifies the *first-degree burn*. The skin is pink or red, dry, and painful. Even a soft sheet or breeze can cause agony, but the pain resolves in a day or two. Regardless of how you treat it, it heals in three or four days without scarring; within a week the burned skin becomes itchy and peels. Severe sunburn can damage deeper layers of skin; *second-degree burns* are signaled by the development of blisters within twelve hours after exposure. Sunburns increase the later risk of skin cancer and premature aging of the skin.

Scald burns are the most common *second-degree* or *partial thickness* burns, accounting for more pediatric hospitalizations than any other type of burn. The peak age for scald burns is between six months and two years of age—another reason toddlers need constant, close supervision. Scalds typically occur when a toddler like Cora pulls a container of boiling water or a cup of coffee off the counter, splashing it onto her face and upper body. Also, dipping braids into boiling water to "set" them can unintentionally scald the scalp, face, or back.

Even tap water can cause burns if the hot water heater thermostat is set too high. Tap water at 130°F takes less than thirty seconds to cause a second-degree burn. Prior to 1978, 80% of homes had hot water heaters set at these dangerous levels. In 1983, Washington State began to require that new hot water heaters be preset at the factory to 120°F. As a result of this simple law, the number of hospital admissions for tap water scald burns was cut in half within five years.

Scalds can also cause deep burns. Nearly five hundred Americans die each year from scald burns; 20% of these deaths are children under five years old. Chemicals, such as corrosive acids, and even vinegar and other household products can cause burns; these can range from superficial to quite deep depending on the strength of the acid, the length of time it is in contact with skin, and the skin thickness.[1] Flame burns, electrical burns, and contact with hot stoves, hot wood stoves, irons, or space heaters are the most common causes of deep *third-degree* or *full thickness* burns. Flame burns from fires are often accompanied by smoke inhalation, which can be even deadlier than the burn itself. *These burns should be evaluated by a health care professional immediately.*

Many small, mild burns such as sunburns can be handled at home. Deeper or more extensive burns should be evaluated by a professional. Your child may need more fluids than she can take at home by mouth and may need stronger pain medications, antibiotic creams, physical therapy, or even surgery to minimize disfiguring scars.

> ### TAKE YOUR CHILD TO YOUR HEALTH CARE PROFESSIONAL IF:
>
> - Any burn (other than a mild sunburn) covers more than 5% of her skin
> - Your child is less than two years old with any kind of burn
> - The burn contains blisters that cover more than a palm-size area of skin (1 percent of total skin surface)
> - A blistering burn occurs on the hands, feet, face, or genitals
> - Any burn encircles the child's arm or leg
> - It is an electrical burn
> - You suspect possible smoke inhalation, regardless of the size of the burn
> - The burn is deep or contains white, charred areas or nonpainful areas
> - The burn looks infected
> - Your child is in severe pain or refuses to eat or drink
> - You are concerned about the appearance of the burn
> - Your child has swallowed a caustic chemical (such as lye or Drano)—you can't tell if the chemical has caused burns in the esophagus or stomach without special tests

*Cora's burn looked like a typical scald burn with a mixture of first- and second-degree burns. It covered about 5% of her total skin area. It was bright pink, and a few spots had blistered and peeled already, leaving raw, tender skin exposed.*

## WHAT IS THE BEST WAY TO PREVENT BURNS?

The best way to prevent burns is to use common sense, create a safe home environment, and supervise your child closely.

> ### PREVENTING SUNBURN
>
> - Minimize sun exposure between 10 A.M. and 2 P.M.
> - Beware of reflective surfaces such as water or snow
> - Don't count on clouds—up to 80% of burning rays can get through
> - Wear protective clothing, such as a hat with a broad brim
> - Use sunscreen with an SPF of 30 or higher

Keep your child out of the sun between 10 A.M. and 2 P.M. Be especially cautious around water or snow because they can reflect burning rays back and intensify the trouble. Don't count on clouds to reduce sun exposure; they let about 80% of burning rays through to the skin. When your child is outdoors, protect her face with a brimmed hat. Use sunscreen generously. The higher the SPF (sun protection factor), the more protection your child has against the sun's burning ultraviolet rays. Choose a sunscreen rated at SPF 30 or higher that protects against UVA and UVB radiation. Zinc oxide (the white cream worn by lifeguards) is the most effective sunscreen. Newer sunscreens containing avobenzone and titanium oxide also protect against the ultraviolet rays that are thought to cause skin cancer. Also, if you're going to apply insect repellent at the same time, put the insect repellent on *first* and *then* apply sunscreen; applying bug spray after the sunscreen dramatically reduces the effectiveness of the sunscreen.[2]

You can also take steps to reduce burn hazards in your home.

Make sure your *hot water heater* is set no higher than 120°F. Your dishwasher and washing machine can still do an excellent job at these temperatures. Many dishwashers now include heat boosters to increase the water temperature in the unit without overheating the rest of the water in the house. By turning

## REDUCING BURN HAZARDS IN THE HOME

- Lower hot water heater temperature to 120°F
- Have smoke detectors and fire extinguishers on every floor
- Cover electrical cords and outlets
- Be careful with space heaters, radiators, woodstoves, and fireplaces
- Practice stove and microwave safety
- Ban baby walkers
- Keep vaporizers and steam machines out of children's reach
- Keep matches and lighters out of children's reach
- Prohibit use of gasoline and fireworks

down your hot water heater, you'll not only reduce the chances of a scald burn, you'll save money on your gas and electric bill, too.

Install a *smoke detector and fire extinguisher* on every floor of your home. A smoke detector is the single most inexpensive investment you can make to protect your family from fire injuries. Most states require landlords to have working smoke detectors in every apartment. Change the batteries regularly; I change mine every fall, the same day I turn the clocks back. I also keep a fire extinguisher in the kitchen and in the living room next to the fireplace.

Toddlers chew everything they can get their hands on. The word *no* just doesn't make sense to an exploring fifteen-month-old. She isn't being bad, she's simply trying to figure out the world. You can't expect toddlers to behave safely; you have to protect them from hazards in the environment. Keep appliances close to outlets, so the cords don't trail across the room. Install *outlet covers*, so your curious toddler isn't tempted to explore electrical outlets with fingers, paper clips, or hair clips.

*Space heaters* get very hot. Clothes or draperies near the space heater can easily catch fire. All too often space heaters are left on when adults fall asleep. Turn off your space heaters when you go to bed. Keep all clothing and fabric well away from them whenever they are on. *Radiators* have caused burns in infants who rolled off beds onto the radiator and toddlers who tried to pull themselves to a stand by holding on to the radiator. Put a barrier between toddlers and woodstoves or fireplaces.

Keep the handles of pots and pans turned away from the edge of the *stove top* to prevent curious toddlers from pulling hot pans onto themselves. Whenever possible, use the back burners of the stove to put more distance between your child and the burner. Do not heat your child's formula in the *microwave*. If you heat any liquids in the microwave, shake the container thoroughly to distribute the heat throughout the contents, and test the temperature on yourself before giving it to your child.

*Baby walkers* are a menace, and they do *not* help children learn to walk any faster. Walkers were the culprits behind many of the scalded children I saw in the Harborview Hospital Burn Unit. The children "walked" over to the stove or table, and quicker than the parent could stop them, pulled pots of boiling water, coffee, or spaghetti down on themselves, resulting in severe burns. If you already have a walker, remove its wheels. Better yet, when friends and relatives want to get you something for the baby, ask for a high chair, a baby gate, a car seat, or an infant swing instead.

*Vaporizers* are a boon for many children struggling with coughs and colds, but steam vaporizers and steam machines can burn curious toddlers. If you have a hot air or steam vaporizer or steam machine, make sure it is safely out of reach of children.

*Matches and lighters* should always be kept out of children's reach. I have seen several tragic house fires in which families lost everything they owned and children were scarred for life because a youngster got hold of his parent's cigarette lighter. Children can unintentionally ignite their clothes while playing with matches or lighters, resulting in severe burns to the face and chest. This is another good reason for parents to stop smoking.

*Gasoline* and kids just don't mix. Some of the worst burns I saw in the Burn Unit were in boys between eight and fifteen years old who were burning leaves and threw gasoline (or lighter fluid) on the fire to get it going. Gasoline spilled on their pants, caught fire, and resulted in severe, disfiguring burns. Don't let a child use gasoline or lighter fluid until he is at least old enough to pay to put it in the family car.

*Fireworks* also cause disproportionate damage among school-age boys. I have seen fingers, hands, feet, and other body parts blown off or burned from fireworks. Do *not* let your children use fireworks without your direct supervision.

*Brian took advantage of his day at home to do a careful inventory of burn and fire safety in his house. He drew up a checklist to show his wife and decided they would review it every year on the anniversary of Cora's burn as a way to remind themselves of the importance of prevention. They also decided to make a fire escape plan and practice that every year as well.*

No matter how safety-conscious their parents are, some children still get burned. What treatments work best for burned children?

## TREATMENTS FOR BURNS

Children who have suffered different kinds of burns (mild vs. deep) require different kinds of therapy. Children who suffer severe burns go through several predictable stages, and they need different therapies at different times.

For the first day or two, they are likely to be in shock, sleepy, and withdrawn from the world. The burned area and other areas may become swollen, and the child requires much more fluid than usual. After a day or two, as the child begins to mobilize reserves to begin healing, the heart rate and blood pressure rise and the child may run a fever. As a burn heals, it gets very itchy. Finally, deep burns tend to leave ugly scars without appropriate therapy. Let's look at the effectiveness of different kinds of therapies for burns. If you want to skip to my bottom-line recommendations, flip to the end of the chapter.

## BIOCHEMICAL THERAPIES: MEDICATIONS, HERBS, NUTRITIONAL SUPPLEMENTS

### *Medications*

#### BURN TREATMENT MEDICATIONS

- Pain medications (prescription and nonprescription)
- Tetanus immunization
- Antibiotic ointments
- Other salves
- Others, such as insulin

Effective *nonprescription analgesic medications* include aspirin, acetaminophen (Tylenol), ibuprofen (Advil), and naproxen (Aleve). These medications are generally safe and effective for mild to moderate pain. If the burn is deep or extensive, your child may need stronger *prescription pain medications*. The most commonly prescribed pain medication is codeine or a combination of codeine and acetaminophen (Tylenol 3). If your child is hospitalized, other pain medications such as morphine may be used. Burns are very painful. Your child will heal much faster if the pain is effectively managed so she can sleep, eat, and drink. No matter how much pain medication your child requires during the early phases of treatment, she will not become a drug addict. In all the years I worked at the Harborview Burn Center, I never saw a child whose pain was effectively managed become addicted. People do crave drugs if they are not given enough medication frequently enough. Far more damage is done by withholding pain medications or undertreating pain than by giving the large doses necessary to make the patient as comfortable as possible.

Burns are highly prone to *tetanus* infection. If your child is burned and has not finished her initial series of immunizations (usually given at two, four, and six months of age), she needs a tetanus shot and a dose of tetanus immune globulin to prevent tetanus. If she has had all of her required immunizations but it has been more than five years since her last tetanus shot, she needs a booster. Nobody likes getting shots, but the risk of tetanus is far worse.

Burn wounds are extremely susceptible to other infections, too. *Antibiotic ointments* help reduce the risk of infection. The most commonly used antibiotic cream is a prescription sulfa drug, silver sulfadiazine (Silvadene). If your child is allergic to sulfa drugs, let your physician know. Other effective antibiotics are available; even simple petrolatum can help soothe burns and reduce infections.[3] Antibiotic ointments are applied once or twice daily following thorough wound cleaning. The process of removing dressings, washing the burn, and replacing the antibiotic ointment can be very painful. Hospitals and burn centers routinely give pain medications before changing dressings. Oral antibiotics are not helpful and are not necessary unless your child has another known infection such as pneumonia.

The most interesting burn salve I have run across is Preparation H. Believe it or not, many people put the famous hemorrhoid medication on minor burns to "soothe inflamed tissues." Even more amazing, someone actually studied the active ingredient, live yeast cell derivative (LYCD), and found that skin grafts did heal faster with it than with a placebo ointment![4] The ointment stings a bit, but nothing that the patients weren't willing to tolerate. These results are intriguing, and I'd like to see more studies in children; you might give Preparation H a try on *minor* burns.

*Cora was up to date on all her immunizations. We gave her some Tylenol 3 in the office and carefully cleaned her burns. The nurse applied antibiotic ointment and covered the whole thing with a large dressing. Brian decided to take the day off from work to stay home with Cora, renting some cartoon videos to distract her from the pain. I gave them a prescription for Tylenol 3 to help keep her comfortable and asked him to return the next day for another assessment and dressing change.*

## Herbs

A number of herbal remedies have been traditionally used to treat minor burns.

### HERBAL REMEDIES FOR BURNS

- Aloe vera
- Calendula, arnica, geranium oil, gotu kola
- *Avoid* raw herbs, tea tree oil, garlic

*Aloe vera* gel first gained popularity during the 1930s with reports of its success as a treatment for radiation burns. It is now a common ingredient in many nonprescription burn remedies. However, due to concerns about potential contamination of commercial products, I recommend that you use the gel from fresh, homegrown leaves. Aloe grows well on windowsills with minimal care. In animal studies, aloe vera is as effective as antibiotic cream in keeping burns free of bacteria.[5] I recommend it to my patients as a remedy for minor burns such as sunburn.

*Gotu kola (Centella asiatica)* is a native herb of Eastern Asia and the Pacific Islands used for numerous skin problems and wounds including burns, skin grafts, and scars.[6] Gotu kola extracts stimulate wound healing by promoting collagen (connective tissue) formation.[7] Excessive collagen, however, can cause disfiguring scars. Gotu kola extracts can also cause irritation and allergic reactions in some people.[8] Gotu kola remains an experimental treatment in the United States; I do *not* recommend it until additional studies of its safety and effectiveness have been completed.

*Calendula,* another popular skin soother, is available in several brands of skin cream sold in health food stores. Calendula seems to have anti-inflammatory properties, and I use it on minor skin irritations. There are *no* studies evaluating its effectiveness in treating burns.

*Arnica* is an ingredient in many herbal salves, creams, ointments, and oils. Applying arnica to broken or irritated skin can lead to a rash. I do *not* recommend arnica applications for burns.

*Geranium oil* is a traditional remedy for cuts, bruises, and burns. Oil of geranium has shown some antibacterial, antiviral, and antifungal properties in the test tube and in experimental mice.[9] There are no studies evaluating its effectiveness in treating burned children. Because of the risk of causing irritation, I do *not* recommend that you apply any aromatherapy or essential oil directly to burned skin.

*Eupolin* ointment is a Vietnamese burn remedy based on an herb known as *Chromolaena odoratum* (previously known as *Eupatorium odoratum*). This herbal extract softens blood clots, blocks bacterial growth, increases the number of wound healing cells (fibroblasts), and speeds the growth of tiny capillaries necessary to grow healthy new tissue.[10] However, no

studies yet show that it helps burn wounds heal faster than any other treatment, and because of the high risk of contamination of herbal products imported from developing countries, I do not recommend this product.

Folk remedies for burns include marshmallow root, plantain, comfrey, and mullein leaves, and slippery elm bark powder. Many of these herbs are added to herbal ointments as skin salve for minor skin irritations or made into poultices. Despite their popularity, they have not been evaluated in scientific studies in the treatment of burns. Because of their potential for contamination with bacteria and fungal toxins, I do *not* recommend raw herbal products as burn treatments unless you have grown, picked, and cleaned the herbs yourself.

Other home remedies include cider vinegar, lemon juice, and baking soda. For minor burns (without blisters), you can use whatever has worked for you. Do *not* use home remedies on second- or third-degree burns.

*Tea tree oil* is an increasingly popular remedy, which contains a potent bacteria killer. However, tea tree oil can be very irritating and cause allergic reactions, especially when used undiluted or straight. It can also be absorbed through the skin, causing severe side effects such as depression, weakness, uncoordination, and tremors. Because of its potential for causing skin irritation, I do *not* recommend it as a treatment for burns.

*Garlic* can also lead to irritation and burns when applied directly to a child's tender skin.[11] Do *not* use garlic poultices on burns.

### Nutritional Supplements

Can vitamins prevent sunburns? Some preliminary studies suggest that certain vitamins may reduce the risk of getting sunburned. In one study, adults who took vitamin C (2,000 milligrams) and vitamin E (1,000 IU) daily for eight days had a lower risk of sunburn than adults who took look-alike placebo pills. That's a lot of those vitamins, and there's no data on long-term use or safety of those kinds of doses for children. Of course, it's a good idea to eat a diet rich in fruits and vegetables that supply these antioxidant vitamins, but I wouldn't throw away the broad-brimmed hat or the sunscreen yet.

Vitamin and mineral supplements are often given to children hospitalized with serious burns. The most commonly supplemented vitamins and minerals are B vitamins, vitamin C, and zinc. Supplementation with trace elements (copper, selenium, and zinc) significantly reduces both hospital stays and infectious complications in burn patients.[12] Some nutritionists have also noted that burn patients tend to run low on magnesium, and have suggested that all patients hospitalized for severe burns should receive magnesium monitoring and supplementation if needed.[13] Iron supplements are avoided because extra iron seems to feed the bacteria that thrive in burn wounds.

## POSSIBLE NUTRITIONAL SUPPLEMENTS FOR BURNS

- Vitamin A (orally)
- Vitamin C (orally)
- Vitamin E (orally or as a salve)
- Zinc, selenium, magnesium copper (orally)
- Honey (salve)
- *No* iron (orally), milk, butter, shortening, or lard (salves)

*Vitamin A* is essential for proper wound healing. Supplemental vitamin A (approximately 10,000 IU daily) seems to decrease the risk of diarrhea that frequently complicates burns.[14] There are no studies evaluating the effectiveness of higher doses of vitamin A. Vit-

amin A overdoses can cause serious side effects. I do *not* recommend vitamin A supplements higher than the doses typically contained in multivitamins (10,000 IU daily) for burned children.

*Vitamin C* is also necessary for healing. Many seriously ill and injured children can tolerate large doses of vitamin C. High doses of vitamin C given immediately after a burn help decrease swelling in animals studies.[15] You can try anywhere from 60 milligrams to 250 milligrams given three to four times daily for a burned child. If your child develops diarrhea (an early side effect of vitamin C overdose), reduce the dose.

*Vitamin E* has been recommended both as a nutritional supplement and as a salve for minor burns. In a study of patients with extensive burns, vitamin E supplements led to higher counts of immune T-cells, possibly improving resistance to infection.[16] On the other hand, vitamin E *salve* does not help burns.[17] Oral vitamin E supplements *may* be useful, but until more studies are done in humans, vitamin E supplements and salves must be regarded as experimental, not proven therapy.

Children with major burns lose a lot of minerals, particularly *zinc and copper.* Zinc is important for immune function and healing. Zinc and copper normally exist in balance, so their replacement needs to be balanced as well. The amount of replacement minerals needed depends on the size of the child and the severity of the burn. For most small burns, foods rich in zinc or a multivitamin/multimineral is sufficient.

*Honey* was cited in an Egyptian papyrus from 2000 B.C. as a treatment for burns; it continues to be used today in many parts of the world as a burn salve. Studies from India show that on minor burns, honey does a better job than the standard antibiotic cream, Silvadene, in reducing infection, speeding healing, and minimizing pain and scarring.[18]

Like all natural products, honey varies in its purity and potency. New Zealand scientists have investigated the antibacterial properties of different kinds of honey against different kinds of bacteria. Manuka honey (from the pollen of *Leptospermum scoparium*) is the most potent honey against *Staphylococcus* bacteria.[19] Despite its killer effects on *Staphylococcus* and fungi, manuka honey has *no* impact on another deadly, burn-infecting bacterium, *Pseudomonas*.[20] Other kinds of honey, including much of what is available in the grocery store, have *no* effect on the usual burn-infecting bacteria and fungi.[21]

Some honey is contaminated with bacterial spores that can cause botulism. People who are allergic to certain flowers or trees can have an allergic reaction to honey made from the pollen of those plants. Honey derived from Turkish rhododendrons *(Rhododendron ponticum)* has been known for centuries as "mad honey" because of its intoxicant effects; it was cited by several Greek historians as playing a key role in military history because of its devastating effects on the invading armies who ate it. Any honey used for medicinal purposes should come from a known source and be tested for purity and potency before being applied to wounds.

Do *not* put *milk, butter,* or *lard* on a burn. Though they may initially feel soothing, they provide a great environment for bacteria to grow and multiply.

## LIFESTYLE THERAPIES: NUTRITION, EXERCISE, ENVIRONMENT, MIND-BODY

### Nutrition

One of the biggest challenges in caring for severely burned children is getting them to eat. Severe burns are a major stress, resulting in metabolic rates (and calorie needs) 50 to 100 percent higher than normal. Children feel miserable and are often nauseated. However, several studies show that hospitalized burned children heal much faster and have fewer infections if they are fed from the day they are admitted to the hospital, even if they aren't hungry. High-protein diets help maintain muscle strength, overall weight, immune function and blood levels of essential amino acids in severely burned children. Some burn centers work with nutritionists to evaluate the optimal balance of the various amino acids that make up proteins. Some favor ornithine alpha-ketoglutarate while others flavor glutamine. This is a complicated and controversial issue. If your child is severely burned, consult a professional nutritionist.

*Extra fluids* are very important, especially in the first few days after a burn. Our bodies are mostly water, and our skin helps prevent our bodily fluids from evaporating. Burns destroy this barrier between body fluids and the environment. Children whose burns cover more than 10% of their skin often lose so much fluid they need intravenous fluid to replace their losses.

*Brian stopped at the grocery store on the way home to pick up extra orange juice and some of Cora's favorite foods (ice cream and peanut butter) to encourage her to eat. He also purchased a chewable children's vitamin to make sure Cora got the vitamins and minerals she needed to help heal her burns.*

### Exercise

Initially, children suffering from burns need to rest, so their body's energy can go into healing the burn. For the first few days, it may help to keep the burned area *elevated*. Just as in a sprained ankle, the injured area is likely to swell. Swelling is not only uncomfortable, but it may impede blood flow and slow the healing process. Elevating an injured extremity means keeping it above the level of the heart.

After the initial healing phase, it is important for children with healing burns to keep *moving their joints,* even though it may be very painful. Burns that extend across joints can cause scars that eventually contract and limit movement. Physical therapists can help a child keep motivated and keep moving, preventing long-term disabilities. Exercise programs improve self-esteem and speed returns to work and school. Slow stretching such as yoga or *Tai Chi* can be very helpful in maintaining limber joints.

## Environment

When a child is burned, the first and most effective therapies are environmental. *Remove the child from the source of the heat.* Usually in scald burns, the hot water or coffee has already run off or evaporated, but if the hot liquid or grease is still on the child's clothes, remove the clothes. If your child's clothes have caught on fire, smother the flames.

Second, *put cool water on the burned area.* Don't use ice. Ice may cause even more damage to the already injured skin. Your child doesn't need to get frostbite on top of the burn. Cool water helps numb the pain. If the burn covers more than 10% of her skin, do not run cold water over her; she will get chilled and be even more uncomfortable. *Large burns need immediate professional treatment.*

Third, *cover the burn with a clean, dry dressing.* You can use bandages or a clean handkerchief, sheet, or towel. Covering the burn reduces pain and lessens the risk of infection.

*Pressure dressings* similar to Ace wraps are used to prevent scars from becoming heaped up and disfiguring. For maximal effectiveness, they should be measured, applied, and monitored by a physical therapist.

*Pigskin* for burns? It's not just for football anymore. Pigskin makes an excellent dressing for minor burns. It is used at major burn centers for some second-degree (blistering) burns. Pigskin immediately reduces pain and the risk of infection and speeds up healing. On the other hand, it is expensive and not widely available in most doctors' offices. It does not work well if the burn has already been treated with any kind of ointment or salve. If you are planning to take your child to a burn center for evaluation and treatment, just wash the burn with cool water, cover it with a clean bandage, handkerchief, or sheet, and bring the child right away. For anything other than a very minor burn, a health care professional should be consulted regarding appropriate burn dressings and dressing changes.

## Mind-Body

*Hypnosis* helps both adults and children to manage the pain of burns and the pain of dressing changes.[22] At the Northwest's regional trauma center, Harborview Medical Center, the staff psychologist who provides hypnotherapy is a key member of the burn team. Hypnotherapy can help decrease pain and improve sleep and appetite. In addition to easing pain, hypnosis also reduces the anxiety and distress associated with dressing changes.[23] Effective hypnotherapy can markedly reduce the need for pain medications in seriously burned children.

*Distraction* with cartoons, stories, and songs can also help burned children deal with the pain of their injuries and dressing changes. Most hospitals have cassette tape players on pediatric wards, so parents can leave recordings of their child's favorite stories and songs to play when the parent can't be there. Computers, video games, and VCRs are favorites among the children on the burn ward. You can also use these simple distraction techniques at home to help your child manage the pain of a burn or other injuries.

At the opposite end of the spectrum from distraction is having the child *fully engaged* in treatment. Some children scream and fight dressing changes despite maximal pain medication and attempts at distraction. Often these children feel wildly out of control. When they are offered the opportunity to help change their dressings, they do much better. Giving children a sense of predictability and control decreases their anxiety and pain, making the whole experience much easier for everyone. Parents know best whether their child will do better with distraction from or increased participation in burn treatments.

## BIOMECHANICAL THERAPIES: MASSAGE, SURGERY

### Massage

Exposing the burn to air or touching it can be excruciating. I do *not* recommend massage directly on burns themselves while they are healing. Some children find massage to other areas comforting, and research studies suggest that massaging the nonburned parts of the body helps patients relax, feel less pain, and have lower levels of stress hormones.[24] Massage is also helpful *after* the burn has healed; it decreases itching, tightness, and pain, improves circulation, and promotes comfort and flexibility.[25] I recommend massage for burn patients; I think it is one of the most underused yet safest therapies around.

### Surgery

If a burn blisters, leave it alone unless the blister is larger than a quarter or has already broken. A small, intact blister helps protect the burn from further injury. Once the blister breaks and the fluid drains out, removing the dead skin on the top of the blister minimizes the chances of infection.

If your child's burn is very deep, *skin grafts* may be necessary to minimize scarring and

maximize function. It takes a few days for the burn to declare itself; that is, to show how severe it really is. Young children can sometimes heal burns that adults can't heal on their own. Most burn surgeons wait at least ten days before doing any skin graft surgery. The child remains in the hospital before surgery to receive fluid therapy, dressings, pain medications, and other necessary treatments. Hospitalization is also required after the surgery to make sure that the skin graft "takes" and the child continues to receive optimal therapy.

## BIOENERGETIC THERAPIES: ACUPUNCTURE, THERAPEUTIC TOUCH, HOMEOPATHY

### Acupuncture

Acupuncture is becoming more and more widely used to treat pain. One comparison study in hospitalized adult burn patients indicated that acupuncture significantly improved their pain.[26] Some researchers are even evaluating acupuncture with electrical stimulation to see if it helps heal burn wounds more quickly; this work is still experimental and is only being tested in wounds that do not heal well with normal treatment.[27] Acupuncture is far from routine in pediatric burn treatments centers.

### Therapeutic Touch

In an excellent double-blind study, Therapeutic Touch (TT) proved to be an effective treatment for skin wounds in adult volunteers. In this study, forty-four healthy men volunteered to undergo a standardized skin wound (made with a skin biopsy instrument). Half the subjects received TT and half did not. The treatment sessions lasted five minutes daily. By means of an elaborate setup of study rooms, subjects did not know whether or not they received TT. A physician who also did not know which men had been treated measured their wounds at the beginning of the experiment and again eight and sixteen days later. The wound sizes in the treated and untreated groups were identical initially (about 59 square millimeters). But eight days later, the wounds in the treated group had healed significantly faster than the untreated group (down to 4 millimeters in the TT-treated group versus 19 millimeters in the comparison group). Sixteen days after the initial injury, thirteen of the twenty-three men in the TT group were completely healed, whereas none of twenty-one men in the comparison group had completely healed.[28] These results are highly significant statistically, although they remain unexplained scientifically.

Therapeutic Touch and Reiki are also effective in helping to ease the pain of burns as well as diminish anxiety in hospitalized burn patients.[29]

*I did Therapeutic Touch with Cora in the office and showed Brian what I was doing. He decided to practice it at home with Cora while she was relaxed and watching cartoons.*

### Homeopathy

Commonly used homeopathic remedies for minor burns include Arnica, Calendula, Causticum, Hypericum, and *Urtica urens.* Only one scientific study evaluated homeopathy's effectiveness for treating burns, and it found that the remedy was no more effective than a placebo.[30] I do *not* recommend homeopathic remedies for burn therapy.

## WHAT I RECOMMEND FOR BURNS

### PREVENTING BURNS

1. *Lifestyle—environment.* Take sensible precautions regarding sun exposure: avoid the hours between 10 A.M. and 2 P.M.; don't count on the clouds, wear a hat; use sunscreen that is at least SPF 30 and provides protection against both UVA and UVB radiation.

Make a burn safety inventory for your house:

    a. Hot water heater temperature 120°F

    b. Smoke detectors and fire extinguishers on every floor

    c. Electrical cords and outlets covered

    d. Space heater, radiator, and steam vaporizer safety

    e. Stove top and microwave safety

    f. No wheeled walkers

    g. Matches and lighters out of reach

    h. Gasoline, fireworks out of reach

    i. Escape plan

*Take your child to a health care professional if:*

- Any burn covers more than 5% of her skin

- It is an electrical burn

- Your child is less than two years old with any burn

- The burn contains blisters

- Any blistering burn occurs on the hands, feet, face, or genitals

- Any burn encircles your child's arm or leg

- There is any chance of smoke inhalation

- The burn contains white, charred areas or nonpainful areas

- Your child is in severe pain

- Your child refuses to eat or drink

- You are concerned about the appearance of the burn

- Your child has swallowed a caustic chemical

## TREATING BURNS

1. *Lifestyle—environment.* Get the child away from the heat, smother flames, remove clothing that has had hot food or liquid spilled on it. Run cool water over the burn.

2. *Biochemical—medications.* Give your child an analgesic medication such as acetaminophen. (Use an antibiotic cream or ointment on the burn.)

3. *Biochemical—herbs.* For minor burns, use nonprescription skin salve containing at least 70% aloe vera.

4. *Biochemical—nutritional supplements.* Consider giving a multivitamin supplement. Consider additional vitamin C, 60 to 250 milligrams three to four times daily.

5. *Lifestyle—nutrition.* Encourage your child to drink plenty of fluids and eat a balanced, high-protein diet.

6. *Lifestyle—mind-body.* Distraction may help make dressing changes more bearable; consider stories, songs, and videos. Other children do better if they can participate in their dressing changes.

7. *Lifestyle—exercise.* As the burn heals, keep your child moving to decrease scarring and limited joint movement.

8. *Bioenergetic—Therapeutic Touch.* Learn how to use Therapeutic Touch to help your child relax and heal faster from burns and other injuries.

## RESOURCES

### Internet

ACH international, a commercial site selling burn treatment products
http://www.burn911.com/

American Medical Association
http://www.ama-assn.org/insight/
spec_con/patient/pat082.htm

Burn Survivors Online Support Network
http://www.alpha-tek.com/burn/

Canadian burn treatment information
http://www.vanserve.org/proinfo.html

International Society for Burn Injuries
http://www.worldburn.org/about.htm

Shriners hospital burn centers
http://www.shrinershq.org/Hospitals/
BurnInst/index.html

# 8
# CHICKEN POX

Julie Frazier called me on a March Monday because her three-year-old, Tom, had come down with the chicken pox. Her six-year-old son, Jeff, had broken out the previous week. Tom had been well until the weekend, when he started to develop cold symptoms and a fever. This morning Tom developed a few little pimples on a reddish base, known as "dewdrops on a rose petal," which are characteristic of chicken pox. Julie bought some diphenhydramine (Benadryl) to treat Jeff's itching and help him sleep, but it just made him more irritable. She wanted to know what else she could try because she did not want two irritable, itching little boys running around the house. She also wanted to know how long this whole thing would last, when the boys could return to school and day care, and if there was any chance that their cousins could have caught it from them over the weekend.

Despite the availability of a vaccine since 1995, many children continue to develop chicken pox. It is the number one cause of vaccine-preventable deaths in children in the United States. Chicken pox is an itchy rash caused by the varicella virus. It is very contagious. No matter how healthy, if they are not immunized, almost all kids will catch it. Currently slightly more than half of eligible American children receive the vaccine, even though it is recommended by the Advisory Committee on Immunization Practices at the U.S. Centers for Disease Control and Prevention and by the American Academy of Pediatrics. Chicken pox can be fatal for adults and for children who have weakened immune systems. Before the vaccine was in widespread use, chicken pox killed between fifty and a hundred people every year; that number has dropped dramatically. Sadly, people continue to die from chicken pox; in 1998, six unvaccinated folks from Florida (including two children) died from chicken pox. These tragedies *can* be prevented.

*What causes chicken pox?*

Chicken pox is caused by the varicella virus, and the disease is often called varicella in medical circles. The varicella virus remains dormant in the body even after the acute illness is over. It can recur in adulthood as the painful disease shingles, or zoster. Children can actually catch the varicella virus from an adult who has an active case of shingles.

A child is *most contagious* in the day or two just *before* he breaks out in the rash. After exposure to chicken pox, a newly infected child develops symptoms in two to three weeks. Usually the rash is preceded by one or two days of cold symptoms and a low-grade fever. Unless you know that chicken pox is going around and your child has been exposed, it's hard to tell if he just has a cold or is having the first chicken pox symptoms. Children are contagious until the last blister has scabbed over, so they should stay out of school or day care until all the blisters have dried up.

The rash itself usually starts on the chest or abdomen as fluid-filled blisters on small patches of red skin. In a day or so the fluid turns cloudy, the blisters break, and they later dry and scab over. The pox are extremely itchy. There may be only one or two on the first day, but they rapidly spread over three to four days to involve the entire body. All of the pox dry up and scab over within ten days.

*The boy's visiting cousins were likely to have been infected over the weekend because Tom was very contagious just before he broke out in the rash. Both Jeff and Tom could return to school and day care as soon as all the pox had dried and scabbed over.*

Children with chicken pox also sometimes suffer from headaches, swollen lymph glands under the neck, fever, tiredness, and irritability. Mood management is an important part of therapy. Seek professional help for chicken pox if your child has any complications, has a weakened immune system, or is an adolescent.

---

**TAKE YOUR CHILD TO THE DOCTOR IF:**

*You suspect he is developing a complication such as:*

- chicken pox on the eyeball itself
- bacterial superinfection of the chicken pox spots
- pneumonia, encephalitis, or Reye's syndrome

*He has a weakened immune system from:*

- taking steroid medications (such as for asthma or arthritis)
- leukemia or AIDS
- an organ transplant

*He is an adolescent*

---

*What kinds of complications can develop from chicken pox?*

In 1 to 4 percent of children, the chicken pox blisters become infected with strep or staph bacteria, leading to problems as minor as a little extra redness and pain to as major as a life-threatening infection. A 1994 outbreak of flesh-eating bacteria (strep) struck several children with chicken pox. Rarely, children with chicken pox develop serious complications such as pneumonia and encephalitis. If your child develops blisters or pain on the eyeballs, take him to an eye doctor quickly to prevent damage to the eye. Children with weakened or suppressed immune systems are at particularly high risk of developing serious complications and dying from chicken pox–related infections. Reye's syndrome is a rare (3 cases per 100,000 children with chicken pox) but serious complication that affects the brain and liver of children with chicken pox and certain other viral diseases, especially if they have been treated with aspirin.

*How can I prevent my child from getting chicken pox?*

Effective *preventive therapies* for chicken pox are now widely available. These include a chicken pox vaccine, acyclovir medication, and immune globulin.

The chicken pox or varicella vaccine is 95% effective in preventing severe chicken pox. Children as young as twelve months old can receive the vaccine, and the Surgeon General's goal is to have 90% of children immunized against chicken pox by the year 2010. The few children for whom the vaccine is not completely protective tend to have much milder cases than unimmunized children. That is, they have fewer than 50 "pox" and they rarely develop a fever.

Children from twelve months to twelve years old receive one injection of the vaccine. Teenagers require two doses, given one to two months apart. The vaccine should *not* be given during pregnancy (because it might cause problems for the fetus). Children who have already had chicken pox do *not* need the vaccine. Since most teenagers have had chicken pox already (even if they didn't have symptoms at the time), they do *not* need the vaccine *unless* they've had a blood test showing that they lack antibodies to chicken pox. Children or adults who have been exposed to a case of chicken pox can cut their chances of getting the disease if they receive the immunization within three days of exposure to a case. The vaccine lasts at least eleven to twenty years,

and possibly even longer. Every time a vaccinated child is exposed to someone with chicken pox, their immune system gets another boost, prolonging the benefits of the immunization.

The three main reasons to immunize are (1) to prevent illness in children who have impaired immunity; (2) to prevent parents from losing work when their child is sick; and (3) prevent the discomfort of having the disease.

Chicken pox can be devastating and even fatal for children whose immune systems are suppressed by leukemia, AIDS, steroid medications, or organ transplants. Families save an average of $50 to $100 per child vaccinated, mostly due to time not lost from work. From a societal perspective, vaccination saves $5 for every dollar spent.

Side effects to the vaccine are rare and mostly mild. Of course, shots hurt, and the injection site may be sore for a few days. Fewer than 5% of vaccinated children develop a rash at the injection site, and another 3 to 5 percent get a rash somewhere else on their body. Out of over 14 million doses of vaccine given in the United States, only three patients developed a chicken pox rash and passed the infection on to someone else, such as their pregnant mom. Some children (mostly older children and adolescents) get a fever as their immune systems go into high gear to respond to the immunization. Severe side effects are rare. The risk of developing shingles (Herpes zoster) actually appears to be lower with the vaccine than with naturally occurring chicken pox.

Acyclovir and immune globulin injections can help prevent chicken pox if given shortly after a susceptible child is exposed to the illness. Acyclovir is very effective in reducing the severity of chicken pox if it is given within one to two weeks of the time the child is exposed to the disease (before the rash breaks out). It works best the earlier it is given. Acyclovir and immune globulin are usually reserved for children with weakened immune systems, premature babies, and infants less than one month old because these children suffer the most serious complications of chicken pox.

*It was too late for preventive therapy for Tom and Jeff; they already had chicken pox. No one in their family had a weakened immune system, so there was no need for preventive therapy for anyone else. It was time to focus on therapies to help make the illness more bearable for Tom, Jeff, and their mother.*

## WHAT IS THE BEST WAY TO TREAT CHICKEN POX?

Although there are no cures for chicken pox, there are a number of therapies that can help you manage your child's symptoms. Let's take a trip around the Therapeutic Mountain and find out what works. If you want my bottom-line recommendations, skip to the end of the chapter.

## BIOCHEMICAL THERAPIES: MEDICATIONS, HERBS, NUTRITIONAL SUPPLEMENTS

### Medications

Several medications help shorten the course of chicken pox, reduce complications, and make the symptoms more bearable.

### MEDICATIONS FOR CHICKEN POX

- Acyclovir (prescription only)
- Antibiotics (if the pox become infected)
- Antihistamines (nonprescription brands are available)
- *Avoid* antihistamine lotions (Caladryl), aspirin, acetaminophen, ibuprofen, and steroid creams

*Acyclovir* effectively treats the illness and prevents complications, *but only if it is started within the first twenty-four hours of the rash*. There is no point in waiting until your child has been sick for three days and you are all miserable before starting acyclovir, because it just doesn't work if it is started late. Acyclovir must be taken four times daily for maximal benefits.

*Antibiotics* are used only if the chicken pox blisters become infected (look redder and become painful as well as itchy). If only one or two blisters are infected, you can use a nonprescription antibiotic ointment, but if the situation doesn't improve in a day or two or if several spots look infected, see your health care professional. Serious bacterial infections spread rapidly. Call your doctor if you have any questions about an infection starting in the chicken pox blisters.

Anti-itch *antihistamine* medicines are somewhat effective and also help children sleep. The most widely used antihistamine, diphenhydramine (Benadryl), is available without a prescription. Antihistamines have 3-D side effects: *D*ry mouth, *D*izziness, and *D*rowsiness. On the other hand, they make some children, like Jeff, more irritable. It is impossible to predict in advance how your child will react. Most kids fall asleep.

You can try Calamine lotion to help dry up the pox and decrease itching, but do *not* use *Caladryl*, the combination of Calamine and Benadryl. Some children absorb a great deal of the Benadryl through their skin, causing an overdose.

Do *not* give *aspirin* to a child with chicken pox. Aspirin has been associated with Reye's syndrome, a serious complication of chicken pox that affects the brain, liver, and other organs. *Acetaminophen* (Tylenol, Panadol, and other brands) is *not* a helpful treatment for children suffering from chicken pox. Although acetaminophen helps kids feel better temporarily, it may actually delay healing from chicken pox. Ibuprofen (Motrin and Advil) has also been linked to a severe complication called necrotizing fasciitis as well as kidney problems and shock. Do *not* put *steroid cream* on chicken pox. Though it is tempting to treat an itch with a nonprescription steroid cream, the steroid suppresses the immune system and may worsen the rash or predispose toward a bacterial infection.

## Herbs

There are no herbal cures for chicken pox. Some herbal poultices are time-honored itch remedies, but there are no scientific studies showing that any of them are more effective than placebo creams or ointments. If you are intent on trying an herbal poultice, the following are traditional remedies.

### TRADITIONAL HERBAL POULTICES FOR ITCHING

- Plantain leaves (can be applied directly)
- Burdock root, peppermint leaves, yarrow sage leaves
- Calendula
- Sedative teas

*Plantain* leaf poultices are traditional remedies for itchy rashes such as chicken pox and poison ivy.[1] Plantain is a common weed growing by roadsides and in abandoned lots. You can apply the leaves directly to the chicken pox. Plantain is very safe.

*Peppermint* tea can be added to bathwater to help soothe itchy skin. Peppermint has a pleasant smell, and your child will probably enjoy playing in this bath for at least fifteen minutes. Some herbalists combine peppermint leaves with other skin softeners such as burdock root, sage, and yarrow leaves.

*Calendula* (pot marigold) has become such a popular skin remedy that many health food stores carry calendula-containing creams and ointments. *Witch hazel* is a traditional liniment used for skin problems. It evaporates quickly, cooling hot, itchy skin.

*Sedative herbal teas* that might calm your itchy, irritable youngster include chamomile, catnip, skullcap, hops, passionflower, and valerian. Combinations of chamomile and mint are commercially available in grocery stores and health food stores. You may have to try an herbalist to obtain some of the others.

*Julie decided to give her boys a combination of chamomile* and *mint tea (available in her grocery store) as an alternative to diphenhydramine (Benadryl). She also found calendula cream to rub into the drying, itchy scabs. She reported that the tea helped them relax at bedtime, and the cream seemed to soothe their dry skin.*

## Nutritional Supplements

There is no evidence that supplementary vitamins or minerals speed healing from chicken pox.

Apple cider vinegar is a widely used home remedy for skin problems. Many parents dab it on sunburns and other minor skin problems. I have some misgivings about using it for chicken pox because of the potential for stinging and burning. If you want to try it, go slowly at first to see how well your child tolerates it before applying it to the whole body. Baking soda can be mixed with a bit of water until it becomes a paste, then dabbed onto the weeping chicken pox to dry them. My sister dumps a boxful of baking soda into the bathtub to banish itchy skin. There's little harm in trying this kind of home remedy.

## LIFESTYLE THERAPIES: NUTRITION, EXERCISE, ENVIRONMENT, MIND-BODY

### Nutrition

Dampened appetites are common during the first few days of chicken pox. You needn't force your child to eat. Keep offering fresh foods, broths, and plenty of liquids. Cool treats such as popsicles, ice pops, and frozen juices are favorites among kids with hot, itchy rashes. Within a few days, your child's appetite will return to normal.

### Exercise

As with other infections, it is helpful to have your child *rest* so that the body's energies can be directed toward healing. Getting overheated from vigorous exercise may make your child even itchier! Most children with chicken pox have normal energy levels within a few days and would just as soon play. That's OK; just don't overdo it.

### Environment

Several environmental therapies can help ease the discomfort of chicken pox.

#### ENVIRONMENTAL THERAPIES

- Tepid baths: *with* oatmeal, barley, cornstarch, arrowroot, or baking soda; *without* bubble bath
- Cool temperatures
- Short fingernails

Heat makes itching worse. *Tepid baths* help ease itching. Daily baths help loosen the crusts and prevent infections. To increase the soothing qualities of the bath, put a double handful of plain, dry *oatmeal* with or without a handful of *barley* into an old stocking or pillow case, tie off the end, and toss it in the bathtub. (Putting the dry oats in a cloth wrap makes cleanup easier.) Alternatively, you can make a watery solution of oatmeal, strain out the oats, and add the leftover water to the bath. Oatmeal is very soothing for all kinds of skin irritations. Commercial oatmeal bathing preparations (such as Aveeno products or Jergens effervescent ActiBath) cost more than breakfast oatmeal and are less messy, but they aren't any more effective than plain old Quaker Oats. Another home remedy is putting a bit of *cornstarch* or *arrowroot* in the bathwater to help dry up the blisters. Alternatively, you might add a handful of *baking soda*.

Do *not* add bubble bath to your child's bathwater; it can further irritate your child's already suffering skin.

Keep your child *cool*. Do not overdress or bundle him. Dress him in loose-fitting clothing to prevent binding and chafing at sore spots. Cool compresses may help. Let him rub the itchy spots with an ice cube. The ice helps numb the itch and isn't messy.

Keep your child's *fingernails short* to prevent scraping and cuts from vigorous scratching. Keep your child's hands, especially his fingernails, clean to minimize the risk of infection. Consider having your child wear soft cotton gloves or socks on his hands to keep from scratching himself during sleep.

### Mind-Body

Distraction can be helpful in keeping your child from scratching. This is a great time to read stories, play games, and sing songs. Your child will be home from day care or school anyway, and after a day or two will probably have plenty of energy for imaginative games to distract him from itching.

## BIOMECHANICAL AND BIOENERGETIC THERAPIES

There are no scientific studies demonstrating the effectiveness of any biomechanical or bioenergetic therapy in treating children suffering from chicken pox.

Several studies have shown that *Therapeutic Touch* is helpful in calming distressed patients, improves wound healing, and is very safe. It may be worthwhile if you would like to try it on your itchy, irritable child, but it has not been specifically evaluated for treating chicken pox. I use Therapeutic Touch or Reiki whenever I treat a child who is uncomfortable for any reason.

*Rhus tox* is the most commonly recommended *homeopathic remedy* for chicken pox—some claim that it is the only remedy needed for this disorder. It has also not been evaluated in comparison trials. It is safe and inexpensive, but there are no scientific studies suggesting that it's any more helpful than home remedies.

# WHAT I RECOMMEND FOR CHICKEN POX

## PREVENTING CHICKEN POX

1. *Biochemical—medications.* Have your child immunized with varicella vaccine.

2. *Lifestyle—environment.* Avoid contact with other children who have chicken pox.

---

*See your health care professional if your child:*

- Develops trouble breathing or other signs of pneumonia

- Becomes disoriented, confused, or has other signs of encephalitis

- Develops a high fever (over 102°F)

- Has a weakened immune system from another illness or medication

- Has signs of infection (redness and pain) in or on the pox

- Complains of eye pain or has chicken pox in or around the eyes

- If you have any other concerns

---

You do *not* need to call or visit your health care professional if your child has a simple case of chicken pox. In fact, visiting a busy waiting room can spread the disease to other children who may not be able to handle it as well as your child. If you want a professional evaluation, please call first and tell the receptionist; there may be a separate waiting room for children with contagious diseases.

## TREATING CHICKEN POX

1. *Lifestyle—environment.* For itching:

- Tepid baths with dry oatmeal, barley, baking soda, arrowroot, or cornstarch

- Cool compresses

- Fingernails short and clean to prevent infection

2. *Lifestyle—mind-body.* Try to distract your child from itching by reading, singing, playing games, or playing his favorite videos. Be patient. Enjoy your time together as much as you can. This, too, shall pass.

3. *Biochemical—medications.* Consider a nonprescription antihistamine medication to help reduce itching. *Avoid* Caladryl lotion, aspirin, acetaminophen (Tylenol), and steroid creams to reduce the risk of medication side effects.

## RESOURCES

*Internet*

American Academy of Family Practice
http://www.familydoctor.org/handouts/
193.html

American Academy of Pediatrics
http://www.aap.org/family/chckpox.htm

Centers for Disease Control and Prevention
http://www.cdc.gov/od/oc/media/fact/
chickenpox.htm

National Institute of Allergy and Infectious
Diseases
http://www.niaid.nih.gov/factsheets/
CHICKPOX.htm

# 9
# COLDS

Janet Black brought her two-year-old son, Jamal, to see me because he was congested and had a fever. His temperature had gone up to 103°F the night before, and at the time of the office visit, it was 101.8°F. He wasn't hungry, but he was drinking juice and playing just as he usually did. It seemed like Jamal had one cold after another since he started attending his new day care center. Janet, who smoked about a pack a day of cigarettes, had suffered from sinus infections all winter; she wanted to make sure Jamal wasn't getting one, too. Jamal's physical exam showed that he didn't have a sinus infection, bronchitis, or pneumonia. He was simply suffering from the common cold. She asked me why kids get so many colds, what she could do to help Jamal get better faster, and what she could do to prevent another bout with the cold bug.

## WHAT CAUSES COLDS?

Sleeping near an open window, getting your feet wet, being in the wind without a hat—none of these cause colds. *Viruses* cause colds in susceptible children. There are over two hundred different kinds of cold-causing viruses. Because so many viruses cause colds, there will probably never be a single vaccine to prevent the common cold.

A person with an experienced, healthy immune system who has a lot of friends and a supportive family can often resist catching a cold whereas someone who is physically or emotionally stressed or isolated falls ill.[1] When study subjects are intentionally exposed to a cold virus, only about half to two-thirds develop symptoms. The others remain well, despite the same exposure. Although some do not get sick, cultures of their noses indicate that they are infected. That is, the virus takes hold, but symptoms do not develop. Those who remain healthy presumably have a more effective immune response to the cold virus.

A child's immune system is less experienced than an adult's immune system. This is one reason children have more colds than adults. The average preschooler has eight to ten colds a year, school-age children have about five colds a year, and the average adult has only four colds a year. When they do get sick, younger children have cold symptoms longer than older children—an average of nine to ten days for infants less than a year old vs. six to seven days for toddlers.

Although colds are rarely serious or life-threatening, they pack a powerful punch in terms of the *cost* they generate for physician visits, medicines, and absence from normal activities. Colds are the leading reason for doctor visits. Nearly a billion dollars a year are spent in the United States on more than 800 varieties of cold medicines. Each year colds cause children to miss 26 million school days and result in adults missing 23 million work days. Colds lead to sinus infections in 5 to 10 percent and ear infections in 30% of children under three years old. Pretty powerful effects from tiny viruses!

At any given moment, 20 to 25 percent of children less than five years old have colds. Children whose *mothers smoke* get 60% more colds than children of nonsmokers. Passive smoking (when the child inhales the fumes of someone else's cigarette) increases the number of infections and the number of symptoms. Children in *day care* experience 70% more colds than children cared for at home. The problem with day care is not the absence of parents so much as the presence of crowds of kids who share viruses.

## COULD IT BE SOMETHING BESIDES A COLD?

There are times when your child's symptoms could be signaling something more serious than a simple cold. A runny nose that lasts for weeks and months is more likely to be an *allergy* than a viral infection, especially if there is sneezing and itching along with the runny nose. A persistent or worsening cold and fever accompanied by facial pain may be signs of a *sinus infection*.

---

### TAKE YOUR CHILD TO THE DOCTOR IF YOUR CHILD HAS:

- A high fever (over 103°F or 39.4°C)
- A sore throat or sore glands in the neck
- Ear pain
- A stiff neck or sore back
- Shortness of breath, wheezing or trouble breathing
- Cold symptoms for longer than seven to ten days
- Or is too sick to drink

---

## WHAT ARE THE BEST WAYS TO PREVENT AND TREAT THE COMMON COLD?

*The only way to treat a cold is with contempt.*
—Sir William Osler, M.D.

Treated or not, most colds resolve on their own within seven to ten days. Let's tour the Therapeutic Mountain to find out the safest symptom relievers. If you want my bottom-line recommendations, skip to the end of the chapter.

### BIOCHEMICAL THERAPIES: MEDICATIONS, HERBS, NUTRITIONAL SUPPLEMENTS

### *Medications*

The 1833 *Mother's Medical Guide* lists leeches as the preferred treatment for childhood chest colds. Leeches were to be applied to the chest until they dropped off or "until fainting takes place." Modern cold medications may be less gruesome, but most are no more effective than leeches. Children get better over several days regardless of whether or not they take a cold medicine. Often parents try a medication in desperation, the child's symptoms eventually improve, and the medication gets the credit.

## COMMON COLD MEDICATIONS

- Antihistamines (Benadryl, Chlortrimeton, Tavist)
- Decongestants (Sudafed)
- Cough suppressants (Dextromethorphan, DM, codeine)
- Expectorants to loosen dry or thick phlegm or mucus (guaifenesin)
- Analgesics (acetaminophen, aspirin, ibuprofen)
- Combinations
- Menthol lozenges
- Antibiotics
- Nedocromil nasal spray
- Ipratropium (Atrovent) nasal spray

Hundreds of nonprescription cold medicines are available, costing desperate consumers nearly $1 billion a year. Most of this money is spent on ineffective remedies. Over 50% of three-year-olds have received nonprescription cold remedies within the last three months.[2]

Though they may be helpful in treating allergies, *antihistamines* such as Benadryl, Chlortrimeton, and Tavist have *not* proven any more helpful than cherry syrup in relieving children's runny noses.[3] There is no theoretical reason to believe they would be helpful. Unlike the runny nose of allergies, which is due to histamine, the runny nose of colds is caused by a class of chemicals called *kinins*. Antihistamines have no effect on kinins. They are somewhat

helpful for adult cold sufferers, probably because they make people sleepy. The active ingredient in Benadryl, diphenhydramine, is so sedating that it is also the active ingredient in many nonprescription sleeping pills. A good night's rest does make people feel better, but kids with colds can do just as well with a dark, quiet room and their favorite stuffed animal with a caring parent nearby. There are some children who have a paradoxical reaction to antihistamines; instead of becoming sleepy, they become awake, active, and irritable. Prescription antihistamines are also not effective in treating kids' colds. Unless your child's symptoms are keeping him awake and you want to try a dose of medication at bedtime to help him sleep, I do not recommend antihistamines.

Many varieties of *decongestants* are available to help unclog stuffy noses. The best known, pseudoephedrine (Sudafed), decreases nasal congestion and sneezing in adults. Many adults also feel a burst of energy after taking decongestants because decongestants are related to caffeine. However, there are no studies documenting any decongestant's effectiveness in treating childhood cold symptoms. Up to 30% of people who take decongestants experience side effects, some of which can be serious: increased heart rate, increased blood pressure, dizziness, hallucinations, psychosis, decreased appetite, and abnormal heart rhythms. I do not recommend oral decongestants for children until they reach school age. Even then, they should only be used during the daytime because they may keep children awake at night.

Decongestant nose drops (¼% Neo-Synephrine) and nose sprays (Afrin, Allerest, Neo-Synephrine 12 hour) have fewer serious side effects and have proved effective in reducing congestion in adults. Use for more than a day or two may result in a side effect called rhinitis medicamentosa. This means that the spray eventually causes symptoms that closely mimic the cold itself. The nose becomes dependent on the spray for normal functioning. Within three or four days, the child's nose gets swollen and inflamed inside if the spray is stopped. To relieve the symptoms, more spray is used, but symptoms reappear when it is stopped—a vicious cycle. There are no studies showing that decongestant nose drops or sprays are any more effective than simple saline nose drops (NaSal) in young children. I do not recommend decongestant drops or sprays unless the child's congestion is so severe that it interferes with drinking or sleeping. Even then, decongestant drops or sprays should be used as little as possible and only for a day or two, to avoid rhinitis medicamentosa. (For more information on breaking your child of the spray habit, see Chapter 4, Allergies.)

Saline nose drops are a completely safe way to loosen sticky nasal secretions. You can make your own saline drops:

## HOMEMADE SALINE NOSE DROPS

DISSOLVE:

- ½ teaspoon of salt in
- 1 cup of tepid water

Put a drop or two of the saline mixture in one nostril. Wait a minute to give the saline a chance to soften and loosen thick or crusted mucus, then remove it with a bulb syringe or nasal aspirator. Repeat on the other side. This process can be safely repeated as often as needed. Some doctors recommend adding *xylitol*, a kind of sugar that makes it very difficult for *Pneumococcus* bacteria to grow and develop into an ear infection. You can find xylitol in your health food store or over the Internet. I have never used it with my son, but he hasn't had a problem with ear infections complicating his colds, either.

Neither of the two most commonly prescribed *cough suppressants*, codeine (prescription only) and dextromethorphan (prescription and nonprescription), are any more effective than placebo cherry syrup in suppressing children's coughs.[4] Save your money. Try a home remedy instead of a cough syrup. (See Chapter 13, Cough).

*Expectorants*, such as guaifenesin, the active ingredient in Robitussin, supposedly loosen secretions so they are easier to cough out. Expectorants are no more helpful than placebo cherry syrup in treating children suffering from coughs and colds.[5]

*Analgesics* such as acetaminophen (Tylenol), ibuprofen (Motrin or Advil) help relieve the discomfort of colds and fevers, but despite popular beliefs, they do *not* cure the common cold. A child doesn't need Tylenol for a fever unless the fever is making him uncomfortable. (See Chapter 19, Fever). If your child is acting OK, you don't even need to take his temperature. Do not wake your child to give him an analgesic. If he's sleeping, he doesn't need it. Fever may be one of the body's best defenses against infections. Nonprescription analgesic medications tend to suppress the immune system and may worsen cold symptoms over time.[6] *Aspirin* has been linked to the sometimes fatal illness Reye's syndrome. I do not recommend treating a child with analgesics unless he is clearly uncomfortable.

Most cold medications contain *combinations* of antihistamines, decongestants, expectorants, cough suppressants, and analgesics. If the individual ingredients aren't effective in reducing cold symptoms or hastening recovery, there's no reason to think combinations will be any more helpful. Combination cold medicines have proven *not* to be helpful in young children, though teenagers may experience some benefit.

Combining several different medications increases the risk of side effects. Many children's cold syrups contain alcohol. Most contain sweeteners, artificial colors, artificial flavors, and preservatives as well as the active ingredients. In 1988, three children died from cold medicine overdoses.

*Menthol* is an ingredient in just about every cough and cold lozenge. Menthol is cooling, soothing, and reduces the sensation of being congested. Adult volunteers who were given menthol lozenges reported marked improvements in their ability to breathe. However, objective measurements of airflow failed to show any change.[7] On the other hand, menthol is safe, inexpensive, and makes cold sufferers feel better. I like it and I use it. Do not put menthol directly under a newborn baby's nose; there are reports of neonates who stopped breathing when menthol was put right under their nostrils.

*Antibiotics* are of no benefit in treating the common cold. Antibiotics kill many common bacteria, but they do nothing at all to the viruses that cause colds. Nor does taking them prevent a child from developing a more serious infection, such as pneumonia.[8] Despite the clear research showing no benefit from antibiotics, nearly half of pediatric office visits for the common cold end up with a prescription for them;[9] this leads to smarter bacteria that are better able to outwit common antibiotics, leading to the need for new and more powerful medicines. We could save ourselves a lot of complications as a nation if we exercised a little restraint when it came to asking for and giving antibiotics!

*Antiviral medications* that have proven useful in treating serious viral infections are under investigation as cold remedies. Pleconaril has proven helpful in test tube studies in slowing down the rampant reproduction of certain cold viruses, but trials in children with colds haven't been completed yet.

A new prescription allergy and asthma medication, *nedocromil*, may benefit children with colds. In a study of adult volunteers who were experimentally infected with two different kinds of cold viruses, nedocromil nasal spray significantly reduced nasal secretions and improved the fuzzy thinking that often accompanies colds.[10] It has not yet been evaluated in children. Nedocromil is safe. If your child has asthma, you should definitely give nedocromil at the first sign of a cold, if not every day.

Among adults with colds, treatment with *ipratropium* (Atrovent) nasal spray reduced runny nose symptoms about 20 to 50 percent compared with placebo spray.[11] Not much has been written in medical journals about Atrovent for children, but some doctors are recommending it to dry up watery noses; it also tends to make the mouth dry as cotton. I don't routinely recommend it.

Although most cold medicines have *not* been demonstrated to be helpful in treating cold symptoms in infants and young children, many parents hopefully purchase them believing that at least they won't do any harm. Wrong. Even nonprescription cold medicines can have powerful and unpleasant side effects.

### SIDE EFFECTS OF COMMON COLD MEDICATIONS

- *Antihistamines:* drowsiness, irritability, dry mouth, fuzzy thinking, thirst
- *Decongestants:* increased heart rate, increased blood pressure, decreased appetite, dizziness, abnormal heart rhythms, hallucinations, psychosis
- *Cough suppressants:* sleepiness, possible addiction
- *Aspirin/acetaminophen:* suppressed immune function

*If medications aren't helpful and may be harmful, why do so many doctors recommend them?*

Good question. Some cold medicines *are* useful for adults, and therefore people assume they'll work for children, too. Two-thirds of parents surveyed in one study were convinced that their children *needed* medicine for their symptoms. Because of this strong parental demand, some doctors fear that if they don't give a prescription, their patients will be dissatisfied and go elsewhere.[12] Please don't pressure your doctor for prescription cold medicines. These products have not been proven to be any more effective than placebos, but they are costly and do run the risk of substantial side effects.

## Herbs

Just as there are a variety of unproven cold medications, there is a similar array of unproven herbal remedies. Most are no more effective than medications for treating children with colds.

### HERBS TRADITIONALLY USED TO TREAT COLD SYMPTOMS

- *Calming:* chamomile
- *Decongestant:* ephedra or *Ma Huang,* eucalyptus, pine oil
- *Expectorant* (to loosen dry or thick phlegm or mucus): angelica, lobelia, hyssop, horehound
- *Anti-inflammatory:* angelica, licorice root, slippery elm bark, hyssop, horehound, bromelain
- *Immune-stimulating:* echinacea, goldenseal, astragalus root
- *Other:* garlic

*Chamomile* tea is soothing and calming and may help your child get the rest he needs, but it has no effect on the actual cold infection itself. *Ephedra* or *Ma Huang* is the original source of the medicinal decongestants ephedrine and pseudoephedrine. There is great variability in the potency of different species and different areas of cultivation of ephedra plants.[13] Dozens of people have died from ephedra overdoses. I do not recommend it for children. *Eucalyptus* or *menthol* (from mint) oil added to a vaporizer or bath will add a soothing smell and may help your child feel less congested, but it doesn't actually affect airflow or the infection itself.

*Angelica* was used by both American Indians and Russians as an expectorant. In animal studies (but not in human beings yet), angelica extracts have anti-inflammatory activity; there are no studies evaluating its use in treating the common cold.

*Hyssop* tea and *horehound* lozenges are safe sore throat soothers but many children dislike their flavor. *Licorice root* tea is soothing for sore throats accompanying colds and boosts the body's own virus-fighting chemical, interferon; however, chronic use can cause problems with blood pressure, swelling, and the balance of salts in the blood.[14]

Tinctures combining *echinacea* and *goldenseal* are available in many health food stores. These herbs seem to boost the body's own immune defenses rather than attacking cold viruses directly. You are less likely to find goldenseal nowadays since it is close to extinction from overharvesting.

*Echinacea* is another matter. Everybody has heard of echinacea, and about 20 to 30 percent of parents have tried giving it to their kids. Numerous studies (mostly from Europe) have demonstrated that echinacea effectively reduces the length of time adults suffer from colds, but it's not very good at preventing them. Studies are under way to see if echinacea can help kids with colds, but until those studies are completed, no one knows what the right plant is (there are at least eight different species), what the right product is, what the right dose is, how often you have to give it, or how long you have to give it. I do not give it to my son when he has a cold. The kind I use for myself is a German product that isn't available in the United States. You can check with the independent testing organization, Consumer Labs, to find out which brands they recommend (http://www.consumerlabs.com).

Used by several Native American tribes, *slippery elm bark* tea has demulcent or mucilaginous qualities that soothe inflamed throats and noses. I often brew a cup if I feel myself coming down with a scratchy throat. You can also find it as an active ingredient in some throat lozenges. There are no scientific studies evaluating its effects on children with colds.

Spices such as ginger, cinnamon, cloves, allspice, and cardamom may also help your child feel less congested. You can brew ⅛ teaspoon of each of these herbs into two cups of water to make a very fragrant tea for your stuffed-up child. Ginger root and cayenne are spicy hot. They may fight the chills and fatigue of fever. In test tube studies, ginger extracts successfully combated one of the common cold viruses.[15] No studies have evaluated the effectiveness of raw, cooked, or powdered ginger or ginger ale in easing cold symptoms in children. But it's easy enough to make a home remedy with ginger: buy a ginger root at the grocery store. Cut up about 1 to 2 inches of the root and boil the pieces in a quart of water for 10 to 20 minutes. Strain out the bits, let it cool, and sweeten as desired. Slowly sip the ginger tea to feel all warm inside.

Some mothers use old-fashioned cold remedies such as onion, comfrey, and eucalyptus poultices or hot flannel packs of fat and camphor. Hot baths with essential oils of eucalyptus, citrus, thyme, rosemary, and tea tree may be soothing and decongesting. Commercial bubble bath products are now available that contain these marvelous fragrances, and I often use and recommend them. There are no studies on the efficacy of poultices or baths in treating children with colds, but if such things are part of your family's healing tradition, they are certainly worth trying. If they irritate your child's skin, discontinue use immediately and consult your doctor.

*Garlic* is another popular home remedy for a variety of ills. Eating a lot of garlic surely helps keep other people at bay, reducing exposure to cold viruses. There are no studies evaluating whether or not garlic helps cure the common cold, but I'm not going to start a fight with my grandmother over it. I try to eat extra garlic when I feel a cold coming on. Garlic poultices can cause severe skin irritation. If you try a poultice, do not leave it in place for more than 20 minutes.

## Nutritional Supplements

### NUTRITIONAL SUPPLEMENTS FOR COLDS

*Unnecessary:* vitamin A
*Yes:* vitamin C
*Maybe:* zinc lozenges
*No:* brandy or bee pollen (propolis)

*Vitamin A deficiency* increases susceptibility to severe lung infections such as pneumonia. A randomized, double-blind, placebo-controlled Australian study showed that in children prone to frequent colds, vitamin A supplements (in doses equivalent to the American Recommended Daily Allowances) decreased the number of colds by about 20%; however, there was no effect on the number of days the children had cold symptoms or on episodes of pneumonia.[16] Studies in Haiti and Indonesia indicate that vitamin A supplements actually increase the risk of developing colds.[17] I prefer that children get their vitamins naturally in the foods they eat. To make sure your child gets plenty of natural vitamin A without getting too much, encourage him to eat vitamin A–rich foods: apricots, cantaloupe, carrots, sweet potatoes, spinach, cheddar cheese, eggs, and fortified milk.

*Vitamin C* is widely used to prevent and treat colds. A 1975 review of scientific studies concluded that vitamin C reduces symptoms and the length of illness.[18] More recent studies confirm the fact that high-dose vitamin C doesn't help prevent colds, but it does help reduce the severity of symptoms and the overall duration of cold symptoms.[19] The long-term effects of taking several grams of vitamin C daily starting in childhood are unknown. The doses many people take for colds (several grams a day) are well beyond natural levels found in fruits and vegetables. Children need 1 to 2 grams per day to relieve symptoms. I take vitamin C supplements (500 to 1,000 milligrams four times daily) when I feel a cold coming on, and I recommend it for my patients when they get colds. Each glass of orange juice contains 60 to 80 milligrams of vitamin C. Your child needs to drink at least four or five glasses of orange juice throughout the day to achieve therapeutic levels of vitamin C, in this case it seems easier to take a vitamin C supplement and wash it down with juice.

*Zinc lozenges* may reduce the severity and length of colds in adults, but they can cause nausea, upset stomach, mouth irritation, and an abnormal sense of taste.[20] An attempt to duplicate the benefits of zinc for children failed; zinc did not help resolve cold symptoms any faster than placebo pills for children and adolescents.[21] Taking high doses of zinc for two weeks or more can actually impair the immune system.[22] I do not recommend zinc supplements to treat the common cold in children.

What about *brandy?* Brandy has been used by parents for ages to soothe sick children, and it may well put a child to sleep. However, brandy (and all other alcoholic beverages) dilates the blood vessels in the nose, compounding nasal congestion. I do not recommend that you give brandy to a sick child.

Several natural health magazines have touted the benefits of *propolis*, a bee product, as an infection fighter because it kills bacteria in test tubes. However, there is no scientific evidence in human adults or children that it is helpful in warding off the common cold. Save your money for effective remedies like chicken soup.

## LIFESTYLE THERAPIES: NUTRITION, EXERCISE, ENVIRONMENT, MIND-BODY

### Nutrition

What about *chicken soup?* Science has proved that chicken soup is helpful in thinning nasal secretions so that they can be more readily cleared.[23] Also, chicken soup blocks the immune reaction that leads to cold symptoms.[24] Nobody knows what the secret ingredient is: the chicken, the vegetables, or love, but chicken soup is definitely better for a cold than steaming hot water. For best results, have your child sip the soup slowly rather than gulp it down. Some of the benefit may lie in inhaling the steaming broth. Effects only last for about half an hour, so it's better to have small amounts of soup throughout the day than one big bowl at suppertime.

Hot chili peppers, horseradish, mustard, Tabasco sauce, salsa, wasabi (Japanese horseradish), and other spicy foods are also thought to be helpful for cold sufferers. Spicy foods thin nasal secretions, make noses run, and open the sinuses even when you're healthy. Such effects may benefit congested children, too. Although there are no scientific studies evaluating chili peppers in the treatment of colds, when eaten in moderation such foods are certainly safe and are probably worth a try if your child tolerates the taste.

When children are congested, they tend to

breathe through their mouths. This dries out the mouth and results in a water loss. The low-grade fevers that often accompany colds also increase water loss. All of this means that your child needs extra fluids when he has a cold. This is why physicians and grandmothers alike admonish parents to give their sick children *plenty of fluids*. How much is plenty? A good rule of thumb is that a child is getting plenty of fluids if he needs to urinate at least every two to three hours while he is awake.

Many children lose their appetite temporarily while they're ill. There's no point in forcing a child with a cold to eat. Keep offering foods that are easily digested such as broths, oatmeal, citrus fruits and juices, grapes, and pears, plums or peaches, lettuce, celery, and carrots.

## Exercise

Make sure your child is resting well during cold and flu season so that his immune system is at full power to fight off attacks by viruses. Fatigue is one of the most common symptoms of the common cold. Some kids continue to play normally. You don't need to force your child to go to bed when he has a cold, but do let him know that it's OK to take an extra nap. Sleeping frees up some of the body's energy to mend itself. It also reduces your child's exposure to other people he might infect.

Moderate exercise may help ward off colds. Several studies indicate that those at the highest risk of colds are either couch potatoes or exercise addicts. Moderation is the key.

Sleeping with an elevated head may help reduce your child's congestion. You may try an extra pillow or letting an infant sleep in his car seat.

## Environment

Keep your child warm and out of drafts, but don't let the bedroom get too stuffy. Eucalyptus, menthol, pennyroyal, pine, rosemary, wintergreen, and tea tree oils placed in the medicine cup of a hot air vaporizer or as part of a steam bath are believed to be helpful by millions of parents, but there is not a single scientific study evaluating their effectiveness.[25] They are safe (if you keep your toddler away from the hot vaporizer itself to avoid burns and away from the essential oils, which can be poisonous if swallowed) and worth a try. *Warning:* Do not take eucalyptus oil or tea tree oil internally; they are for inhalation only.

Tobacco smoke paralyzes the cilia that sweep cold viruses out of the nose and throat. Exposure to cigarette smoke increases the chance that your child will get a cold and will make it more difficult for him to fight it off. Please, do not smoke and do not allow others to smoke around your child.

Steam has been used by countless people to combat congestion. Most studies suggest that steam treatment is helpful for adults with colds.[26] None of these studies tell us about the effect of steam or mist on children's colds, whether repeated (as opposed to the one-time treatments tested in the studies) steam treatments are helpful, or how much time a child must spend with the vaporizer or steam treatment to benefit from it. A cool mist vaporizer is probably just as helpful, and is less likely to cause unintentional burns. At this point the jury is still out. Until it comes in, give vaporizers a try. If your child benefits, keep it up; if not, discontinue treatment.

A word about vaporizers and humidifiers: If you use one, clean it daily. Mold and bacteria love the moist environment in a vaporizer and will quickly grow inside. Follow the manufacturer's instructions for regular cleaning.

Most kids under four years old just can't blow their noses the way adults can. To help infants and toddlers clear their secretions, remove them with a bulb syringe or nasal aspirator. Squeeze the bulb syringe, then insert the small end in your child's nostril. Release the bulb and allow the suction to draw the mucus out. If the mucus is dry or thick, you can loosen it with a drop or two of water or saline drops (NaSal). Wait a few minutes for the mucus to soften and then use the bulb syringe. Do one nostril at a time.

Wash your hands! Washing your hands and having your child wash his hands are the best ways to cut down the spread of colds and other infectious illnesses.

## Mind-Body

Psychological stress lowers resistance to colds. The more stress, the higher the risk of catching a cold. Among volunteers who were intentionally infected with cold viruses, those with the most stress were the most likely to develop symptoms; those with less stress had almost no symptoms despite having similar infections. Interestingly, the chance of getting symptoms was most strongly related to the actual stresses the subjects experienced rather than whether they interpreted these experiences as stressful. One easily avoided stress is lack of sleep. Cuddling and reassuring your child that you love him are great antidotes to stress.

The power of a variety of placebos to improve cold symptoms also suggests that our minds have powerful effects on both getting colds and the amount we suffer from them once infected. Given these facts, it is important to reinforce the idea that the child is strong and has the power and ability to overcome his cold symptoms. If you give your child the message that he is weak or susceptible to illness, you may be creating a self-fulfilling prophecy.

## BIOMECHANICAL THERAPIES: MASSAGE, SPINAL MANIPULATION

## Massage

One of the fondest memories of my childhood is receiving a Vicks VapoRub massage when I had a cold. I have been unable to find a single study evaluating the efficacy of this time-tested technique, but I'm sure that the combination of parental love, a warm bed, and Vicks has made colds more bearable for thousands of children, and I heartily recommend them. Other massage oils that help open up a clogged nose include camphor, camphorated olive oil, eucalyptus, menthol, and pine. Tiger balm, a fragrant balm found in many health food stores, contains a combination of camphor, menthol, cajeput, and clove oils.

Massage the face by pressing on cheekbones and following the contours of the bone in a downward movement. Also massage feet, especially the big toe. Massage the back of the child's head, downward over the base of the skull, the spine, chest, and abdomen. This can be done on infants as young as one month old. If the lymph glands in the neck are enlarged, gently massage the glands downward (to help them drain toward the heart). Folk remedies include massaging the soles of the feet with mustard powder. If you try this, you must be careful to wash off the mustard afterward to avoid burns.

## Spinal Manipulation

Osteopathic manipulation of the neck and upper back to aid the lymphatic drainage of the head and neck has been recommended, but has not been scientifically evaluated, so remains unproven. I do not routinely recommend spinal adjustments as cold remedies.

## BIOENERGETIC THERAPIES: ACUPUNCTURE, HOMEOPATHY

## Acupuncture

There are no studies comparing acupuncture to any other treatment in children with colds. One series of cases of adults treated with acupuncture for respiratory illnesses reported improved symptoms, but there was no untreated comparison group, so it's hard to tell how many would have improved without treatment.[27] I do not generally recommend acupuncture for children with colds.

### Homeopathy

Homeopathic remedies for the common cold include Aconitum, Allium, Arsenicum, Belladonna, Bryonia, Euphrasia, Gelsemium, Kali bichromium, *Nux vomica,* Phosphorus, and Pulsatilla. The homeopathic remedy, Oscillococcinum seems helpful for adults suffering from influenza.[28] However, there are no published studies showing that homeopathy benefits children with colds.

## WHAT ABOUT JANET AND JAMAL?

*Janet had just enrolled Jamal in his new day care and didn't think she could transfer him any time soon. The first thing I advised her to do was to quit smoking. Quitting now would help reduce Jamal's frequent colds and minimize her recurrent bouts with bronchitis and sinusitis. I had her choose a date she would quit, gave her the name of an internist who could prescribe a nicotine patch to battle her cravings, and called her in a week to see how it was going. I recommended that until her quit date, she avoid smoking in Jamal's presence—especially indoors or in the car.*

*Second, I recommended that she make a big pot of chicken soup that she and Jamal could sip over the next few days. While she was at the grocery store, she decided to try the ready-made chamomile and slippery elm bark herbal teas.*

*Third, we discussed the home vaporizer. Janet wanted to try adding eucalyptus oil to the medicine cup to see if that helped. She said that when she was a little girl, her mother always rubbed mentholatum on her chest, and that it made her feel much better. She decided to continue the family tradition.*

*Both Janet and Jamal were back to normal within three days. Janet quit smoking, but she relapsed two weeks later. I reassured her that relapses are common and that one slip did not mean she was doomed to failure. Three tries later, she has finally quit for good. She and Jamal enjoy making their cold remedy (chicken soup) together, and have had fewer colds every year for the last three years.*

✳

# WHAT I RECOMMEND FOR COLDS

## PREVENTING COLDS

1. *Lifestyle—environment.* Do not smoke and do not allow others to smoke around your child. If your child must be in day care, try to make sure he is in a setting with small groups of children or in small classes in separate rooms to minimize his exposure to cold viruses. Wash your hands and make sure your child washes his.

2. *Lifestyle—exercise.* Regular moderate exercise helps to keep the immune system in top shape.

---

*See your health care provider if your child has:*

- A high fever (over 103°F or 39.4°C)

- A sore throat, sore glands in the neck

- Ear pain

- A stiff neck or sore back

- Shortness of breath, wheezing, or trouble breathing

- Cold symptoms for longer than 7 to 10 days

- Or is too sick to drink

---

## TREATING COLDS

1. *Biochemical—medications.* Use saline nose drops. Do not use antihistamines, cough syrups, decongestants, or expectorants in children less than five years old. Older children may benefit from decongestants. Avoid decongestant nasal sprays unless your child is having so much trouble breathing that he can't eat or sleep. Use analgesics only to treat discomfort. Treat the child, not the thermometer.

2. *Biochemical—nutritional supplements.* Give vitamin C, 1 to 2 grams divided into several doses over the course of the day.

3. *Lifestyle—nutrition.* Give plenty of fluids, chicken soup (sipped slowly through the day), raw or baked garlic, ginger, spicy foods.

4. *Lifestyle—exercise.* Ensure sufficient rest, encourage extra naps.

5. *Lifestyle—environment.* Use a steam or cool mist vaporizer, especially with menthol or eucalyptus oils in the medicine cup.

6. *Lifestyle—mind-body.* Give extra hugs and encouragement, and encourage positive thoughts.

7. *Biochemical—massage.* Give massages using mentholatum, Tiger Balm, or Vicks VapoRub.

## RESOURCES

### Internet

U.S. Center for Disease Control and Prevention
http://www.cdc.gov/

Common Cold Center's page on Alternative medicines for the common cold
http://www.cf.ac.uk/biosi/associates/cold/alt.html

National Institutes of Health (NIH) National Institute on Allergy and Infectious Diseases
http://www.niaid.nih.gov/factsheets/cold.htm

New York Online Access to Health (NOAH)
http://www.noah.cuny.edu/respiratory/cold.html

# 10
# COLIC

Ken Johnson called one evening about his baby girl, Nancy. He had just arrived home after a hard day at the office; his wife, Erica, was cooking dinner, and six-week-old Nancy was crying again. He had tried feeding her, rocking her, singing to her, carrying her, and bouncing her. Nothing seemed to work for more than a minute before she started crying again, and she looked as if her tummy hurt. He wondered how Erica had coped with this all day, but she said that Nancy was not that fussy until about the time he came home. He wondered if the baby didn't like him, if he did something to cause the crying, or if she had a medical problem. He called his mother for advice; she said it sounded like colic. He wanted to know what I thought, whether he should bring her in for an evaluation, and if there were any natural remedies that would help.

All babies cry. By the time she's six weeks old, the average baby (even without colic) cries for one and a half to two and a half hours a day. Colic is intense or excessive crying (more than three hours a day for three or more days a week) in babies who are between three weeks and three months old. It is *not* a sign of serious illness, bad temperament, misbehavior, or inadequate parenting, but it *is* distressing for parents.

Most parents quickly learn the difference between a hungry cry, a pain cry, an angry cry, and a bored cry. Colic is different. It sounds like a cry of pain—intense, high-pitched, and continuous. Colic is usually worse in the evenings when parents are getting home, trying to fix dinner, and unwind from the day. Colic usually peaks around the time the baby is six weeks old and is almost always over by three months. Sometimes the screaming and crying are accompanied by vigorous kicking, and the baby is difficult to console. While crying, babies with colic often pull their legs up, make tight fists, have swollen or distended tummies, appear to be in pain, and burp or pass gas.

About 10 to 20 percent of babies develop colic. Colic is more common in firstborn babies than in subsequent children. It is most common among babies whose parents are professionals and least common among babies whose parents are unskilled laborers. It may be that these babies really have different amounts of colic or it could be that their parents just have different expectations about how much babies should cry. An interesting study from Sweden found that the rate of reported colic was lower when moms kept track of babies' behavior using daily diaries than when they were interviewed after the fact.[1] It may be that we tend to remember the crying as even worse than it seemed at the time.

Babies with colic may appear to be totally miserable, but they are generally healthy from every other standpoint. They eat well and gain weight; they don't have fevers, diarrhea, or any other symptoms.

---

### WHEN TO TAKE A COLICKY BABY TO A HEALTH CARE PROFESSIONAL

- Poor feeding, diarrhea, or weight loss
- Fever
- Crying is unusually severe or more than three hours daily
- Colic starts before two weeks of age or persists beyond three months of age

---

If your child has any of these signs, take her to the doctor for an evaluation. She may be suffering from another problem such as a bladder infection, ear infection, or other serious health problem.

*What causes colic?*

No one has come up with one right answer for what causes colic in all babies, but there are lots of theories.

---

### THEORIES FOR CAUSES OF COLIC

RESULT OF:

- Developmental stage
- Emotions and family stress
- Differences in infant temperament and physiology
- Food intolerance

---

Infants *develop* rapidly after birth. The coordination between swallowing, digestion, and peristalsis (waves of contraction that move food through the intestines) is still developing. The nervous system is also developing, and the baby may be plain old worn out or overstimulated by the time evening comes—at least until she has learned to pace her arousal and sleep cycles over the course of the day.

*Emotions* can also affect digestion and gas formation. Family tensions often precipitate increased infant crying. Mothers who feel they have plenty of help and support in caring for the baby and who feel they had a good childbirth experience are less likely to have colicky babies. Confident mothers are less likely to have colicky babies than mothers who are anxious about their parenting abilities. On the other hand, having a colicky baby can make even a calm, happy mother lose confidence and feel anxious and depressed. (Sorry, dads, there just aren't very many studies about how fathers' moods and expectations affect infant colic.) Having a baby with colic doesn't mean you are a bad parent, but it can surely make you feel like a failure.

Even very young babies definitely have different *temperaments* and physical makeups. Some babies may just be naturally fussier and have different digestive dynamics than others. Babies who have difficult temperaments (for example, irregular sleep patterns, oversensitive, more squirmy, etc.) in the first two weeks of life cry and fuss more at six weeks than other babies.[2] Higher levels of motilin, (a molecule that increases intestinal activity) are present in newborn babies who eventually develop colic than those who do not.[3] Colicky babies also produce more gas and digest milk sugar (lactose) less well than babies who are not colicky.[4] Some colicky babies seem to be suffering from reflux or heartburn. Having colic doesn't necessarily mean that the child will have a difficult disposition later on. One of my former mentors, Dr. Peter Karofsky, frequently assures parents that the fussiest babies become the sweetest toddlers.

## DIETARY RISK FACTORS: DO THEY OR DON'T THEY CAUSE COLIC?

- Formula vs. breast-milk
- Iron-fortified vs. low-iron formulas
- Frequency of feeding
- Cow's milk sensitivity
- Diet of the nursing mother

There is no difference in the risk of developing colic between babies who are *breast-fed* and those who drink *formula*. Breast-fed babies tend to cry and fuss more often than babies who are fed formula, but they do not cry more total hours overall. Breast-fed babies' stomachs empty faster after a feeding, and they are hungry again sooner. Once their hunger is attended to, they usually stop crying.

The risk of having colic is twice as high among infants fed *low-iron formula* as among the babies fed *iron-fortified formula*. Several studies have shown that iron supplementation does *not* make colic (or spitting up or diarrhea or gas) worse, old folklore notwithstanding. Anemic children have far more behavior problems than children who receive enough dietary iron.

Breast-fed babies who are fed *less often* (every three to four hours) tend to cry more than babies who are fed *more often* (every two hours). Feeding your baby every two hours may seem exhausting, but over the first few weeks of life it may result in less crying.

Babies whose parents *respond to their cries more quickly* fret much less than babies whose parents wait a bit longer to see if the baby will stop crying on its own. You can't spoil a young baby! In fact, you may make your life easier if you respond to the baby quickly and feed the baby more often in the first two to three months of life.

There is a small group of babies whose colic improves when they no longer drink *cow's milk formulas* or their breast-feeding mothers abstain from drinking cow's milk. About 25% of colicky babies seem to be sensitive to cow's milk protein.[5] Cow's milk proteins are absorbed by mothers and concentrated in breast milk; in fact, the levels of some of these proteins are higher in the breast milk of mothers who drink cow's milk than they are in cow's milk itself.[6] Several scientific studies of fomula-fed infants who seemed to be sensitive to cow's milk showed that colic disappeared when infants were fed a formula free of cow's milk protein; when the protein was reintroduced, the babies became colicky again. *For most babies, what the mother drinks makes no difference at all*. If you decide to stop drinking milk, be prepared to wait a week or more to see an improvement in your baby's symptoms; it may take that long for all of the cow's milk proteins to be totally flushed out of your system. And make sure you're getting enough protein and calcium from other foods.

Some nursing mothers notice that when they eat certain foods, their baby has more colic. A New Zealand study showed that the only foods eaten by nursing mothers that were consistently associated with colic in their babies were fruit and chocolate. Chocolate, as well as coffee, tea, and cola, contains caffeine. Some babies are sensitive to other foods in the nursing mother's diet, such as soy, corn, wheat, and eggs. These foods are also the most common food allergens in infants and young children (see Chapter 4, Allergies). Other foods that find their way into breast milk and seem to distress some babies are cabbage, broccoli, onions, peppers, and beans. On the other hand, many babies like the taste of their mother's milk better if she's eaten garlic.

You can probably do well without some of these items in your diet, but if you omit milk, be sure you get enough calcium from other sources. It is important that the nursing mother's diet be well balanced, with plenty of green vegetables and other sources of calcium, vitamin D, and protein (such as calcium-fortified orange juice, canned fish, or tofu). If you decide to omit or restrict your intake of dairy or other major food groups, please check with your health care professional to make sure you are getting all of the nutrients you and your baby need.

Do *not* try to treat your child's colic by offering her a variety of solids. Feeding a baby a variety of foods early in life is a definite risk factor for developing food allergies as well as colic. Solids (such as rice cereal) have been proven *not* to be helpful in treating colic. Hold off on solids until your baby is at least four months old to minimize her chances of developing food allergies.

## CAN COLIC BE PREVENTED?

Some babies are going to get colic no matter what you do. However, there are things you can try to reduce the likelihood that your baby will develop colic. All of the effective prevention techniques are from the lifestyle side of the Therapeutic Mountain.

1. *Nutrition.* If you are *nursing* your baby, *feed at least every two hours* rather than every three to four hours. If you are feeding your baby formula, choose one that is iron-fortified to reduce the risk of colic and anemia. Do *not* introduce solids in your baby's diet until she is at least four to six months old.

2. *Behavior. Carry your baby* as much as possible. Several years ago, a Canadian study showed that parents who carried their babies four to five hours a day were rewarded by a 50% reduction in infant crying at six weeks of age compared with parents who carried their babies two to three hours a day.[7] The improvement was especially noticeable in the evening hours when colic tends to be worse. Unfortunately, more recent studies have been unable to duplicate the benefits of increased carrying on infant colic. Despite these studies, I still advocate carrying your baby at least three hours daily because I believe it helps promote bonding between parents and infants and facilitates quicker responses to babies' needs.

   *Respond to your young baby's cry quickly* (within ninety seconds). This reduces crying both in the short run and in the long run as your baby learns that you are ready, willing, and able to meet her needs. "Spoiling" the young baby (under four months old) actually improves his behavior. You don't make a two-month-old tougher, stronger, or more self-sufficient by expecting her to cry it out; you just get more crying.

*Don't smoke.* Smoking parents are more likely to have babies who cry a lot during infancy, and their children are more likely to suffer from colds, ear infections, and other problems later on.

*Relax.* The more you and your spouse do to remain calm, to gain the support and confidence you feel you need to be good parents, and to nurture your own relationship, the less likely you are to have a baby who develops colic, and the better you will be able to cope with colic or any other problem that comes along. Make sure you get enough sleep and support to cope with a crying baby. Many parents find it helpful to join a parent support group so they can hear how other parents deal with the same issues they face and so they can feel less alone in learning how to be good parents.[8]

## WHAT CAN YOU DO TO TREAT A BABY WITH COLIC?

All babies outgrow colic. Colic doesn't do any long-term or serious damage to babies unless the parents become very frustrated and lash out at the defenseless child. Remember that having a baby with colic doesn't mean that you are a bad parent or that you have a bad baby. Colic is definitely distressing to the baby and the baby's family and it is worth trying safe remedies. The best remedies involve *lifestyle therapies*. If you don't feel you can cope, get help. Let's go around the Therapeutic Mountain to find what works in treating colic. If you want to skip to the bottom-line summary, flip to the end of the chapter.

## BIOCHEMICAL THERAPIES: MEDICATIONS, HERBS, NUTRITIONAL SUPPLEMENTS

### *Medications*

#### MEDICATIONS (NONE PROVEN SAFE AND EFFECTIVE)

- Simethicone (nonprescription Mylicon)
- Lactase
- Sedatives (prescription), antihistamines, alcohol
- Dicyclomine (Bentyl)

One of the most commonly used medications to treat infant colic is *simethicone* (Mylicon), which seems to reduce gas. Simethicone reduced the number of crying attacks and was preferred by 20 of the 26 study parents in one study.[9] However, a European study showed no benefits of simethicone compared with placebo,[10] and a large study conducted in pediatric clinics from North Carolina to Utah showed that simethicone was not more helpful than placebo in reducing infant colic.[11] Babies improve at the same rate regardless of whether they receive placebo or simethicone. I do not routinely recommend simethicone for treating colic.

Because some babies seem to be sensitive to lactose (milk sugar), some folks recommend using supplemental *lactase* (the enzyme that helps us digest lactose) for treating colic. Unfortunately, two studies have failed to show that lactase is any more helpful than a placebo.[12] I do not routinely recommend it.

*Sedatives, antihistamines,* and motion-sickness medications, including *dicyclomine (Bentyl)* are outdated and potentially harmful colic remedies.[13] These treatments have some potentially serious side effects, including Sudden Infant Death Syndrome.[14] Like these old-fashioned medications, old-fashioned remedies such as giving the baby wine or other *alcoholic beverages* are dangerous and are now discouraged by most pediatricians. I do *not* recommend *any* medications as colic remedies.

## Herbs

### HERBAL REMEDIES FOR COLIC

- *Effective:* combination of balm-mint, chamomile, fennel, licorice, vervain
- *Other traditional remedies:* mint family, anise, caraway, catnip, chamomile, cumin, dill, fennel, ginger

A 1993 study documented that three to four ounces per day of an herbal tea (cont`aining chamomile, fennel, vervain, licorice, and balm-mint) was significantly more effective than a placebo (a tea with simple sugar and flavoring but no herbs) in eliminating infant colic.[15] It is not known which of the herbs in the herbal tea is the effective ingredient. Many of my Eastern European and Mexican parents bring chamomile tea with them, asking if it is safe to give the baby. Chamomile is a traditional tummy-settling tea in many parts of the world. Although no babies in this study had any side effects, it is possible that some babies might. Some babies are even allergic to chamomile. A California baby developed botulism from contaminated homegrown chamomile tea. Despite this one report, I think chamomile tea is one of the safest remedies around and I regularly recommend it to parents who have a colicky baby.

Other traditional herbal recommendations include anise, catnip, peppermint leaf, fennel, caraway seed, chamomile, and ginger root. The old remedy, gripe water, which is still available in Britain and Canada is made from dill. Dill, fennel, and caraway are all from the same family of plants. Although they have not undergone extensive, rigorous scientific study, they appear to be safe and I often recommend them.

*Warning:* Do not give your baby more than 4 to 6 ounces per day of herbal tea. Filling up on tea means there is less room for the milk your baby needs to grow. Start slowly, say one ounce at first, and watch the baby for several hours for any side effects or reactions before trying more. Be sure you obtain your herbs from a trusted source and that you know exactly what you are giving your baby. The side effects of contaminated herbs can be deadly.

## Nutritional Supplements

A favorite British remedy for colic is onion tea. Slice one or two yellow onions into two cups of water. Bring to a boil and simmer for 15 minutes. Strain the onion. Cool the tea to room temperature. Try giving it a teaspoon at a time. Many babies do not like the flavor of onion tea, but some respond immediately. Although I like the idea of this simple home remedy (and some of my British friends swear by it), it has *not* been evaluated in a formal study. No other nutritional supplements have been scientifically evaluated as colic treatments.

## LIFESTYLE THERAPIES: NUTRITION, ENVIRONMENT, MIND-BODY

## Nutrition

### NUTRITIONAL APPROACHES TO COLIC

- Formula: cow's milk–free
- Rice cereal
- Fiber
- Frequent burping

Although there is no difference in the rate of colic between breast-fed and formula-fed infants, colic improves for some formula-fed babies if they are switched to a formula that does not contain cow's milk, such as soy formula or Nutramigen.[16] A favorable response to a diet free of cow's milk does *not* necessarily mean that your baby is allergic to cow's milk; she may tolerate it easily when she gets a little older. After a month or two on an alternative formula such as Nutramigen, many babies can return to their previous (less expensive) formula without difficulty.

For years, parents have believed that giving the baby a little *rice cereal* helps with crying. A study from Johns Hopkins disproved this common myth.[17] It turns out that most parents started the solids about the time their baby was getting over colic anyway, and the cereal got the credit for improvement. There's no scientific evidence that cereal cures colic.

Because babies with colic look as if they're in the same kind of pain as adults with irritable bowel syndrome (who are often helped by increased fiber), some people have tried treating colicky babies with *fiber*. However, a comparison study showed that adding fiber does not improve colic.[18] Another nice-sounding theory bites the dust!

Another old-fashioned, safe (and still scientifically untested) therapy is *frequent burping*. Some babies eat very fast and swallow a lot of air. All that gas in the tummy may make colic worse. Try burping your baby every five to ten minutes during feeding.

## Environment

A *warm pack* or *hot water bottle* on the baby's tummy is an old-fashioned colic remedy. Others recommend a warm bath as a way to relax an upset baby. There are also lots of recommendations in old medical texts about placing the baby on her tummy over your knees or over a rolled-up towel to increase pressure on the abdomen. Some parents put the baby's tummy across their knees and then gently bounce the baby to help break up gas bubbles and relieve pressure. There are no scientific studies evaluating the effectiveness of these time-honored remedies. Because they are safe, you may want to try them. Just be sure that if you use a warm pack or hot water bottle, you test the temperature and make sure it is not too hot for a baby's sensitive skin.

*Music* has also proven useful in treating infant colic. In one study, psychologists trained parents in classical conditioning. When the colicky baby was quiet, calm, and not crying, the parents played a recording of the baby's favorite music (selected by the parents) and paid extra attention to the baby. When the infant started to cry, the parents turned off the tape and withdrew attention briefly. This procedure was followed throughout the day. Within days, crying and colic had significantly decreased. When the parents returned to their old way of dealing with crying, the crying again increased.[19] Music therapy is definitely safe and worth trying, but it takes a fair amount of good observational skills and discipline for parents to carry it off.

## Mind-Body

Behavioral strategies are the keys to effective colic management. Many parents have found it useful to get into a rhythm of responses to a colicky baby.[20]

### BEHAVIORAL RESPONSES TO COLIC

1. Check to make sure that she isn't hungry (has she been fed in the last two hours?)
2. Check to make sure nothing is causing pain (an open diaper pin or a hair wrapped around a finger, toe, etc.)
3. Check to see if the diaper needs changing

4. Think about her level of stimulation and activity

a. Is she bored?
b. Is she overstimulated? Too much playing, singing, rocking, or any other visual, auditory, tactile, or other stimulation can overwhelm a baby.

Still no luck? After you have checked these things, you may find the following helpful.[21]

- Slow, rhythmic rocking (not jiggling or shaking)
- Going for a walk in a stroller
- Swaddling or wrapping her snugly and placing her in a dark, quiet room
- Letting her suck her fist or fingers
- Going for a ride in the car
- Putting her in her car seat and putting the car seat on top of the dryer while it is running on "fluff" (no heat). This provides vibration and white noise that soothes many babies. Please make sure someone stays with the baby to make sure the car seat doesn't vibrate right off the dryer!
- Running the vacuum cleaner or a hair dryer next to the baby while she's in the car seat. This is simply a source of "white noise," which some babies find strangely soothing.

Because so many parents have found a car ride an effective way to reduce infant crying, manufacturers have devised a product to simulate the effects of going on a car ride. This device, called SleepTight, can be attached to the infant's crib, and has resulted in decreased crying in many infants.[22] Because you are likely to use such a device for only a short time, I recommend that you talk with other parents or your child care provider about buying one together and then renting it out as families need it. Some insurance companies will help with reimbursement for part of the cost if you have a physician prescription. You can reach the manufacturer at: (800) 662-6542 (800 NO-COLIC).

As a last resort, you can let your baby cry himself to sleep. This is very hard for most parents to do. Most parents feel guilty and also worry that the neighbors will be annoyed at hearing the baby cry or worry that the neighbors will think they are bad parents. You may want to take turns taking responsibility for the baby for an hour or two so you can get a break. If you are a single parent, try to find another trustworthy adult to care for the baby for an hour so you can take the time to recenter yourself.

## BIOMECHANICAL THERAPIES: MASSAGE, SPINAL MANIPULATION

### Massage

Danish custom includes massage treatment for infant colic.[23] The baby is held on her side, supported by the parent's arm, with the head somewhat down and the bottom elevated. The tummy is then massaged in a circular, clockwise fashion, starting with small circles at the belly button, and gradually increasing the size of the circles outward. You can do the tummy rub through the baby's clothes, or if she is naked use warmed olive oil, almond oil, castor oil, or cocoa butter. Massage oils that include chamomile, lavender, and geranium are thought to be especially soothing. The massage should be given about twenty to thirty minutes after a meal so the baby's stomach has had a little time to empty (and she doesn't spit up all over you!). You can extend the massage to include the baby's whole body. Other massage therapists recommend variations on this technique.[24] I think massage is terrific, feels wonderful, helps bonding between parents and babies, and probably does not have a single bad side effect when it is done gently and lovingly. Give it a try!

## Spinal Manipulation

You may have heard that chiropractic manipulation helps babies with colic. One study showed that six-week-old babies who were treated with three sessions of chiropractic manipulation cried less over the course of the next two weeks.[25] However, treatment started just about the time most colic was at its worst, and babies tended to improve over time with or without treatment. Since this study did not include a group of babies who were not treated (control group), we can't say that chiropractic was any more helpful than no treatment.

A study from Denmark compared chiropractic adjustment to dimethicone drops for colicky babies; the investigators concluded that two weeks of chiropractic treatment (typically three to five treatments total) was significantly better than two weeks of dimethicone treatment, cutting crying time more than twice as much (two to three hours less daily in the chiropractic group compared with one hour less daily in the dimethicone group).[26] These results are promising, but it's awfully hard to "blind" the parents and the baby as to which treatment the child is getting. The next step is repeating the study and evaluating the overall costs compared with the benefits of other treatments.

## BIOENERGETIC THERAPIES: THERAPEUTIC TOUCH, HOMEOPATHY

### Therapeutic Touch

Therapeutic Touch has been reported to be helpful for crying babies and children.[27] Although there are no studies on colic specifically, I know from my own clinical experience that TT relaxes and calms both the giver and receiver, and I use it in the clinic when confronted with a baby who is crying for any reason.

### Homeopathy

The most common remedies are Chamomilla, Colocynth (from the herb bitter cucumber), Dioscorea (wild yam), *Magnesia phosphorica*, *Nux vomica,* and Pulsatilla. There are no scientific studies evaluating the effectiveness of these remedies in treating infant colic. I do not recommend them.

✳

# WHAT I RECOMMEND FOR COLIC

## PREVENTING COLIC

1. *Lifestyle—mind-body.* Respond to your baby's cries quickly. Carry your baby in your arms as much as possible. Surround yourself with supportive family and friends. Take care of yourself, too. Learn and practice stress management techniques; you'll need them to handle toddler temper tantrums later on anyway!

2. *Lifestyle—nutrition.* If you are nursing your baby, nurse often (every two to three hours). If you are formula feeding, use iron-fortified formula.

3. *Lifestyle—environment.* Don't smoke.

---

*When to see your doctor:*

- If the colic persists or recurs daily, talk with your doctor about a temporary change in formulas to one that does not contain cow's milk; if you are nursing, consider altering your diet to omit suspect foods.

- If home remedies do not work, if your baby has other symptoms, or if she is over three months old and still has colic, see your health care professional. Severe, persistent crying may be a sign that your child has an infection (like an ear, bladder, or kidney infection) or other treatable condition. Other worrisome symptoms include black or bloody stools, vomiting, diarrhea, or fever in an infant less than two months old.

---

## TREATING COLIC

1. *Lifestyle—mind-body.* Check to make sure she's not hungry, not in pain, not in a wet or dirty diaper, and not bored or overstimulated.

Try a ride in the car seat, five to ten minutes in a swing or rocker, or SleepTight.

If you've done all of the above, and the baby is still crying, ask for help, put the baby in her crib for ten minutes, close the door, and take time to get calm and regroup before you try again.

2. *Biomechanical—massage.* Consider a tummy massage or a warm hot water bottle.

3. *Lifestyle—environment.* Try music therapy: when she's quiet, play her favorite music and praise her; when she starts crying, stop the music and ignore her for a minute or two.

4. *Biochemical—herbs.* Try herbal tea containing chamomile, mint, fennel, licorice, and vervain.

RESOURCES

*Internet*

American Academy of Family Practice
http://www.aafp.org/afp/20010115/tips/
10.html

Directions for a massage for a colicky baby
http://www.alternativeparenting.com/
health/colic_infant_massage.htm

More on massage and other resources
http://www.infantmassage.com/
colic.htm

# 11
# CONJUCTIVITIS (PINKEYE)

Jose Fernandez came into the clinic on a Thursday afternoon with his three-year-old daughter, Maria, bearing a note from her day care center. He'd been called at work to come pick her up and take her to the doctor because she had pinkeye; they wanted her to be seen and treated before she returned to the center. Maria had been fine except for a runny nose. She awoke that morning with some yellowish crusting that matted her eyelashes together, but she was happy and playful. She had also begun tugging at her left ear. Jose wanted to know how to help Maria get well soon and how to prevent the disease from spreading to his infant son, George.

Pinkeye or conjunctivitis is an inflammation of the conjunctiva, the transparent covering that lines the inner surface of the eyelids and the front of the eyeball. It is very common. Different things cause conjunctivitis at different ages. Newborns can catch it from their mothers during delivery; their eyes can also be irritated by the antibiotic drops used to prevent infections. Toddlers typically catch it from other toddlers. Conjunctivitis in older children and adults can be caused by allergies and irritants as well as infections. Occasionally red eyes can be a sign of a serious illness affecting other parts of the body, such as measles.

## SYMPTOMS OF CONJUNCTIVITIS

- Red or pink eye with watery discharge
- Dry matter in eyelashes or gooey yellowish-green discharge
- Swollen eyelid
- Itchy feeling or irritation that feels like sand in the eye
- Swollen lymph nodes under the chin or in front of the ear

## WHAT CAUSES CONJUNCTIVITIS?

### CAUSES OF CONJUNCTIVITIS
### IN CHILDREN

- Infection
- Irritants or allergies
- Injuries
- Other illnesses

Conjunctivitis in the *newborn* may be caused by gonorrhea or chlamydia (the two most common sexually transmitted diseases). These infections are serious. Gonorrhea conjunctivitis can cause blindness if it is not recognized and treated quickly. Chlamydia infections can cause pneumonia. Symptoms starting on the third or fourth day of life are usually due to gonorrhea, and those that start when the baby is a week or two old are more likely to be due to chlamydia. The initial treatment (antibiotics) is always aimed at them since their consequences are so serious.

The eye drops given at birth help prevent newborn eye infections; they are given routinely (and in some states by law) to all babies. The eye medicines given to most newborns (erythromycin and tetracycline) are safe, effective, and nonirritating. However, the older medicine, silver nitrate, sometimes irritates eyes for two to three days. Conjunctivitis on the first day of life is usually due to eye drops.

Among *older children*, the viruses and bacteria that cause conjunctivitis are the same culprits that cause colds, ear infections, sinus infections, bronchitis, and pneumonia. *Hemophilus influenza*, the most common cause of bacterial conjunctivitis, is notorious for causing the combination of conjunctivitis and ear infection (see Chapter 17, Ear Infections). Bacterial conjunctivitis typically lasts about a week or ten days (that length can be cut by three to five days with antibiotics) while viral infections tend to last two to three weeks (and do not improve with antibiotics). The Herpes virus causes cold sores, and genital infections can cause serious damage if it spreads to the eye. If your child has signs of a herpes infection (tiny blisters on red skin) near the eye, the eyelid, or the tip of the nose, take her to be evaluated immediately so appropriate treatment can be started promptly. In the summer and autumn, *Adenovirus* commonly causes conjunctivitis and a sore throat.

The most common eye *irritants* in older children and adults are cigarette smoke, wood smoke, and pollution. Swimmers' eyes often become irritated with chlorine. Allergies such as hay fever commonly cause red, irritated, itchy, watery eyes during pollen season. Allergies usually cause other symptoms as well, such as runny nose, cough, and an itchy mouth (see Chapter 4, Allergies).

The most common causes of minor eye *injuries* are insect bites, accidental pokes from stray fingers, and scratches from overuse of contact lenses. Rarely, children get glue in their eyes. SuperGlue is one of the worst offenders. Chemical injuries from bleach splashes, lye, or other cleaning agents can cause serious damage.

More serious eye diseases, such as glaucoma, are also characterized by red, painful eyes, but they don't cause as much discharge or matting as with infectious conjunctivitis. If your child's eyes are not getting better after a few days of treatment, if the eye is painful, or your child is having trouble seeing, don't wait around trying home remedies. Seek professional help. Conjunctivitis can also be a symptom of other serious illnesses such as measles, Lyme disease, or rheumatoid arthritis. In these cases, your child will have other symptoms besides an irritated eye. When in doubt, see your doctor.

## DIAGNOSING CONJUNCTIVITIS

Usually, diagnosing the different causes of pinkeye is pretty straightforward based on the child's symptoms and a physical examination. For example, itching is usually due to allergies. Insect bites usually affect the eyelid around the eye rather than the eye itself. Infectious conjunctivitis caused by viruses is usually accompanied by cold symptoms. Viral and bacterial eye infections are sometimes difficult to distinguish from each other without additional tests.

*Laboratory tests* can help sort out the cause of conjunctivitis. These tests include taking a swab of the inner eyelid for a culture, measuring the pressure inside the eye, checking the eye's reaction to light, using a special stain to look for scratches on the eyeball, and looking deep inside the eye with a special instrument. Newborns require a culture to help distinguish between different kinds of serious infections. Children who have red, painful eyes need to have their vision tested and to have the pressure inside their eyes measured to make sure they don't have glaucoma.

*On physical examination, Maria had an infected left ear as well as a gooey, yellow discharge and redness in both eyes. Because she had signs of another infection (ear), it was most likely that bacteria were the cause of her conjunctivitis. No other tests were necessary.*

---

### SEE YOUR HEALTH CARE PROFESSIONAL IF YOUR CHILD HAS:

- Eye symptoms any time in the first two months of life
- Any injury to the eye
- Pinkeye and ear pain
- Severe pain in the eye
- Trouble seeing from the eye
- Cloudy spots on the eyeball
- Abnormal or irregular pupil ( the black disk in the middle of the eye)
- A bulging eye
- Symptoms that don't improve within two weeks

---

These symptoms may signify a more serious condition requiring medical care.

## WHAT CAN YOU DO TO PREVENT CONJUNCTIVITIS?

There are several things you can do to reduce the chances that your child will develop conjunctivitis.

---

### PREVENTING CONJUNCTIVITIS

- Regular prenatal care
- Avoid eye irritants: *no smoking around children*
- Avoid allergens
- Minimize exposure to other ill children
- Practice good hygiene
- Plenty of sleep

---

Mothers who receive regular *prenatal care* are less likely to have an infection when they deliver their babies. This reduces the chance that the baby will catch an infection during delivery.

*Don't smoke* and don't let others smoke around your child. Cigarette smoke not only irritates the eyes but also predisposes to colds, ear infections, and asthma. *Avoid allergens*. If your child has hay fever or other allergies to pollen, keep the windows closed between 5 A.M. and 10 A.M. when pollen counts are highest. (See Chapter 4 for more tips on preventing allergic symptoms.)

Most children who have infectious conjunctivitis catch it from *other kids*. Crowding is one of the surest ways to spread infectious illnesses. If you have options in your choice of day care provider, choose one that has fewer children or smaller classrooms rather than a large, crowded environment. If your child has infectious conjunctivitis, try to keep her away from other kids so she doesn't spread it to them.

*Good hygiene* helps prevent the spread of infectious conjunctivitis. Don't let your youngsters share towels, washcloths, pillows, or bedding with each other. Wash your hands frequently. Have your child wash her hands after each trip to the bathroom, before every meal, and before bed.

Make sure your child gets *plenty of sleep.* Sleep boosts immunity and calms allergic reactions. Sleeping also rests the eyes and gives them a chance to heal if they become irritated.

## WHAT IS THE BEST WAY TO TREAT CONJUNCTIVITIS?

Even without treatment, infectious conjunctivitis usually resolves on its own in seven to ten days. Let's tour the Therapeutic Mountain to find out what works and what doesn't. If you want to skip to my bottom-line recommendations, flip to the end of this chapter.

## BIOCHEMICAL THERAPIES: MEDICATIONS, HERBS

### Medications

Different medications are indicated for different kinds of conjunctivitis. The medicine used to prevent or treat a serious infection in the newborn is different from that used to soothe irritated or allergic eyes in older children.

### MEDICATIONS FOR CONJUNCTIVITIS

- *Newborns:* antibiotics
- *Infectious conjunctivitis:* antibiotics
- *Irritated eyes:* nonprescription drops or eye washes
- *Allergies:* several types of medication

Newborns who have infectious conjunctivitis must be treated with *antibiotics* by mouth or injection to prevent serious complications such as blindness and pneumonia. All of these medications require a prescription. They include ceftriaxone (injection or intravenous), cefotaxime (intravenous), and erythromycin (by mouth).

Ceftriaxone is a powerful antibiotic that can be given as a single injection to eliminate gonorrhea conjunctivitis. Another antibiotic, cefotaxime, is used for jaundiced babies in whom ceftriaxone is contraindicated. If there is a lot of discharge, the infant's eyes need to be thoroughly washed several times daily to eliminate all of the infectious goo. This should be done by professionals. Erythromycin, clarithromycin, and azithromycin kill chlamydia and help prevent the infected infant from developing pneumonia. If a child is diagnosed with either gonorrhea or chlamydia conjunctivitis, both parents should be tested and treated as well. *Eye drops alone are insufficient treatment for a newborn with conjunctivitis* unless cultures have proven that neither gonorrhea nor chlamydia are to blame for the symptoms.

If an older child has an ear infection, sinus infection, or pneumonia at the same time she has pinkeye, the culprit is almost certainly *bacteria.* The combination of an ear infection and pinkeye, known as the *otitis-conjunctivitis syndrome,* is especially common in the winter months. It can be effectively treated with prescription antibiotics such as amoxicillin clavulanate (Augmentin).

*Because Maria had an ear infection plus conjunctivitis, I gave her a prescription for amoxicillin to cover both infections. After twenty-four hours of antibiotic therapy, Maria could return to her day care center without the risk of infecting other children.*

Prescription antibiotic eye medications work well for conjunctivitis caused by bacteria in children beyond the newborn period. These prescription antibiotics include ciprofloxacin, polymixin B, tetracycline, erythromycin, gentamicin, tobramycin, combinations (Polytrim), and others. The antibiotics are placed in the eye three to four times daily. Eye drops can be tricky to give young children. Eye ointments are easier and last longer but can cause blurry vision. I recommend eye ointments to treat infants and toddlers and eye drops to treat school-age children and teenagers. My nurse always demonstrates the best technique for giving eye drops and ointment for parents who have never done it before. Pull down the lower eyelid and place the medication in the dip between the eyeball and the eyelid, as close to the outer corner of the eye as you can. The body's natural tears will spread the medication over the eye before flushing it through the tear duct located at the inner eye near the nose. This is much harder than it sounds. Antibiotic eye drops often sting when they are first applied. The stinging usually stops within sixty seconds. However, if you get the medicine into the eye, you should start to see some improvement within twenty-four hours.

*If your child has been sent home from day care, as Maria was, she can return to school after she has completed twenty-four hours of treatment for a bacterial conjunctivitis.*

There are also prescription antiviral medications to treat the serious eye infections caused by the Herpes virus. These medications work only against herpes, not pinkeye due to other viruses. Herpes is serious and should be monitored by an eye specialist (ophthalmologist).

For children and teenagers whose eyes are simply irritated due to smoke or overuse, several nonprescription medications are available. If your child's eyes are not better after three days of nonprescription medication, take her to a health care professional to make sure the problem doesn't require prescription.

## EYE DROPS FOR IRRITATED EYES

| GENERIC NAME | BRAND NAME | DURATION OF EFFECT |
|---|---|---|
| Phenylephrine | AK-Nephrin, Isopto-Frin, Prefrin | 30 to 90 minutes |
| Tetrahydrozyline | Visine, Mallazine, Murine Plus | 1 to 4 hours |
| Naphazoline | Allerest, Clear Eyes, Naphcon | 2 to 3 hours |
| Oxymetazoline | OcuClear, Visine LR | Up to 6 hours |

These eye drops can make your child feel better while the body is healing the underlying problem, but they do *not* cure the problem. They shrink the blood vessels and dilate the pupil, reducing the swelling and irritation. If your child has blurry or painful vision, have her examined first by a physician before using any eye drops; these symptoms could signal a more serious condition, and you do *not* want to simply cover them up. Drops should also *not* be used if there has been an injury (such as a cut or scrape) to the eye, because they can slow the blood flow needed for healing; in children suffering from glaucoma or high blood pressure; or in children under two years old. Do not use any eye drops for more than three days in a row without seeing a health care professional. Using them longer could result in dependence on the medication; that is, when you stop the drops, the eyes will become even redder than before. Read the package directions carefully and do not exceed the recommended doses.

Artificial tears are simply saline solutions that help wash irritants out of the eye and help keep eyes moisturized when they feel dry. There are numerous brands. They are very safe. Rarely, children are allergic to one of the buffers or preservatives used to maintain the shelf life or sterility of these products. Many nonprescription eye washes contain boric acid and salt. Even though acid sounds scary, boric acid solutions are very gentle and have been used safely for many years. Check the label for precise directions.

Several kinds of prescription medication can help ease the discomfort of allergic conjunctivitis, easing the itching, tearing, and redness triggered by pets and pollens. These drops work best if you wash the eye first with saline drops to clear out pollen and other irritants.

Eye drops containing *nedocromil* (Tilade) or *lodoxamide* (Alomide) reduce sensitivity to allergens such as ragweed. They are most helpful when used to *prevent* allergic symptoms; they are less effective after your child has already developed red, itchy eyes. Administer them before your child goes outside during pollen season or before going to a home with a cat or dog if animal dander causes allergy flare-ups. They are also useful for treating conjunctivitis due to chronic irritation, such as irritation from contact lenses. They are my first choice for preventing allergic conjunctivitis. Two new prescription products help in both preventing and treating allergic conjunctivitis in children three years and older: *olopatadine* and *ketotifen*.

### PRESCRIPTION EYE MEDICATION FOR ALLERGIC CONJUNCTIVITIS

- Nedocromil, lodoxamide (Tilade, Alomide); olopatidine, ketotifen
- Anti-irritant plus antihistamine (Naphcon-A, Vasocon-A)
- Ketorolac (Acular)
- Steroid drops
- Oral antihistamines

If your child already has symptoms, eye drops containing *antihistamines* may help ease the itching and watering. Most antihistamine eye drops also contain phenylephrine or naphazoline, which help shrink swollen blood vessels and dilate the pupil, thereby reducing redness and swelling. Do not use them for more than three days without seeing a physician. Prescription antihistamines include *emadastine* (Emadine) and *levocabastine* (Livostin). The strong prescription anti-inflammatory and pain medicine *ketorolac* (Acular) relieves eye itching caused by allergies. It is expensive and causes severe stinging in 40 percent of children, but it lasts up to six hours.

Antihistamine pills, capsules, and syrups can help prevent and treat many allergic symptoms, including itchy conjunctivitis. New prescription antihistamines don't cause as much drowsiness as the older nonprescription products, but they are very expensive. They can be used at the same time as antihistamine eye drops. Prescription *steroid eye drops* reduce inflammation. However, they may increase the risk of developing an eye infection, so you must be very sure that symptoms aren't really due to an infection before using them. I never prescribe steroid eye drops without consulting an eye specialist.

### Herbs

There are *no* scientific studies comparing herbs to medical treatments for children with conjunctivitis. Natural remedies are not necessarily safe. Some are dangerous. There is one case report of a child who had a severe allergic reaction to chamomile tea wash.[1] Common house and garden plants can cause severe irritation. The Euphorbia family (poinsettia, mole plant, and others) produces an irritating milky sap that actually causes conjunctivitis if it comes in contact with the eye.

Common traditional herbal remedies for

conjunctivitis are chamomile flowers, euphrasia, eyebright, and pot marigold (calendula).[2] Less commonly recommended are complex concoctions containing chickweed, comfrey, elderflowers, goldenseal, marshmallow, plantain, raspberry leaves, and/or rosemary. Rose water or a compress or poultice made of rose petals, witch hazel, and oil of chamomile is believed to be soothing and cooling to irritated eyes. In test tube and animal studies, goldenseal *(Hydrastis canadensis)* has antibacterial and anti-inflammatory properties, but it has *not* yet been studied in children. I do *not* recommend that you place any herbal products directly into your child's eye.

Folk remedies for conjunctivitis include *poultices* made from castor oil, grated raw Irish potato, cucumber slices, violet leaves, or yogurt. If your child's eyes do not improve within three days of home remedies, consult your health care professional.

Some herbalists also recommend drinking certain *herbal teas* such as eyebright, chrysanthemum (available in many Chinese groceries), goldenseal, and marshmallow. Again, there are *no* studies evaluating their effectiveness in treating conjunctivitis. My favorite herbal home remedy for conjunctivitis involves chamomile tea. Put two tea bags of chamomile tea in a cup with boiling water. Steep for twenty minutes then drink. Have your child lay down and put the cooled tea bags over closed eyes. Let her rest for twenty minutes. Then toss out the tea bags and wash hands. Do *not* use this remedy for anyone who is allergic to chamomile or its close relatives in the daisy family.

## LIFESTYLE THERAPIES: NUTRITION, EXERCISE, ENVIRONMENT, MIND-BODY

### Nutrition

No particular diet has proven helpful in preventing or treating conjunctivitis. Many parents feed extra carrots to children with eye problems because carrots are good for the eyes. Most of carrots' benefit comes from their high concentration of vitamin A, which is important in preventing blindness. Eating a well-balanced diet with an emphasis on fresh, organic fruits, vegetables, and grains is helpful in maintaining health and overcoming illness, no matter what the cause. But extra carrots will *not* help your child heal her conjunctivitis any faster.

### Exercise

It's almost impossible to keep a child from rubbing his eyes when they're irritated, but this is one time it's helpful to support your child's efforts to exercise some restraint. Rubbing and itching aggravate the irritation and increase the risk of spreading an infection.

Help your child *rest her eyes*. Turn off the television. Turn on the radio. Read her a story. Sing her a song. Have her close her eyes, and go on an imaginary journey together.

### Environment

Wash your hands every time you touch the area around your child's eye. Encourage her to wash her hands frequently. She will inevitably touch her irritated eyes frequently. Handwashing helps stop the spread of disease, and it is a good habit in general. Infectious conjunctivitis is very contagious, so be sure that no one else uses the washcloths, pillowcases, and towels used by the child with pinkeye. Don't let a teenager with conjunctivitis share cosmetics with anyone else. It's a good idea to refrain from sharing eye makeup even when your child and her friends are completely well; viruses can hang around on makeup for long periods just waiting for someone to place them near a vulnerable eye.

Washing the eye with warm water, salt water, or artificial tears is soothing and helps loosen the crusts that adhere to eyelashes. Warm, wet compresses applied four or five times a day will help increase circulation to the eye, hastening healing. For children who have pinkeye because of exposure to a caustic chemical such as bleach, lye, or SuperGlue, the most important treatment is to flush the eye with plenty of water (several quarts), followed by immediate evaluation by an eye specialist.

Contact lenses should not be worn until pinkeye has completely resolved.

## Mind-Body

In any illness, the child can be helped to feel more comfortable by calm, reassuring parents. I encourage parents to spend extra time with their child when she is ill. This helps the child rest, so other treatments and the body's own regenerative powers can work.

## BIOMECHANICAL THERAPIES: MASSAGE, CHIROPRACTIC, SURGERY

### Massage

Although massage is great for most conditions, rubbing the eyes just aggravates the irritation. Do *not* massage irritated eyes.

### Chiropractic

There are no studies showing that chiropractic or osteopathic adjustments help heal conjunctivitis.

### Surgery

Surgery is not necessary for simple pinkeye. If your child has suffered an eye injury, especially if a sharp object has penetrated the eye, see an ophthalmologist (eye specialist) immediately.

## BIOENERGETIC THERAPIES: THERAPEUTIC TOUCH, PRAYER, HOMEOPATHY

### Therapeutic Touch

In my practice I have found that *non-contact* Therapeutic Touch is helpful in reducing inflammation and surgery in the eyes and sinuses, but there are no studies specifically evaluating it for these conditions.

### Prayer

Likewise, there are no studies specifically evaluating the power of prayer to calm conjunctivitis, but there are no side effects, either, so I recommend prayer if it is consistent with your family's beliefs.

### Homeopathy

The most commonly used homeopathic remedies for pinkeye are Apis, Belladona (homeopathic doses *only*), a combination of Calendula and Hypericum (Hypercal), Euphrasia (eyebright), Mercurius, and Pulsatilla. There are no studies documenting their effectiveness, although they are inexpensive and safe.

# WHAT I RECOMMEND FOR CONJUNCTIVITIS

## PREVENTING CONJUNCTIVITIS

1. Prospective mothers should receive regular prenatal care to detect and treat any infections early and avoid passing them on to their infants.

2. *Lifestyle—environment.* Do not smoke and do not allow others to smoke around your child to prevent eye irritation.

   Avoid allergens or seek professional help to prevent allergic symptoms (see Chapter 4).

   Maintain good hygiene to avoid catching conjunctivitis. Wash hands frequently. Do *not* share eye makeup.

---

*Seek professional help immediately for:*

- Redness or discharge from the eye in the first two months of life

- Eye pain

- Loss of vision in either eye

- A history of injury to the eye or chemical contact with the eye

- Pain in the eye with exposure to light

- Bleeding from the eye

- A swollen or bulging eye

- A pupil (the black disk in center of eye) that is irregular or does not get smaller when a light is shined in the eye

---

## TREATING CONJUNCTIVITIS

1. *Biochemical—medications.* If you suspect that the symptoms are due to an *infection*, see your health care provider to consider using an antibiotic.

2. *Biochemical—medications.* If the symptoms are due to *allergies*, avoid the allergen, use cool compresses, and consider nonprescription eye drops to help reduce symptoms. If your child's eyes are still irritated, see your physician about prescription medications.

3. *Lifestyle—exercise.* Rest the eyes; avoid rubbing them.

4. *Lifestyle—environment.* Gently wash the crusty or gooey matter around the eyes and eyelashes with warm water, sterile saline, or a boric acid solution using a clean washcloth or cotton ball.

Try warm compresses several times daily. Read a story or sing to your child while the compresses are in place.

Remove contact lenses and do not use them again until symptoms have resolved.

RESOURCES

*Internet*

American Academy of Family Practice
  http://familydoctor.org/handouts/183.html
  http://aafp.org/patientinfo/conjunct.html

Prevent Blindness America
  http://www.preventblindness.org/children/
  conjunctivitisFAQ.html

# 12

# CONSTIPATION

Belle Zagorski called about her four-week-old grandson, Walter, who was having a bowel movement every two days. She thought a breast-fed baby should have a stool every time he nursed. She was worried that Walter was constipated, although his stools were soft and he wasn't straining to have them. Belle's daughter wasn't worried, but Belle wanted my opinion about what was normal and whether she should be concerned.

Penny Brandenburg, a local nurse practitioner, called me to ask my advice about Karo syrup. She had been taught that adding a little corn syrup to a bottle of formula was a good remedy for constipation in babies; recently she'd seen a child suffering from botulism contracted from eating honey. She knew that honey could harbor botulism spores, and she wondered if corn syrup, a similar sweetener, held the same hazard.

Eric Kay came in with his three-year-old daughter, Susan, because of her severe constipation. Susan had been doing fine until she was being toilet trained, but then she'd started having less frequent stools. Because she'd held them so long, they were hard and painful when they passed, so she was even more reluctant to sit on the potty. Eric wanted to know what to do.

There's a great deal of variability in the normal frequency of bowel movements. Almost all babies (98.5%) have their first bowel movement within the first day of life; those that don't may have an anatomical problem leading to blocked bowels. Breast-fed babies can have a stool every time they nurse. Others have a stool every day or two. Among older children, more than 95% have bowel movements between three times a day and once every two days. Anything more than three times a day (diarrhea) or less often than every four days (constipation) calls for a professional evaluation.

Constipation simply means that your child is having stools less frequently than is normal for her, has hard or dry stools, or is having difficulty passing them. Encopresis is the technical term for prolonged, severe constipation with stool buildup (impaction) in the rectum and occasional leaking of stool into the underwear (soiling).

Occasional constipation is a fairly frequent childhood complaint; it becomes even more common during adulthood and is practically epidemic among those over sixty-five. Chronic constipation increases the risk of colon cancer in later life. There is an inverse association between the intake of fruits and vegetables and the risk of developing colon cancer; the more fruits and vegetables you eat, the lower the risk of cancer.

## What Causes Constipation?

The commonest cause of constipation is *insufficient fiber* in the diet.[1] Americans and Western Europeans eat the least fiber and have the highest rates of constipation and bowel cancer in the world. Fast foods are typically low-fiber foods. If Americans doubled the amount of fiber in the diet, we could dramatically reduce problems with constipation and colon cancer.

Constipation is a more common complaint in the summertime because children sweat more and may get dehydrated. *Dehydration*

## COMMON CAUSES OF CONSTIPATION

- Insufficient fiber in the diet
- Insufficient water or other fluids, especially in hot weather or with a fever
- Changes in diet or routine
- Ignoring the urge to defecate, postponing defecation
- Prolonged bed rest
- Severe dieting, anorexia nervosa
- Medication side effects

makes stools dry and harder to pass. Feverish children also lose more fluid than normal, increasing their risk of dehydration and constipation. Faced with dehydration, the body starts to draw on water wherever it can, including the bowels, resulting in drier, smaller stools, and constipation. Another reason to give plenty of fluids to a feverish child!

*Dietary changes* are often accompanied by changes in stool frequency. Many babies who are switched from mother's milk to formula are constipated for a few days before they adjust to the new food; this difficulty is probably due to the fatty acid content of most formulas. It may be eased by providing a little extra vitamin A.[2] Breaks in the regular routine of eating, sleeping, and playing, such as traveling, moving, or the arrival of a new baby in the house frequently provoke temporary constipation. Bowel movements usually return to normal when the child becomes adjusted to the new routine or life returns to normal.

Some children are just so busy and preoccupied that they *postpone* going to the toilet until after the urge has passed. The stool remains in the rectum, and the body gradually reabsorbs more and more water from it until the stool becomes hard and dry. Dry, hard stool is more difficult to pass, and it may be uncomfortable or even cause tiny tears in the delicate skin around the anus. A vicious cycle sets in, wherein the child postpones defecating, the stool becomes hard, defecation becomes painful, and the child delays further. It's best to avoid this cycle altogether by having a regular toilet time every day during which the child sits for five minutes, regardless of the outcome.

*Bed rest* slows down many bodily functions. Sedentary or wheelchair-bound children are more prone to constipation than their active counterparts. Even a little mild to moderate exercise keeps blood flowing to all the organs. Don't let your child spend hours glued to the television. Have her get up and play.

Teenage girls who *diet* intensively or have *anorexia nervosa* frequently have problems with constipation. Interestingly, teenage girls are more prone to constipation during certain phases of their menstrual cycle. Due to hormonal fluctuations, they are most likely to suffer from constipation about sixteen to twenty-one days after the start of their periods.

Widely used *medications* such as antacids containing aluminum (Amphogel, for example) and prescription painkillers containing codeine also slow down the intestinal flow. Overuse of laxatives results in dependence on them; when the child stops taking the laxative (even natural ones such as senna and cascara), the bowels slow down.

*Unusual causes of constipation* in children are Hirschprung's disease (in which part of the bowel does not have a proper nerve supply and doesn't move the stool along), botulism, spinal cord tumor, and hypothyroidism. Milk allergy may present as constipation during the toddler years;[3] in fact, allergies to cow's milk can be so severe that doctors think the problem requires surgery![4] If you suspect any of these problems, see your doctor for a definitive diagnosis.

Constipated children often suffer from other symptoms such as irritability, tiredness, headaches, depression, and just feeling out of sorts. The ongoing pressure from large amounts of stool in the colon irritates the bladder; this makes children who suffer from chronic constipation prone to bed-wetting and bladder infections as well. (See Chapter 6, Bed-Wetting.)

---

**WHEN TO SEEK PROFESSIONAL HELP FOR A CONSTIPATED CHILD**

- No stools for four or more days
- Swollen, distended, or painful abdomen
- Vomiting as well as constipation
- Pain when passing a stool
- Blood in the stool
- Dark black stools
- Constipation alternating with diarrhea
- Frequent, painful, or rushed urination

---

These symptoms may indicate a more serious problem such as an intestinal blockage, intestinal bleeding, impaction, irritable bowel syndrome, or a bladder infection.

## How Can You Prevent Constipation?

**FIVE TIPS FOR PREVENTING CONSTIPATION**

1. Begin by breast-feeding
2. High-fiber diet (whole grains, fruits, and vegetables)
3. Plenty of fluids (six to eight glasses per day)
4. Exercise
5. Regular routine

*Breast-fed* babies tend to have softer, more frequent stools than babies who are fed formula. Formula-fed babies do just fine in general, but they are slightly more prone to constipation. Babies on soy formulas in particular tend to have harder, less frequent stools than babies who are nursed or who are fed cow's milk–based formulas.[5] In the summertime, formula-fed babies may benefit from water supplements between feedings.

For older infants and children whose diet includes solids, the top remedy for preventing constipation is eating a diet high in natural *fiber* or roughage. Fiber increases the bulk of stools, draws water into the bowel, softens stools and makes them easier to pass, and stimulates contractions in the colon that move the stool along. Eating a diet that is high in whole grains, fruits, and vegetables is the best way to prevent constipation.

Drinking plenty of *fluids* is also important for maintaining healthy bowels. Fiber draws water into the intestines, softening the stool. If there is not enough water in the system, the fiber can just clog up and make things worse. Water helps soften stools so they are easier to pass. Adding extra water substantially increases the benefits of extra fiber.[6]

Regular *exercise* also helps keep things flowing. Children who are confined to bed for long periods (such as after surgery) have more trouble with constipation than children who are up and running around. On the other hand, if your child is normally active, adding a new, strenuous exercise routine won't necessarily improve her constipation.[7]

Keeping a *regular schedule* is helpful in preventing constipation. Most adults have experienced the temporary constipation that accompanies a trip in which the normal daily routine is disrupted. Children who are being potty trained benefit from having a regular life schedule, including sleep, meals, and scheduled time on the toilet. It is best to schedule potty time after a meal to take advantage of the gastro-colic reflex. This is a physiologic reflex (on which most housebreaking routines are based for puppies): when the stomach is full, a nerve reflex stimulates the bowels to move. This is why so many babies have a bowel movement right after they nurse. Children who are so constipated they no longer feel the urge to go need a routine time in which they sit on the toilet whether they feel they have to go or not. Just sitting on the toilet stimulates thoughts and reflexes that enhance regular bowel movements.

## WHAT IS THE BEST WAY TO TREAT CONSTIPATION?

The best way to treat constipation is to prevent it by living a healthy lifestyle—high-fiber diet, fluids, exercise, and a regular routine. If the problem persists, there are additional proven remedies. Let's consider a variety of therapies to find out what works. If you want my bottom-line recommendations (so to speak), flip to the end of the chapter.

## BIOCHEMICAL THERAPIES: MEDICATIONS, HERBS, NUTRITIONAL SUPPLEMENTS

### *Medications*

Though many medications are effective, do *not* use them until you've tried dietary changes first. A variety of nonprescription medications are available to treat constipation. Do *not* use any of them for more than a week without checking with your child's doctor. Do *not* use them if your child has severe abdominal pain, nausea, vomiting, blood in the stools, or cramping, because they could worsen a serious underlying condition.

The mainstay of prevention and treatment for constipation is increased *fiber*. Fiber is the safest, most natural treatment for constipation. The two principal natural types of fiber medications are based on *psyllium* (from psyllium seeds) and *methylcellulose* (plant fiber). There is also an effective synthetic fiber, *polycarbophil.*

Psyllium is the fiber in Metamucil and many other bulk laxatives. These medications come in a variety of forms: fruit-flavored, sweetened or unsweetened powder to mix with water or juice, or as wafers. Allergic reactions to psyllium are rare. Each teaspoon of Metamucil contains about 2.2 grams of fiber. This is the same amount of fiber found in one dark Finn crisp cracker (2.5 grams) and less than the amount in two Fiber Rich Bran Crackers (6 grams). Methylcellulose is the fiber in Citrucel. Each rounded teaspoon of Citrucel contains approximately 2 grams of fiber. *Read labels* to find out how much fiber each remedy (or food) contains.

## NONPRESCRIPTION MEDICATIONS TO TREAT CONSTIPATION

- *Fiber or bulk agents:* Psyllium (Metamucil and others), Methylcellulose (Citrucel), Polycarbophil (Fiberall chewable tablets and others)

- *Stool softeners:* Docusate (Colace)

- *Lubricants*: Mineral oil

- *Stimulants:* Bisacodyl (Dulcolax), Cascara (Nature's Remedy Natural Vegetable Laxatives), Senna (Senokot, Fletcher's Castoria), Castor oil

- *Magnesium salts:* Milk of Magnesia, Epsom salts

- *Others:* Maltsupex, glycerin suppositories (Babylax), lactulose (Cephulac)

*Fiber* works best if it is taken with lots of fluid. The liquid combines with the fiber, swelling up and creating the bulking effect that expands the colon and softens the stool. You may need to repeat doses two to three times daily for one to three days before you see results. Fiber-containing laxatives should *not* be used by children who have blocked bowels, because they can make the blockage worse. Fiber laxatives are too harsh for children under three years old.

*Docusate (Colace)* is one of the most frequently used stool softeners in hospitals. Colace draws water into the bowel, softening the stool and making it easier to pass. Aspirin, ibuprofen, and other anti-inflammatory medicines may interfere with it. Colace is helpful when stools are hard and dry or when passage of a firm stool is painful, as in children suffering from anal fissures (tiny tears in the skin around the anus from passing hard stools). Colace is available as capsules, syrup, and as infant drops. It is one of the safest medicines around, though some children do not like the taste and complain of nausea when they have to swallow the liquid form.

*Mineral oil* has long been used to "grease the skids" of children suffering from severe, chronic constipation. The dose for children with mild constipation is 1 teaspoon to 1 tablespoon given at bedtime. For children with severe encopresis, higher doses can be used; check with your doctor for the proper amount for your child. It generally works in six to eight hours. Mineral oil tastes awful, but please do *not* hold your child's nose while getting him to swallow it. If it is accidentally inhaled (aspirated), it produces a nasty pneumonia, and you may end up with a gasping, choking child whose symptoms are far worse than simple constipation. Mineral oil is much more palatable if it is cold, emulsified, or mixed with frozen yogurt or ice cream, peanut butter, or chocolate syrup. Despite concerns that prolonged use of mineral oil may lead to loss of vitamins and minerals in the stool, a study that actually measured the levels of beta-carotene, vitamin A, and vitamin E showed that even prolonged (four months) use of mineral oil did not lower blood levels of these vitamins.[8] If your child has severe, chronic constipation, mineral oil can be safely given for several months to get things back on track.

*Bowel stimulants* work directly on the intestines to stimulate peristalsis, the waves of contractions that move food and waste through the bowel. Stimulants generally produce results in six to ten hours when taken by mouth. They can work in as little as an hour if given as suppositories. Bowel stimulants can lead to dependence if they are used on a regular basis. They can be very powerful and cause cramping pain and diarrhea if too much is given. Several kinds are available.

*Bisacodyl (Dulcolax)* is the most widely used bowel stimulant in hospitals. It is available as tablets or suppositories. Like fiber, it should *not* be used in children who may have blocked bowels or appendicitis, because it could aggravate these conditions.

*Yellow phenolphthalein* is a bowel stimulant that used to be the active ingredient in several widely used nonprescription stool softeners such as Ex-Lax and Correctol. However, its use as a laxative was banned by the U.S. government in 1997 because large doses caused cancer in lab animals. Laxatives that used to contain this compound have been reformulated to rely on other bowel stimulants such as senna (ExLax) and bisacodyl (Correctol).

*Cascara sagrada (Nature's Remedy Natural Vegetable Laxative)* is a natural bowel stimulant. Cascara is secreted in breast milk, so if you take it while you are nursing, your baby may get diarrhea. *Senna (Senokot, Fletcher's Castoria*, and others) is another potent natural bowel stimulant, which is safe even for nursing mothers. *Castor oil* is an old-fashioned natural bowel stimulant extracted from castor beans; several brands contain sweeteners and flavorings that may make castor oil more palatable. Frequent use of these natural bowel stimulants may result in dependence on them. Do *not* use them for more than two or three days in a row without professional consultation.

*Magnesium salts* are the active ingredient in *Milk of Magnesia* and *Epsom salts*. Many families keep them on hand to treat indigestion, heartburn, and upset stomach. By drawing water into the intestines, magnesium salts soften the stool and increase peristalsis. They generally work in one to three hours. The dose of Epsom salts for children is 1 to 2 teaspoons in a glass of water. Magnesium salts can impair the absorption of other prescription medicines. If your child is taking a prescription medicine, check with your doctor or pharmacist to make sure that Milk of Magnesia will not interfere with it. Ibuprofen and aspirin can interfere with magnesium's effect on the bowel. Do *not* go overboard on magnesium; too much can be fatal.[9]

*Maltsupex* is a natural extract of barley malt, which helps draw water into the bowel, softening stools. Like fiber laxatives, Maltsupex should be taken with plenty of liquids. *Glycerin suppositories (Fleet Babylax)* are among the safest remedies for constipated infants. They work within half an hour by stimulating the defecation reflex. *Lactulose (Cephulac* and other brands) is an artificial sugar that is not digested by humans. It is broken down by the normal gut bacteria, resulting in carbon dioxide and other compounds that stimulate bowel movements. Lactulose can cause gas, belching, nausea, and discomfort. It should *not* be used with other laxatives.

There are many varieties of nonprescription laxatives. The similarities in names can be confusing. Some products made by the same manufacturer contain different kinds of ingredients. *Read labels carefully*. To treat mild constipation start with fiber; consider Maltsupex or Milk of Magnesia because they have great safety records. Do not use bowel stimulants (synthetic or natural) without professional consultation; relying on bowel stimulants for more than a week could result in dependence.

## Enemas

The vast majority of constipated children can be effectively treated without resorting to enemas. However, children who have severe stool buildup or impaction may need enema therapy to clean out the problem before starting on other treatments to restore normal bowel patterns. Enemas are *not* helpful for children who have a decrease in bowel movements because they have not eaten. Once impacted stool has been evacuated from the rectum, enemas do not have any advantage over oral laxatives in maintaining normal bowel function. I do *not* recommend them except for children whose severe constipation has not responded to other therapies.

Pediatric enemas contain a variety of ingredients. The most widely used are *Pediatric Fleet* products. Do not use phosphate enemas repeatedly except under the supervision of a health care professional, because they can result in abnormalities in the body's normal salt and water balance. Homemade enema solutions include milk and molasses, detergent, milk alone, coffee, and a variety of other substances. These solutions have *not* undergone rigorous safety evaluations and may cause severe side effects. Do *not* give your child coffee enemas, because they can also upset the body's delicate balance of salt and water if used repeatedly.

Many specialists in treating severe constipation recommend a combined approach: enemas initially to clean out impacted stool, followed by a high-fiber diet, daily mineral oil, a stool softener (such as Colace) to help retrain the bowel, and counseling to address possible causes and consequences of this problem. Despite concerns that this regimen might deplete blood levels of vitamins and impair growth, recent studies have shown that with proper medical supervision, these combination regimens are safe and effective.[10]

## Herbs

### HERBS TO TREAT CONSTIPATION

- Cascara sagrada (buckthorn)
- Senna
- Aloe
- Dong Quai
- Others

*Do not rely on herbs or medicines that are bowel stimulants* until after you've tried dietary therapy, increased water, increased exercise, and regular time on the toilet. Do *not* use herbal laxatives for more than two days without consulting your health care professional. Chronic use can lead to dependence on the laxative for normal function and disturbances in blood chemistry.

*Cascara* and *senna* are powerful laxatives. Senna is one of the safest and most physiological of all laxatives.[11] It generally works in eight to ten hours; bedtime doses should achieve results by breakfast. You can find these herbs in the grocery store or health food store as commercially prepared teas. They are sometimes combined with fennel and peppermint—two traditional tummy soothers that may ease the cramps provoked by strong bowel stimulants. *Aloe juice,* prepared from the inner surface of aloe leaves, is a more potent cathartic (bowel stimulator) than aloe gel, which is typically used as a skin soother rather than a laxative. Aloe tends to cause more cramping than other herbal laxatives. Overuse of aloe and cascara has been linked with bowel cancer.[12] Treatments are not necessarily safer just because they're natural.

*Dong Quai* (from the root of *Angelica sinensis*), which is often used to treat menstrual cramps, is also a mild laxative. Other herbs that may help relieve the intestinal spasms that sometimes accompany constipation are chamomile, ginger, lemon balm, licorice root, mulberry, and wild yam.[13] Herbs that may help soothe an irritated intestine are marshmallow root and slippery elm bark tea. (See Chapter 16, Diarrhea.) None have been tested as constipation remedies for children.

## Nutritional Supplements

*Vitamin C* overdoses can cause diarrhea. You can safely give vitamin C supplements to a child who is constipated, but the primary treatment for constipation should be diet, not supplements.

*Avoid aluminum.* Aluminum can make constipation worse. Aluminum is found in some antacids such as Amphogel in the form of aluminum hydroxide. Read labels before you give your child an antacid for an upset stomach related to constipation. Also avoid cooking acidic foods (such as tomato sauce) in aluminum saucepans, because the acid tends to leach aluminum into the food.

## LIFESTYLE THERAPIES: NUTRITION, EXERCISE, MIND-BODY

A healthy lifestyle is the cornerstone of therapy for constipation.

## Nutrition

What are the top three remedies to prevent and treat constipation? Fiber, fiber, and more fiber! Fiber also decreases blood cholesterol and evens out blood sugar levels. An Australian community education effort to increase the intake of whole grain bread led to a 58% increase in the sale of whole grain bread and a 49% decrease in laxative sales![14] It takes about a week for increased fiber intake to show results. There are several different kinds of dietary fiber. You may want to combine different kinds to achieve the most balanced effect.

| TYPE OF FIBER | FOOD SOURCE |
|---|---|
| Cellulose and hemicellulose | Wheat, rice, or oat bran |
| Mucilages | Psyllium seeds, legumes, guar |
| Pectin | Apple peel, carrots |
| Others | Food thickeners and additives: gum arabic, xanthan gum, algin, carrageenan |

Fiber is not digested by humans but is partially broken down by the bacteria that normally live in the intestines. The bacterial breakdown releases chemicals that help stimulate peristalsis. *Cellulose* (the fiber in bran) is present in all plants. It helps draw water into the intestine, making stools larger, softer, and easier to pass. Wheat bran increases the volume of stool and decreases the time it takes to move through the intestines. *Psyllium seed (Plantago ovata)* is one of the most powerful laxatives from the plant kingdom. *Guar* and *pectin* are good for the bowel and help to lower cholesterol. *Gums*, such as xanthan gum, gum arabic, algin, and carrageenan, are used in many prepared foods to help stabilize them and give them substance; they are also mild laxatives.

Start slowly and gradually increase your

child's fiber intake. For kids who are used to a steady diet of white flour, fat, and sugar (such as doughnuts or bagels and cream cheese for breakfast), suddenly switching to a high-fiber menu can spell flatulence, cramping, and diarrhea. Start by replacing doughnuts or white bread with whole grain bread or bran cereal. Then add one or two fresh fruits or vegetables a day. Then add high-fiber snacks such as Ry-Krisp crackers (7 grams per serving), Kavli 5 grain, RyVita Crisp Bread or Finn crisp crackers (6 grams per serving) or Wasa Fiber, Hearty of Light Rye Crisp Bread (5 grams per serving). If foods alone don't do the trick, consider adding wheat or rice bran to your child's cereal or sprinkled on top of toast. Go slowly. Try adding one high-fiber food every few days. Do *not* give bran supplements to children under three years old without a doctor's advice. It could cause bowel blockages in young children who don't drink enough fluid.

## HIGH-FIBER FOODS

- Bran, wheat, or rice
- Bran cereals, puffed whole grain cereals, muesli
- Bran muffins, bran cookies, bran crackers, whole grain pancakes
- Beans, peas, lentils
- Dried fruit (prunes are best; figs, apricots, raisins, and dates are also good)
- Fresh fruit and vegetables, especially cabbage, carrots, apples, and celery
- Seeds and nuts (for children over four who are unlikely to choke)
- Popcorn

Prunes have a well-deserved reputation as laxative food. Other excellent dried fruits include figs and dates. You can make a yummy jam that will help keep your child regular:

## RIGHT AND REGULAR JAM

2 cups water
1 ¼ cup dried, chopped pitted dates
1 ¼ cup dried, chopped figs
1 tablespoon corn meal

Combine all ingredients in a glass, ceramic, or stainless steel pot. Bring to a boil. Simmer and stir until thickened. Cool to room temperature before serving. Keep refrigerated. Use as desired on whole grain toast, pancakes, waffles, etc.

Most kids love fruit, and fresh fruits and vegetables are excellent sources of fiber. The most fiber is provided by bran, followed by cabbage, carrots, and apples—cole slaw anyone? Medicinal rhubarb root is a traditional remedy for constipation, but there are no scientific studies evaluating the effectiveness of plain old garden rhubarb stalks. If your kids like it, go ahead and let them have it, but it is probably no more potent than any other fresh fruit or vegetable. If your child doesn't like eating fruit, you can make a delicious fruit smoothie.

## FRUIT SMOOTHIE FOR EXTRA FIBER

IN A BLENDER COMBINE:

1 banana
½ apple (with peel, but without seeds or core)
½ cup of yogurt with active cultures
½ to 1 teaspoon of wheat or rice bran (optional)
½ cup of pear, apple, or black cherry juice

You can add other fruits as you wish and adjust the amount of fruit and juice until you achieve the consistency your child prefers. This makes a delicious shake, and it contains all the fiber and fruit sugar your child needs to get going in the morning.

*Psyllium* seeds are the source of several laxative medications. Rather than give your child a medication, look for psyllium seeds at the health food store. Try small amounts (¼ teaspoon) sprinkled on breakfast cereal. Alternatively, to make sure your child gets fluid along with the seeds, soak the seeds in a cup of water to soften them and allow them to start to swell; have your child swallow the whole thing—water and seeds. Some children develop severe allergic reactions to psyllium seed. If your child develops a rash, hives, or any other symptoms, stop the psyllium. Alternatively you could try flaxseed. Flaxseed is one ingredient in Uncle Sam cereal, which also contains bran flakes. This is an excellent cereal for children prone to constipation. You can find flaxseed in most health food stores. It tastes fine. You can add ½ teaspoon to your child's regular cereal or sprinkle it on toast.

Plain popcorn is an excellent and fun source of fiber. Don't wipe out the nutritional benefits by adding butter or salt. Stick to plain popcorn, flavored with a bit of your favorite herbs, Brewer's yeast, or Parmesan cheese.

Following fiber, the most important dietary component is *water*. Fiber draws water into the bowel to increase its bulk, stretch the colon, stimulate bowel action, and soften the stools. If there is not enough water, the fiber can become hardened and stuck, causing complete bowel blockage. On the other hand, pushing fluids beyond the body's basic needs doesn't offer any particular advantage. Offer your child fluids, but don't hound her into drinking more than she is comfortable with.

Fruit juice helps promote regular bowel movements. Fruit juices contain the fruit sugar fructose, and another sugar that is not well absorbed by the body, sorbitol. Fruit juice is so potent at loosening the bowels, it is often an unsuspected cause of chronic diarrhea. The most potent fruit juices are pear, apple, black cherry, prune, and syrup of figs. Fruit juices in moderation are safe even for children less than three years old, but too much fruit juice can lead to diarrhea and poor growth. Remember tooth brushing after fruit juice!

Many "sugar-free" candies and gums also contain fructose and sorbitol as sweeteners. Both of these sugar substitutes are poorly absorbed by many children and adults. Because they are not well absorbed, they draw water into the intestines, softening the stool and making it easier to pass. They are also broken down by normal gut bacteria, creating gas and further stimulating the bowel. Sorbitol is so good at moving things along it is used in an emergency medication to help speed the elimination of poisons. Thus, children with sloppy stools may benefit from cutting back on sugarless foods, while constipated kids might benefit from having a few more "sugar-free" sweets.

Like Penny Brandenburg, I was taught to add 1 to 2 tablespoons of Karo corn syrup to each bottle of formula for babies suffering from constipation. Since we now know that botulism spores have been found in corn syrup as well as honey, many practitioners strenuously recommended *avoiding* these products for infants under a year of age.

*I advised Penny Brandenburg not to recommend Karo syrup but to stick with syrup made from simmering dried figs, dates, raisins, and prunes in plain water: 1 to 2 teaspoons with each meal. She was relieved to have an alternative remedy.*

Many adults notice that their morning cup of *coffee* can really get things moving. Coffee stimulates the bowel, and it does so quickly. Even decaffeinated coffee can provoke bowel action in as little as four minutes.[15] I am *not* advocating coffee as a regular beverage for children; but for occasional use when a child is constipated due to travel or a disruption in schedule, a small cup of coffee just might do the trick.

Cheese is frequently blamed for constipation, and many practitioners recommend avoiding cheese if a child is constipated. Despite widespread injunctions against cheese, a study in older adults showed that even a tenfold increase in cheese intake had no effect on stool volume or frequency.[16] In fact one dairy product, yogurt, may actually be helpful in restoring healthy bowel bacteria and reducing constipation.[17] Try adding yogurt (with active cultures) to your child's regular diet.

## Exercise

Bed rest slows down bowel activity. Mild to moderate exercise helps keep things moving. Exercise also helps reduce stress. Strenuous endurance sports such as long-distance running and cycling are associated with an increased risk of diarrhea, especially in girls. The best idea for maintaining balance and regularity is to keep moderately active—neither too much time in front of the TV nor running marathons. Make sure that your child has access to plenty of fluid during exercise to avoid dehydration.

## Mind-Body

Stress upsets the stomach and aggravates all kinds of bowel problems. Some children react to stress with headaches, some have diarrhea, some have sleep problems, and some suffer from constipation. Anticipate the possible consequences of unavoidable stress (such as starting school, moving, death of a pet or family member) by increasing your child's intake of fiber-rich foods during stressful periods.

To keep the gastrointestinal system functioning smoothly, try to keep meal times and toileting times low key. Make sure that your child's time on the toilet is pleasant; don't

demand performance. Simply allow it to happen naturally. When your child does have the desired results, positive reinforcement such as praise and stickers can work wonders. Behavior management techniques are most effective when combined with fiber and stool softeners.

Much of childhood constipation is a result of the child ignoring the urge to defecate because she is preoccupied with something else. Ignoring the urge to go allows the colon time to reabsorb more water from the stool, making it dry and difficult to pass. Habitually suppressing the urge to defecate actually changes the bowel's normal dynamics and makes it more difficult to go once the child is willing. Remind your child *not* to postpone the urge to defecate.

*Hypnosis* and *biofeedback* have proven effective in treating chronic, severe constipation and encopresis and for patients with irritable bowel syndrome. They are *unnecessary* and *ineffective* for the vast majority of children with short-term or mild constipation.[18] Biofeedback helps retrain the defecation reflex, leading to improved control of bowel function that can last for months after the training is completed. It is most effective if used in the context of increased fiber, stool softeners, and behavioral techniques such as regular toilet-sitting times. Biofeedback therapy should be reserved for children with severe constipation who have not benefited from other lifestyle therapies. New technologies have made it possible to develop biofeedback using interactive computer games and portable devices to help children relearn how to use the muscles used to poop.[19]

## BIOMECHANICAL THERAPIES: MASSAGE, SURGERY

### Massage

Despite its widespread use, massage did *not* prove helpful in the only scientific study of its effectiveness in treating constipation.[20] Still, massage is safe and can improve communication and attachment between parents and their children. As long as you are gentle, there is probably no harm in giving your child a tummy rub when she is constipated.

## Surgery

Surgery is *not* needed to treat garden-variety constipation. It *is* necessary for illnesses such as Hirschprung's disease, in which part of the bowel has an abnormal nerve supply. It is also lifesaving in cases of intestinal obstruction. If you suspect either of these problems, see your doctor.

## BIOENERGETIC THERAPIES: ACUPUNCTURE, THERAPEUTIC TOUCH/REIKI, HOMEOPATHY

### Acupuncture

Acupuncture was *not* found to be effective for treating constipation in the only scientific study evaluating it.[21] This study was done on adults; no studies have been done on children. Given its known effects on the entire GI tract, it would not be surprising if acupuncture was helpful; it may be worth trying if better known and less expensive measures haven't worked.[22]

### Therapeutic Touch/Reiki

Although there are no scientific studies specifically evaluating the effectiveness of Therapeutic Touch/Reiki and other types of healing as therapies for constipation, I have used them for several hospitalized patients over the last few years. All patients who had complained of constipation who were treated with Reiki or Therapeutic Touch (usually for other medical problems as well as constipation) had a bowel movement within twelve hours of the treatment. In fact, I'm starting to get something of a reputation—not one that I'm sure I'm seeking. All of these patients were also receiving numerous other therapies as well, so it is hard to give the credit entirely to "energy healing." However, because this type of healing work is so valued by patients and so safe, I continue to use it, pending the results of formal scientific studies.

### Homeopathy

There are no scientific studies evaluating the effectiveness of homeopathic remedies in treating adults or children suffering from constipation. Commonly used remedies include *Alumina, Bryonia, Calcarea carb, Lycopodium,* and *Nux vomica* (especially if the child has vomiting as well as constipation). Although they haven't been formally tested, they are probably safe.

*Susan had impacted stool in her rectum. Eric began giving her 2 tablespoons of mineral oil at night (mixed with chocolate frozen yogurt) and in the morning (followed by pear juice). We gave her Colace to take twice daily as well to soften her stools. Her mom also began making fruit-bran-yogurt smoothies for breakfast and sending Susan to day care with a container of pear juice and bran crackers for snacks. Susan had a sticker chart that she filled in with a new sticker each time she had a bowel movement. Six months later, she was regular as a clock on her new high-fiber diet without any medications or herbal treatments. She never needed another enema or referral for biofeedback. Her parents were delighted and felt that the changes in Susan's diet had spilled over to theirs, benefiting the whole family.*

✳

# WHAT I RECOMMEND FOR CONSTIPATION

## PREVENTING CONSTIPATION

1. *Lifestyle—nutrition.* Start your infant's life out right by breast-feeding. If you are feeding your baby formula, you may need to give her water supplements in the summer. Feed your toddler or older child a diet rich in whole grains, fresh fruits, vegetables, yogurt, and plenty of water. The goal in terms of number of grams of dietary fiber is: age in years + 5 = total grams of dietary fiber per day. Make sure your child gets plenty of fluids.

2. *Lifestyle—exercise.* Encourage your child to get some exercise or outdoor play. Keep a regular scheduled potty time (after meals works best) every day.

3. *Lifestyle—mind-body.* Give positive rewards for positive results. Avoid embarrassing or punishing your child for "misses."

4. *Biochemical—medications.* Avoid codeine-containing pain relievers and antacids that contain aluminum.

---

*When to seek professional help for constipation:*

- No stools for four or more days despite home remedies described below

- Swollen or distended belly

- Vomiting as well as constipation

- Pain with passing a stool or pain in the abdomen, especially on the lower right side

- Blood in the stool

- Dark black stools

- Constipation alternating with diarrhea

- Frequent, painful, or urgent urination

---

## TREATING CONSTIPATION

1. *Lifestyle—nutrition.* For constipated *infants* try a little extra water, fruit juice (apple, pear, black cherry, or prune juice), or the juice from stewed figs, dates, raisins, or prunes. For constipated *toddlers* or *older children*, increase fiber intake: high-fiber crackers and cookies, more fruits, vegetables, dried fruit, beans, popcorn, flax or psyllium seeds; add pear, apple, prune, or black cherry juice; consider sugarless gums or candies that contain sorbitol as treats; try a teaspoon of flaxseeds on bran cereal or whole grain toast; add high-fiber crackers as treats. Make sure she's getting plenty of fluids. Consider a possible allergy to cow's milk and have her evaluated if you suspect this is the problem.

2. *Lifestyle—exercise.* Encourage regular exercise. Have a regular time to sit on the toilet after meals.

3. *Lifestyle—mind-body.* Give positive rewards (such as stickers) for positive results.

4. *Biochemical—herbs.* Try laxatives such as cascara or senna (Fletcher's Castoria or Senokot) given in divided doses over the course of the day. Do *not* use for more than two days without seeing your health care professional.

5. *Biochemical—medications.* Try fiber-based medications (Metamucil), stool softeners (Colace), or mineral oil. For infants, try a glycerin suppository. If all else fails and your child is severely blocked up, consider a Fleet's enema to clear out the impaction in the rectum initially.

NOTE: Coincidentally, a multidisciplinary group from the University of Michigan came up with almost identical guidelines, including the use of herbal-based senna to treat chronic constipation.[23]

RESOURCES

*Internet*

Children's Medical Center of the University of Virginia
http://www.med.virginia.edu/docs/cmc/tutorials/constipation/

National Digestive Diseases Information Clearinghouse (NIH)
http://www.niddk.nih.gov/health/digest/pubs/const/const.htm

North American Society of Pediatric Gastroenterology and Nutrition
http://www.naspgn.org/constipation.pdf

Keep Kids Healthy.com
http://www.keepkidshealthy.com/welcome/treatmentguides/constipation.html

# 13
# COUGH

Nine-month-old Philip Koshi started coughing two days ago when he developed a cold. He sounded like a seal barking, and his cough was worse at night. His parents started to bring him to the emergency room at 2 A.M., but on the way, he improved so much they thought the doctors would think they were crazy, so they sheepishly returned home. Philip seemed better this morning, but his parents wanted to make sure he didn't have another night like that one.

Terri Nguyen was a pale, tired-looking fourteen-year-old who had been coughing for several days. She had recently returned from a trip to visit her grandmother in Vietnam. The last two days she had noticed more phlegm and had developed a fever. This morning she had coughed up some yellow-green mucus, flecked with blood. She wanted a shot of antibiotics so she could participate in a swim meet the next day.

Kris Masterson brought in his fourteen-month-old daughter, Emily, who had been coughing off and on for weeks, ever since she had bronchiolitis. Emily's lungs seemed to be extra sensitive; every cold she caught brought on more coughing spasms. Chris wanted to know if this was normal or if he should worry about cystic fibrosis.

Coughing is the body's natural method for clearing the airway. Anything that irritates or blocks the air passages stimulates a cough reflex. Generally the cough happens for a good reason. It is a mistake to suppress a cough unless you know for certain what is causing it and that it is not serving a useful function.

**TAKE YOUR CHILD TO A HEALTH CARE PROFESSIONAL IF SHE IS:**

- Persistently coughing for more than a week despite home therapies
- Coughing so hard she can't catch her breath
- Coughing up blood
- Wheezing
- Breathing very fast
- Turning blue in lips or fingernails
- Lethargic
- Complaining of pain in the chest
- Complaining of headache or facial pain as well as coughing
- Has a fever over 103.9°F

## What Causes Coughs?

Coughs have many causes.

### CAUSES OF COUGH

- Infections (see Chapter 9, Colds)
- Reflux or aspiration
- Allergies, smoke, irritants (see Chapter 4, Allergies)
- Asthma (see Chapter 5)
- Cold air
- Heart failure
- Reflex, nerves, habit
- Serious illness—cystic fibrosis

Most coughs in children are due to *colds* and tend to get better over the course of a few days (see Chapter 9). However, some viruses such as pertussis, influenza, and respiratory synctitial virus (RSV) cause coughs that last for weeks or even months. Other cough-causing infections include croup, sinus infection, bronchitis, and pneumonia.

Coughs in infants may be due to a condition called *gastroesophageal reflux*. Reflux means that some of the baby's stomach (gastric) contents come back up the esophagus and a little is inhaled into the airway, causing cough and irritation. *Aspiration* is when a piece of food goes down the wrong way and gets in the lungs.

Other cough causes are: allergies (Chapter 4), cigarette smoke and other irritants, asthma (Chapter 5), cold air, and even heart failure (when fluid from the heart backs up into the lungs). Sometimes tickling the ear canal (when we look inside to see if there is an ear infection) provokes the cough reflex. Most adults have experienced a nervous cough. Children can develop a chronic coughing habit following an illness in which their cough was rewarded by extra attention. Serious illnesses such as cystic fibrosis are also characterized by recurrent coughing.

Despite modern myths to the contrary, immunizations do *not* weaken the immune system or cause coughing. Literally hundreds of studies on millions of children have shown that while immunizations are often uncomfortable, they actually boost immunity and prevent many serious illnesses such as whooping cough.

*Dry coughs* are usually due to irritants, allergies, a foreign body (such as a piece of food that got stuck down the wrong way), or asthma. *Rattlelike coughs* stem from phlegm in the back of the nose or throat and are usually due to simple colds. *Productive coughs* indicate that mucus is present in the airways and needs to be cleared. Most children under the age of eight swallow their mucus instead of spitting it out. The swallowed mucus usually passes through the intestines uneventfully. However, if a lot of mucus is swallowed, it can irritate the stomach, producing nausea and even vomiting.

### DIAGNOSING COUGHS

- Symptoms
- Physical examination

- Chest X rays
- Other: blood tests, skin tests

Most of the time, the reason for the cough can be determined by its characteristics, other symptoms (such as fever and wheezing), and a physical examination. Croup coughs are dry, worse at night, and usually affect children between the ages of six months and three years during the fall and winter. Croup is caused by a virus. The cough sounds like a seal barking. It is relieved by mist, steam, or going out in the cool night air. Croup sounds terrible as the child struggles for breath and then coughs and coughs and coughs. The child's sudden improvement on the way to the emergency room is embarrassing for many parents who were sure their child was on the brink of death, but it is a completely normal response to the cool night air. If the child doesn't improve on the way to the doctor's office or hospital, medical treatments are effective. Croup usually lasts for three to four days and is worse on the second and third nights of the illness.

*Philip Koshi's cough was due to croup. Emily Masterson had the typical, unfortunate, prolonged cough that follows a bout with respiratory synctitial virus (RSV). Though you might think that a cough from bacterial pneumonia would be worse, it usually resolves with a few days of antibiotics. Viruses, on the other hand, can damage the cells lining the air passages, leaving the child's lungs weakened for weeks or months. Kris was right to think about cystic fibrosis (CF). Infants with recurrent coughs or pneumonia (especially infants who are not growing well) should be tested for CF. Emily's tests turned out to be negative; she did not have CF. Emily eventually overcame her cough.*

Sometimes an X ray of the chest or sinuses is helpful. Less commonly, blood tests (to check for white blood cells fighting pneumonia) and skin tests (to check for tuberculosis, TB) are needed. If the child is old enough to spit out the phlegm he coughs up, it can be checked for bacteria and TB.

*Terri Nguyen's cough sounded like pneumonia because of her fever, cough, fatigue, and blood-flecked yellow-green sputum. We did an X ray of her chest, took some of her sputum to the laboratory for a culture, and did a skin test for tuberculosis before starting her treatment.*

## WHAT'S THE BEST WAY TO PREVENT COUGHS?

### PREVENTING COUGHS

- Avoid cigarette smoke
- Immunize against pertussis (whooping cough), pneumococcus (pneumonia), and influenza
- Treat underlying illnesses
- Minimize exposure to sick children

*Avoid exposure to cigarette smoke.* Smoke irritates the airways and makes even healthy kids cough. Do not smoke and do not allow others to smoke around your child, especially in enclosed spaces such as your home or car.

Make sure your child is *immunized against pertussis* (whooping cough). Despite its detractors, the highly effective pertussis vaccine has practically eliminated the old scourge of whooping cough. Pertussis can be fatal to infants and young children; those who survive often have lifelong lung damage.[1] The new vaccine has about 90% fewer side effects than the old vaccine. Whooping cough epidemics have reemerged in countries where governments stopped pertussis immunization programs due to public fears about the vaccine. Immunization is very effective in preventing this potentially fatal illness during childhood. Protection wanes over the years. By twenty years of age, 90% of those who were fully immunized as children are again susceptible to pertussis. Nowadays, the biggest outbreaks of pertussis are among teenagers and adults. Most adults who get pertussis are only moderately ill and never even go to the doctor. This is why pertussis will probably never be completely eradicated and why childhood immunization programs must continue. Many physicians are urging that we begin a program to re-immunize adults as well to eliminate the reservoir of whooping cough.

*I caught pertussis from one-month-old Dedra Shapiro (who hadn't yet received her first immunizations) during my residency training. Dedra was hospitalized with a severe cough. Soon after admission she stopped breathing. I immediately began mouth-to-mouth resuscitation. She did well, but an hour later her laboratory tests came back positive for pertussis. Two days later, I was coughing and had positive tests for pertussis. I took antibiotics for a week and continued to cough for six months. Even years later, my lungs were extra sensitive to infection. Like most young infants, Dedra caught pertussis from a parent who was sick with what he thought was simple bronchitis.*

Vaccines are also available to prevent two other coughing diseases. The pneumococcal vaccine (Prevnar) is available for babies as young as two months old. It helps protect against the bacteria that is the most common cause of ear infections, sinus infections, and pneumonia. The influenza vaccine is available for babies six months and older. Many physicians, including me, believe it is a good thing for all eligible kids to get this vaccine to prevent illness in children and missing days of work for parents. I'm especially in favor of kids getting it if there's anyone at home who has a chronic illness, such as asthma, who could get really sick from influenza. The flu vaccine must be taken every year because different strains of the virus appear each year to cause problems.

Treat any underlying allergies and asthma (see Chapters 4 and 5) to reduce the risk of asthma attacks and the coughing that accompanies them.

As much as you can, minimize your child's exposure to other children who are sick. The more time spent with young children, the more exposure to infections. If your child is in day care, select a situation with fewer rather than more children, if possible.

## WHAT IS THE BEST WAY TO TREAT A COUGH?

Treatment should always aim at helping the child's body heal the underlying illness rather than just suppressing the cough. Coughs can indicate a serious problem that should be treated (such as asthma or pneumonia); nighttime coughs can also be very annoying and lead to sleep loss for the whole family. On the other hand, coughing may be the body's best defense and protection against pneumonia. Let's tour the Therapeutic Mountain to find out what works for most coughs; if you want to skip to my bottom-line recommendations, flip to the end of the chapter.

## BIOCHEMICAL THERAPIES: MEDICATIONS, HERBS, NUTRITIONAL SUPPLEMENTS

### Medications

There are three main types of cough medicines: cough suppressants, expectorants (to help loosen secretions), and throat soothers such as cough drops.

There is good news and bad news about *cough suppressants*. The good news is that you can save a lot of money. The bad news is that none of them are very helpful, which is why you can save your money.[2] The two most commonly used cough medicines (dextromethorphan, the DM ingredient in many nonprescription cough medicines, and codeine, the most common prescription cough medicine) are no more effective than placebo syrup in reducing coughs in children under twelve years old.[3]

Placebos make us feel that we are doing something to help ourselves; some children (and adults) feel better and have fewer symptoms even with a placebo. Cough medicines are *not* any better than placebos, and they may have serious side effects such as irritability, fussiness, lethargy, and high blood pressure. Recently, some teenagers have started abusing dextromethorphan as a cheap way to get "high"; in fact, it just makes them feel "weird." *The American Academy of Pediatrics Committee on Drugs says that cough medicines should not be used for children.*[4]

*Expectorants* supposedly loosen secretions so they are easier to cough out. The most common one is guaifenesin (Robitussin). Although guaifenesin helps thin secretions, it is no more helpful than placebo syrup in reducing the frequency or severity of coughs.[5] I do *not* recommend expectorants.

*Cough drops* work mostly by stimulating saliva, coating and soothing an irritated throat. Any hard candy will do the same thing; lemon and other citrus flavors are particularly potent saliva stimulators. Do *not* give cough drops or hard candy to children under four years old who might choke on them. Cough drops with menthol or eucalyptus oils also help a congested nose feel less stuffy. Sucking on a vitamin C lozenge also stimulates saliva and may help fight the cold behind your child's cough.

The ineffectiveness of cough suppressants and expectorants does not mean that other medicines for specific types of cough are not helpful. *If your child is coughing because of croup, asthma, or allergies, use the treatments your health care professional has recommended and any others you have found to be helpful.*

For example, children suffering from severe croup that has not responded to home therapies can be helped by two prescription medications.

## CROUP MEDICATIONS

- Racemic epinephrine (epi)
- Steroids

*Racemic epinephrine* is given by a mist machine (called a nebulizer) in a doctor's office or emergency room. Racemic epinephrine helps shrink the swollen and inflamed blood vessels that line the airways, blocking airflow and causing coughs. Racemic epinephrine can be lifesaving. It works within minutes, providing rapid relief of breathing difficulties, but it only works for one to two hours, so it may need to be repeated several times. Rather than risk sending home a child who may need another treatment within an hour, many doctors automatically hospitalize a child who needs one racemic epinephrine treatment to be sure additional treatments are readily available if needed. Like caffeine (to which it is related), racemic epinephrine can cause a rapid heartbeat, shaky hands, agitation, and trembling. These side effects quickly disappear as the medicine wears off.

*Steroids* help reduce inflammation and swelling. Although they can have serious side effects when used over long periods of time (weeks or months), steroids are safe when used on a short-term basis (less than five days). The steroids that are used for children's illnesses are *not* the same kind of steroids athletes use to build muscles. Steroids given by mist machine (nebulizer) or with a face mask and spacer provide significant symptomatic improvement for several hours. Steroids are also effective when given by injection.[6] Though a shot is more painful than a mist treatment, you can be sure your child is actually receiving the medication; some children do not cooperate with the mist machine, and the parent ends up getting most of the dose! Steroid syrups taken by mouth are also helpful, even in children suffering from severe, life-threatening croup. A short round of steroid treatment might very well spare you several days in the hospital.

*We started Philip Koshi on a three-day course of a steroid syrup to help prevent more serious symptoms and a possible hospitalization. His parents were pleased to tell me at his next checkup that his croup symptoms rapidly improved, and there were no more midnight trips to the hospital.*

Antibiotics have *no* role in the treatment of coughs due to viruses. However, if your child's cough is caused by bacterial pneumonia, bronchitis, or a sinus infection, antibiotics such as erythromycin, azithromycin, clarithromycin, and doxycycline can help clear the underlying cause. If you suspect that your child has one of these illnesses, have her evaluated by a health care professional.

Children whose lungs have been damaged by viral or bacterial infections early in life may need asthma-type medicines to manage their symptoms for several years to keep them from coughing and wheezing.[7] If your infant or toddler has had a cough lasting for more than two weeks, see your doctor to see if prescription medicines might help.

## Herbs

Different kinds of herbs are used for different kinds of cough, but *only* menthol (extracted from mint) has proven useful in the lab in terms of reducing irritant coughs. There are lots of historical anecdotes and rich cultural traditions supporting a variety of herbal remedies. There are infection-fighting herbs, expectorants, herbs that soothe an irritated throat, herbs to warm and stimulate a child who is fatigued and chilled, and herbs to sedate a child who has been kept awake by a cough. Herbal remedies are usually taken as tea. Doses vary by age, and are usually made up according to the "seat of the pants" rule! *There have not been any studies showing that any herbal remedies are useful treatments for coughing children.*

### "SEAT OF THE PANTS" RULE FOR DOSES OF HERBAL TEA FOR COUGHS

- Children *under a year:* no more than 1 teaspoon three to four times daily
- Children *one to three years old:* up to 1 ounce four times daily
- Children *four to six years old:* up to 2 ounces four times daily
- Children *seven to twelve years old:* up to 3 ounces four times daily
- *Teenagers and adults:* 3 to 4 ounces every four to six hours

The heat from hot tea helps increase circulation to the throat, hastening healing to the whole area.

### HERBAL COUGH REMEDIES

- *Infection-fighting herbs:* eucalyptus, garlic, hyssop, plantain, thyme
- *Herbs to stimulate the immune system:* borage, dandelion root, echinacea, garlic, marigold, nettles, and wild indigo
- *Herbs to help loosen mucus so that it is easier to cough up (expectorants):* angelica root, anise seed, cowslip, elecampane, fennel, white horehound, hyssop, mullein, plantain, sage, senega snakeroot, thyme
- *Herbs to soothe a dry cough (demulcents):* anise, comfrey, elecampane, horehound, licorice,

lobelia, marshmallow root, mullein, slippery elm bark, wild cherry bark
- *Herbs to stimulate and warm a weak and chilled child:* anise, cinnamon, cloves, fennel, ginger, ginseng, hyssop, sarsaparilla root, thyme
- *Relaxing herbs to help a coughing child sleep:* chamomile, catnip, lime flowers

*Warning:* Although coltsfoot has been used in Europe, Asia, and America for many years as an herbal remedy for coughs, coltsfoot flowers (the most commonly used part of the plant) are highly toxic to the liver and may cause cancer. Senega snakeroot can cause severe stomach upset. Overdoses of licorice tea can adversely affect the body's salt and water balance. No scientific studies document the effectiveness of any of these remedies in treating children with coughs.

### POULTICES FOR COUGHS

- Mustard, garlic, or onion
- Turpentine or camphor
- Castor oil

A time-honored treatment for chest colds is the *mustard poultice.* Mustard poultices apparently increase circulation to your child's chest, creating a soothing sense of warmth. Do not let the mustard come in direct contact with your child's skin. It is irritating and could cause a burn. This same sense of heat and increased circulation can be achieved with a *garlic* or *onion poultice.* Do not use a garlic poultice for more than twenty minutes at a time or it can cause severe skin irritation. Some herbalists recommend that the garlic poultice be placed over the soles of the feet to draw heat downward.

Other folk remedies placed on the feet to draw the circulation downward are *turpentine* and *camphor.* A North Carolina woman who was my patient during medical school swore that her homemade turpentine poultices were what was really curing her but asked me not to tell her doctor, because she didn't want him to be disappointed in his antibiotics!

*Castor oil poultices* are also used in many parts of the country and were recommend by the psychic Edgar Cayce as a remedy for many illnesses. Castor oil is very soothing, so it can be applied directly to the skin or as a poultice for the chest, abdomen, or back.

None of these folk remedies has undergone scientific evaluation. There is a huge potential of getting ripped off or getting dangerous products until the FDA starts regulating herbal products more carefully. If your child fails to improve in a day or two or becomes more ill, consult your health care professional to make sure there is not a serious and easily treated condition causing the cough.

## Nutritional Supplements

*Vitamin A* protects the mucous membranes of the nose, throat, and lungs, but it is *not* helpful against ordinary coughs. Among malnourished children, vitamin A supplements are helpful for treating measles pneumonia. However, vitamin A supplements do *not* reduce cough or pneumonia in well-nourished infants or children. Too much vitamin A may *increase* the risk of respiratory infections.[8] If your child eats a healthy diet, he does *not* need supplemental vitamin A.

*Vitamin C* has proved effective in reducing the symptoms of the common cold in adults (see Chapter 9). Vitamin C also makes coughing and wheezing less likely.[9] One large Dutch study suggested that adults who consumed more vitamin C were less likely to suffer from coughs and had better tests of lung function;[10] this is encouraging. However, studies on children have not yet been done.

*Garlic-honey* is a combination of two common folk remedies. It is made by combining 4 to 5 cloves of minced garlic with 3 ounces of honey in a blender. You can give a teaspoon several times daily—that is, if you can get your child to swallow it! Both garlic and honey have antibacterial properties, but there are *no* scientific studies evaluating their effectiveness in treating coughs. Both ingredients are safe, readily available, and have a long history of use.

A favorite British remedy is *onion-honey* cough syrup. This is made by combining 2 to 3 cups of chopped onions with ½ cup of honey and cooking slowly for two or three hours over low heat. This combination is safe and can be given by teaspoon every one to two hours as needed, but when I've tried it, I've decided I'd rather have the cough than swallow the stuff.

A better-tasting combination for dry, tickly coughs is *honey and lemon*. You can combine them as a syrup or add a bit of each (to taste) to hot water or an herbal tea. It tastes much better than garlic or onion remedies, too. To avoid the risk of botulism, do *not* give honey remedies to children less than one year old. Honey remedies have *not* been scientifically tested for treating coughing children.

*Red pepper, hot pepper, and curries* that make your eyes water will also make your nose water and loosen secretions. If your child feels like eating, try spicy foods to help thin the phlegm in the lungs and throat.

## LIFESTYLE THERAPIES: NUTRITION, EXERCISE, ENVIRONMENT, MIND-BODY

### Nutrition

*Kris was frustrated with Emily's chronic cough. He'd read that milk made mucus worse and should be avoided when a child has a cough or cold. Millions of Americans avoid dairy products when they have a cough or cold. Does milk make mucus thicker?*

An Australian study divided 169 adults into two groups: one was given a milk drink and the other was given a soy drink disguised so as to be indistinguishable in appearance or taste from the cow's milk drink. Before the study started, nearly half of the adults believed that milk made mucus worse. *Both* test drinks (cow's milk and soy) made some subjects' tongues and throats feel "coated" and made their saliva feel thicker.[11] So the culprit may not be the cow's milk itself so much as any beverage that is thicker than juice or water. Milk does *not* increase mucus production in adults with colds.[12] I have not found a single scientific study that answers the question of whether milk increases lung secretions or makes coughing worse in children.

Do give your child plenty of *fluids* when she has a cough. Fluids help soothe irritated airways and help clear the bacteria, viruses, or irritants that are causing the cough. Fluids also help keep phlegm loose so it is easier to cough out.

Feel like fish? One study showed that young adults in Norway who ate fish regularly (more than twice weekly) had a much lower risk of having a nighttime cough than those who didn't eat much fish.[13] I'm not aware of any studies testing how well fish fixes a cough once you have one, but fish contain fatty acids known to combat the kind of inflammation that triggers many coughs. I recommend fish as part of a healthy diet.

### Exercise

*Despite her fatigue, Terri wanted to participate in a swim meet the following day.*

When the body is fighting a serious infection, it needs all of its reserves to win the battle. I generally recommend that kids take it easy until their fever and cough have been gone for twenty-four hours before resuming their normal activities. Even then they should take it slow and be gentle with themselves. They may feel well enough to walk around the house but find that they tire and their cough returns when they resume more vigorous activities. Children tend to cough more with exercise, especially when exercising in cold, dry air (such as speed skating or sledding).

*I advised Terri to sleep in and take naps rather than push herself to compete the following day.*

If your child has a wet, productive cough, you can help secretions drain with a simple exercise. Have your child lay face down on a bed and slide forward until the head and chest are hanging down off the bed. Your child can rest her head and arms on the floor or on a pillow on the floor. Being upside down helps the mucus drain out. In medicine, this is called *postural drainage* because it is the hanging-down posture that helps the lungs drain. It may also make your child feel light-headed, so don't do it for more than five to ten minutes at a time. After the child has been upside down for a minute or two, encourage her to cough to help bring out the mucus and phlegm. Studies of children with severe coughing due to cystic fibrosis have shown that this simple exercise results in a fivefold increase in the amount of mucus cleared compared with simply resting.[14]

When your child is resting, prop her head on a pillow or have her lie on her side to minimize postnasal drip, the source of many a nighttime cough.

## Environment

### ENVIRONMENTAL THERAPIES

- Avoid smoke
- Avoid damp, moldy environments
- Try mist or steam
- Suction nose with bulb syringe

*Do not smoke* and do not allow others to smoke around your child. Tobacco smoke, wood smoke, and air pollution aggravate respiratory problems such as coughing. Keep your child warm, away from cold drafts. If you keep the window open in your child's bedroom to provide fresh air, make sure she has plenty of covers to prevent her from feeling chilled.

Although mist or steam may be helpful in treating a child with a cough, living in a damp house with mold growing on the walls is not. Coughs are 80 to 90 percent more common among children living in homes parents describe as *damp or moldy* than among children in homes parents say are without damp or mold. Nasty mold and irritating dust mites prefer to live in damp environments. Remove mold thoroughly with a 10% bleach solution. To discourage mold and dust mites from living in your home, consider using a dehumidifier, vacuum regularly, and use an electrostatic air filter.

On the other hand, very *dry* air aggravates most coughs because it dries the secretions that normally soothe the air passages in the throat and lungs. *Mist, steam, and vaporizers* increase the moisture in the air passages and help loosen secretions. Despite the lack of controlled trials evaluating its effectiveness, mist is recommended by most health care providers because of its history of helping children with croup. One of my favorite home remedies for croupy kids is to run the hot water in the shower until the bathroom is very steamy. Then sit with the child on your lap in the steam and tell him stories or sing songs.

Despite years of use, *cool mist* has not proved helpful in treating croupy coughs.[15] The cool mist tents previously used in hospitals caused chills and made it difficult for parents to cuddle their child. If you use a vaporizer, clean it regularly to prevent a buildup of mold or fungus in the unit. A seldom-cleaned print shop humidifier harboring fungi and bacteria was responsible for a serious coughing illness in sixteen out of twenty-eight workers in the shop.[16] Be careful with steam vaporizers to avoid accidental burns to curious toddlers.

If your child's cough is due to a runny nose (postnasal drip) and he is too young to blow his nose, you can try *suctioning* his nose *with a bulb syringe.* Suctioning may need to be repeated every few hours. If your child's secretions are too thick to be removed easily with a bulb syringe, place a few drops of saltwater solution (½ teaspoon of salt in 8 ounces of water) in each nostril before suctioning. Do one nostril at a time so your child doesn't feel as if she's drowning.

## Mind-Body

As with any illness, it is helpful for the parent to remain calm and stay with the child to reassure him. Extra attention, such as reading stories, will help distract your child from whatever is ailing him and remind him that he is loved. Crying and being upset increase your child's need for oxygen. This is not a problem under normal circumstances, but if your child is having trouble breathing, crying may make matters worse.

Coughs often keep everyone in the house awake, especially as parents lie in bed wondering if their child is going to stop coughing or even stop breathing. If your child is having a hard time breathing, you and your spouse might want to take turns staying with him. If you know that someone is responsible, you can more easily relax and sleep yourself, so that you are better able to care for your child when your "shift" comes.

Some coughs are simply a kind of bad *habit,* which lingers on long after the initial cause for the cough is gone. In children with asthma, coughing can become a kind of conditioned response to any kind of stress. This kind of cough is dry, harsh, and *very* frequent; it usually stops when the child falls asleep. Children who have these coughs don't usually have any other behavioral or emotional problems, but

they can often be helped with behavioral techniques, such as relaxation, self-hypnosis, and guided imagery.[17]

*Hypnosis* has also proven useful in treating the child with a habitual cough. An eleven-year-old boy who had such a severe, persistent cough that he missed a month of school was able to stop coughing with the help of a psychologist who taught him to use mental imagery and self-hypnosis.[18] The imagery involved characters from *Star Wars* who had a special medicine that would eliminate the cough. His cough quickly subsided, and he was able to return to school. When coughing recurred, he returned to his *Star Wars* companions, whose imaginary ministrations restored his health.

Another behavioral technique is to simply *count and record* the number of coughs per half hour. This is done several times over the course of the day. Sometimes the coughing will decrease with counting alone. You can also give your child stickers or other rewards for reducing the number of times he coughs per hour. As he achieves the goal, praise him, reward him, and set a new goal.

## BIOMECHANICAL THERAPIES: MASSAGE, SPINAL ADJUSTMENT, SURGERY

## Massage

Millions of parents and children around the world can attest to the healing power of a chest rub when a child has a cough or cold. If you haven't tried it yet, do. The old standbys are Vicks VapoRub and mentholatum. Alternatively, consider mixing vegetable oil (5 teaspoons) with 2 to 3 drops of essential oils of eucalyptus, lavender, pine, or thyme for a pleasant-smelling rub. Place a bit of the oil in your palm, and rub your hands together until they are warm. Massage your child's chest, neck, and upper back with this mixture.

## Spinal Adjustment

There are no studies showing that chiropractic or osteopathic adjustments benefit children suffering from any kind of cough. Stick with massage; if parents provide it, it is far less expensive than a visit to any kind of health care professional, and there are better data to support massage than spinal adjustment.

## Surgery

Surgery is rarely necessary *unless* your child has gotten food (such as a peanut, raisin, or piece of hot dog) or a toy down the wrong pipe (aspirated it), and it has landed in the lungs. In this case, bronchoscopic surgery (in which a fiber-optic tube is placed down the airway so that the object can be seen and removed) might be necessary. *If your child aspirates (chokes on) something, take him to an emergency room immediately.*

## BIOENERGETIC THERAPIES: ACUPUNCTURE, THERAPEUTIC TOUCH/REIKI/HEALING TOUCH, PRAYER, HOMEOPATHY

## Acupuncture

In China, coughs have been treated with acupuncture for many years. In one series of patients with different kinds of cough, cupping (a variation of acupuncture treatment) for five to ten minutes was helpful.[19] However, this study did not include a control (comparison) group of untreated patients, so it is impossible to tell how many would have improved anyway. I do *not* regularly recommend acupuncture as therapy for common coughs. On the other hand, I've seen a number of patients with cystic fibrosis whose breathing improved remarkably after acupuncture treatments; these patients now request acupuncture whenever they're admitted to the hospital with pneumonia because they know it makes them feel better.

## Therapeutic Touch/Reiki/Healing Touch

Similarly, there are no studies evaluating the impact of any kind of hands-on healing technique in treating children's coughs. However, I've watched kids with asthma, pneumonia, and even kids on breathing machines (ventilators) have an easier time breathing when I treated them with these techniques. One young woman who had cystic fibrosis had such severe coughing following a bronchoscopy that the anesthesiologist was forced to put her back under anesthesia to help her breathe again; the woman's mother insisted that the anesthesiologist call me because she'd seen her daughter improve when I'd treated her. Within minutes of my arrival, the young woman no longer required the powerful medicines to quell her coughing spasms and was able to breathe and talk easily. Was it the Therapeutic Touch, a conditioned response, or just good timing? More research is needed to answer this question for sure; in the meantime, I'm going to continue to offer these hands on healing techniques because they seem helpful and calming and have no serious side effects.

## Prayer

Similarly, despite the lack of randomized controlled clinical trials, I recommend prayer for folks who have values that support prayer. People who pray tend to be healthier and more confident and to experience less suffering. I've seen many children respond to the calm presence of people praying for them. Faith is a balm for the weary spirit and body.

## Homeopathy

Commonly recommended homeopathic treatments for *dry, barky coughs* (such as croup) are *Aconitum, Belladonna* (use homeopathic doses only; more concentrated doses can be poisonous), *Ipecac, Phosphorous, Rumex,* and

*Spongia.* For *productive (wet) coughs* with much mucus *Euphrasia* (eyebright) and *Natrum sulphuricum* (sodium sulphate) are used. *Pulsatilla* is recommended for several types of childhood coughs. None has undergone comparison studies in children with coughs. They are very safe, but should not be used as a substitute for proven medical therapies for serious coughing problems like tuberculosis, asthma, or cystic fibrosis.

## WHAT I RECOMMEND FOR COUGHS

### PREVENTING COUGHS

1. *Lifestyle—environment.* Avoid exposure to cigarette smoke and other irritants. Avoid exposure to sick, coughing children. Discourage cough-causing mold and dust mites by keeping the humidity under 50% and thoroughly cleaning your home weekly.

2. *Biochemical—medications.* Have your child immunized against pertussis (whooping cough), pneumococcus, and influenza. Treat underlying illnesses such as asthma and allergies (see Chapters 4 and 5).

3. *Lifestyle—nutrition.* Make sure your child eats a diet rich in fish and fruits that contain vitamin C.

---

*Take your child to a health care provider if he is:*

- Coughing so hard he can't catch his breath

- Coughing up blood

- Wheezing

- Breathing very fast

- Turning blue in lips or fingernails

- Lethargic

*Or if he has:*

- Pain in the chest for more than a day

- Headache or facial pain as well as coughing

- A fever over 103.9°F

- A persistent cough that has not improved with home remedies

---

## TREATING COUGHS

1. *Lifestyle—nutrition.* Encourage your child to drink plenty of fluids to keep the mucus and phlegm loose so it is easier to cough up.

2. *Lifestyle—exercise.* Encourage your child to rest. To help drain phlegm from the lungs of a child with a wet cough, have her lie with her head and chest hanging down off the edge of the bed for five to ten minutes. Then have her cough hard to clear the phlegm.

3. *Lifestyle—environment.* Try a humidifier, vaporizer, or steam treatment. Consider adding essential oils of menthol (mint).

4. *Biochemical—medications, herbs.* Hard candy, herbal cough syrups, cough drops, and hot tea with honey may help soothe a throat irritated by coughing. Antibiotics may be necessary for pneumonia. Other medications as needed depending on the underlying cause. There is no need for guaifenesin, dextromethorphan, or codeine in kids less than twelve years old.

5. *Bioenergetic—Therapeutic Touch/Reiki.* Try Therapeutic Touch, Reiki, or other forms of hands-on healing.

6. *Bioenergetic—prayer.* If it is consistent with your family's beliefs, pray. Prayer helps calm the mind and spirit and can ease many symptoms.

RESOURCES

*Internet*

American Academy of Family Practice
http://www.aafp.org/afp/981015ap/
dowell.html

Kids Health (Nemours Foundation)
http://kidshealth.org/parent/general/sick/
childs_cough.html

University of Cincinnati Medical Center
http://medcenter.uc.edu/news/
99whooping.ucm

University of Pittsburgh
http://www.hsls.pitt.edu/curric/camc/
cough/cough.html

# 14

# CRADLE CAP

*Joan Andrews brought in her son, Jeremy, for a two-month checkup, frantic at his appearance. "He's being christened next week, and just look at his head," she lamented. Jeremy had a large patch of cradle cap on his scalp. Joan wanted to know if there was anything she could do or if he would have to wear a hat until he graduated from college.*

Cradle cap is a thick, greasy-looking yellow or white crusting rash on the baby's scalp. The skin underneath is often red and irritated-looking. It is also known as infantile seborrheic dermatitis—red, flaking skin on the forehead, scalp, behind the ears, under the armpits, and in the groin. As awful as it looks, it is not itchy or painful. It usually bothers parents much more than it bothers the baby.

Cradle cap often begins unnoticed behind the ears and spreads to the scalp and eyebrows. It usually starts when the baby is two weeks to three months old and can last into the toddler years. Some studies suggest that babies who develop cradle cap have a slightly increased risk of developing seborrhea when they are older. Seborrhea is caused by an overactivity of the skin's sebum glands and sometimes by a yeast called *Pityrosporum ovale*. It seems to be more common where the skin is slightly warmer, such as the scalp.[1] It is *not* caused by poor hygiene or poor parenting, and it is *not* caused by vitamin deficiencies. Washing more frequently or with harsh soaps often just makes seborrhea worse and definitely irritates the child.

Rarely children have cradle cap as a symptom of a severe defect in their immune system. These babies also grow poorly and have diarrhea. If your baby has other problems besides cradle cap, please have him evaluated by a health care professional.

## TREATMENTS FOR CRADLE CAP

Cradle cap eventually resolves on its own regardless of what you do. Though there are a few time-honored home remedies, the primary modern treatments are medicated shampoos, moisturizers, oils, and patience. Let's tour the Therapeutic Mountain to find out what works and what doesn't. If you want to skip to my bottom-line recommendations, flip to the end of the chapter.

## BIOCHEMICAL THERAPIES: MEDICATIONS, HERBS, NUTRITIONAL SUPPLEMENTS

### Medications

The main medical therapies are medicated shampoos, hydrocortisone cream, and anti-yeast medications.

#### MEDICATED SHAMPOOS AND CREAMS

- Selenium sulfide (Selsun Blue and others)
- Pyrithione zinc (Danex and others)
- Coal tar derivatives (Tegrin Medicated and others)
- Combinations (Sebulex—sulfur and salicylic acid, Neutrogena T/Sal—coal tar and salicylic acid, Sebex T—coal tar, colloidal sulfur, salicylic acid)

Selenium sulfide shampoo (such as Selsun Blue) and pyrithione zinc (Danex) slow skin turnover on the scalp, reducing the flaking and scaling symptoms. Coal tar derivatives (such as pine tar soap) are commonly used folk remedies for scaling skin conditions such as seborrhea, but they can irritate the skin and may make it more sun sensisive; they also smell awful. Coal tar is *not* recommended for children under two years old. Be careful not to get any of these products in your child's eyes. If they make the scalp more irritated, discontinue use and consult your health care professional.

For infants whose cradle cap does not respond to medicated shampoos, a mild hydrocortisone cream often does the trick. You don't need anything stronger than 0.5% or 1% hydrocortisone (available without a prescription) applied two or three times daily. Although it helped with the skin rash in my son, I stopped using it because I didn't like how his hair looked when it was all goopy with cream. I ended up washing his hair more often, and I didn't think it was worth it to treat what is essentially a cosmetic problem rather than a health problem.

Because the yeast *P. ovale* is more common on the scalps of babies with cradle cap, some dermatologists recommend prescription antiyeast medications such as ketoconazole (Nizoral) cream or shampoo. It works well and is not absorbed into the system, so it has few, if any, side effects.[2] Ketoconazole shampoo is now available without a prescription.

### Herbs

Some herbalists recommend washing the baby's scalp with a tepid tea made from burdock, chamomile, comfrey root, meadow sweet, slippery elm bark, or plain tea. Others put goldenseal tincture directly on the rash. Cocoa butter is another old-fashioned home remedy to rub into the scalp of babies suffering from cradle cap; cocoa butter may soften the crusting so it is easier to remove. Swedish herbalists use borage oil massage for cradle cap.[3] This makes more sense than any other herbal remedy, but has not been thoroughly evaluated in American scientific studies. If you want to try an herbal home remedy, go ahead, but if your baby develops any increased irritation, stop the remedy and see your health care professional.

### Nutritional Supplements

The old theory that biotin deficiency caused cradle cap has been proved false. Some practitioners also recommend supplementing the diet with essential fatty acids such as evening primrose oil. This has also *not* proven helpful. If your baby is growing well and does not have other symptoms, he does *not* need nutritional supplements for cradle cap.

## LIFESTYLE THERAPIES: ENVIRONMENT, MIND-BODY

### Environment

My favorite treatment for seborrhea was taught me by an Italian pediatrician. After washing the baby's scalp with plain water, massage in a little extra virgin olive oil. The olive oil softens the scales so they are easier to remove. Gently comb out the loose scales or flakes of skin. Do *not* try to remove scales that still adhere to the skin, because you could cause further irritation and bleeding. There are no scientific studies of this time-honored treatment, and I honestly can't say that extra virgin oil is more effective than plain olive oil, but I have recommended this traditional treatment for years. It is safe, relatively inexpensive, and readily available. Other practitioners recommend wheat germ oil or other oils. Use what you have on hand; discontinue any treatment if your baby's rash becomes worse or looks irritated.

### Mind-Body

The only effective mind-body therapy for cradle cap is patience!

## BIOMECHANICAL THERAPIES

### Massage

Aromatherapists recommend adding a drop or two of essential oil of lavender to one teaspoon of vegetable oil as a massage oil for the scalp. There are no scientific studies evaluating the effectiveness of essential oils in treating this or any other pediatric problem, but lavender oil is probably safe and is easily obtained from health food stores. Many aromatic oils kill bacteria and fungi that may contribute to rashes. If you would like to give lavender a try, go ahead, but discontinue use if your baby's scalp gets worse or becomes irritated.

There's no role for *spinal adjustment* or *surgery* in caring for cradle cap.

## BIOENERGETIC THERAPIES

There are no studies evaluating the effectiveness of any of these therapies in treating babies suffering from cradle cap. This is one situation where I did *not* find that Therapeutic Touch, Reiki, or any other hands-on healing technique was particularly helpful. Though I believe that prayer helped me feel calmer and more confident about my son's scalp, I never saw any direct impact on his skin.

# WHAT I RECOMMEND FOR CRADLE CAP

---

*See your health care professional if:*

- The rash does not improve with home remedies

- The rash gets worse, spreads, or looks infected

- Your baby has other symptoms such as poor growth or diarrhea

- You are concerned about the rash or other symptoms

---

1. *Lifestyle—environment.* Use only water or olive oil to wash your baby's scalp. Avoid irritating soaps.

2. *Biomechanical—massage.* Massage the scalp with pure olive oil or other vegetable oil or borage oil. Consider adding a drop of lavender oil to one teaspoon of vegetable oil. Then gently comb out the loosened flakes, or rub them loose with a soft toothbrush.

3. *Biochemical—medications.* Consider using a medicated shampoo such as Sebulex. Be careful not to get it in the baby's eyes. If there's no improvement in two weeks, consider a trial of nonprescription 0.5% or 1% hydrocortisone cream. If there's no improvement after two weeks, see your health care practitioner about the possibility of prescription medications such as ketoconazole cream or shampoo.

## RESOURCES

### Internet

American Academy of Dermatology
http://www.aad.org/pamphlets/
seborrhe.html

American Academy of Family Practice
http://www.aafp.org/afp/20000501/
2713ph.html

National Library of Medicine
http://medlineplus.adam.com/ency/
article/000963.htm

National Eczema Association
http://www.eczema-assn.org/
seborrheic.html

# 15
# DIAPER RASH

During his twelve-month checkup, Carmen Morales asked about a
diaper rash her son, Marco, had developed. He had been on antibiotics
for an ear infection for the past week and had developed a bright red,
irritated rash that was worst on his scrotum and the creases in his
thighs. Red patches and spots led up to his belly button. Carmen had
been using cloth diapers, changing them five or six times a day. Her
mother thought Marco had a yeast infection on his bottom. Carmen
wanted to know if the antibiotics caused Marco's yeast infection; if she
should avoid giving Marco bread and other foods containing yeast, and
what was the best way to prevent and treat a diaper rash.

Very few babies escape infancy without at least one bout of diaper rash. Diaper rashes can be caused by several different things. All cases do better with good hygiene, yet individual management is guided by individual considerations.

## WHAT CAUSES DIAPER RASH?

### CAUSES OF DIAPER RASH

- Irritation from contact with stool and urine
- Yeast (*Candida albicans*)
- Less commonly—allergy, eczema, seborrhea, psoriasis, infection

*Irritation diaper rashes* are pink or red; they look a bit like a sunburn. They appear only in the diaper area and are usually more severe in the skin that directly touches the diaper than in creases and folds. Irritation rashes occur when the bacteria that are normally present in stool break down the chemicals present in urine, forming ammonia—an alkaline (high pH) irritant to babies' delicate skin. Prolonged exposure to wet, dirty diapers is the chief cause of irritation diaper rashes; many are also complicated by yeast infections.

*Yeast diaper rashes* are usually bright or dark red and are worst in warm, damp skin folds or creases. Typically, yeast diaper rashes extend out from the main rash in red spots. The yeast that cause these rashes, *Candida albicans*, is *not* the same as brewer's yeast, nutritional yeast, or baking yeast; it is passed from person to person, not from food or soil. Yeast infections are *not* aggravated by eating yeast. Food yeast and infectious yeast are completely different organisms. Candida also causes infant thrush (a white rash in the mouth) and vaginal yeast infections in teenagers and adult women. Candida yeast can be carried on mothers' nipples, reinfecting the baby every time he nurses.

Candida yeast are usually kept in check by the normal bacteria that reside in babies' stool, intestines, and skin. When a child takes antibiotics, the normal bacteria are reduced, making way for Candida to take over. Thus, children who take antibiotics risk developing thrush and Candida diaper rashes.

Less commonly, diaper rashes are caused by allergies to soaps, detergents, diaper wipe chemicals, or fabric softeners. Eczema (see Chapter 18), seborrhea (see Chapter 14, Cradle Cap), or bacterial infections can also cause diaper rashes. Bacterial infections usually start at either the belly buton or the anus and spread from there. They tend to be painful and red, and the skin is tight-looking. If you think your baby has one of these unusual causes of diaper rash, see your health care professional.

Several things increase the odds of developing diaper rashes. Diaper rashes are more common among babies who drink formula than those who breast-feed. Rashes are most common in nine- to twelve-month olds than in newborns or toddlers, although Candida diapers rashes often appear much earlier. They are very common when babies have diarrhea.

Diaper rashes are most common in babies who are kept in cloth diapers (especially if plastic covers are used) and least common in babies in super-absorbent disposable diapers; commercial disposable diapers that contain water-resistant petrolatum ointments may prove even more effective in preventing diaper rashes. Babies who have more Candida yeast in their stool tend to have more frequent and severe rashes. Antibiotics such as amoxicillin suppress the body's normal protective bacteria, allowing yeast to multiply and precipitating diaper rashes. Diarrhea-inducing antibiotics (such as Augmentin) are double jeopardy—they reduce protective bacteria and increase dirty diapers.

### DIAPER RASH RISKS

- Feeding formula instead of nursing
- Age: nine to twelve months old
- Diarrhea
- Cloth diapers with plastic covers
- Antibiotics, especially those that cause diarrhea

*Carmen's mother was right. Marco had a typical yeast diaper rash, which may have been precipitated by the antibiotics he was taking for his ear infection. Carmen did not have to withhold yeast-containing foods.*

## TREATMENTS FOR DIAPER RASH

Irritant diaper rashes usually resolve within two to three days if treated promptly. *The best treatment for diaper rash is environmental: keep the diaper changed regularly and keep the bottom clean and dry.* Let's tour the Therapeutic Mountain to find out what works. If you want to skip to my bottom-line recommendations (so to speak), flip to the end of the chapter.

## BIOCHEMICAL THERAPIES: MEDICATIONS, HERBS, NUTRITIONAL SUPPLEMENTS

### Medications

Medications help heal yeast diaper rashes faster.

#### NONPRESCRIPTION OINTMENTS FOR IRRITANT DIAPER RASH

- *Barrier ointments:* petrolatum (A&D, Vaseline), lanolin
- *Drying agents:* zinc oxide (Desitin, Dyprotex)
- *Antibacterial:* methylbenzethonium chloride (Diaparene, A&D Medicated)
- *Don't use:* clioquinol (Vioform) or iodoquinol (Vytone, Yodoxin)

I recommend ointments rather than powders or creams because they are less likely to wash off when the baby urinates. Barrier ointments, such as A&D ointment, help keep urine and stool away from the baby's skin. If the baby's diaper is changed regularly, a barrier ointment such as A&D ointment or Vaseline may be all you need to prevent diaper rashes. Drying agents such as zinc oxide, the active ingredient in Desitin, help dry up weepy, oozing skin. The active ingredient in Diaparene is mild for babies, but it kills the bacteria that breaks down urine into ammonia. Thoroughly clean and dry the baby's bottom before applying any medication.

Read labels carefully for skin-care products. Do *not* apply any products containing clioquinol or iodoquinol to your baby's skin. These two compounds have severe toxic effects on the brain and nervous system. Both the World Health Organization and the American Academy of Pediatrics recommend that they *not* be used to treat diaper rashes.

Antifungal medications can help cure diaper rashes caused by yeast.

#### NONPRESCRIPTION CREAMS AND OINTMENTS FOR YEAST DIAPER RASH

- Nystatin (generic brands, Mycostatin, Nilstat)
- Undecylenic acid (Caldesene, Desenex)
- Miconazole (Micatin, Monistat)
- Clotrimazole (Lotrimin)
- Gentian violet

I recommend *nystatin* ointment for yeast infections. Nystatin is a natural yeast killer derived from *Streptomyces* bacteria; it was discovered in New York State, which gave its name to the yeast killer. It is safe, effective, and inexpensive; it has been used for over forty years to treat yeast infections of the mouth (thrush), vagina, and diaper area. Side effects are extremely rare, even if it is used recurrently or for long periods of time. Nystatin can be given by mouth to eradicate thrush and to kill the yeast hiding in the intestines, preventing reinfection and repeated diaper rashes.

*Undecylenic acid* (Caldesene) is effective against yeast diaper rash, prickly heat, and jock itch (which is also caused by a fungus). *Miconazole* and *clotrimazole* kill many common fungi and yeast, including Candida. They are very effective and generally safe, but allergic reactions and mild irritation, burning, and stinging have been reported. Symptoms tend to improve within two to three days, but it takes a full two weeks of treatment to completely eradicate the yeast.

*Gentian violet* is an old remedy for yeast infections. (NOTE: It is *not* derived from the herb gentian, which is a bitter-tasting appetite stimulant.) It is very effective for both oral yeast (thrush) and diaper yeast infections. Because it is so messy, stains clothing a deep purple, and can cause skin and mouth sores, it is no longer widely used. Still, because it is so effective, many grandmothers request gentian violet when more modern treatments fail to do the job.

More powerful (and more expensive) antifungal medications such as amphotericin B (which was also derived from *Streptomyces* bacteria), itraconazole, ketoconazole, and fluconazole are available with a prescription. If nonprescription treatments have not worked within two to three weeks, take your child to be evaluated by a health care professional to make sure you are not dealing with something more complicated than a simple irritation or yeast. Your baby may benefit from a prescription medication.

Be cautious about what you put on your baby's skin. Infants' skin is very thin and can easily absorb medicines. For example, a midwestern baby treated with a veterinary salve, Phillip's Corona Ointment, absorbed enough of the active ingredient (a hormone) through her skin to develop early puberty, with pubic hair and breast development.[1]

## Herbs

Many grandmothers, some herbalists, and even some physicians recommend chamomile tea as a wash for the diaper area.[2] Other herbal teas sometimes used to wash an irritated bottom include chickweed, comfrey, elder flowers, lavender, marigold, marshmallow root, and rosemary. These herbs can also be mixed with almond oil (then strained out) to make a soothing bottom rub. Other herbal remedies for diaper rash are tinctures of calendula, goldenseal, or myrrh (available in health food stores and some pharmacies). Ointments containing calendula, comfrey, or marshmallow (found in many health food stores and herbal catalogs) are also used to soothe irritated skin such as diaper rashes. This is another case where there are *no* scientific studies, but herbal remedies are generally inexpensive and have a low rate of side effects. There are rare children who are allergic to chamomile and other herbs. If any treatment makes your child worse, discontinue it and seek the help of a health care professional.

Another old-fashioned bottom wash is witch hazel (which is drying, as is rubbing alcohol). You can find witch hazel in your local pharmacy. Apple cider vinegar and lemon juice are also used as washes for the diaper area to create a more acid (lower pH) environment, which is less hospitable to yeast infection. Although lowering pH to reduce yeast infection is a good theory, there are no studies evaluating the effectiveness of these home remedies; they may cause stinging if applied to broken or irritated skin.

Garlic has antifungal properties in test tubes and animal studies.[3] However, garlic is irritating, and putting a garlic poultice on too long can cause allergic reactions, irritation, and even minor burns.[4] Do *not* put garlic on a baby's bottom. Berberine, the active ingredient in goldenseal, has also been shown to have antifungal effects in test-tube studies.[5] None of these herbal remedies have been evaluated for their safety or effectiveness in human infants suffering from diaper rashes.

Beware of applying egg white to your baby's bottom as a treatment for diaper rash. Although this home remedy is widely used in Britain, it has caused severe egg allergies. Eggs are a fairly common allergen among infants under one year old; it is not surprising that applying a potential allergen to broken skin causes problems.

## Nutritional Supplements

Babies with frequent diaper rashes have lower levels of zinc in their systems than infants with less frequent rashes.[6] This has led to trials of zinc supplements to reduce the risk of diaper rash. Zinc supplements (10 milligrams per day) may prevent yeast diaper rashes in some formula-fed babies, but they are not helpful in preventing diaper rashes in nursing babies. Breast-fed babies get all the zinc they need from mother's milk. If your baby drinks formula and has already had several yeast infections, you might want to give zinc a try to prevent future episodes. Overdoses of zinc can suppress the immune system. Do not give more than 10 milligrams daily and do not give it for more than two weeks without checking with your doctor.

Vitamin A is used to treat a number of skin conditions. In a Spanish study, vitamin A cream (such as that used in A&D ointment) was evaluated as a preventive therapy for diaper rash.[7] It failed to reduce the number or severity of diaper rashes compared with placebo cream. Although it is widely used and recommended, vitamin A is no more effective than simple ointments such as Vaseline.

Some parents simply break open a vitamin E capsule and rub the oil on their baby's irritated skin. This may be worth a try if you have vitamin E capsules on hand; there are no studies evaluating its effectiveness or safety.

Very rarely, nutritional deficiencies can cause diaper rashes. For example, one sign of biotin deficiency is a severe diaper rash. For babies suffering from biotin deficiency, supplemental biotin may clear up the rash. If you suspect biotin deficiency, check with your doctor. It's pretty rare.

## LIFESTYLE THERAPIES: NUTRITION, ENVIRONMENT

### Nutrition

For babies over six months old, some mothers supplement their child's diet with yogurt (with active cultures) when he is taking antibiotics. The live *Acidophilus* bacteria in the yogurt help replace the yeast on the baby's skin, preventing diaper rashes. The yogurt must contain active cultures to have any chance of being helpful. Check the label; most commercial brands do *not* contain active cultures. The brand with the highest concentration of active healthy bacteria is Stonyfield Farms. Some mothers apply the *Acidophilus* or yogurt directly to the baby's bottom. Others buy probiotic supplements at the health food store and make a cream by mixing the supplements with water or petroleum jelly, applying the mixture to the baby's bottom. I have not heard of any side effects from this treatment, and it makes sense to me.

Many parents have heard that excessive sugar in the diet predisposes to yeast infections such as diaper rash. While it is true that diabetic adults are more prone to yeast infections, it is not clear that altering a child's diet changes his risk of having a diaper rash. Most nine- to twelve-month-old babies do not need and do not eat sugar, yet this is the peak age of diaper rashes. Sugar is unlikely to be a major factor in diaper rashes. On the other hand, sugar intake *does* increase the risk of tooth decay.

### Environment

The most effective treatment for diaper rashes is to keep the baby's bottom clean and dry. The best ways to accomplish this are by:

- Changing the diaper frequently (at least eight times daily)
- Avoiding plastic pants, which reduce air circulation to the diaper area
- Allowing the baby's bottom to be exposed to air

Change your baby's diaper immediately after he has a bowel movement or urinates to minimize the time his tender skin is in contact with urine or stool. If he already has a diaper rash, check his diaper every hour, and change it immediately if it is wet or soiled. After cleaning his bottom with plain water or a hypoallergenic wipe, allow him to air-dry before you put the next diaper on him. You can lay a diaper or towel under him so he doesn't wet his bed or the floor or wherever he is lying. The best times for air-drying are during naps and right after diaper changes. Some parents make sure their baby's bottom is really dry by using a hair dryer (set on low) to blow-dry the bottom. Be very careful; unintentionally, overzealous parents have severely burned their baby's bottom with hair dryers.

*Be careful with the diaper wipes.* Many of them contain alcohol, which can sting broken or irritated skin. Some wipes also contain perfumes and other chemicals that could further irritate your baby's tender skin. Stick with hypoallergenic wipes or plain water and mild soap.

There is conflict between the values of health, convenience, and ecology over which is better—*cloth vs. disposable diapers.* There are fewer and less severe rashes in babies diapered exclusively in disposable diapers than in those using cloth diapers. The new super-absorbent diapers are even more effective in keeping babies dry and reducing diaper rash. Many parents are surprised to learn that disposable diapers take up less than 1% of space in landfills. The main thing is to keep the baby clean and dry with frequent changes rather than worrying about what the diaper is made of. If you use cloth diapers and wash them at home, use chlorine bleach to sterilize them and double-rinse them to make sure all of the potentially irritating detergent, bleach, and softener residues are removed before putting them in the dryer.

You can add ¼ cup of vinegar to the final rinse to make the diaper more acidic (discouraging the growth of yeast), but remember that vinegar does not kill germs as effectively as bleach.

Longtime home remedies for diaper rash include the use of *cornstarch or arrowroot powder* sprinkled on the baby at diaper changes. There are many testimonials to the effectiveness of cornstarch, but there are *no* scientific studies showing that it is any more effective than simply changing the diaper frequently and keeping the baby clean and dry. There's actually one sad case in which a baby died after inhaling a cloud of cornstarch.

*Do not use talcum powder;* talc creates a dust cloud when it is applied, and inhaling the powder has caused serious lung problems in some babies.

## BIOMECHANICAL THERAPIES

None has any proven benefit in treating infants with diaper rash.

## BIOENERGETIC THERAPIES: ACUPUNCTURE, THERAPEUTIC TOUCH, PRAYER, HOMEOPATHY

No studies have evaluated acupuncture, Therapeutic Touch, Reiki, or prayer in treating diaper rash. I wouldn't subject a baby to acupuncture needles, but I might give prayer and healing touch therapies a chance alongside more commonly used treatments.

Homeopathic remedies for diaper rash include creams, ointments, and sprays made from calendula and arnica. Extremely dilute homeopathic remedies given by mouth for yeast diaper rashes are *Arsenicum, Belladonna, Chamomile, Graphite, Hepar sulfur, Symphytum,* and the combination of *Hypericum* and *Calendula* known as *Hypercal.* There are *no* scientific studies showing that these remedies are any more effective than other creams or ointments. There are also no reported side effects.

# WHAT I RECOMMEND FOR DIAPER RASH

## PREVENTING DIAPER RASH

1. *Lifestyle—nutrition.* Breast-feed your baby for at least one year.

2. *Lifestyle—environment.* Change your baby's diapers at least six to eight times a day, more often if he has diarrhea. Keep the baby's bottom clean and dry. Consider using disposable diapers, especially the super-absorbent brands or those that contain a petrolatum layer on the side touching the baby. If you use cloth diapers, double-rinse them. Use vinegar in the last rinse to make them mildly acidic and discourage yeast from living there. Do not use plastic diaper covers. It is better to allow some air circulation.

3. *Biochemical—medications.* Consider using a barrier ointment (such as Desitin, A&D ointment, or Vaseline) with each diaper change, especially when your child has diarrhea, to protect his skin from stool and urine.

---

*Take your child to a health care professional if:*

- The rash looks as if it may be infected (blisters or other symptoms)

- The rash spreads outside the diaper area

- Your child has a fever, decreased appetite, or other symptoms

- The rash is not improving or is getting worse with home treatment

- You are concerned about the rash or any other symptoms

---

## TREATING DIAPER RASH (A, B, C'S—AIR, BREAST-FEEDING, AND BARRIER OINTMENTS, CLEANING THOROUGHLY)

1. *Lifestyle—environment.* As above. Allow your baby to go for a period without any diapers on at all to allow the bottom to air-dry completely. Do not use commercial baby wipes containing alcohol, fragrances, or other chemicals, because these may further irritate your baby's skin. Use a clean washcloth and plain water. Do *not* use talcum powder; inhaling it can cause lung problems.

2. *Lifestyle—nutrition.* Breast-feed your baby for at least a year. If you are feeding your baby formula, consider supplementing his diet with 10 milligrams per day of

zinc. Consider using yogurt with live cultures to restore the "good" bacteria to the diaper area. Try giving it by mouth (½ to 1 cup daily), or apply directly to the baby's bottom. Alternatively, you can provide *Lactobacillus* supplements mixed in with baby's other food.

3. *Biochemical—medications.* For yeast diaper rashes, try nonprescription barrier ointments containing nystatin (Mycostatin, Nilstat), undecylenic acid (Caldesene), clotrimazole (Lotrimin), or miconazole (Monistat). If none of these are helpful, see your health care professional about prescription medications.

## RESOURCES

### *Internet*

American Academy of Family Practice
http://www.aafp.org/afp/20000115/
20000115b.html

American Academy of Pediatrics
http://www.aap.org/family/diapr.htm

David and Lucile Packard Children's Hospital
http://www.kidsource.com/lspchs/
diaper.rash.html

The Longwood Herbal Task Force
(information about herbal remedies)
http://www.mcp.edu/herbal/

The Mayo Clinic
http://www.mayohealth.org/mayo/9905/
htm/rash.htm

Pampers
http://www.pampers.com/primer/
3321.html

# 16
# DIARRHEA

The morning after her family picnic, Suzanne Cooper awoke with diarrhea. Her stools were so watery they ran out of her diaper and down her leg. What a mess! No one else was sick, and she wasn't vomiting. Her parents wondered if it was something she ate or one of those viruses that made weekly rounds at her day care center. Her grandmother encouraged them to feed her flat soda. Their neighbor said to stop all milk products. Her aunt said to feed her whatever she wanted. Her father, Joe, had several questions for me:

• Did Suzanne need to come in to the office to be seen?
• How would he know if she was dehydrated?
• Besides food poisoning and the flu, why do children get diarrhea?
• How could he prevent Suzanne from getting it again?
• What was the best way to treat her now that she was sick?

Sooner or later all parents deal with diarrhea. The average child younger than five years old has two to three episodes a year. Diarrhea is simply when children have more stools than is normal for them, especially if the stools are runny or watery. The normal number of stools varies from child to child; it also varies with the child's diet. Breast-fed babies can have a bowel movement as often as after every meal.

Diarrhea is the body's way of getting rid of toxins, bacteria, and parasites. It usually lasts a day or two, but it may last for a week. Diarrhea is not life-threatening unless the child becomes severely dehydrated or the diarrhea is a symptom of an underlying problem.

This chapter is about *acute diarrhea* (diarrhea that lasts less than ten days). If your child has *chronic diarrhea* (diarrhea that has lasted weeks to months) and is not growing well or gaining weight, please take her to a health care provider for a complete evaluation. Your child could have a problem absorbing nutrients (such as milk sugar or wheat gluten), serious inflammation in some part of the intestinal tract (such as Crohn's disease), a genetic problem affecting intestinal contractions or a problem that requires surgery (such as Hirschprung's disease).

Worldwide, diarrhea is the leading cause of childhood death; fatal cases almost always occur in malnourished children under five years old. There are many fewer deaths due to diarrhea in the United States (about 300 per year) than in most other parts of the world, but diarrhea causes plenty of suffering even here in the land of plenty. Almost all diarrhea deaths are due to dehydration. What are the most worrisome symptoms?

These may be signs that your child has something other than simple diarrhea or needs more therapy than you can provide at home.

## HOW DO YOU KNOW IF YOUR CHILD IS BECOMING DEHYDRATED?

- She voids (pees/urinates) less than four times per day or less than half of what is normal for her
- She doesn't have tears when she cries
- She loses weight
- She has sunken eyes, sunken fontanel (soft spot on baby's head)
- Her lips and tongue are dry, she has stringy saliva
- Her hands and feet are much cooler than her arms and legs

---

### WHEN TO CALL YOUR CHILD'S HEALTH CARE PROVIDER

- The diarrhea lasts longer than a week or there are more than ten stools per day
- Your child has a fever higher than 101°F for more than one day
- She has pain in the lower right part of her abdomen
- There is blood in the stools
- Your child is less than six weeks old
- She is losing weight
- She is vomiting for more than one day
- Your child is lethargic, disoriented, confused, or doesn't recognize you
- She is not acting like herself
- She has a high fever (over 103°F) at any time or has a seizure
- She refuses to drink or isn't thirsty (NOTE: it's normal for children to refuse solids when they're sick, but they should still be thirsty)
- She looks dehydrated

---

If your child has any of these signs, she needs more fluid. Children who are *vomiting* (see Chapter 26) are more likely to become dehydrated than children who have diarrhea alone.

*Suzanne did not have any signs of dehydration; she could be treated safely at home.*

## WHAT CAUSES DIARRHEA?

There are many causes for diarrhea. Below are the most common ones. The leading cause of diarrhea in young children is a *viral infection*, most commonly rotavirus. Rotavirus is the number-one cause of diarrhea worldwide among children who are between three and fifteen months old. Every year, rotavirus infections among American children under the age of three cost approximately $1 billion in parents' missed work, doctor visits, laboratory tests, treatments, and extra diapers.

## COMMON CAUSES OF DIARRHEA

*Infections from viruses, bacteria, or
   parasites*

*Reactions to food:*

- Food poisoning (e.g., *Staphylococcus* bacteria)
- Food intolerance, sensitivities, allergies
- Excessive intake of fruit or "sugarless" gum

*Reactions to vitamins or medications:*

- Excessive vitamin C
- Excessive use of laxatives
- Side effect of antibiotics, antacids, or other medications

*Other causes:*

- Nervous diarrhea
- Miscellaneous: teething, ear and bladder infections
- Irritable bowel syndrome or inflammatory bowel diseases

*Bacteria* cause diarrhea in several ways. A few bacteria, such as cholera, attack the intestinal walls, while others, such as *Staphylococcus* (the cause of most food poisoning), indirectly cause symptoms by producing toxins which poison the gut. Other common diarrhea-causing bacteria include *Salmonella, Shigella,* and *E. coli.* Viruses and bacteria are usually passed from person to person, but they can also be transmitted by contaminated meat, poultry, and water. When you go camping and drink from a stream, you risk picking up a diarrhea-causing parasite, *Giardia. Giardia* can also be passed from person to person, especially in day care centers with insufficient handwashing.

*Suzanne could easily have caught rotavirus at her day care. Food poisoning was a less likely cause of her diarrhea because no one else was sick who ate the same foods.*

Overindulgence in hot dogs and other greasy foods accounts for post–ball game diarrhea, but even healthy foods can cause diarrhea if consumed in excess. Lactose (milk sugar) intolerance is a common cause of crampy abdominal pain, bloating, and diarrhea in those who lack the enzyme necessary to digest it (lactase). Cow's milk, eggs, soy protein, and other allergenic foods cause diarrhea in fewer than 10% of children. Children who are sensitive to cow's milk usually develop symptoms within the first six months of life. Undercooked hamburgers resulted in a deadly epidemic of *E. coli* diarrhea in Washington State in 1993. Every year there's an outbreak of severe diarrhea illness from some type of food or water; most of these are due to undercooking, insufficient washing, pasteurization, or sterilization. A recent outbreak of infectious diarrhea from fresh-pressed apple cider emphasizes the importance of good hygiene even in natural products. Drinking too much pear or apple juice accounts for astonishing amounts of toddler diarrhea; these fruit juices contain the stool-loosening sugars sorbitol and fructose. Chewing a lot of sorbitol-containing "sugarless" gum can also induce diarrhea.

Diarrhea is one of the early signs of a *vitamin C overdose.* Children or adults who suddenly start taking 500 to 1,000 milligrams of vitamin C several times a day to treat a cold may find they are having more frequent and looser stools. Children can usually tolerate higher doses of vitamin C when they are ill or if they gradually build up tolerance.

Many *medications* cause diarrhea, either as a direct effect (e.g., chocolate-flavored Ex-Lax, which children may mistake for candy) or as a side effect. The antibiotics prescribed for many ear infections kill the normal bacteria in the gut as well as the bacteria in the ear, resulting in diarrhea. Sugar-free medications such as sugar-free theophylline are sometimes sweetened with sorbitol, which can cause diarrhea. Antacids can also cause diarrhea by drawing water into the intestines.

Several other unrelated factors can also trigger diarrhea. Diarrhea due to *stress* is exemplified by the long lines to the bathroom right before a test in school. For reasons we do not fully understand, some children also get diarrhea when they are cutting *teeth* and when they get *ear infections*. *Bladder infections* cause sympathetic bowel irritation, occasionally resulting in diarrhea.

Unusual, serious *bowel diseases* and enzyme deficiencies can also cause diarrhea. Irritable bowel syndrome causes alternating diarrhea and constipation as well as belly pain; inflammatory bowel diseases such as ulcerative colitis and Crohn's disease can cause diarrhea as well as poor growth and a host of other problems, but these types of diarrhea are usually chronic (long-term) rather than acute (short-term).

The best treatment for your child's diarrhea depends on what is causing it. Regardless of the cause, give your child extra fluids to replace what she is losing with all those runny stools.

## How to Prevent Diarrhea

### TO PREVENT YOUR CHILD FROM GETTING DIARRHEA

- Use good hygiene: frequent handwashing, especially after diaper changes, when cooking poultry, and with toddlers who are toilet-training
- Thoroughly cook all meat, poultry, and eggs
- Use pasteurized products when possible
- Breast-feed for at least three months
- Make sure your drinking water is pure

Because most diarrhea is caused by viruses that are passed from person to person, the best prevention strategy is *frequent handwashing*. Toilet-training toddlers need reminders to wash their hands after using the potty and before eating. Frequent handwashing is absolutely essential in day care centers where there are children in diapers. Diarrhea outbreaks are more common in crowded day care settings than in those with fewer children. Handwashing is also important in the home before, during, and after food preparation. Much of the poultry in this country is contaminated with diarrhea-causing *Salmonella* bacteria. *Salmonella* is killed when the poultry is thoroughly cooked (eliminating the risk from the meat itself), but be sure to clean your cutting board, counter, knife, and hands before preparing other foods, especially raw salads. I recommend that you clean your cutting board and counter daily with a 10% bleach solution.

*Breast-feed* your baby for at least the first three months of life. Formula feeding markedly increases an infant's chances of getting diarrhea. Formula-fed babies have ten times the risk of getting rotavirus diarrhea compared with breast-fed babies.[1] Breast-feeding can also decrease the duration of diarrhea if your child does get sick. Nursing effectively reduces the risk and severity of diarrhea from outbreaks of even very aggressive bacteria and parasites.[2] Breast milk contains immune factors (immunoglobulin A) that help prevent bacteria from attacking the intestines and help reduce symptoms of diarrhea even when bacteria and parasites do get into the system.

Consider feeding yogurt to your child regularly to prevent diarrhea. A study at Johns Hopkins showed that regularly giving infants the "good bacteria" contained in yogurt markedly reduced their chances of getting rotavirus diarrhea. You can get these benefits only with yogurt containing live cultures or by giving supplements of *Bifidobacteria* or *Strep thermophilus* (available at health food stores).

Always *boil your water* or use a special filter when you go camping. When you travel abroad, use bottled, boiled, or filtered water if there is any question about its purity. Be sure that the "natural" fruit juices that you buy have been properly pasteurized, and wash all fresh fruit to make sure it's free of bacteria.

Researchers are working on a *vaccine* to prevent diarrhea due to rotavirus. The one that came out in the late 1990s caused some serious problems, was withdrawn, and so it's back to the drawing board with the rotavirus vaccine. Scientists are also evaluating the effectiveness of rotavirus immune globulin (molecules that fight rotavirus). Preliminary studies show that immune globulin cuts in half the number of days children suffer from diarrhea.[3]

## WHAT'S THE BEST WAY TO TREAT DIARRHEA?

The two principles of treatment are:

1. Address the underlying cause
2. Give fluids to prevent dehydration

If your child has diarrhea from drinking too much pear juice, the obvious treatment is to cut back on the juice. Even if the cause is not so obvious, you can still help prevent dehydration by making sure your child drinks plenty of fluids. Offer something to drink every fifteen to thirty minutes while she is awake. Over the course of a day the frequent fluids add up, preventing dehydration. Let's consider the whole range of therapies to find out what works best. If you want to skip to the bottom line, flip to the end of the chapter.

## BIOCHEMICAL THERAPIES: MEDICATIONS, HERBS, NUTRITIONAL SUPPLEMENTS

### *Medications*

#### MEDICATIONS FOR DIARRHEA

*Do use:* bismuth subsalicylate (Pepto-Bismol)

*Don't use:* paregoric, loperamide (Imodium), diphenoxylate (Lomotil)

*Sometimes use:* kaolin-pectin (Kao-Pectate), antibiotics, immune globulin

*Someday use:* vaccines for diarrhea

Good old-fashioned Pepto-Bismol *(bismuth subsalicylate)* given every four hours has been shown to be a helpful treatment for sudden, watery diarrhea, even when the diarrhea is caused by a bacterial infection.[4] Bismuth subsalicylate contains the active ingredient in aspirin (salicylate); to minimize the risk of developing the serious complication Reye's syndrome, do not give Pepto-Bismol or other aspirin-containing remedies when your child has influenza. Although their names are similar, influenza is not the same as intestinal flu. Influenza symptoms are usually high fever, exhaustion, weakness, headache, muscle aches, and coughing. Diarrhea is not a typical part of the influenza picture, but there's no guarantee that a child can't get influenza and a rotavirus infection at the same time. When in doubt, skip the Pepto-Bismol or consult a health care professional.

Avoid the strong adult diarrhea medicines *paregoric, loperamide* (Imodium), or *diphenoxylate* (Lomotil). These medicines are from the same drug family as codeine and morphine. Although one of their main side effects is constipation, other side effects include sleepiness, nausea, and distended bellies. Some children have become comatose and died from taking loperamide (Imodium). Keep these medicines out of reach of children.

Another commonly used medication is *kaolin-pectin* (Kao-Pectate). Pectin is found in apple peels and is used to thicken jams and jellies. Pectin thickens stools and makes them less sloppy, but it does *not* decrease the overall amount of fluid lost or speed up the child's recovery from diarrhea. It gives the appearance that the child is better when she may still be battling the problem.

*Joe had already given Suzanne some Kao-Pectate by the time he called me. Kao-Pectate is not actually harmful, but the improved consistency of the stools can be deceiving. I urged Joe to continue to offer Suzanne frequent sips of fluid to avoid dehydration even though her stools appeared to be less watery.*

The vast majority of American children with diarrhea do not need and do not benefit from *antibiotics.* Many antibiotics actually cause diarrhea because they wipe out the "good" bacteria that normally live in the intestines as well as the "bad" bacteria that cause ear infections, sore throats, and other infections. Antibiotic treatment for diarrhea is only indicated for children who have diarrhea due to certain bacteria or parasites, such as cholera, shigella, amebiasis, or persistent *Giardia.* If your child is severely dehydrated or has bloody stools, a stool test is necessary to determine if she needs antibiotics. In some cases, antibiotics can actually make the picture much worse, resulting in more complications. For example, in the late 1990s, children with certain serious *E. coli* infections who were treated with antibiotics actually did worse than children with the same infection who battled the disease without antibiotics.

A recent experiment showed that infection-fighting *immune globulin,* helped hospitalized children get over their diarrhea and get out of the hospital faster.[5] Immune globulin treatment is unnecessary for children who have the typical diarrhea that lasts for just a few days and who can drink enough fluids to keep from getting dehydrated. It is still considered an experimental therapy and is not widely available.

A few years after the first edition of *The Holistic Pediatrician* was published, a new vaccine against *rotavirus* was developed and heralded as a potential savior for thousands of children worldwide. However, within a year of its widespread use, a serious side effect was observed—intussusception. This occurs when part of the bowel slides into the next part, kind of like one part of a telescope sliding into another; this can cut off the blood supply to the bowel, causing serious problems, even death. The vaccine was withdrawn. Scientists are still trying to come up with an effective, safe vaccine.

## Herbs

### HERBAL REMEDIES FOR DIARRHEA

*Do not use:* carob, other tannin-containing herbs, Chinese herbal patent medicines

*Maybe use:* goldenseal, barberry, oregon grape, chamomile, cinnamon, garlic, ginger, mint, raspberry leaf, slippery elm bark

There are no randomized, controlled studies demonstrating that any herbal remedies safely reduce the length or severity of childhood diarrhea. Nonetheless, many herbal remedies have been used for generations. Their main benefit is probably due to the fact that they are taken as tea, which helps prevent dehydration.

*Carob* powder is an old-time Mediterranean folk remedy for diarrhea, because it contains *tannin*. Carob reduces the growth of bacteria and binds some of the toxins produced by bacteria. In a Dutch study, carob pod powder (1 tablespoon per day) was significantly better than placebo in shortening the course of diarrhea.[6] Dosages in different studies vary up to tenfold. Because carob is a biological substance, its potency varies, and it is not regulated by the FDA the same way that medicines are. I do not recommend that you rely solely on carob treatment for simple childhood diarrhea until there are better studies documenting its safety.

Many of the other herbal remedies commonly recommended for treating mild diarrhea also contain a substantial (5 to 8 percent) amount of cancer-causing tannin. Herbal remedies that have a high tannin content include agrimony or cocklebur, alder, and the leaves and tops of betony. Avoid herbal diarrhea remedies that contain these herbs.

*Goldenseal, barberry,* and *Oregon grape* all contain the chemical berberine. Berberine kills many of the bacteria and parasites that cause diarrhea.[7] Goldenseal was used by Native Americans to treat diarrhea. Goldenseal is generally the easiest of the berberine-containing plants to obtain. However, because of overharvesting goldenseal is endangered, and most herbalists no longer recommend it.

Several herbal remedies do not contain tannin: *chamomile tea* and *red raspberry leaf tea,* widely used in Europe as an aid to digestion, and *cinnamon,* which is commonly recommended for digestive disturbances. You can add a pinch of cinnamon to yogurt to help soothe the intestines of a child suffering from diarrhea. *Garlic* is believed to help the immune system fight whatever bacteria or virus is causing the diarrhea. You can flavor rice with a bit of garlic. *Ginger* (the basis for old-fashioned ginger ale) is recommended worldwide for treating upset stomachs. Ginger (¼ teaspoon chopped or grated), combined with the juice of half a lemon and 1 teaspoon of honey in a cup of hot water, makes a lovely tea for children with an upset stomach. *Peppermint leaf tea* and *catnip tea* are also recommended for all sorts of stomach pains, cramps, indigestion, and diarrhea. You can also add a leaf or two of mint to flavor yogurt and calm the stomach.

I do *not* recommend Chinese patent medicines to treat diarrhea. Chinese patent medicines are herbal mixtures formulated into pills. There are huge variations in the amount of active ingredients, and about one-third of the products tested have shown contamination with drugs, mercury, lead, or arsenic. They are not safe; they are not regulated by the FDA. If you decide to use Chinese herbs, please see a reputable pharmacist, preferably one at a large Chinese medicine training program with a lot of students looking over his shoulder!

## Nutritional Supplements

### NUTRITIONAL SUPPLEMENTS FOR CHILDREN WITH DIARRHEA

*Do use:* zinc if you suspect zinc deficiency or the diarrhea is protracted; probiotics supplements such as *lactobacillus* or *bifidobacterium*

*Don't use:* vitamin C, copper

*Maybe use:* vitamin A

When children have prolonged diarrhea (more than seven to ten days), they lose a lot of nutrients in their stools. One of the important minerals lost this way is *zinc*. Zinc deficiency can also cause diarrhea. Studies from India, Bangladesh, Pakistan, and Peru indicate that zinc supplements help speed recovery from diarrhea.[8] Zinc deficiency is not common among American children. If you believe your child has a zinc deficiency, a reasonable dosage for children six to eighteen months old is: 10 milligrams of elemental zinc twice daily for one to two weeks. If your child is younger than six months old, please consult your health care professional for a proper dose.

Recent research has highlighted the effectiveness of so-called probiotic bacteria such as *Lactobacillus GG, Bifidobacterium bifidum* and *Streptococcus thermophilus*.[9] These are the healthy bacteria that normally live in our intestines. They can be wiped out be antibiotic treatment and some infections. Giving supplemental probiotics to treat diarrhea episodes can cut their duration by two days.[10] Giving probiotics to hospitalized children significantly reduces their risks of catching diarrhea in the hospital.[11] Probiotics are also helpful in preventing traveler's diarrhea. I recommend yogurt and other probiotics to just about every child I see. Typical doses of the capsule form of *Lactobacillus GG* are one capsule daily for children less than 25 pounds (the capsule can be broken and the contents poured into water, milk, or infant cereal) and two capsules daily for children over 25 pounds. If your child doesn't like pills, you can use yogurt or kefir that contain active cultures.

Diarrhea is one of the side effects of too much *vitamin C*. Do not give your child supplemental vitamin C when she has diarrhea. Excessive *copper* can interfere with zinc absorption and increase elimination of zinc. Do not give your child copper supplements while she has diarrhea.

The data on *vitamin A* treatment for diarrhea have been conflicting. Initial reports from Thailand and Brazil indicated that supplemental vitamin A might reduce the risks of severe diarrhea.[12] Subsequent research in India showed that it did not reduce the number of episodes, the severity, or length of diarrhea.[13] Until research is done using vitamin A to treat American children with diarrhea, its effectiveness remains unproved.

## LIFESTYLE THERAPIES: NUTRITION, ENVIRONMENT, MIND-BODY

### Nutrition

Nutritional therapy is the mainstay of diarrhea treatment.

DO:

- Continue to breast-feed
- Give electrolyte-balanced fluids
- Continue full-strength milk or formula unless diarrhea is severe
- Give yogurt, rice, lentils, potatoes

DON'T:

- Give plain water alone without other fluids or foods
- Give apple or pear juice
- Feed your child snacks containing Olestra

*Breast milk* is the best food for an infant with diarrhea. If your infant is dehydrated, breast-feed more often and consider adding other liquids that have a balanced solution of water, salt, and sugar.

The World Health Organization recommends that children with diarrhea be treated with *oral rehydration solution* (ORS). The most convenient, *electrolyte-balanced liquids* to replace fluid losses from diarrhea are premixed water-sugar-salt solutions such as Pedialyte and Lytren. A new option in the ready-made electrolyte market is frozen popsicles; these are not regular popsicles. They are specially made with electrolyte solution and enticing flavors. Both the liquid and the frozen varieties have been formulated with just the right amount of salt and sugar (glucose) to help your child replace the fluids she's losing with her diarrhea. Rehydration solutions are much better than half-strength Jell-O, soft drinks, or fruit juices, which have too much sugar (glucose) and not enough salt.

*I asked Joe not to replace Suzanne's fluid losses with soda or apple juice, despite his mother-in-law's advice. These fluids just don't have the proper balance of salts and sugar that a child suffering from diarrhea needs.*

You can make your own rehydration solution at home:[14]

## HOMEMADE REHYDRATION SOLUTION

- 1 quart (1 liter) of clean water
- ½ teaspoon (2.5 grams) of salt *or* ¼ tsp salt and ¼ tsp baking soda *or* ¼ tsp salt and ¼ tsp salt substitute (with potassium)
- 4 to 8 teaspoons (20 to 40 grams) of sugar
- Optional: Add ¼ tsp to 1 tablespoon of flavored gelatin for color and flavor

Measure the ingredients with measuring cups and spoons, and use pure water.

Very little salt is needed, and some doctors recommend that some of the salt be replaced with baking soda (usually for children with more severe dehydration) or salt substitute (which supplies potassium).[15] In many parts of the world, *rice water* is used to treat dehydration in infants with diarrhea. Several studies have shown it to be at least as effective as

standard rehydration solutions, if not more effective.[16] In other parts of the world, cereal powders such as corn, millet, and sorghum are mixed with water and salt to make the rehydration solution. An alternative recipe replaces the sugar with rice cereal. A commercial formulation, Ricelyte, is available or you can make your own.

## HOMEMADE REHYDRATION SOLUTION: ALTERNATIVE

- 1 quart of water
- ½ teaspoon of salt *or* ¼ tsp salt and ¼ tsp baking soda *or* ¼ tsp salt and ¼ tsp salt substitute (with potassium)
- 2 ounces (50 to 80 grams) or about 1 cup of rice cereal for babies

*Joe decided that they would make their own rehydration solution at home. Because they had infant rice cereal on hand for the baby anyway, he decided to use the rice cereal–based solution. That way he could avoid giving his children straight sugar and save money. He wanted to know exactly how much rehydration solution he needed to give Suzanne. How much was enough?*

A good rule of thumb is four ounces of extra fluid for each diarrhea stool. Give the fluid a little at a time. If your child is vomiting and you give her a large amount to drink at once, it could all be vomited back up. Giving a large amount at a time can also stimulate another bowel movement, making the diarrhea and dehydration worse. If your child is vomiting, try giving just a tablespoon (15 milliliters) or an ounce (30 milliliters) every fifteen to thirty minutes, and increasing the amount gradually as your child tolerates it. If your child is thirsty, give fluid more frequently.

Despite the neighbor's advice, you do not need to dilute milk, stop milk, or switch to a different formula. Most children recover quite nicely from their diarrhea within a few days regardless of the type of milk they drink. When I was in training to be a pediatrician, I was taught that babies who had diarrhea should be fed clear liquids, advancing to quarter-strength formula, then half-strength formula, and finally full-strength formula. Now we know that diluting milk or formula for children with diarrhea is unnecessary and may even be counterproductive. Recent studies showed that children who were fed full-strength milk regained weight faster than those who were fed diluted milk.[17] Diluting formula will not help your child recover from the diarrhea any faster and deprives your child of needed calories.

There have been at least twenty-nine studies involving a total of over two thousand children with diarrhea to see if feeding a lactose-free diet is helpful. Lactose is the sugar found in cow's milk. Children who are mildly or moderately ill do just as well on cow's milk (or formulas based on cow's milk) as those who are taken off of cow's milk products.[18] That said, there *are* times when it *is helpful to stop milk*.

## STOP MILK AND MILK PRODUCTS IF YOUR CHILD HAS:

- Severe diarrhea requiring hospitalization
- Diarrhea for more than two weeks
- Doesn't tolerate lactose (milk sugar) even when well
- Was malnourished even before developing diarrhea

Physicians used to tell parents to stop all *solids* until the child was tolerating milk, and then restart solids slowly with *B*ananas, *R*ice cereal, *A*pple sauce, and *T*oast or *T*ea, the BRAT diet. We were also told to avoid high-fat or fried foods. There are no scientific studies showing that this conventional medical wisdom is right. Most children do just as well by continuing their usual diet as children who are put on special diets. A study in Pakistan showed that children with diarrhea who were fed their traditional diet of rice, lentils, and yogurt did better than children fed only rehydration fluids and soy formula.[19] A study in Mexico showed that severely malnourished children with persistent diarrhea actually did quite well on a chicken-based diet, and did not need special formulas.[20] Mexican, Guatemalan, and Peruvian studies showed that even beans can safely be included in the diet of children with diarrhea.[21] The World Health Organization recommends that regular feeding should be continued during diarrhea episodes; the BRAT diet is unnecessary and possibly counterproductive.[22] Another medical myth bites the dust.

*Rice* and *yogurt* are the most easily digested foods for children recovering from acute diarrhea.[23] Rice, other cereals, potatoes, and other starchy vegetables are easy to digest and help reduce the duration of diarrhea. Children with persistent diarrhea who were fed yogurt did better than those who were fed plain cow's milk.[24] A Finnish study showed that the secret is the active *acidophilus* cultures: children who ate yogurt with active cultures recovered a day faster than children who ate yogurt with inactive cultures.[25] A French study compared children given jellied milk vs. those given yogurt every day for lunch: those given the yogurt (some of which was fortified with extra *Lactobacillus*) had *much* shorter spells of diarrhea—three days shorter, on average.[26] Homemade yogurt contains active cultures and avoids the artificial colors, flavors, and sugars contained in many commercial brands. More and more studies suggest that giving *acidophilus* and other healthy bacteria (known collectively as probiotics) is an effective way to cut down on diarrhea episodes and to reduce the severity and duration of diarrhea when it does occur.

Extra *fiber* may make the stools look more solid, but it doesn't prevent dehydration or shorten the course of illness. Some parents who are tired of dealing with the mess of sloppy diapers may want to consider fiber supplements. Fiber doesn't affect your child's illness, but it may reduce the mess of watery stools.

Plain *water* is OK as a supplement, but it should not be the only fluid you give. When your child has diarrhea, she is losing water and salt, so both need to be replaced. The intestines actually absorb water better if it contains a little sugar. Plain water does not contain any salt or sugar and is not absorbed as well as solutions that contain them. If a child gets too much water without replacing the salt lost because of the diarrhea, there can be blood cell damage, seizures, and even coma.

*Fruit juices* and flat soda are not as helpful as the rehydration recipes described above. No one would treat diarrhea with prune juice, but many parents don't realize that as little as 5 to 8 ounces of pear juice causes loose stools in many children. Apple juice and grape juice can also make diarrhea worse. White grape juice may be a little better and makes for far less colorful diapers. If you want to give fruit juice and avoid the mess, try white grape juice.

Ah, progress. Now we have chips and other snacks that promise us calorie free indulgences. Thanks to the advent of Olestra, we have yet another contributor to diarrhea. Not that many kids choose fat-free chips for fun, but with the current obesity epidemic in America, more and more weight-wary parents are buying fat-free products. Please don't give them to a child who is suffering from diarrhea; you're likely to make things worse.

*Joe realized that it was time to stop giving Suzanne soda. He put her back on milk, giving her ½ cup of rehydration solution to sip over fif-* *teen minutes every time she had a diarrhea stool. He went to the store to buy some yogurt with active cultures. He made a big batch of rice as a side dish for supper. He was concerned that Suzanne was starting to get a diaper rash from all the diarrhea, and wondered what he could do for that.*

## Environment

You can reduce the risk of diaper rash that often accompanies diarrhea by changing your child's diaper frequently and putting an ointment such as Vaseline, A&D, or Desitin on the skin with each diaper change. Diaper rashes occur when the bacteria in the stool interact with urine, forming a compound that is very irritating to babies' tender skin. If you can keep the skin clean and dry, you can reduce the risk of rash. If possible, have your baby take naps with the diaper *under* her rather than around her, exposing her bottom to air, and allowing it to dry out. Some parents also use a fan or a hair dryer set at a very low setting to help dry their babies' bottoms more thoroughly. Be sure you don't burn the skin! (For more information about diaper rash, see Chapter 15.)

## Mind-Body

Although mind-body therapies are rarely used to treat short-term diarrhea problems in children, therapies such as hypnosis can be helpful in treating older children and adolescents who suffer from nervous diarrhea and irritable bowel syndrome.[27]

## BIOMECHANICAL THERAPIES

There are no studies documenting the effectiveness of any biomechanical therapies in treating ordinary childhood diarrhea.

## BIOENERGETIC THERAPIES: ACUPUNCTURE, HOMEOPATHY

### Acupuncture

In a series of 170 infants who were treated with acupuncture for diarrhea, most children recovered in two to three days.[28] However, there was not a comparison group of children who did not receive acupuncture. It is impossible to tell how fast the children would have improved without acupuncture or with a different treatment. Until comparative studies are done, acupuncture remains an unproven effective remedy for children with diarrhea.

### Homeopathy

A recent randomized, controlled trial demonstrated the effectiveness of individualized homeopathic treatment for Nicaraguan children with diarrhea.[29] This study was repeated in children from Nepal; children treated with individualized homeopathic remedies had fewer stools and their diarrhea didn't last as long as children who got placebo remedies.[30] Common recommendations for homeopathic remedies for diarrhea are:

*Arsenicum album (arsenic trioxide)* for children who are vomiting, have tummy pain, and severe, foul-smelling, burning, watery diarrhea that is worse at night. Arsenicum is recommended for the child who is very anxious and restless. Children with this type of diarrhea also like to be cuddled under warm blankets and do not want to be left alone. Arsenicum is the most commonly recommended homeopathic remedy for diarrhea due to food poisoning.

*Calcarea carbonica (calcium carbonate)* for the diarrhea that accompanies teething. The child is afraid of the dark and doesn't like to be alone; there is a lot of sweating during sleep and the stools smell sour.

*Chamomilla (chamomile)* for children whose diarrhea is related to cutting teeth. The child is restless, whining, or irritable or clinging. He may ask for something and then reject it.

*Podophyllum (May apple)* for children who are very thirsty for cold water. The diarrhea is worse in the morning, and there isn't much vomiting.

*Ipecac* (the very diluted, homeopathic form only!) for children who have intractable vomiting along with their diarrhea.

*Pulsatilla* for diarrhea from eating excessive amounts of rich foods.

*Sulfur* for children whose diarrhea is worse at night or very early in the morning, the diarrhea smells like rotten eggs, or there is redness around the child's anus.

Use only *one* remedy at a time. Do *not* combine remedies without the advice of a licensed homeopathic practitioner. If you decide to use homeopathic remedies, seek the help of a homeopathic practitioner who is experienced in treating children. Remember that the most important therapy is hydration.

✳

# WHAT I RECOMMEND FOR DIARRHEA

## PREVENTING DIARRHEA

1. *Lifestyle—nutrition.* Breast-feed your child for at least the first three to four months of life. Don't feed them snacks containing Olestra or other fat substitutes.

2. *Biochemical—nutritional supplements.* After weaning, consider daily doses of yogurt with live cultures or healthy bacteria or supplements of *Bifidobacteria* or *Strep thermophilus.* Whenever your child takes antibiotics, make sure they eat yogurt every day, and consider using a dietary supplement containing *Lactobacillus GG, Bifidobacterium bifidum,* and/or *Streptococcus thermophilus.*

3. *Lifestyle—environment.* Use good hygiene to prevent the spread of viruses and bacteria that cause diarrhea:

- Wash your hands

- Wash food preparation surfaces using bleach

- Thoroughly cook all meat products

- If your child is in day care, choose one with just a few children in uncrowded settings to prevent infectious illnesses, including diarrhea

- When traveling, drink bottled or filtered water. Do not drink out of streams when you are camping unless you boil, filter, or treat the water

---

*Take your child to your health care professional if she:*

- Is less than six months old

- Has vomiting as well as diarrhea

- Isn't drinking well

- Looks dehydrated (no tears when crying, less urine/wet diapers, dry mouth, sunken eyes)

- Has a fever higher than 102°F or is breathing faster than usual

- Has diarrhea for longer than a week

- Has blood in stools

- Looks sicker than you would expect with a simple virus—lethargic, irritable

- Has ingested a drug or known toxic substance

---

## TREATING DIARRHEA

1. *Lifestyle—nutrition.* Give plenty of fluids (Do not give apple, pear, or prune juice; avoid cola, boiled milk, and homemade soft drinks.)

Give one of the commercial rehydration solutions such as Cerealyte, Equalyte, Infalyte, KaoLectrolyte, Pedialyte, or make your own:

> 4 cups of water (1 quart)
>
> ½ teaspoon of salt (or ¼ tsp salt and ¼ tsp baking soda)
>
> 1–1½ cups (50–80 grams) of rice cereal for babies or 2 tablespoons of sugar
>
> Add a half teaspoon of instant Jell-O powder for flavor/color

Offer 1 tablespoon to 1 ounce every fifteen to thirty minutes; increase as tolerated so that the child is drinking 4 to 8 ounces of fluid for each diarrheal stool in the past hour.

If your child is breast-feeding, continue to breast-feed. Supplement with rehydration fluids. If your child did not have any problems with milk before, continue it or try a lactose-free soy milk or enriched rice milk. You do not need to stop milk, formula, or solids unless the diarrhea is so severe that the child is hospitalized. If any foods seem to make the diarrhea worse, stop them for a day or two, then try again.

Do not force your child to eat; offer her solids if she's hungry and not vomiting.

If your child is hungry for solids, try yogurt (with active cultures) or rice. You can flavor them with cinnamon, ginger, or mint leaves.

2. *Biochemical—medications.* Pepto-Bismol—every four hours (see label for dosing information).

3. *Biochemical—nutritional supplements.* Consider dietary supplements with *Lactobacillus GG* or *Bifidobacterium bifidum* or *Streptococcus thermophilus.*

4. *Bioenergetic—homeopathy.* Homeopathic remedies must be individualized to a child's particular symptoms; consult a homeopathic physician.

## RESOURCES

### *Internet*

American Academy of Pediatrics
http://www.aap.org/policy/gastro.htm

National Digestive Diseases Clearinghouse
http://www.niddk.nih.gov/health/digest/
pubs/diarrhea/diarrhea.htm

National Library of Medicine
http://medlineplus.adam.com/ency/
article/003126trt.htm

# 17

# EAR
# INFECTIONS

Sheryl Wu brought in her three-year-old, Nathan, because she was concerned that he might have another ear infection. He had a cold for a few days and then became more fussy and clingy. He had a fever when he was put to bed at 8 P.M., and awoke at midnight, crying and holding his right ear; he was restless and irritable most of the night. He seemed better in the morning, but he'd already had three ear infections this year. Sheryl was concerned that Nathan had another ear infection and she was frustrated that the infections kept coming back. She wanted to know why Nathan had so many ear infections, what she could do to prevent them, and the best ways to treat them. She didn't like the idea of giving him antibiotics all the time, but she didn't want Nathan to suffer and she didn't want to jeopardize his hearing.

If your child suffers from ear infections, you are far from alone; over 80% of children develop at least one ear infection by the time they're three years old and about one-third of children have had three or more infections. Ear infections account for about 25% of all doctor visits for children under five years old and account for more antibiotic use than any other childhood disease.[1] The cost of treating ear infections runs about $3.5 billion a year in the United States, not counting parents' time away from work or extra day care. About 25% of children less than two years old have had six or more doctor visits for ear infections—that adds up to a lot of pain and suffering for the kids and a lot of time out of work for the parents.

What we usually think of as an ear infection is actually an infection of the *middle ear (otitis media)*. The infection occurs between the eardrum and the inner ear, not in the ear canal. A middle ear infection that comes on suddenly is called *acute otitis media* (AOM). In AOM, the middle ear is filled with pus. After the acute infection is over, the bacteria are gone, but some fluid persists for several weeks or months; 90% of kids are free of fluid within 90 days. The chronic or persistent presence of fluid is called *chronic otitis media* or *serous otitis* or *otitis media with effusion* (OME). Colds and allergies can also cause middle ear fluid; even food allergies can cause fluid in the ears. OME is usually painless, but it can decrease hearing (which can lead to delayed speech development) and predispose a child to another bout of acute otitis media. When children suffer from repeated ear infections, it is called *recurrent otitis media* (ROM). Confusing, isn't it?

Inside the Human Ear

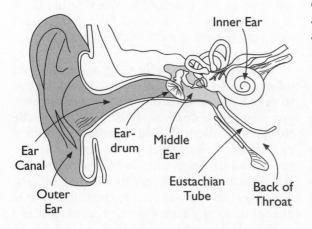

AOM causes a wide range of symptoms. Some children have *no symptoms* at all. These infections are usually discovered during a routine physical exam; the kids don't require treatment unless they have significant ongoing hearing loss or there's some other problem. Most children with AOM have *pain* in the

infected ear, especially when they lie down. Lying down increases the blood flow to the head, resulting in more pressure in the infected ear. This is why children with ear infections are often most fussy at night. Sick children tend to be more *whiny, clingy,* or *withdrawn* regardless of why they are ill. They also tend to *behave as if they are younger than they are;* this is called *regression,* and is a normal response to stress. For example, a sick child may start sucking his thumb even though he stopped sucking it six months previously. Ear infections usually are accompanied by *fever* and a *decreased appetite.* Older children may also report that they *cannot hear as well* in the infected ear or that it feels full or stuffy. If the pressure in the middle ear builds too high, it *can rupture the eardrum,* allowing the pus to drain into the ear canal and leading to scars on the eardrum. If this happens, you can see bloody, waxy, or milky white drainage from the ear. If the fluid presses on the inner ear, it can affect the sense of balance, creating *clumsiness* and leading kids to complain of *dizziness.*

### POSSIBLE SYMPTOMS OF MIDDLE EAR INFECTIONS

- None
- Pain in the ear, especially when the child lies down
- Pulling at ear
- Fever
- Irritability, whining, crying, sleeping less
- Clinging, withdrawn, wanting to be held
- Decreased activity, lethargy, sleeping more, decreased appetite
- Acting younger (regression)
- Decreased hearing
- Pus draining from ear
- Swollen lymph nodes in the neck
- Dizziness and clumsiness

## DIAGNOSIS

It is easier to diagnose an ear infection in a four-year-old who can tell you that his ear hurts than in a four-month-old who is simply feverish and irritable. Ear pain is a pretty reliable sign of an ear infection, but not always! Other causes of ear pain include sudden pressure changes (such as riding a high-speed elevator or an airplane), headaches, infections in the sinuses, teeth, or throat, problems with the jaw joint (tempero-mandibular joint, TMJ) and objects (such as crayons, pebbles, or beads) stuck in the ear. You can't depend on the color of the outer ear to diagnose an ear infection, because the infection is actually deep inside the ear canal behind the eardrum. The only way to be sure your child has an ear infection is to check for fluid behind the eardrum.

### DIAGNOSING EAR INFECTIONS

- Otoscopy
- Pneumatoscopy
- Tympanometry and acoustic reflectometry
- Tympanocentesis

A special device, an *otoscope,* is used to look into the ear canal and see the eardrum. Looking at the eardrum is called *otoscopy.* You can buy an otoscope to look yourself, but it is difficult to do without training and an unusually cooperative child. Medical students spend months and years learning to diagnose ear infections accurately. Exams can be tricky, especially when the child is squirming, there is wax in the canal or the child is crying. When a child cries so hard that his face turns red, the eardrum usually turns red, too, and this redness can be mistaken for an infection. Redness doesn't predict the course of the child's illness.

Health care professionals use several additional techniques to diagnosis ear infections.

*Pneumatoscopy* (or pneumatic otoscopy) is the fancy name for seeing if the eardrum moves back and forth with mild air pressure. If there is pus or other fluid in the middle ear, the eardrum doesn't move very well. I use pneumatoscopy whenever I look in ears. Accurate diagnosis depends on the combination of otoscopy and pneumatoscopy.

*Before I did pneumatoscopy in Nathan's ears, I told him that I was looking for birds in his ear, and that he might feel their wings softly tickling him. He sat still during the exam, absorbed in the idea of birds in his ears.*

Fancier tests such as *tympanometry* and *acoustic reflectometry,* in which sound waves are bounced off the eardrum to see whether or not it moves, are also available to help confirm the diagnosis, but they aren't necessary for most children. If your child has had persistent fluid (chronic otitis) for three months or more, he should have a *hearing test* to determine whether or not the fluid is affecting his hearing. Children with persistent fluid and hearing loss may benefit from therapy with antibiotics or surgery.

The gold standard for diagnosing an acute infection of the middle ear is obtaining pus from behind the eardrum. This procedure, *tympanocentesis,* is done by sticking a small needle through the eardrum and withdrawing middle ear fluid into a syringe. It was routine in the pre-antibiotic era because it helped relieve the pressure in the middle ear by drawing off pus. Nowadays, it is used in research studies, but is almost never necessary for routine diagnosis. I recommend tympanocentesis only for diagnosing ear infections in:

- Children less than one month old
- Children whose immune systems are weakened or suppressed
- Children whose infections have not responded to the usual antibiotics

Blood tests are not useful in diagnosing ear infections or in distinguishing simple ear infections from other serious illnesses such as meningitis.

Ear infections are caused by the interaction of three factors.

## WHAT CAUSES EAR INFECTIONS

- Blockage of the eustachian tube, which drains the middle ear
- Bacteria buildup
- The body's white blood cells' reaction to the bacteria (inflammation)

Under normal circumstances, the eustachian tube drains the middle ear into the back of the throat, equalizing pressure and draining bacteria and viruses out of the middle ear. Several things can block normal eustachian tube drainage.

### EUSTACHIAN TUBE BLOCKERS

- Swelling (from an allergy or a cold)
- Swollen adenoids or tonsils
- An unfavorable position or weak muscles around the eustachian tube
- Bottle propping

When children have colds or allergies, their noses aren't the only things that swell and feel stuffy. The lining of the eustachian tube also swells and may block drainage. Swollen tonsils or adenoids near its outlet at the back of the throat can also block drainage from the eustachian tube. The tonsils and adenoids are large lymph node–like structures located near the eustachian tube opening. If they are larger than average or they swell up during an infection or allergy, they can obstruct eustachian tube drainage.

The eustachian tube is narrow in young infants and grows as the body grows. In infancy, the tube lies almost horizontally between the middle ear and the back of the throat, making it fairly easy for bacteria from the nose and throat to migrate to the ear. As children grow, the eustachian tube becomes longer and more vertical, and it is more difficult for bacteria to migrate from the back of the throat to the middle ear. This is why ear infections are much less common in older children and adults. Some children have less developed muscles around the eustachian tube, and it falls shut easily. Breast-fed babies have about half the risk of ear infections as formula fed babies.[2] Breast-feeding takes a little more muscles than bottle-feeding, and helps develop the muscles around the eustachian tube as well as building a really strong immune system.

Propping a bottle with the baby on his back to feed him allows milk to flow back into the back of the throat, blocking the eustachian tube. Babies who are fed flat on their backs with their bottles propped up have more ear infections than infants who are held while they're fed.

The body patrols the middle ear with *immune molecules* called immunoglobin A. It takes some experience with a particular strain of bacteria to develop the specific kind of immunoglobin needed to manage those bacteria. As children grow older, their immune systems develop more experience and respond more quickly and efficiently. This is one reason why older children tend to have fewer ear infections than infants.

When the eustachian tube is blocked, bacteria have no easy way out of the middle ear. They proceed to set up housekeeping, multiplying like mad. When the immune system gets wind of the situation, it rushes in to clean up the problem that should have been taken care of by an open eustachian tube. The white blood cells release chemicals to kill the bacteria, but these chemicals also cause swelling and irritation. With such pitched battle going on in the tiny space of the middle ear, it's no wonder the child is in pain.

## WHICH CHILDREN ARE MOST LIKELY TO GET EAR INFECTIONS?

By the time they're six months old, nearly 40% of children will have had at least one ear infection, and 20% will have had two or more infections. There are two kinds of risk factors for ear infections: the kind you can do something about (modifiable), and the kind you can't do anything about (non-modifiable).

| RISK FACTORS FOR EAR INFECTIONS | |
|---|---|
| NONMODIFIABLE | MODIFIABLE |
| Age less than two | Exposure to lots of kids |
| Boys more than girls | Formula feeding |
| Race: Caucasian, Indian, Eskimo | Feeding flat on back, or propping the bottle |
| Family trait | Exposure to tobacco smoke |
| Season: winter and fall | No immunizations |
| | Pacifiers |

Several non-modifiable factors increase the risk of having ear infections. Because of the position of the eustachian tube and their inexperienced immune systems, younger children (under two years old) are at higher risk than older children are. No one know why, but boys are more likely than girls to have ear infections. Caucasian, Native American, and Eskimo children are at higher risk than are African-American or Hispanic children. Like many other characteristics, the tendency for recurrent ear infections runs in families. Ear infections are much more common during the cold and flu seasons of fall and winter.

There are also several modifiable factors that influence the risk of ear infections. Children who are *exposed to lots of other children* are much more likely to get ear infections than children who are spared exposure to other children's colds. Child care in large groups (ten or more children) increases the risk of getting an ear infection by about 50% compared with keeping a child at home or being in a small family day care setting. Nowadays, it is almost impossible to avoid day care of some kind. However, if your child has been getting a lot of ear infections, you may want to look into a setting with fewer children.

Infants who are fed *formula* have a higher risk of getting ear infections in the first six months of life compared with infants who are fed mother's milk. One study showed that the risk of recurrent ear infections in babies' first year was about 12% in infants exclusively breast-fed for the first four months of life compared with 20% among infants who were breast-fed for less than four months.[3] Breast-feeding helps protect your child because breast milk contains immune factors that can help fight infections, and it spares your child exposure to potential allergens in formulas. Breast milk is protective even for children at very high risk of ear infections, such as those with cleft palates.

Infants who are fed while *flat on their back* are more likely to get ear infections early in life than children who are fed with their heads elevated. If you feed your child from a bottle, keep the child's head up to keep the milk from getting into the eustachian tube. Putting a child to bed at night with a bottle of milk in his mouth increases the risk of both ear infections and cavities.

Children whose *parents smoke* get about 50% more ear infections than children whose parents do not smoke.[4] *Do not smoke* and do not allow other people to smoke around your child, especially in enclosed places such as cars and homes.

*Sheryl's mother-in-law lived with her family and was a smoker. Sheryl didn't like the fact that her children were around tobacco smoke, but she didn't feel that she could change her mother-in-law's behavior. I wrote a prescription for Nathan saying that he should not be around tobacco smoke because it increased his risk of getting ear infections, colds, and asthma. Sheryl gave this prescription to her husband who gave it to his mother, who agreed to smoke only outside the house.*

*Pneumococcus* bacteria are responsible for many childhood ear infections. Immunization with *pneumococcal vaccine (Prevnar)* and daily treatment with the antibiotic sulfisoxazole results in a 90% reduction in ear infections in children with recurrent ear infections.[5] The pneumococcal vaccine is now recommended for infants as young as two months old. It prevents ear infections and other serious infections caused by this nasty bacteria; it is also recommended for toddlers and preschoolers who are in day care or who have any other risk for pneumococcal disease. Not all ear infections are caused by *Pneumococcus,* so the vaccine doesn't completely eliminate the risk of getting ear infections, but it does decrease the risk significantly, and I think that's worth it.

*Influenza vaccine* is not just for senior citizens anymore. Influenza vaccine was traditionally given to seniors to prevent deadly wintertime infections, but recent studies have shown that lots of kids get influenza, too, and ear infections are a common complication of influenza in children. The vaccine effectively prevents influenza in over 90% of children, cutting the number of ear infections by 30%. Infants as young as six months old are eligible to receive the vaccine. I recommend it, especially for those children in day care who are exposed to more germs than kids who stay at home. And there's good news on the horizon as scientists perfect an influenza vaccine that can be given by nasal spray instead of the old shot. Hurray! Good medicine that's easy to take.

Preliminary evidence implicates *pacifiers* as risk factors for recurrent ear infections.[6] Pacifiers may also interfere with breast feeding. Although I used to think pacifiers were harmless, I do not encourage their use except for soothing children who are in pain (such as newborns in the intensive care unit or babies getting an immunization or circumcision). And I hold out hope that future studies will exonerate pacifiers because so many children are really soothed by using them *and* there is at least one study indicating that they may reduce the risk of Sudden Infant Death Syndrome (SIDS).[7] *Chewing sugarless gum* may actually help prevent both cavities and ear infections (see section below on *xylitol*).

A note about recurrent ear infections: For children who get an ear infection within one month of a previous infection, don't blame yourself or your treatment. Most of the time (75%) the recurrence is due to a new bacteria altogether. Recurrences are rarely due to giving the wrong antibiotic or an insufficient length of treatment. They are more likely to reflect problems in the environment, such as crowding or cigarette smoke, or problems in the child's anatomy or physiology, such as large adenoids or allergies.

## WHAT IS THE BEST WAY TO TREAT AN EAR INFECTION?

Even without any specific treatment, most children (70% to 80%) will get over ear infections on their own. Then why treat? There are two main reasons: ear infections hurt and they can sometimes lead to more serious problems ranging from ruptured eardrum to hearing loss, to infections of the bones around the ear (mastoiditis).

About 30% of children under two years old with recurrent middle ear infections have some mild to moderate *hearing loss*. Hearing usually improves when the middle ear fluid finally dissipates. It takes an average of one month for the fluid to clear out even with optimal treatment. However, the period before two years of age is the time of major language development, and hearing loss during this period may put children behind in their language skills.

Several long-term studies have examined the impact of middle ear infections on children's language development and school performance. Doctors and psychologists in North Carolina followed a large group of children from birth until school-age, checking them frequently for ear infections and monitoring their development.[8] There was *no* relationship between the number of ear infections in the first three years of life and subsequent scores on any of several IQ tests or academic achievements in kindergarten. There *was* an association between the number of days a child had fluid in the middle ear and subsequent teacher reports of decreased attention. Children with more ear infections tend to be less able to pay attention to their tasks and less able to work independently.[9] However, a *much* bigger factor in children's language development and school performance is parental responsiveness to the child and the creation of a stimulating home environment. These results have been duplicated in large studies in Pennsylvania.

If you suspect that your child has a middle ear infection, you may try home treatments for twelve to twenty-four hours before consulting a health care professional *unless:*

- Your child is under 12 months old
- The pain is severe
- The fever is higher than 103°F
- Your child seems sicker than usual or you are concerned about his appearance or behavior

In these cases, see your health care professional without delay. Let's consider all the therapies to find out what works best. If you want to skip to my bottom-line recommendations, flip to the end of the chapter.

## BIOCHEMICAL THERAPIES: MEDICATIONS, HERBS, NUTRITIONAL SUPPLEMENTS

### *Medications*

#### MEDICATIONS FOR EAR INFECTIONS

- Analgesics or pain medicines
- Antibiotics
- Steroids
- Antihistamines and decongestants

*Pain* is one of the worst symptoms for most children suffering from ear infections. Even the most powerful antibiotics take 24 hours or so to improve symptoms; in the meantime, you'll want to help your child manage his pain. The most commonly used pain relievers are *acetaminophen* (the active ingredient in Tylenol, Panadol, and other non-aspirin pain relievers) and *ibuprofen* (the active ingredient in Motrin and Advil). Both are effective pain relievers and fever fighters; and both are available without a prescription. Acetaminophen takes about 45 minutes to start working; each dose lasts about four hours. Ibuprofen starts working a few minutes sooner and lasts six to eight hours. Ibuprofen has another benefit; it can actually decrease the inflammation in the ear that's causing the pain, not just cover it up. This may help decrease the amount of fluid in the middle ear and allow healing and normal hearing to occur faster. Do not give your child aspirin. Aspirin suppresses the immune system, and it can cause a sometimes fatal illness called Reye's syndrome.

*Anesthetic eardrops* can also help reduce pain in the ear. The most commonly prescribed anesthetic eardrop is Auralgan. These medications do not help the ear infection go away any faster, but they can help your child feel more comfortable while he fights off the infection. A 1997 study reported that Auralgan was significantly better than olive oil drops, relieving pain within 30 minutes.[10] Do not put drops of any kind *in* your child's ear if there is anything draining *out* of your child's ear; if you see drainage, see your doctor.

Since the dawn of the *antibiotic* era, the frequency of complications due to ear infections has fallen dramatically.[11] In 1938 (before antibiotics), 20% of cases of severe ear infections resulted in mastoidectomy (removal of the mastoid bone behind the ear). After the introduction of antibiotics, the rate of mastoidectomy dropped to less than 1%. Is this because antibiotics work so well or have the bacteria become more tame? The standard of care in the United States and most European countries is to treat ear infections with antibiotics. On the other hand, doctors in the Netherlands and Iceland mostly focus on helping the child through the pain and other symptoms of an ear infection, while they wait for the body's own immune system to take care of the problem. Fewer than 2% of children with ear infections in these countries get prescriptions for antibiotics. The rate of mastoiditis is about the same as in countries that rely more heavily on antibiotics; complication rates are virtually identical to those in countries that routinely use antibiotics. Countries that use fewer antibiotics also have much lower rates of "smart" (drug-resistant) bacteria; in fact, they have about 90% less drug-resistant bacteria than countries that use antibiotics more freely.[12]

Studies of the effectiveness of antibiotics have been conflicting. Some suggest that antibiotics are not helpful, particularly for older children who are less likely to have severe infections.[13] In the 1950s, studies in Europe and America showed that antibiotics were significantly more effective than placebo in decreasing drainage from the ear[14] resulting in fewer complications such as meningitis and mastoiditis.[15] By the late 1960s, one study showed that 90 percent of children treated with antibiotics improved in one to two days, compared with 75% of those who received placebo medication.[16]

However, an analysis published in 1997 in the prestigious *British Medical Journal* showed that the benefits of antibiotics in children over six months old were questionable. Their analysis showed that antibiotic treatment had no significant impact on pain at 24 hours, and no impact on the number of subsequent bouts of infection or hearing loss a month later. The antibiotic group tended to have less pain at 48 hours, but in order to prevent one child from having pain, seventeen children needed antibiotic treatment.[17] This means that sixteen children got antibiotics unnecessarily for every one child who benefited from them. Children less than two years old are more likely to benefit from antibiotics than those three years and older. In a Dutch study, seven or eight toddlers needed to be treated for each one who really benefited from antibiotics (about half the number in older kids).[18] The tough part about these decisions is that we simply do not know if your child is one of the many who won't benefit from antibiotics or the one who will. One alternative is to let parents make the choice when the situation is not life-threatening. That is, give parents a prescription and ask them not to fill it unless the child does not improve within 72 hours or if the child seems to be getting worse. In a British study, this strategy resulted in parents giving antibiotics far less often while still being satisfied that their child's health was not endangered.[19] I like this approach because it empowers parents while providing support and backup.

*If you decide to go for antibiotics, how do you know which one to choose?*

Overall, the commonly used antibiotics have similar effectiveness. That is, there is no major advantage of the newer, more expensive antibiotics over plain old amoxicillin. And amoxicillin tastes better than most of the expensive new alternatives, too. A large study in Colorado looked at what happened to over 10,000 children who were treated with antibiotics for ear infections. Among those who were given amoxicillin, about 12% needed another antibiotic within three weeks; among those given more expensive antibiotics, 13% needed a different antibiotic within three weeks.[20] The side effects from amoxicillin and expensive antibiotics were practically identical, and if anything, the amoxicillin group actually did a little better! Nevertheless, the rapidly rising number of infections, intense marketing and parental demand have led to skyrocketing prescriptions for powerful, expensive antibiotics.

Amoxicillin can cause upset stomach, diarrhea, allergic reactions, and diaper rashes in about 6% of children; more expensive antibiotics cause a bit more side effects. (See Chapter 15, Diaper Rash) Amoxicillin is still one of the safest antibiotics, and is the first-line medication for children who are not allergic to it. Several recent studies suggest that giving larger doses of amoxicillin twice a day for only five days works just as well as more frequent and longer treatments.[21] Fewer doses are not only easier to remember and provide, they also seem to result in fewer side effects such as diarrhea; in one study, 27% of children given antibiotics three times daily had diarrhea, compared with only 10% of those given antibiotics twice daily.[22] So, for the last several years, I have routinely recommended a five-day course of antibiotics for children who need them.

For children with allergies to amoxicillin, those whose infection does not respond to amoxicillin, or families without refrigerators (amoxicillin needs to be refrigerated), several alternative antibiotics are available. They include trimethoprim-sulfamethoxazole (Bactrim or Septra), trimethoprim alone (Primsol), clarithromycin (Biaxin), azithromycin (Zithromax), cefixime (Suprax), cefpodoxime (Vantin), cefuroxime (Ceftin), amoxicillin-clavulanate (Augmentin), erythromycin-sulfisoxazole (Pediazole), and others. Augmentin has emerged as the leading contender for antibiotic of second choice following amoxicillin. If your child's infection does not respond to a particular antibiotic one time, he may respond to it well the next time. Don't give up on amoxicillin just because it didn't work one time; it may work just fine the second time around, especially if a bigger dose is used. Side effects occur in 20 to 30 percent of children treated with antibiotics. If your child has a reaction to one antibiotic, remember that others are available.

For children who are vomiting or cannot take medicine by mouth for some other reason, a single shot of a powerful and expensive antibiotic, ceftriaxone, is as effective as ten days of amoxicillin.[23] A single shot of ceftriaxone costs about four times as much as ten days' worth of amoxicillin ($40 vs. $10). In an emergency room survey of parents of children seen for ear infections, parents favored the one-time shot of ceftriaxone over ten days of home antibiotics by 4 to 1. For children infected with highly resistant bacteria, three daily shots of ceftriaxone kill 100% of the bacteria causing otitis media. I think this treatment is a little drastic and definitely the most expensive option, but if your child has a very bad ear infection *and* has some underlying problem with his health or immune system, it may be your best bet.

Unless your child has recurrent infections, please don't ask your doctor for a prescription for antibiotics to *prevent* ear infections. Antibiotics do *not* keep colds from turning into ear infections.

Although many children get well regardless of whether or not they receive medication for their ear infections, the current standard of medical care in the United States is to treat them (especially those less than two years old) with an antibiotic. This is not necessarily true in other parts of the world. In Switzerland, the Netherlands, and Britain, antibiotics are reserved for children who are not better in two to three days or in those with severe or complicated cases.[24] In these countries, 92 to 96 percent of children suffering from ear infections reportedly recover within three days without antibiotic therapy.

I often recommend that parents give their child supplemental *acidophilus* or *yogurt* while they are taking antibiotics for ear infections. The antibiotics kill many of the body's normal bacteria, and can lead to yeast infections in the mouth (called *thrush*), the diaper area, and the vagina (*Candidiasis*). The *Lactobacillus* bacteria in acidophilus and yogurt help replace the body's normal bacteria and prevent yeast infections. There are no studies specifically evaluating yogurt in preventing diaper rashes in children taking antibiotics for ear infections, but it is harmless, and many parents report that it is helpful.

A bigger problem with the common use of antibiotics is the development of bacteria that are resistant to them. The same bacteria that cause ear infections also cause sinus infections, bronchitis, and pneumonia. As antibiotics are used more widely, the bacteria start to figure out how to work around them and eventually become totally resistant to the medications. In one suburban day care center, a strain of ear infection bacteria became resistant to four different antibiotics that were used in that community.[25] The development of resistance means that infections that do require antibiotics become harder and harder to treat, requiring ever newer and more powerful drugs to work.

Recurrent ear infections affect over 10% of young children. For children with recurrent infections, taking antibiotics daily is an effective way to reduce the risk of future infections.[26] Prophylactic antibiotics cut the risk of recurrent infections from 40 to 80 percent, but they only work as long as the antibiotic is taken.[27] Once the child stops taking it, his risk of getting an ear infection returns to what it would have been had he never taken any and he is probably at higher risk of being infected with "smarter" antibiotic-resistant bacteria. The American Academy of Pediatrics recommends prophylactic antibiotics for children who meet any of the following criteria:

- One or more infections in the first six months of life
- Two or more infections in the first year of life
- Three or more infections in one year, regardless of age
- Four or more infections within six months, regardless of age

The most commonly prescribed preventive antibiotics are amoxicillin or sulfisoxazole *(Gantrisin),* given once a day at bedtime.

Although I have subscribed to this rule for years, recent studies are casting some doubt on the ironclad necessity of giving antibiotics to prevent ear infections. First, it's well known that the more antibiotics are used, the better bacteria get at outsmarting them, making infections much harder to treat. The greatest risk factor for having resistant bacteria is having been recently treated with antibiotics. Second, lots of times people forget to give the child the medication, and it doesn't do any good if it stays in the bottle. Third, recent studies suggest that amoxicillin may not be as effective as we used to think in preventing those recurrent infections; in fact, it may not be any better than placebo pills.[28] Fourth, the more antibiotics kids get, the more likely they are to lose their normal bowel bacteria and instead become colonized with really nasty bacteria that can cause serious diarrhea. It's a tough call, but nowadays, more and more doctors turn to antibiotic prophylaxis as a last resort rather than a front line.

When fluid stays in the middle ear for six weeks or more following an acute ear infection, it is called a *chronic* ear infection or chronic otitis media with effusion (OME). Chronic ear infections impair hearing and predispose to repeated infections. In this situation, treatment with a *combination of an antibiotic* and *prednisone* (a steroid that decreases inflammation), followed by a second course of antibiotics may help clear up the middle ear.[29] While the antibiotic kills the bacteria, the steroid helps decrease eustachian tube swelling, thereby promoting middle ear drainage. Although steroids can have harmful effects when given over long periods of time, they have few side effects when they are taken for less than a week.

*Steroid nasal sprays* are more effective than placebo sprays in clearing middle ear fluid and they avoid the potential body-wide side effects of taking steroids by mouth because very little of the medicine is absorbed into the blood stream.[30] They reduce swelling in the adenoids and eustachian tube and promote middle ear drainage. I recommend steroid nasal sprays for patients whose middle ear fluid has persisted for six to twelve weeks despite other treatments.

*Antibiotic eardrops* are *not* effective against middle ear infection because they do not cross into the middle ear space (the eardrum is in their way). Eardrops containing neosporin and polymixin may actually damage the inner ear if they are given to a child with a punctured eardrum.[31] I do not recommend antibiotic eardrops for children with acute or chronic ear infections unless the infection is in the ear canal (external otitis or swimmer's ear).

*Antihistamines* and *decongestants (common cold medicines)* are not effective treatments for children who have persistent fluid in the middle ear (OME).[32] Antihistamines usually make children sleepy and dry their secretions. Paradoxically, some children react to antihistamines by becoming agitated. Decongestant nasal sprays do not reach the eustachian tube where they are needed to help drain the middle ear and are not helpful in treating ear infections. Decongestants taken by mouth raise blood pressure and make people feel wound up, tense, and less hungry. Many adults who take decongestants report feeling much better, but decongestants are like coffee. When you drink coffee, you may feel more awake and energetic, but you haven't really given you body any more energy. When the effect wears off, you feel exhausted and need to either rest or take more of the drug to feel better again. Obviously, this is not a cycle you want to start in a sick child. Overall, decongestants and antihistamines offer no advantage over antibiotics alone, and they demand a high price in terms of side effects. I do *not* recommend them.

## Herbs

Several herbal *teas* have been used for children with ear infections, but none has yet proved effective and safe in preventing or treating ear infections. These include echinacea, goldenseal, and licorice root. Other herbal teas or tinctures for children with ear infections include calendula, chamomile, elderflower, goldenrod, ground ivy, hops, hyssop, lobelia, peppermint, passionflower, red clover, skullcap, St. John's wort, and wintergreen. Chamomile, hops, and passionflower are recommended because of their powers to sedate. St. John's wort fights viruses, at least in test tubes. Echinacea may help speed healing from the common cold, but studies of its effects in treating ear infections haven't been published yet.

Herbs come in a variety of forms (dried, alcohol extracts, water extracts), and there is not much standardization in terms of dosage and frequency. This means that the product you buy may be a complete rip-off, containing little or none of the active herb. It might also be contaminated with pesticides, herbicides, heavy metals, or the wrong herb or even medications! Although many of these preparations have been used for many years as part of traditional herbal healing, there is no scientific evidence evaluating their effectiveness in children with ear infections, and I do *not* recommend them as specific treatments to help cure ear infections. On the other hand, a nice cup of chamomile tea can be a gentle sedative for an upset child (or stressed-out parent!). Do *not* give your child ephedra (Ma Huang) as a decongestant; it can cause heart problems, high blood pressure, and other serious side effects.

Parents from many different parts of the world swear by herbal eardrops such as *garlic oil eardrops* to treat their child's pain. To make garlic oil, soak 4 to 5 crushed cloves of garlic in ¼ cup of olive oil overnight. Strain out the garlic bits. Gently warm the oil, and place one to two drops in the painful ear. Please do *not* put chunks of garlic in the ear. Garlic pieces can get stuck in the ear canal. If your child's ear hurts when you wiggle the outer ear or there is any discharge from the ear, *do not* place garlic oil or anything else in the ear canal without checking with a health care professional. Other herbal eardrops include mullein oil (mullein flowers, covered with olive oil overnight, then strained), St. John's wort oil (St. John's wort flowers, mixed with olive oil and strained) or tincture of plantain or witch hazel. Other home eardrop remedies include supersaturated solutions of *sugar* or *Epsom salts*. To make a supersaturated solution, heat a cup of water and stir in sugar (or Epsom salts) a teaspoon at a time until no more will dissolve. Gradually cool the solution until it is comfortable, and put a drop or two in the painful ear. If your child suffers *any* discomfort with any of these drops, flush the ear with warm water or hydrogen peroxide and discontinue their use.

## Nutritional Supplements

Some practitioners recommend dietary supplements or foods containing high levels of vitamins A, B-complex, C, and E, zinc and evening primrose oil to boost the immune system during an acute infection. These supplements are probably harmless, but there is no scientific evidence that they speed healing of ear infections.

I know it's unusual for a doctor to recommend sugar, but the sugar from birch trees, *xylitol*, seems to have impressive effects in preventing ear infections. In fact, xylitol is so good at blocking bacteria, it is used in some "sugar free" chewing gums to help prevent cavities.[33] In test tubes, it stops the growth of *Streptococcus pneumoniae*, the bacteria most commonly responsible for serious ear infections; it also helps prevent nasty bacteria from sticking to the cells lining the eustachian tube, so it's easier to slough off the bacteria.[34] In two studies involving nearly 1,200 Finnish preschoolers, those who received chewing gum (kids old enough to chew gum) or syrup (younger kids) sweetened with xylitol (8 to 9 grams daily) had 30 to 40 percent fewer ear infections than the children who received regular gum or syrup.[35] This is terrific news. The only problem is that we don't know exactly how much xylitol kids have to take or how often they have to take it in order for it to work. We also don't know if it works well when started at the first sign of a cold or in the early stages of an acute infection.

While the studies are being done, I recommend that kids who have frequent ear infections start chewing at least three to five sticks a day of chewing gum sweetened with xylitol. Some doctors are also recommending nose sprays that contain xylitol; but since most kids hate nose sprays, I'm going to stick with the chewing gum. Read the labels; I've found that several major brands of "sugarless" chewing gum (bubble gum flavor) are actually sweetened with xylitol. You can also find xylitol in the health food store and on the Internet.

## LIFESTYLE THERAPIES: NUTRITION, EXERCISE, ENVIRONMENT, MIND-BODY

### Nutrition

If your child has frequent middle ear infections, consider having him evaluated for allergies. Food allergies can cause swelling and inflammation of the eustachian tube and the nose and lead to fluid buildup in the middle ear. By omitting allergy-inducing foods, you may reduce the frequency of ear infections. In one study, children who had persistent middle ear fluid and documented food allergies went on a diet eliminating those foods for 16 weeks; middle ear fluid resolved in nearly 90% of them. When they were rechallenged with the problem food, 94% had recurrent middle ear fluid.[36] Don't restrict your child's diet for more than a week without consulting a health care professional, or he could end up with inadequate amounts of calcium, protein, or other essential nutrients.

Many parents reduce their children's intake of dairy products when they have a cold or ear infection, because they believe that milk increases mucus production. Also, some parents restrict sugar, honey, and sources of concentrated fruit sugar when their child has an infection; based on the theory that sugar inhibits the immune system. No studies have documented that reducing milk or sugar during an ear infection speeds recovery.

Do make sure that your child gets plenty of fluids; your child will feel even worse if he gets dehydrated.

### Exercise

Because one of the underlying causes of ear infections is blockage of the eustachian tube, exercises that help open the eustachian tube may be helpful. How do you exercise the eustachian tube? Think of the ways you pop your ears after a sudden change in altitude: yawning, bearing down, blowing your nose with the nostrils pinched shut, and chewing gum. Probably the easiest of these for children is chewing gum or blowing up balloons. Obviously it's difficult, if not impossible, to have an infant chew gum, but most children over the age of about two and a half are delighted to try. Sugarless gum is best. Beware: too much sugarless gum can cause diarrhea. Don't let your child go to bed with gum or he could awaken in the morning with a gooey mess in his hair. Is there any scientific evidence as to whether chewing gum is effective? Not yet, but it would sure be fun to find out!

Is *air travel* safe for children with ear infections? Yes. In a study of fourteen children with middle ear fluid who flew in commercial pressurized airplanes, none developed complications. Children who are on the verge of getting an ear infection or who have colds or allergies that intermittently block the eustachian tube may experience some pain, especially during landings. If your child has a cold and is prone to ear infections, let him breast-feed, suck on something, or chew gum during takeoff and landings to help keep the eustachian tube open.

It's also helpful to prop the child's head up on a pillow, especially when he goes to sleep. Propping the head up also helps the eustachian tube drain the middle ear.[37]

## Environment

For many years, people have used *heat packs* or *ice packs* to treat the pain of ear infections. Ice packs take the heat out of an inflamed tissue; heat packs increase circulation and theoretically remove toxins more quickly. I have patients who use both. Some parents apply an ice pack or a bag of frozen peas or corn to a child's ear when the child complains of ear pain. Other parents put a hot water bottle, heating pad, or warm washcloth on the painful ear while waiting for more definitive therapy. If your child doesn't respond to warm compresses, you can try ice packs and vice versa. I don't know which of these is more effective (there are good reasons to believe in both) or if the main benefit is simply doing something for and spending time with the child. Please don't use heat packs or cold packs for more than twenty minutes at a time. Commonsense precautions can prevent burns and frostbite.

Another time-honored technique is instilling *warm mineral oil* or *olive oil* in your child's ear (see section on herbal treatments above). Heat the oil as you would for a baby's bottle and make sure it is not too hot before dropping in your child's ear. The heat speeds circulation and comfort, but no scientific studies have evaluated its effectiveness.

Do *not* try to remove earwax or anything else from your child's ear. Earwax, bathwater, and other things in the ear canal do not cause middle ear infections. If you see pus or any kind of drainage from your child's ear, the eardrum may have ruptured. If there is drainage from the ear, do not put *anything* in the ear until you have consulted a health care practitioner.

A therapy that was popular a few years back was *ear candles*. These were special hollow candles used only to help draw toxins out of the ear. The bottom was placed in the ear canal (violating the old rule of never putting anything smaller than your elbow in your ear!) and the top was lighted. The theory was that the heat would melt ear wax and allow it and other bad things to drain out. The problem was that they didn't work; candle wax dripped into the ear and some kids got burned or received other injuries. Overall they were much more trouble than they were worth.[38] I do *not* recommend them.

## Mind-Body

Whenever a child is in pain, it is helpful to keep him calm. The best approach to keeping your child calm is to stay calm yourself. Visualize yourself as competent and able to care for and help your child; visualize your child as healthy and able to heal whatever is ailing him. Once you are in a calm frame of mind, you can distract your child from the pain by singing favorite songs, telling stories, playing quiet games, and reminding him of how much you love him.

*Nathan was so distracted by the idea of having birds in his ear, he was eager for the previously dreaded ear exam.*

## Biomechanical Therapies: Massage, Spinal Manipulation, Surgery

### Massage

Many parents naturally massage an area affected by illness or injury. Gentle massage of the upper back, neck, and around the ears and back of the head with cocoa butter, camphorated oil, Tiger Balm, or Vicks VapoRub is soothing and relaxing. Some parents also gently massage the enlarged lymph glands in the neck. Massaging downward toward the chest may help drain the lymph glands that are swollen with white blood cells fighting the infection. Foot massage may also be relaxing and less uncomfortable if the child is very sensitive around the ears and neck. There are no studies evaluating the effectiveness of massage in treating children with ear infections, but I can't think of contraindications and would love to see a study evaluating it.

## Spinal Manipulation

Osteopaths claim that their treatment, particularly cranial manipulation, is effective in both preventing and treating ear infections. Osteopathic manipulation was one of the most frequent recommendations made by the American psychic Edgar Cayce for children suffering from recurrent ear infections. The idea of treating a fundamentally anatomic problem (eustachian tube drainage) with an anatomic therapy (spinal or cranial manipulation) is appealing, but not well researched.

One of the most common reasons that families take their children to chiropractors is to help prevent recurrent ear infections. Chiropractors have reported numerous anecdotes about recurrent infections that finally stopped after a course of three to five sessions of chiropractic adjustments. In 1999, there was a report evaluating the feasibility of doing a randomized controlled, blinded study of chiropractic spinal manipulative therapy for children with chronic fluid in their ears—those most prone to recurrent infections. It concluded that such studies are possible, but very difficult.[39] The University of Arizona received a federal grant in 1998 to undertake a five-year study to evaluate this question. But even after the results of that study are in, it will be a while before we know how cost-effective it is to try to prevent ear infections using chiropractic vs. antibiotics vs. immunizations vs. stopping exposure to other kids by changing day care arrangements. Even after the scientists are done, the tough questions will always be in the hands of parents. Until more data are in, I don't recommend chiropractic as a way to prevent recurrent ear infections.

## Surgery: Myringotomy, Tympanocentesis, Tympanostomy Tubes, Adenoidectomy

My grandfather practiced medicine in the days before antibiotics. He specialized in performing *myringotomies* on children with severe ear infections. A myringotomy involves taking a tiny scalpel and cutting a hole in the eardrum so that the pus from the middle ear can drain out. Myringotomies help relieve the pain-causing pressure, but they often leave permanent holes and scars in the eardrum. Studies performed since antibiotics became available show that antibiotics are a better choice, and now myringotomies are rarely done—gone the way of the horse and buggy.[40]

Another one of the oldest treatments for ear infections is *tympanocentesis*, puncturing a hole in the eardrum with a needle and removing the pus. Unlike myringotomies, removing pus with a tympanocentesis needle rarely leaves a permanent hole in the eardrum or leads to scarring. However, as antibiotics have become more popular, fewer doctors have learned how to do tympanocentesis. It is mostly done nowadays by ear-nose-throat (ENT) doctors and is rarely necessary except for infants less than a month old who develop ear infections (because they often have unusual bacteria that need different antibiotics) or for older children whose infections are not improving with the usual antibiotics.

Placement of *tympanostomy tubes* (ear tubes) is the most common operation performed on children.[41] This procedure involves placing a tiny plastic tube (which the British call grommet) through the eardrum. The tube allows drainage from the middle ear to the ear canal, functioning like a backup eustachian tube. Tubes improve hearing among children who have persistent fluid for six months or more which could theoretically improve their hearing and hence, speech development and school performance and all kinds of important things. However, there's really no need to rush to place ear tubes; in a study of over 6,000 children, ear tubes provided some short-term benefits in terms of hearing, but the kids who *didn't* get ear tubes placed right away ended up doing just as well by the time they were three years old in terms of speech, language, and behavior as those who immediately got the tubes placed.[42] This is still a complicated issue; we don't know if there are benefits that crop up after the kids are three years old.[43] In the meantime, I think it's reassuring that there's no evident harm of waiting to put in ear tubes, even if your child has persistent fluid in his ear for more than three to six months.

Ear tubes only work until the tube becomes plugged up or comes out (usually within six to twelve months).[44] Two recent studies show that children with ear tubes can safely swim even without ear plugs. But ear tubes can scar the eardrum and cause other complications. No one knows for sure what the very long impact (fifty to seventy years down the road) is of putting a foreign body in the eardrum at age two.

Recurrent and persistent ear infections are frustrating, and placement of ear tubes offers hope for quick relief from a chronic problem. Like many quick solutions to long-term problems, it is usually not the miracle that had been hoped for. Long-term problems usually require long-term solutions. If adequate alternative treatments have been tried for six months and the child has persistent middle ear fluid that interferes with hearing, families might consider surgery. Children who are almost certain to have frequent and severe ear infections, such as children with cleft palate, are definite candidates for ear tubes because they help maintain hearing and developing speech.

Because swollen adenoids can block the eustachian tubes, *adenoidectomy* (removal of the adenoid lymph tissue) with or without *tonsillectomy* is another surgical therapy for children with recurrent ear infections. These additional surgeries done at the same time that ear tubes are placed is more effective than ear tubes alone in preventing recurrent infections and may reduce the risk of requiring subsequent surgery.[45] This surgery should not be sought unless your child has had middle ear fluid for at least six consecutive months despite other therapies.

## BIOENERGETIC THERAPIES: ACUPUNCTURE, THERAPEUTIC TOUCH/PRAYER, HOMEOPATHY

### Acupuncture

Acupuncture has been recommended for treating ear infections, but there are no studies evaluating the effectiveness of acupuncture treatment compared with antibiotics or other therapies for children with ear infections. I do not recommend acupuncture for this condition.

### Therapeutic Touch/Prayer

I use Therapeutic Touch to help me diagnose ear infections before I look in the ear, and I have found it highly accurate in predicting what I find when I look with an otoscope. Still, the otoscope is the gold standard, and I haven't thrown mine away. I also use Therapeutic Touch to treat children with ear infections, but have not found it to be an instant cure or any better than the child's own immune system. There are no studies systematically evaluating the effectivenss of these "energy healing" techniques, but they are very safe and often valued by families, so I continue to use them until scientific studies have had conclusive results.

## Homeopathy

Scientific data about the effectiveness of homeopathy to treat ear infections has been accumulating over the last dozen years. In a German study, children who went to homeopathic practitioners were compared to those who went to ear, nose, throat (ENT) specialists; those who were treated homeopathically tended to get better more quickly and to have fewer recurrences than those who went to the specialists. Only five out of about 100 children who were treated homeopathically ended up needing antibiotics.[46] On the other hand, this was a self-selected group of children whose average age was five years old (when most ear infections go away on their own without any treatment). It is possible (in fact, it seems pretty likely) that those who went to the specialists were sicker and less likely to do as well as those who went to homeopaths. An intriguing result, but a poor study design left more questions than answers.

A British study reported that children who had fluid in their ears who were treated with homeopathic remedies did better than those who didn't receive homeopathy. The differences were not statistically significant, and the authors concluded that a much larger study would be necessary to determine whether or not homeopathy is beneficial.[47] Similarly, a preliminary study done in Boston followed twenty-four children who were more than six months old and who were treated by physicians with homeopathic remedies for an acute ear infection. Most (67%) of these children ended up receiving another homeopathic remedy within a month and two ended up taking antibiotics.[48] This seems like a pretty good track record except that the children treated in this study were the kind of kids who are most likely to do well without *any* medical therapy; for example, 95% of them were breast-fed on average for fifteen months! A randomized, controlled trial is clearly in order here.

It arrived, in the February 2001 issue of *Pediatric Infectious Disease Journal*, rocking the world of conventional doctors by describing a randomized, double-blind trial comparing homeopathy to placebo in seventy-five children diagnosed with ear infections. Despite the expectation that homeopathy would not offer any benefits beyond sugar pills, the results indicated that homeopathy was better; there were fewer symptoms and fewer treatment failures with homeopathy than with placebo.[49] A lot of folks are scratching their heads wondering how this could be, while others (the ones who decided to hold off on antibiotics for a while) are wondering if homeopathy might not represent a nice alternative to watching and waiting to see if things get better on their own.

Homeopathic practitioners use a variety of remedies for children with ear infections depending on their exact symptoms. Most professional homeopaths rely on a single remedy, carefully selected for the patient's individual temperament and symptoms. The remedies most commonly used to treat children with ear infections include Aconitum, Apis, Arsenicum Album, Belladonna, *Calcarea carbonica,* Capsicum, Chamomilla, *Hepar sulphuris calcareum, Kalium bichromium,* Lachesis, Lycopodium, *Mercurius solubilis,* Pulsatilla, and Silicea. In the randomized trial, for example, the most frequently used remedies were Pulsatilla, Chamomilla, Sulfur, and *Calcarea carbonica.* Most parents, on the other hand, simply choose a remedy off the grocery store shelf; many of these products contain combinations of the most commonly used individual remedies. For example, ABC is a homeopathic mixture containing minute amounts of Aconite, Belladonna, and Chamomilla; it covers all the major types of acute ear infect ions in children. Homeopathic remedies are typically given one to three times daily for less than five days.

As far as I'm concerned, homeopathy looks like a promising approach for parents who are willing to hold off on antibiotics but who want to try *something* while their child is ill. Seeing a homeopathic practitioner takes longer than seeing a regular physician, and the costs may not be covered by your insurance unless your homeopathic practitioner is an M.D. or chiropractor. Self-treatment with homeopathic remedies may be fine for children over two years old who have been breast-fed for at least a year, who are not in day care, whose parents do not smoke, and who have had all their immunizations.

If you decide to use homeopathy and *if your child is not better after 24 hours of homeopathic treatment, please have him examined by a health care professional.* Also, if your child's earache is accompanied by a headache or stiff neck, do not try homeopathic remedies or any other home treatment. Go directly to a health care facility to make sure your child does not have meningitis or another serious infection that requires antibiotics.

❋

# WHAT I RECOMMEND FOR EAR INFECTIONS

## PREVENTING EAR INFECTIONS

1. *Lifestyle*—nutrition. Breast-feed your infant for at least twelve months; do not feed your infant while he is lying on his back; do not put a child to bed with a bottle of juice or milk.

2. *Lifestyle*—*environment.* Do not smoke, and do not allow others to smoke around your child; avoid exposure to wood smoke, other irritants, and allergens. Avoid putting your child in day care until he's at least 12 months old; if your child is in day care, avoid crowded settings (more than six children per room) especially during the fall and winter when cold viruses abound. Minimize pacifier use; encourage sugarless gum sweetened with xylitol.

3. *Biochemical*—*medications.* Get your child immunized against *Pneumococcus* (starting at two months old) and against influenza (starting at six months old).

---

*Take your child for a professional evaluation if he:*

- Is less than twelve months old

- Has a temperature higher than 103°F

- Refuses to drink liquids

- Has severe ear pain for more than one day

- Seems sicker than usual, or you are concerned about his appearance or behavior

- Has ear pain that has not improved within one or two days with home remedies

---

## TREATING EAR INFECTIONS

1. *Biochemical*—*medications.* Consider pain medication such as acetaminophen or ibuprofen; consider antibiotics for an acute infection, especially if your child is less than two years old. If your child has recurrent ear infections (more than three infections within six months), consider a trial of three months of preventive antibiotics. After six months of persistent fluid in the middle ear, consider adding steroid nasal sprays.

2. *Biochemical—herbs or medications.* Try warm oil of garlic eardrops or anesthetic eardrops such as Auralgan.

3. *Lifestyle—mind-body.* Comfort or distract your child (rocking, holding, telling stories, etc.).

4. *Lifestyle—exercise.* Have your child exercise his eustachian tube by blowing up balloons, chewing gum, or sucking on something. Prop his head on a pillow when he goes to sleep to minimize the pressure buildup in his ear.

5. *Lifestyle—environment.* If your child has frequent colds and ear infections, have him evaluated and treated for allergies (see Chapter 4, Allergies). Try putting a warm pack or an ice pack over his ear for ten minutes to reduce ear pain. Definitely stop smoking and do not allow anyone to smoke around your child! Try to get your child into a day care with fewer kids and less crowding. Do not use ear candles.

6. *Biomechanical—surgery.* If antibiotics, allergy treatments, and steroids haven't worked within six months, it's time to consider surgery for ear tubes.

7. *Bioenergetic—homeopathy.* Consider a trial of a homeopathic remedy containing pulsatilla.

❉

RESOURCES

*Internet*

American Academy of Pediatrics
http://www.aap.org/policy/otitis.htm

American Academy of Family Practice
http://www.aafp.org/policy/camp/
otitis.html

National Institutes of Health
http://www.nih.gov/nidcd/health/
pubs_hb/otitism.htm

# 18
# ECZEMA

Wendy Fowler brought in her ten-month-old, James, because of his skin rash. He had been seen in the clinic four months ago by another doctor who had diagnosed eczema and recommended hydrocortisone cream. Although the rash initially improved, it was now back; James's itching was driving Wendy crazy, and she was concerned that the rash on his chest was becoming infected. James's father suffered from asthma and allergies, and James had had two ear infections already. He was otherwise healthy. Wendy wondered:

- What causes eczema?
- What else could she do to rid James of this rash?

Whether it's called eczema or atopic dermatitis, this rash is itchy and it keeps coming back. Eczema is "the itch that rashes." Anything that provokes itching and scratching (such as an insect bite) can trigger an eczema flare-up. It starts out red, dry, and itchy. As it gets worse, it contains little blisters that break down into scabs, provoking more itching. Over time, the skin may become thickened and rough like tree bark, and the skin color may get darker or lighter than in unaffected areas. When the rash is well managed, the skin color and texture improve over several months.

Eczema affects different areas of the skin as children grow and develop. In young infants, it usually appears on the cheeks. Drooling often irritates the skin around the mouth. During toddler years, the rash tends to occur on the backs of the arms and legs. In older children and adults, the worst symptoms are on the inside of the elbows and the backs of the knees. High-top sneakers and other shoes that make the feet sweat can aggravate eczema on the feet. The backs of the hands can be real trouble spots for dishwashers, cooks, and others who frequently have their hands in water.

Eczema is very common. By seven years old, about 1 in 5 children have been diagnosed as having eczema; 85% of cases appear by five years of age. As with James, it is more common in firstborn children, those who were especially large as newborns, and those who have eczema or asthma in the family. People who have eczema are prone to symptoms for their whole lives, but they often improve during adolescence and early adulthood.

As if severely itchy, dry red skin wasn't enough, children with eczema frequently suffer from other problems. *Asthma* (Chapter 5) and *allergies* (Chapter 4) are much more common in eczema sufferers. Infants with *cradle cap* are also prone to eczema (Chapter 14). Children with eczema often put so much energy into healing their skin that there is not enough left over to grow well; thus, they may be *thin and short*. The *lymph nodes* in the neck, the armpits, and the groin can become quite *swollen* in children suffering from eczema. The neck lymph nodes swell when eczema affects the face; the armpit nodes swell when eczema affects the arms; and the groin nodes swell when eczema affects the legs. Miserable and itchy, children with eczema also frequently suffer from *sleep problems*, *behavior problems*, and *difficult temperaments*. They are also prone to developing *skin infections* and *warts*. Scratched and irritated skin is easily infected with viruses (such as Herpes) and bacteria (such as *Staphylococcus*). If your child's eczema suddenly takes a turn for the worse, especially if it becomes *painful*, take him to a health care professional to be evaluated for an infection.

*It looked as if James had a typical case of hereditary eczema. He had scratched it vigorously, and a few spots were starting to look infected.*

## Other Illnesses That Can Be Mistaken for Eczema

Many things besides eczema cause childhood rashes. For example, newborn *seborrhea* is frequently mistaken for eczema. Seborrhea is less itchy, and it usually appears before the infant is two months old, whereas eczema is very itchy and usually starts after three months of age. Like eczema, seborrhea tends to occur on the face and scalp, but unlike eczema, it often affects the diaper area as well. *Scabies* are tiny mites that cause a very itchy rash which is quite contagious; its treatment is very different from the treatment for eczema. *Skin allergies* and *contact dermatitis* also look like eczema and are treated similarly. Children can have red, itchy skin from allergies to soap, detergent, fabric softeners, dryer sheets, and nickel jewelry. *Fungal infections* such as ringworm also look like eczema. *Rare immunological diseases* and serious nutritional deficiencies also cause symptoms that look like eczema, but they have other, more serious symptoms as well. If you aren't sure what's causing your child's rash, consult your health care professional.

### RISK FACTORS FOR ECZEMA

- *Heredity:* sensitive immune system
- *Environment:* overbathing, drying soaps, allergies, irritants
- *Diet:* early feeding of solids, food allergies
- *Mind-Body:* stress

Like asthma and hay fever, eczema tends to *run in families*. If one twin has eczema, chances are that the other twin has it, too. A particular problem on chromosome 11 is characteristic of the sensitive immune system found in eczema, asthma, and allergies. Many eczema sufferers appear to have a problem transforming the essential dietary fatty acids, such as linoleic and linolenic acid, to prostaglandin $E_1$. Prostaglandins affect the immune system and many other bodily functions. Abnormal immune function may account for the oversensitivity of children who suffer from eczema, asthma, and allergies.

Paradoxically, one of the most common triggers of eczema is overzealous *bathing* in hot water, if it's not followed immediately by applying emollient creams and ointments. Just as hot, soapy water helps remove grease from the dishes, it also removes the natural oils that protect the skin. They must be replaced immediately to avoid drying and cracking. Soap is generally unnecessary for babies because babies don't make the smelly sweat that older children and adults do. Soap is only necessary for removing greasy dirt. *Soaps* and *detergents* trigger eczema in many children. In my experience, Tide detergent and Ivory soap are two of the most common culprits. On the other hand, insufficient bathing is not the answer, and dirty skin can make the child prone to painful and aggravating infections.

*I advised Wendy to switch to Dove, Camay, or another moisturizing soap. I also encouraged her to consider a milder laundry detergent without fragrances or softeners.*

Other environmental triggers include *skin infections* (such as impetigo), *sweating*, *stress*, *irritants* (such as tobacco smoke and wool sweaters), and *allergies*. Allergies can be either from something that touches the child's skin or from something inhaled or eaten. Children who are allergic to animal fur, dust, and dust mites have fewer eczema symptoms when their environment is cleaned up.[1] Although some parents have long suspected that molds, grass, and other allergy triggers might cause

eczema flare-ups, pediatricians were reluctant to believe that inhaling a compound could cause a skin reaction. However, the scientific data are beginning to support the parents' view: dust mites, cockroaches, house dust, molds, and grasses can all trigger eczema as well as sneezing, watery eyes, and coughing.

Early introduction of a variety of solid foods triples infants' risk of developing eczema.[2] A healthy baby does not need any food other than mother's milk or formula in the first four to six months of life. Children can learn to like a variety of foods later in childhood; please do *not* start your baby on solids before he is four months old.

## FOODS ASSOCIATED WITH ALLERGIC ECZEMA[3]

- Acidic foods, such as oranges, tomatoes, pineapple
- Proteins, such as eggs, nuts (especially peanuts), milk, soy, shellfish
- Wheat and corn
- Sweets, chocolate, soft drinks preserved with sulfur dioxide
- Artificial flavors, possibly salt

*Food allergies* worsen symptoms in about 10 to 20 percent of children with eczema.[4] The foods that trigger eczema are the same as those that trigger other allergic symptoms such as wheezing, runny nose, sneezing, and an upset stomach.[5] Nursing babies whose mothers abstain from allergenic foods may have a lower subsequent risk of eczema than those whose mothers eat these foods. *Acidic foods* such as citrus and tomatoes commonly cause a rash around the mouth in sensitive children. There are a couple of case reports of reduced eczema symptoms in children who were switched to low-salt diets, but there have not been any controlled trials documenting salt's detrimental effect on eczema.[6] On the other hand, there's plenty of salt in the typical diet, and I generally counsel families to toss the salt shaker.

Unfortunately, skin tests and blood tests are not very helpful in diagnosing food allergies. Keep a diary to record your child's symptoms and any foods that seem to make them worse. If the child's previous reactions have been mild, parents can withhold a suspected food for several days, then give it and watch for symptoms. The problem with this approach is that the parents and child know that the child is getting the suspected trigger, and negative expectations are powerful triggers of adverse effects. It is very difficult for families to test and treat their child for food allergies without professional assistance. A strong placebo effect comes into play whenever a challenging, costly treatment is recommended; this certainly applies to elimination diets. It is imperative that such an effort be undertaken only under rigorous, placebo-controlled conditions.

The best test is a double-blind challenge. In a double-blind challenge, the child avoids eating any of the suspected food for a week before the test. The health care practitioner gives the child one of two different capsules—one contains the suspected allergen and the other contains an inert placebo. Neither the professional, the parents, nor the child know the contents of the capsule. Parents and professional watch the child for several hours (up to two days) to see if symptoms develop. If a child has had a previous severe reaction (including wheezing, shortness of breath, shock, or low blood pressure) to a particular food, the double-blind food challenge should only be done in a facility capable of managing pediatric emergencies.

Even children who have proven severe food allergies often outgrow them within a year or two. No one knows exactly why, but you don't have to worry that a current sensitivity (or even a severe allergy) means a lifetime of restrictive diets.

For a while there was a rumor that having measles as a child protected children from developing eczema. According to this rumor, measles vaccination programs were making eczema more common. Not true. Several scientists in Finland actually went to the trouble of studying over 500,000 individuals to assess the association between having measles and developing eczema or asthma; they found that having had real, natural measles actually *increased* the risk of developing eczema by about 30% and increased the risk of developing asthma by 67%.[7] Yet another good reason to get your child immunized against measles—a substantially lower risk of developing eczema!

## How to Treat Eczema

Let's tour the Therapeutic Mountain to find out what works. If you want to skip to my bottom-line recommendations on eczema, flip to the end of the chapter.

## Biochemical Therapies: Medications, Herbs, Nutritional Supplements

### *Medications*

#### MEDICATIONS FOR ECZEMA

- Emollients or moisturizers
- Urea and coal tar
- Immunomodulators: steroids, tacrolimus, and others
- Antihistamines to relieve the itch
- Antibiotics to fight infections complicating the rash
- Other

The mainstay of medical treatment is to apply *emollients* or *moisturizers* to the skin several times daily. Avoid products that contain alcohol because alcohol can dry the skin. Effective, inexpensive emollients include Eucerin ointment, Vaseline petrolatum jelly, and even plain vegetable oils from your kitchen cabinet. Ointments and oils generally work better than creams or lotions because they don't wash off as easily. Hand creams containing urea are also very effective.[8] As awful as they sound, coal tar creams, such as Clinitar, are effective in treating chronic eczema when the skin has become thick and rough like tree bark;[9] newer formulations don't smell as bad as older preparations.

*Immunomodulators* are a class of medications that affect immune system function. The most well known are steroids, but newer medications are invented every day. For example, strong medicines have been developed to keep the immune system from destroying transplanted organs. One of these medicines, *tacrolimus* (Protopic), is useful when applied to eczematous skin. It is very effective, even for severe eczema that has not been effectively treated with steroids. Tacrolimus has been FDA approved for short-term use in children two years and older to treat eczema that has not responded to other therapies. It is expensive and it causes a brief period of stinging, burning, and itching in many children who use it, and it increases sun sensitivity; don't use it before sunbathing.[10] *Ascomycin* is a similar drug under development. *Recombinant interferon gamma* is another treatment under investigation for severe eczema; it is expensive and requires regular injections which will probably dissuade most families from even considering it. Other potent immunosuppressive medications include *cyclosporine, methotrexate,* and *azathioprine* (Imuran).

*Steroid creams* or *ointments* are probably the most widely used eczema medications. They come in many varieties and strengths.

The mildest, 0.5% and 1.0% hydrocortisone cream, are available without a prescription. Most physicians recommend applying steroid ointments after a bath when the skin is warm and the pores are open to absorb the medicine. This application needs to occur within three minutes of stepping out of the tub in order to get through the top layers of the skin before they dry out. If you want to skip the stopwatch, just remember that you need to get the remedy on while the child's fingertips still look like wrinkled raisins. After applying the steroid, cover it with an oily emollient (such as petrolatum, vegetable oil, or Crisco) to seal it in. Stronger, prescription steroids can cause side effects such as weakening and thinning of the skin. They should be used only under professional supervision and only as long as necessary to treat severe symptoms. When symptoms are under control, return to milder preparations. Your health care professional will help you determine the best regimen for your child.

Steroids often improve symptoms dramatically, but they do not "cure" eczema. When treatment stops, symptoms recur. On the other hand, there is *no* evidence that treating eczema with steroid creams (or any other treatment) "drives" the problem deeper into the body or that eczema treatment "causes" asthma or other problems.

*Antihistamines*, such as Benadryl (a nonprescription brand of diphenhydramine), reduce itching and scratching. Your doctor can prescribe stronger antihistamines to help your child sleep when the itching is particularly fierce. Daytime antihistamine use is for those children who can't stop itching and who are willing to be a little sleepy. NOTE: A few children have just the opposite reaction to antihistamines; they get hyper. Kids who react one way to one of these medicines won't necessarily react the same way to all of them. If you don't like the side effects with one antihistamine, bear in mind that there are several other options. Although antihistamines don't cure the underlying cause of eczema, they can help interrupt the itch-scratch-itch-scratch cycle and help improve symptoms.

Prescription *antibiotics* are useful for treating skin infections that frequently accompany eczema. Usually a five- to ten-day course of an oral antibiotic that kills *Staphylococcus* bacteria is sufficient to get the infection under control. Antibiotic ointments are useful if the infected area is small; they cause fewer side effects than antibiotics that are taken by mouth. Occasionally, eczema is complicated by yeast or a fungal infection. In this situation, the combination of a steroid and an antiyeast, antifungal medication may be helpful.

When they can't find anything else to put on eczema, some parents have resorted to *Calamine* lotion. Though it may provide temporary relief, Calamine's drying effect makes it a poor choice for long-term use.

## Herbs

Randomized, controlled trials of a *Chinese herbal tea* showed a significant improvement in eczema symptoms for both children and adults.[11] In test-tube studies, these herbs affect a variety of chemicals involved in immunologic reactions.[12] Traditional Chinese medicinal herbal teas contain ten or more ingredients, and the potency of different ingredients can vary as much as fivefold between different batches. There are several reports of patients who developed severe liver toxicity while taking Chinese herbal remedies for eczema; the liver toxicity markedly improved once patients stopped taking the tea, but it returned when the tea was resumed.[13] There is also a worrisome report about an adult who developed severe heart problems after taking Chinese herbs to treat eczema (for two weeks).[14] Many of these teas taste bad, and children cannot

easily be persuaded to drink them. If you decide to try Chinese herbs, consult an herbalist who is trained in traditional Chinese medicine *and* have your child's liver function tested regularly to avoid harmful side effects. Do *not* use Chinese patent medicines (herbs in pill form) because these products have the greatest risk of being contaminated and causing problems.

*Licorice root's* active ingredient, *glycyrrhetinic acid*, has anti-inflammatory properties similar to those of steroids.[15] Several case reports in the 1950s British dermatology journals claimed benefits from ointments containing glycyrrhetinic acid.[16] Unfortunately, other studies failed to reproduce these promising results, possibly because of the natural variation in the potency of licorice extracts.[17] Consequently, licorice root never caught on as an eczema remedy. Still, some herbalists recommend compresses containing licorice root tea as a soothing home remedy for mild eczema. I think this is a safe home remedy, and I often recommend licorice tea compresses instead of wet wraps for children with severe eczema.

I'm much more comfortable recommending that patients drink familiar, recognizable teas rather than exotic blends. That's why I was pleased to read a report in a 2001 issue of *Archives of Dermatology* noting that 63% patients with eczema who drank three cups daily of oolong tea reported moderate or marked improvements in their skin symptoms; the benefits were first noticeable within a week after starting to drink the tea regularly, and over 50% of persons continued to note benefits for up to six months.[18]

Other herbs used to treat eczema include aloe vera, calendula, chamomile, lemon balm, coleus root (recommended for asthma and allergies as well), gotu kola, and St. John's wort oil (used for skin wounds and infections), yellow dock root, Oregon grape, and echinacea. I like the idea of aloe vera because it helps heal wounds and kills bacteria that cause skin infections; I'm skeptical about St. John's wort because it can cause serious sun sensitivity. Sage, nettle, and burdock tea added to the bath are drying teas said to be helpful for weepy, blistery rashes. Poultices made from plantain, strawberry leaves, goldenseal, and violet are traditional cures for eczema. Whatever the cause of the itch, oatmeal compresses or oatmeal baths are soothing. Despite years of anecdotal experience, all of these herbs remain *untested* scientifically as treatments for childhood eczema. I do not recommend most of them except for trials of topical use.

Beware of tea tree oil, *Melaleuca alternifolia*. Although it is a proven antiseptic, it is irritating and can actually *cause* allergic, eczema-like rashes.[19]

## Nutritional Supplements

### HELPFUL SUPPLEMENTS FOR ECZEMA

- Essential fatty acids: evening primrose oil
- Vitamin C
- Probiotics: yogurt, kefir, and supplements

Because of the presumed defect in metabolizing *essential fatty acids* in children with eczema, supplemental essential fatty acids may be helpful.[20] Evening primrose oil (EPO, Efamol), borage oil, and black currant oil contain high amounts of one of these essential fatty acids, gamma linolenic acid (GLA). A randomized, controlled crossover trial in Italian children showed a significant improvement in eczema symptoms when the children received 3 grams daily of EPO compared with children who received placebo olive oil.[21] A 1989 summary of nine controlled trials concluded that EPO improves eczema symptoms.[22] Recent studies have had mixed results.[23] EPO is very safe and it has been licensed in several European countries as an eczema treatment.[24] You might want to try EPO supplements if your child has severe, recurrent eczema. However, it takes four to twelve weeks for EPO to achieve maximal benefits. If you don't see any improvement in eight weeks, I'd stop the supplements and try another approach.

Other sources of *essential fatty acids* can be found in both the plant and animal kingdoms. Flaxseed, herring, mackerel, and salmon contain other essential fatty acids (from the omega-3 series of fatty acids), which offer intriguing possibilities for eczema treatment.[25] Still, there are not enough studies to recommend their routine use. I recommend that children prone to eczema, allergies, and asthma eat these kinds of fish at least once a week as part of a healthy diet. Unless, of course, they're allergic to fish!

In a double-blind, placebo-controlled crossover trial, supplemental *vitamin C* (50 to 75 milligrams per day—or the amount in one tall glass of orange juice) significantly improved eczema in children.[26] At these doses, it is safe and worth a try.

*Yogurt* is good for the gut. Eating yogurt (and the healthy bacteria used to make it) also appears to be good for the skin. Our intestines are lined with millions of immune cells, ready to fight infectious diseases that might invade through the intestinal walls. It turns out that by keeping the intestines and their immunologic guards healthy with "good bacteria" such as *Lactobacillus GG, L. casei,* and *Bifidobacterium* (the same kinds of bacteria used to make yogurt, kefir, and other fermented dairy products), we can reduce the risk of food allergies, eczema, arthritis, and many other conditions associated with an imbalanced immune system. Mothers who consume these healthy bacteria for two weeks before delivery and then for the subsequent six months have half the risk of having a baby develop eczema as mothers who don't consume a diet rich in probiotics; this is because babies pick up the bacteria living on their mom's skin and if the mom has good bacteria, chances are the baby will, too.[27] If your child has been weaned or is drinking formula instead of breast milk, consider supplementing the formula with *Lactobacillus GG, L. casei,* and/or *Bifidobacteria* twice daily. Even if your baby already has eczema, these supplements may help soothe his skin.[28]

*I suggested that Wendy start giving James evening primrose oil and 100 milligrams of vitamin C mixed in applesauce and that she start feeding him yogurt every day and giving him* Lactobacillus GG, L. casei, *or* Bifidobacterium *supplements twice daily.*

Despite initially hopeful case reports, subsequent studies have shown that vitamin E and selenium are *not* helpful for most people with eczema. Vitamin A supplements are also *not* helpful. Zinc supplementation was *not* helpful for children with eczema in a British randomized, controlled double-blind trial.[29] If anything, the children taking extra zinc had a little worse itching. I do not recommend vitamin A, vitamin E, or zinc supplements for children with eczema unless they have a deficiency.

## LIFESTYLE THERAPIES: NUTRITION, EXERCISE, ENVIRONMENT, MIND-BODY

### Nutrition

Food allergies trigger symptoms in 20 to 40 percent of children who have eczema.[30] Allergies to milk protein are among the most common; other common triggers include eggs, peanuts, walnuts, wheat, corn, soy, fish, shellfish, and acidic foods such as tomatoes and strawberries. Some food-sensitive children notice big improvements if they totally eliminate food triggers.[31] (See Chapter 4, Allergies.) Complete elimination of all possible food aller-

gies can result in marked improvements in skin symptoms.[32]

Breast-feeding protects babies from developing eczema, and the protection lasts decades.[33] Some moms try to avoid particularly allergenic foods during pregnancy and while nursing their babies to provide additional protection to their offspring, but this has not necessarily been proven to help.[34] Still, if food sensitivities run in your family, it might be worth restricting the most common allergens and taking probiotic supplements during the latter part of pregnancy and while breast-feeding.

Eliminating dietary staples such as milk runs the risk of starvation, or at least severe nutritional imbalance.[35] Up to 75% of children on cow's milk elimination diets receive insufficient calcium.[36] Despite the occasionally impressive short-term benefits of elimination diets, ongoing studies have shown that a year after starting them, even children who initially improved with the diet were no better off than children who maintained their usual diet.[37] The emotional and financial costs to the family of a child following a strict elimination diet are high. Even highly motivated families of children who have well-defined food allergies frequently find it impossible to maintain elimination diets.[38] Only try the food elimination diets if your child has severe, extensive (more than 20% of the skin affected) eczema that is not controlled by other regimens *and* you seek the help of a nutritionist or dietitian.

Many children outgrow their sensitivity to foods. Even if your child's eczema is clearly worse with a certain food, it doesn't mean she can never have it again. You may carefully reintroduce it in six to twelve months. If there is still a reaction, wait another few months and try again.

*We decided not to pursue possible food allergies at our initial visit and to wait to see how well James responded to other therapies. We held an elimination diet open as a possibility later if the initial therapies didn't do the trick.*

## Exercise

Eczema not only interrupts *sleep* due to itching and scratching, it is also worsened by insufficient sleep. Keep bedrooms cool to minimize itching. Don't overdress the child. Make sure he has plenty of opportunities to sleep at night and even nap during the day. Sufficient sleep helps keep the immune system on an even keel.

## Environment

In general, heat makes all itching worse. Sweating washes the protective, lubricating natural oils off the skin. Cold relieves itch. I advise many of my patients with a small itchy area to rub an ice cube on it rather than scratching. Avoid overdressing your child, and avoid giving him baths in very hot water.

On the other hand, sunlight may improve eczema symptoms. Ultraviolet light, UVA and UVB, are established treatments for psoriasis and eczema, but their long-term risks (excessive wrinkling, skin damage, and skin cancer) must be weighed against short-term benefits. Although sunlight therapy has been used for years, there are *no* comparison trials assessing its effectiveness. Sweating can definitely aggravate eczema, and excessive sunlight increases the risk of developing skin cancer later on. Avoid the most intense rays between 10 A.M. and 2 P.M.; use a sunscreen.

Make sure your child's fingernails are cut short and kept clean to reduce the risk of infection from constant scratching. You may want to put a pair of gloves or socks over your child's hands at night to keep him from scratching himself in his sleep.

Too much bathing without sufficient lubrication afterward dries the skin and makes eczema worse. Although harsh soaps can remove protective oils from the skin, antibacterial soaps such as Hibiclens can rid the skin of bacteria that aggravate eczema.

### BATH-TIME HINTS FOR CHILDREN WITH ECZEMA

- Give your child a bath two to three times weekly rather than daily
- Use tepid (not hot) water
- Avoid soaps or use only moisturizing types such as Dove
- Soap only the armpits, groin, feet, diaper area, and greasy, dirty areas
- Put a tablespoon of vegetable oil in the bathwater to soothe the skin; *or* put 2 cups of oatmeal in an old stocking or pillowcase, tie the end in a knot, and throw it in the bathwater for a soothing soak; *or* add a cupful of baking soda to the bathwater
- After the bath, pat, rather than rub, the skin dry
- Apply an emollient, such as Eucerin, Crisco, or Vaseline, immediately after bathing

*Avoid bubble baths* because they can dry the skin and may cause an allergic reaction.

Many children with eczema have worse symptoms in the winter, when indoor air is dry. You might keep a *humidifier* going in the child's bedroom to add moisture to the air.

One study showed that some children with eczema had markedly improved symptoms when careful attention was paid to cleaning their environment.[39] The culprit here isn't dirt itself, but a microscopic critter called the *dust mite*. This bug also aggravates asthma and allergies in sensitive children (see Chapters 4 and 5). Ridding the house of dust mites by thorough dusting and using special hypoallergenic bed covers and high filtration rate vacuums can significantly improve eczema symptoms.[40] Dust and dirt themselves do *not* cause eczema. In fact, one study showed that children who grow up in farming families and who are exposed to lots of dirt and animals, actually had about half the risk of developing eczema as their urban counterparts.[41] Obviously, for some children, animal dander is associated with severe allergic symptoms; farm life is not for everyone, nor should itchy children take to sleeping with the family furry pet in hopes of driving the demon of itch away.

Avoid using detergents, soaps, fabric softeners, and dryer sheets that contain *perfume*. Nearly 4% of eczema patients are allergic to perfumes. Interestingly, those who react to the fragrances in dishwashing detergent seem to be most sensitive when the dishwater is very hot; washing in more tepid water causes less of an allergic reaction.[42]

The most effective environmental therapies involve a *combination* of all the above *plus* avoiding smoking around your child *plus* the Nutrition and Biochemical therapies described above.[43]

*Wendy decided to decrease James's bathing from daily to twice a week, stop using soap, and use a milder detergent. She decided to add a cup of oatmeal to James's bathwater and to apply Eucerin and steroid cream immediately after the bath. She also went on a cleanup campaign to destroy dust-mite strongholds in James's room.*

Another environmental technique for treating eczema involves wet/dry wraps. You can do this with or without other treatments, such as steroid creams and with or without herbal remedies. Start with just one part of the body—say an arm or a leg. If you want to do it along with a steroid cream, apply the cream before starting the wrap. Then soak some cotton flannel or old cotton diapers in water (or herbal tea such as chamomile or licorice) and wring it out so it's still damp, but not dripping. Wrap the moistened dressing around the limb.

Then add one more layer of *dry* cotton. Leave this on for 20 minutes to two hours. Then move on to another affected area. Do *not* wrap the whole body at once, or your child may become overheated and uncomfortable; you may do both arms at once or both legs at once. Do *not* leave the wraps on overnight. Do *not* wrap too tightly—avoid cutting off the circulation! Do *not* use this technique if the eczema is complicated by a herpes infection or impetigo. Experiment to find out what combination works best for you and your child.

## Mind-Body

Eczema can both contribute to stress and be worsened by stress. *Hypnosis* can effectively alter skin sensations such as itch and pain. Hypnosis has proven effective in reducing pain in adults with eczema.[44] Hypnosis, autogenic training, and behavioral therapies that focus on relaxation and stress management may help children learn to manage the stressors that make their symptoms worse *and* help them cope with the stress of having an uncomfortable chronic condition. They can lead to significant improvements in itching and in the severity of the rash itself.[45]

*Biofeedback* aimed at relaxation and hand warming has also proved effective in a study of five patients with severe eczema.[46] Other mind-body techniques such as visualization, progressive relaxation, meditation, or deep breathing that help children relax and manage stress may also be helpful. Such techniques affect the oversensitive immune system itself--the source of eczema symptoms.

## BIOMECHANICAL THERAPIES: MASSAGE

## Massage

Massage is a natural way to apply emollients and other skin treatments for eczema.

Vegetable oil, evening primrose oil, jojoba oil, and even plain old Vaseline and Eucerin have all been recommended as excellent emollients. Some herbalists recommend adding a drop or two of chamomile or yarrow oil to one teaspoon of vegetable oil to enhance its healing effects. There is one study suggesting that massage itself actually heals eczema.[47] We know that massage benefits the immune system and helps children relax. Sounds to me like a win-win situation.

## BIOENERGETIC THERAPIES: ACUPUNCTURE, THERAPEUTIC TOUCH, HOMEOPATHY

### Acupuncture

Although one case report indicated that transcutaneous electrical nerve stimulation (TENS) was helpful in treating an adult with eczema, there are no scientific trials evaluating acupuncture's effectiveness in treating childhood eczema.[48] I do not recommend it.

### Therapeutic Touch

Therapeutic Touch reduces pain, improves wound healing, and is calming. I use Therapeutic Touch when I see patients with eczema, although it remains scientifically untested as a specific eczema remedy.

### Homeopathy

The most commonly recommended homeopathic remedies for eczema are: *Carcinosin, Housedust, Medorrhinum, Oleander, Pulsatilla, Sulfur,* and *Tub bov*. Homeopathy was reported helpful in a series of ninety children treated with these and other remedies.[49] Unfortunately, there was no comparison group of children who did not receive homeopathic remedies. This makes it impossible to tell if symptoms improved because of patients' expectations, by chance, or as the natural course of the illness over time. Although homeopathic remedies may be safe, they are still unproved for eczema. I do not recommend them.

✳

# WHAT I RECOMMEND FOR ECZEMA

## PREVENTING ECZEMA

1. *Lifestyle—nutrition.* Start your child off right by breast-feeding for at least 12 months. Once your baby is eating solids regularly, make yogurt a daily part of the diet and gradually add fatty fish once a week. Do *not* introduce any solids in the first four to six months of life; after four months, introduce no more than one new food per week. While you are pregnant and nursing, consume yogurt or kefir with active cultures daily.

2. *Lifestyle—environment.* Do not smoke, and do not allow others to smoke around your child. Minimize your child's exposure to allergens such as dust, dust mites, furry pets, and pollens. Do not use drying soaps on your baby or bathe her too frequently. Use tepid water in her baths.

---

*Take your child to a health care professional if:*

- You are concerned that the rash could be caused by something else

- The eczema takes a turn for the worse, becomes painful, or looks infected

- There is no improvement after four weeks of home therapy

---

## TREATING ECZEMA

1. *Lifestyle—environment.* Bathe your child less often. Avoid drying or perfumed soaps. If you do use soaps, try a moisturizing type. Avoid strong, scented detergents. Make sure that all clothing has been rinsed well to remove soap residues before drying. Try putting 10 cups of dry oatmeal in an old stocking and drop it in your child's bathwater. Alternatively, put 2 tablespoons of vegetable oil in your child's bathwater. Let your youngster "scratch" with an ice cube. Use a high filtration vacuum, install hypoallergenic mattress covers and dust thoroughly to remove dust mites and other airborne eczema triggers.

2. *Lifestyle—diet.* Eat yogurt, kefir, or other healthy bacteria–containing foods daily and eat fatty fish or flaxseed at least once a week. If your child has severe, extensive eczema, talk with a nutritionist about trying an elimination diet.

3. *Biochemical—medications*. Use Eucerin, Vaseline, or vegetable oil as a moisturizer or emollient after baths and before bed. Avoid "moisturizers" that contain alcohol. Talk with your health care provider about treatment with a steroid cream or ointment. Follow recommendations exactly. Consider using an antihistamine at night to reduce nighttime scratching. If the rash looks infected, try an antibiotic ointment or see your doctor.

4. *Biochemical—nutritional supplements*. Supplement your child's diet with at least 50 to 75 milligrams per day of vitamin C. Consider supplementation with 3 grams daily of evening primrose oil. Consider giving your child *Lactobacillus GG* or *L. casei* or *bifidobacterium* supplements twice daily.

5. *Lifestyle—mind-body*. Consider taking your child for hypnotherapy or biofeedback to help him learn to desensitize his skin and to learn to deal with stressful triggers. Consider using guided imagery or meditation techniques to learn to manage the stress of having a chronic, uncomfortable condition.

6. *Biomechanical—massage*. Give your child a massage at least three times a week using a vegetable oil to help soothe the skin and the soul.

7. *Biochemical—herbs*. Consider consulting a practitioner of Traditional Chinese Medicine to discuss herbal tea. Do *not* use Chinese patent medicines. Consider using an herbal emollient such as aloe vera or an herbal compress containing licorice, chamomile, calendula, or slippery elm bark tea.

## RESOURCES

### Internet

American Academy of Dermatology
http://www.aad.org/atopicderm.html

Eczema Network
http://www.eczema.net/

Longwood Herbal Task Force
http://www.mcp.edu/herbal/

National Eczema Association for Science and Education (NEASE)
http://www.eczema-assn.org

National Eczema Association
http://www.eczema.org/

# 19
# FEVER

Greg Edgecomb called me one Sunday evening because his three-week-old daughter, Nicole, had developed a fever of 102°F (39°C) and was not interested in breast-feeding. She was also sleepier than usual. I asked Greg to bring Nicole to the emergency room, so we could make sure she did not have a serious infection.

Sarah Klein called before work to ask if she should bring in Jacob, her two-year-old son, for an evaluation of his fever of 103°F (39.4°C). Jacob had had a cold for several days but had been drinking, playing, and sleeping normally until that morning when he awoke with a fever and rapid breathing. Sarah had given Tylenol and sponged Jacob, but his temperature was still 101°F (38.4°C). Sarah was concerned that Jacob might have pneumonia, and I agreed to see him as the first patient that day. On the way into the clinic, Jacob had a seizure. Sarah wanted to know if a seizure could be caused by a fever alone or if it meant that Jacob had meningitis.

Frank LittleBear brought in his eighteen month old, Tara, for a checkup and immunizations. The nurse noticed that Tara felt warm and checked her temperature: 101.5°F (38.7°C). Frank said Tara had a cold but had been behaving completely normally. He wondered if Tara could still get her scheduled immunizations or if they would have to make another visit.

Although they are frightening for many parents, fevers are a natural defense against infections. Even cold-blooded animals such as fish and reptiles seek warmer surroundings to boost their temperatures when they are fighting infections. Those that are allowed to raise their temperatures have higher survival rates than those that are kept cool.

Fevers are a leading cause of children's doctor visits. When winter's blizzards blow, fever reaches its peak season. Fever is not a disease itself, but it is a symptom of many common childhood illnesses. Most children who have fevers can be safely managed at home. Knowing a few basic facts about fevers may save you a trip to the doctor's office.

## What Is a Fever?

Temperatures normally vary up to one full degree over the course of a day, with lower readings in the morning and higher ones in the afternoon. Children tend to run slightly higher temperatures than adults. Normal temperatures range from 97.1°F (36.2°C) to 99.5°F (37.5°C) when measured in the mouth or ear. Temperatures vary depending on where they are measured. Rectal measurements are generally higher than oral, underarm, or ear measurements.

### TEMPERATURES CONSIDERED FEVERS

- *In the mouth or the ear:* above 99.4°F (37.5°C)
- *Under the arm (axillary):* above 98.6°F (37°C)
- *Rectally:* above 100.4°F (38°C)
- *Low-grade fevers:* less than 102°F (38.9°C), measured rectally
- *Moderate-grade fevers:* between 102°F (38.9°C) and 104°F (40°C), measured rectally
- *High fevers:* greater than 104°F (40°C), measured rectally

Even among children with temperatures higher than 105°F (40.5°C), only about one-third have a serious bacterial illness. It is not until temperatures exceed 106°F (41°C) that the majority of children have a serious illness such as pneumonia. Infections rarely cause a fever of 106°F and *never* cause a fever over 107°F. Only heatstrokes or rare medical conditions cause temperatures higher than 107°F.

## What Causes Fever?

Infections such as colds, flu, ear infections, and sore throats are the most common causes of fever. Rheumatoid arthritis and cancer are uncommon childhood illnesses, but they can cause fevers. Teething does not raise the temperature above 101°F (38.4°C).[1] Overbundling can cause fevers in babies. The temperature in a closed car in summer sunshine can easily exceed 110°F (43.2°C) and cause heat illness, stroke, or even death in a child left inside while the parent makes a "quick stop" at the store.

Our temperature is normally controlled by a "thermostat" in the hypothalamus, a small area in the middle of the brain close to the pituitary gland. When a child has an infection, the white blood cells fighting the infection send chemical messengers called interleukins to the hypothalamus. The thermostat, normally set at 98.6°F (37°C), is raised to help the white blood cells fight the infection. The hypothalamus sends orders to the rest of the body to raise the temperature. The body responds by seeking a warm room, putting on more clothes, and shivering. When the set-point returns to normal, new orders go out; the body reduces the temperature by sweating, throwing off covers, and drinking cool water.

This explains the "chills and fever" when a fever builds and the sweating when a fever "breaks." When our body temperature is lower than the brain's thermostat, we feel chilled and try to warm up. Shivering is one of the most effective ways to warm up quickly. This is what happens when someone has the "shaking chills." When the set-point returns to normal and our temperature remains high, we feel hot and start to sweat. Sweating is a sign that the set-point has been lowered and the fever has "broken."

When a child is overbundled, the temperature may rise even though the thermostat remains set at 98.6°F (37°C). Babies can't easily remove their own clothes, move to a cooler place, or sweat enough to cool off, so they can get overheated and have a higher temperature just from being overdressed or in a hot environment.

Fever raises the heart rate and breathing rate and increases the loss of fluids. Blood levels of zinc and iron fall, while copper levels rise. Levels of the stress hormone, cortisol, double.[2]

## DO FEVERS CAUSE BRAIN DAMAGE?

There is *no* risk of brain damage unless the temperature rises above 107°F (41.7°C) and stays there. Fevers even from serious illnesses such as pneumonia and kidney infections do not cause temperatures high enough to cause brain damage. The only thing that causes that kind of temperature is *heatstroke*. Heatstroke occurs when someone overexercises or overdresses in a hot environment and cannot cool off. During heatstroke, the internal thermostat remains set at 98.6°F (37°C), but the body can't dissipate the heat from exercise and the environment. Eventually it gives up.

*I saw heatstroke bring down a North Carolina teenager who was playing basketball indoors in August and who didn't stop to rest or get a drink of water until he passed out with a temperature of 107.6°F (42°C). He was fine once we got some fluids into him and cooled him off.*

Many parents worry that fevers less than 102°F can cause brain damage. This fear has created an epidemic of over-treatment even when the child has a low-grade fever, which may be helping him fight an infection. Many physicians and pharmacists have perpetuated fever phobia by fixating on the child's temperature when inquiring about symptoms. Fever phobia contributes to a lot of unnecessary medication for children with low-grade fevers. Remember, we care for the *child,* not the temperature!

## DO FEVERS CAUSE SEIZURES?

Sometimes. Between the ages of six months and five years, about 2 to 5 percent of children have seizures when they have a fever; of those who have one fever-triggered seizure, about one third have another seizure within two years. This is *not* the same as epilepsy. Seizures triggered by fevers last less than fifteen minutes and typically involve jerking movements of the whole body, not just one side or one part.

*Sarah's son, Jacob, fit this picture.*

Seizures triggered by fevers run in families, are more common in children who have epilepsy, and are more common among children who attend day care. Why are they more common in day care attendees? Probably because children in day care get more infections and more fevers. In children who are otherwise healthy and developing normally, a typical fever-triggered seizure does *not* damage IQ or cause later school problems or epilepsy.

Seizures look scary. Most parents who see their child have a seizure are afraid the child is going to die, even though the typical seizure stops within a few minutes and does not cause any long-term harm. If your child has a seizure with a fever, remain calm, check your watch to see how long the seizure actually lasts (even though it seems like hours, it probably will be less than five minutes), make sure he is lying on his side on the floor or bed in a safe place away from sharp objects. Do not try to put anything in his mouth. Old-fashioned beliefs that seizures make people swallow their tongues are just plain wrong. If the seizure lasts longer than four minutes, call 911 or take him immediately to the nearest emergency room. If it lasts less than four minutes, take him to your regular health care provider or the emergency room.

*When I examined Jacob fifteen minutes after his seizure, he was sleepy and had pneumonia. Sarah was scared by the seizure, which had lasted about two and a half minutes. She said she finally understood what her mother had gone through when Sarah had fever-triggered seizures as a child. We treated Jacob with an injection of antibiotics for his pneumonia. He was better by the next day. Like most children who suffer a fever-triggered seizure, Jacob has never had another one. Note: Giving your child Tylenol at the first sign of illness will not necessarily prevent seizures.*

Fevers are uncommon in children under six months old. It's hard to tell just by looking at them whether or not young babies are ill; special tests may be needed, depending on your child's other symptoms. If your child is under three months old and gets any fever, have her evaluated by a health care professional. Do *not* try to treat a fever in an infant yourself without having her professionally evaluated. Feverish children under six weeks of age may need to be hospitalized while the cause of the fever is being sorted out.

Several tests used to be routine for children having their first seizure. Children up to a year of age will probably need to have a spinal tap if they have a fever-triggered seizure, just to make sure that meningitis hasn't caused the fever and the seizure. An EEG test and brain scans are *not* necessary for most children with their first uncomplicated fever-triggered seizures.

Nor do most children need blood tests to evaluate electrolytes, blood sugar, or levels of different minerals or white blood cells unless there are specific findings on their physical examination that lead the doctor to suspect a problem in one of these areas.

*Nicole's tests showed that she had a kidney infection. She was hospitalized and received antibiotics by vein. Later tests showed that the infection had been caught in time and there was no permanent kidney damage. Her parents were relieved that their quick response to Nicole's fever spared her problems she might have developed if they had delayed care.*

Fevers can be signs of serious illness.

---

### SEEK PROFESSIONAL HELP FOR FEVER IF THE CHILD:

- Is less than three months old
- Is lethargic, refuses to drink fluids, is not interested in play
- Has a seizure, stiff neck, limb, or abdominal pain
- Has trouble breathing or swallowing her own saliva
- Has pain when she urinates, is vomiting or not keeping down liquids
- Looks sicker than you'd expect from a viral illness

---

## DO FEVERS DO ANY GOOD?

Yes. Fevers kill many germs. *Streptococcus pneumonia*, the bacteria responsible for many ear infections and pneumonia, is killed at temperatures over 104°F. In the pre-antibiotic era, practitioners often *caused* fevers in patients (e.g.,with steam baths) to cure disease. I do *not* recommend that you give your child a fever on purpose, but you don't need to worry about the fever either. Instead, try to figure out why your child's body may be creating one. Treat the child, *not* the thermometer.

## CAN CHILDREN WITH FEVERS RECEIVE THEIR REGULAR IMMUNIZATIONS?

Yes. Children with fevers and minor illnesses such as colds and ear infections can receive immunizations safely.

*Frank's daughter, Tara, could have her scheduled immunizations even though she had a fever.*

## WHAT'S THE BEST WAY TO TAKE A CHILD'S TEMPERATURE?

The new *digital thermometers* work quickly (in less than thirty seconds) and are accurate and easy to read. Check *Consumer Reports* for the best values. Many doctors' offices now use electronic thermometers that measure the temperature in the ear. Even if your child has an ear infection, the reading in that ear will be less than half a degree higher than the child's real (core) temperature. Ear wax doesn't affect the accuracy of temperatures measured by ear thermometers. *Glass thermometers* can be difficult to read and take several minutes to reach core temperature. They also contain mercury, which is poisonous for people and the environment (when the glass breaks and the mercury runs out). I do not recommend them.

The new *temperature strips* and *temperature-sensitive pacifiers* are easy to use, but they tend to underestimate the true temperature. Newer models may be more accurate than the older ones available in the early 1990s, but they still tend to read about half a degree lower than rectal thermometers and it may take several minutes to get a reading.

Our hands are also not too accurate in judging fevers. Most parents and health care professionals tend to overestimate a child's temperature when feeling the forehead; on the other hand, they seldom miss a real fever. However, I still feel foreheads on my patients because I often get a sense of the child by touching him and most children feel soothed when someone who cares about them strokes their forehead. And if I don't detect an increased temperature with my hand, a real fever is extremely unlikely.

Measuring the temperatures *under the armpit* is the safest and easiest for most parents. The temperature under the armpit usually is a little lower (about one degree lower) than the temperature inside the body. Do *not* leave your child alone with a thermometer under the arm. It can break (if it's an old glass one) or slide out, resulting in an inaccurately low reading.

Temperatures measured *rectally* are the most accurate, especially in children under five years old, but taking a rectal temperature can be tricky. Please ask your health care provider to show you how. Be sure to clean the thermometer carefully with rubbing alcohol and wash it in cool water before and after measuring a rectal temperature. Use a lubricant such as petroleum jelly on the thermometer before trying to insert it. The tip of the thermometer should be about one inch inside the rectum for the most accurate temperature; don't force it in. You will need to hold your child still with his "cheeks" (buttocks) together to hold the thermometer in place. Do *not* leave your child alone, even for a minute, with a rectal thermometer in place. The thermometer can slide in too deep or slide out completely. Glass thermometers can break if your child moves suddenly.

Temperatures can be measured in the *mouth (orally)* with the thermometer under the tongue in older children. It is difficult to obtain an accurate reading in children whose noses are so stuffy that they have to breathe through their mouths. In these cases, an armpit (axillary) temperature may be better. For the most accurate reading with an oral thermometer, don't start to measure until several minutes after your child has eaten or drunk anything cold or hot. Be sure to clean the thermometer with rubbing alcohol and rinse it in cool water before and after using it. Let it dry thoroughly before putting it in the mouth. Place the tip of the thermometer under the tongue and have the child close her mouth, holding the thermometer in place with her hand, *not* her teeth. Glass thermometers need to stay in place for at least three minutes to be accurate. You can read an electronic thermometer as soon as it beeps (usually in thirty seconds or less).

Do *not* leave a child alone with an oral thermometer in place. Sick children may be distracted easily and forget to keep the thermometer under their tongue, resulting in an inaccurately low reading. Older children may have learned that they can create a "fever" (and thereby avoid an unwanted activity such as school) by holding a thermometer near a lightbulb, rubbing it between their hands, or running it under hot water. Don't tempt your child to use one of these common tricks by leaving her alone with the thermometer.

## WHAT'S THE BEST WAY TO TREAT A FEVER?

Most parents can tell when their child is sick because the child doesn't eat, sleep, or play as she normally does. The child may whine, cling, and regress to more babylike behavior or become quiet and withdrawn. If your child isn't acting sick, there's no reason to take or treat her temperature. The only reason to treat the child's fever is to help her feel more comfortable. Let's tour the Therapeutic Mountain to learn what works safely; if you want to skip to my bottom-line recommendations, flip to the end of the chapter.

## BIOCHEMICAL THERAPIES: MEDICATIONS, HERBS, NUTRITIONAL SUPPLEMENTS

### *Medications*

#### PROVEN SAFE AND EFFECTIVE

- Acetaminophen (Panadol, Tylenol, Tempra, nonaspirin pain reliever)
- Ibuprofen (Pediaprofen, Children's Advil, Children's Motrin)

How does *acetaminophen* (the active ingredient in Tylenol, Panadol, Tempra, and other nonaspirin fever medications) work? It resets the brain's temperature thermostat. Acetaminophen also helps the child feel more comfortable with her other symptoms. It does *not* make the illness go away any faster. You can't tell how sick your child is (that is, whether you are dealing with a cold or pneumonia) by how much the temperature goes down when taking Tylenol. A child with a high fever is unlikely to achieve a completely normal temperature from Tylenol, but she may well feel more comfortable. *Don't watch the temperature, watch the child.*

If you decide to use acetaminophen, read the package instructions carefully for the correct dosage for your child. Do not give it more often than every four hours. Overdoses can cause liver damage. There is no benefit to dividing doses every two hours. There is no benefit to alternating acetaminophen and ibuprofen. Keep medicine out of your child's reach (in a childproof or locked cabinet) between doses. It takes about forty-five minutes to an hour for acetaminophen to start working. The effects wear off in four to six hours, so if your child is uncomfortable again in that time you can repeat the dose. Please do *not* wake up your child to give her acetaminophen. If she's sleeping, the medicine is much less important than the rest she needs to fight the infection.

Acetaminophen is very safe when taken in recommended doses. I've never seen a child experience side effects from it when it was taken as recommended. Acetaminophen does not prolong most illnesses or other symptoms or suppress the immune system. Generic or store brands are just as effective and safe as name brand acetaminophen.

Do *not* use *aspirin* without talking to your child's doctor. Giving aspirin when a child has influenza or chicken pox is associated with a sometimes fatal condition called Reye's syndrome. Other side effects of aspirin include upset stomach, prolonged bleeding, and allergic reactions, especially in asthmatic children. It is not worth the risks when good alternatives are available.

*Ibuprofen* (Children's Motrin or Advil), works a bit faster, a bit longer (six to eight hours instead of four hours for acetaminophen), and may reduce fever a bit more than acetaminophen (by about one degree Fahrenheit).[3] However, ibuprofen is more likely than acetaminophen to cause an upset stomach. Because of its rapid onset and prolonged effects, ibuprofen has become my number-one choice when a child needs medication to treat her discomforts caused by fever.

What about alternating acetaminophen and ibuprofen? There is no evidence that this is helpful, and it doubles the risks of side effects. If your child's discomfort is not better with either acetaminophen or ibuprofen, it's time to call the doctor and get some help figuring out what's making the child so uncomfortable. Don't experiment by combining medicines on your own.

## Herbs

A number of herbs used in other parts of the world have proven effective as fever fighters in animal studies. These include the East Indian plant known as Akra (*Calotropis pro-*

*cera*),[4] the African and Chinese fever remedy rhinoceros horn,[5] and the herb *Euphorbia hirta*.[6] A German combination containing ash tree, poplar, and goldenrod, known as STW 1, was shown in animal studies to be as effective as aspirin in reducing fever.[7] Despite their effectiveness in animal studies, I do *not* recommend any of these herbal remedies for treating feverish children until additional studies have evaluated their safety and effectiveness in humans. And until herbal remedies are better regulated (providing better consumer protection) in the United States. Right now you run the risk of being ripped off or of giving your child some unintended contaminant.

*White willow bark* is the original source of common aspirin. It has been used since ancient times around the world to treat fever and the aches and pains of a variety of illnesses. Willow bark tea does not taste very good. Because the active ingredient in willow bark is metabolized in the body to salicylic acid (aspirin), it may cause the same problems as aspirin—upset stomach, suppressed immune system, possible allergies, and Reye's syndrome.

Other traditional remedies have not been evaluated in comparison studies, although they have been used for centuries. Bitters, such as Angostura bitters or gentian, have long been recommended to reduce fever, especially in illnesses characterized by upset stomach and diarrhea. Boneset tea was used by Native Americans to break the bone-breaking fevers and chills of influenza. It is bitter and may cause nausea and vomiting. Catnip tea is used in treating low-grade fevers to help a child relax and to induce sweating. Echinacea helps bolster the immune system and is used to treat the common cold. Elderflower tea is sometimes used in combination with catnip or peppermint and yarrow to treat fevers. Licorice root has some antibacterial and anti-inflammatory properties and is used to treat fevers accompanying inflammation. Bitter-tasting yarrow flowers were said to have been used by the Greek hero Achilles to staunch the flow of blood from his battle wounds. Modern herbalists recommend a tea from its flowers to reduce fever and as a general tonic. There are *no* scientific studies evaluating the effectiveness of any of these herbal remedies in treating fever in children.

Herbal remedies are not necessarily safe just because they are natural. A traditional Asian remedy for fever, star anise (*Illicium verum*), proved an effective fever fighter in rodents but also caused seizures.[8] Feverfew is used primarily as a painkiller for headaches and arthritis, but it can cause allergic reactions.[9] Beware of possible contamination in herbal products. Most have been used for many years and generally are considered safe if given in small doses over a few days. If a child does not respond within a day or two to home remedies, her temperature exceeds 103.9°F, or she is lethargic, having trouble breathing, or acts very ill, take her to be evaluated by a health care professional.

## Nutritional Supplements

### NUTRITIONAL SUPPLEMENTS AND FEVER

*No:* vitamin A

*Maybe:* vitamin C. zinc, ginger, bee products, garlic, beet juice

Chronic *vitamin A* overdoses can actually *cause* fevers. So can overdoses of a number of minerals.

Blood levels of *vitamin C* decline during fever. High doses (1 gram or more in adult volunteers) of vitamin C temporarily *raise* the temperature by almost one degree.[10] In animals, giving vitamin C supplements along with acetaminophen (Tylenol) boosts Tylenol's antifever effects and decreases its potentially toxic effects on the liver. It has not yet been studied as a fever fighter in humans. You may want to give your child vitamin C–rich juice to wash down ibuprofen or acetaminophen.

Children with Down's syndrome have weak immune systems and tend to get a lot of fevers. Among children with Down's syndrome, daily *zinc* supplements of 25 to 50 milligrams significantly reduce episodes of cough and fever compared with similar children given placebos. Zinc supplements have not been studied as preventive therapy in healthy children.

In animals, *ginger* has proven to have fever-fighting properties.[11] There are *no* studies evaluating ginger's effectiveness in treating fevers in children, but I often recommend it as an antinausea remedy. *Bee products* such as propolis have also gained popularity recently for treating a variety of illnesses, but studies have *not* demonstrated any antifever effects of propolis and there are *no* studies evaluating its effectiveness in feverish children. *Garlic* has been used to treat infectious illnesses since ancient times by Egyptians, Greeks, and Romans and is known as Russian penicillin. *Beet juice*, sometimes combined with carrot juice, is a British folk remedy for fever. There are *no* studies on the effectiveness of garlic or beets for reducing fever in children.

## LIFESTYLE THERAPIES: NUTRITION, EXERCISE, ENVIRONMENT, MIND-BODY

### Nutrition

Feed a cold and starve a fever? Most children with fevers are not hungry. Neither force-feed nor withhold food from a feverish child. Let appetite be the guide. Offer her foods that are easy to digest (such as rice, crackers, yogurt, and broth) several times a day, but let her appetite guide what and when she eats.

Do give your child *extra fluids* while she has a fever. Higher body heat causes extra sweating, and this fluid needs to be replaced. Fresh fruit juices are excellent. Carrot and beet juices are good choices as vegetable juices for feverish children. Some children like to suck on ice cubes or fruit juice popsicles when they have a fever. Others like to sip simple chicken broth.

## Exercise

Having a fever takes a lot of energy. Let your feverish child *rest*. Athletes also should take rest breaks and drink plenty of fluids to avoid becoming overheated on hot days. Gentle exercises, such as swimming, yoga, and *Tai Chi*, may be better exercise alternatives in August, and even these may be too strenuous for a child fighting a fever.

## Environment

When a child has a fever, the body's thermostat is set higher temporarily and the body will try to maintain the new higher temperature. Children maintain a higher temperature by shivering, moving to a warm room, or asking for extra blankets or to be held close. Removing all the child's clothes or giving sponge baths will make her uncomfortable and more likely to shiver because it does *not* reset the internal thermostat. Sponging does *not* affect the underlying cause of the fever. By artificially lowering body temperature without resetting the internal thermostat, sponging may make things worse. If your child is already sweating because her fever set-point has been reduced (the fever has "broken"), sponging away the sweat with tepid water may help her feel more comfortable.

Do *not* sponge your child with rubbing alcohol. Rubbing alcohol can be absorbed through the skin, causing low blood sugar, seizures, and even coma.

## Mind-Body

Remain calm. Keep your child company. Read her stories while she is awake. Cuddle her and let her know she is loved. Remind her that she will be feeling better soon and that while she is sick it is OK for her to rest. The behavior of many children regresses when they are sick. Your child may want to cuddle an old favorite teddy bear or prefer stories that were outgrown months previously; she may start talking in baby-talk again. This is normal; your child will be back to her usual self soon. You may want to play soothing music or children's books on tape. You can play videos that you have approved as appropriate for your child. Do not give in to the temptation to let the TV be your sick child's baby-sitter.

## BIOMECHANICAL THERAPIES

*Massage* feels wonderful and can be soothing for a sick child, but there are *no* scientific studies evaluating its effectiveness in treating fevers. There are no studies evaluating the effectiveness of *chiropractic* or other types of spinal adjustment in treating fevers. I do not recommend chiropractic treatment for feverish children. There is *no* role for surgery in the treatment of simple fevers, but it may be needed if the underlying problem is appendicitis.

## BIOENERGETIC THERAPIES: ACUPUNCTURE, THERAPEUTIC TOUCH/HEALING TOUCH/ PRAYER, HOMEOPATHY

### Acupuncture

Acupuncture treatment effectively reduces fever in arthritis-like disorders in animals.[12] Until such studies have been performed on human children, I do *not* recommend acupuncture as a primary treatment for typical fevers.

### Therapeutic Touch/Healing Touch/ Prayer

There are no studies specifically evaluating the impact of any type of healing touch therapy or prayer in treating feverish children. However, I always use healing touch when working with a feverish child, and most children and their parents seem to find it comforting. There are no side effects to prayer, and I recommend it for all kinds of conditions if it is consistent with your family's beliefs and values.

### Homeopathy

Several remedies are traditionally used by homeopathic practitioners in extremely dilute doses (more concentrated doses can be poisonous) for treating various kinds of fever: Aconitum, Arsenicum, Belladonna, Bryonia, *Ferrum phos,* Gelsemium, *Nux vomica,* Pulsatilla, and Sulfur. The primary Bach flower remedy for fever is Rescue Remedy. There are *no* scientific studies evaluating the effectiveness of homeopathic remedies in treating children with fever.

## WHAT I RECOMMEND FOR FEVER

*Seek immediate professional help if your child:*

- Is under three months old and has any degree of fever

- Is any age and the temperature is over 104°F

- Looks very sick

- Is more difficult than usual to awaken

- Won't stop crying with your usual loving care

- Is confused or delirious

- Loses consciousness or has a seizure

- Has a stiff neck

- Has painful or frequent urination

- Is unable to keep down clear fluids

- Has trouble breathing or can't swallow her own saliva

- Cries when you touch or move her

- Has a rash with deep red or purple spots that don't fade or blanch when you press on the skin

## WHAT TO AVOID WHEN YOUR CHILD HAS A FEVER

1. *Lifestyle—environment. Don't* sponge your child with alcohol or ice water. Sponge only when the fever is breaking, use tepid (not ice) water, and sponge only as long as it helps her feel comfortable. Neither overdress nor completely undress your child. Her body will find its own proper temperature if you dress her as usual and offer a light blanket or two.

2. *Biochemical—medications. Avoid* aspirin. Do *not* awaken your child to give anti-fever medicines.

---

*When to call or visit your health care provider:*

- If your child is less than two years old and the temperature is above 102°F

- If your child is urinating less often than usual (fewer than four wet diapers a day). This may be a sign that your child is becoming dehydrated. Offer additional fluids

- If the fever lasts more than a day or two, especially if it's not clearly associated with a simple cold or flu

---

## TREATING A FEVER AT HOME

Remember, treat the child, not the thermometer reading.

1. *Biochemical—medications.* Try acetaminophen or ibuprofen to reduce your child's discomfort. Do not exceed the doses recommended on the package label. Do not alternate acetaminophen and aspirin every two hours.

2. *Lifestyle—nutrition.* Give your child plenty of extra fluids to drink. Juices and broth are excellent and easily digested.

3. *Lifestyle—environment.* You may give a tepid water sponge bath if your child is sweating (the fever has "broken").

4. *Lifestyle—exercise.* Encourage your child to rest.

5. *Lifestyle—mind-body.* Stay with your child, offering love, support, and encouragement. Remember that most fevers resolve in two to three days on their own.

6. *Bioenergetic—Therapeutic Touch.* If it is consistent with your family's beliefs, pray and offer healing touch therapies.

## RESOURCES

### *Internet*

**American Academy of Pediatrics**
http://www.aap.org/family/febseiz.htm

**American Academy of Family Practice**
http://www.familydoctor.org/healthfacts/
069/nav.html

**YourHealth**
http://www.yourhealth.com/ahl/1266.html

# 20
# HEADACHE

Michael Fahnestock called me shortly after he and his wife moved to town. Their eleven-year-old daughter, Kim, had started having headaches a few weeks before they moved. She was now having them almost twice a month. She had told her father that she knew when she was getting a headache because she saw flashing lights. Shortly afterward, she complained of terrible pain, usually on the left side of her head. She had tried aspirin, but that didn't help very much. She felt better after a long nap. Mike initially attributed the headaches to the stress of the move, and then he thought Kim might be getting migraines like her mother and grandmother. He called me to see if there were any new treatments for migraine and to make sure Kim didn't have something more serious, like a brain tumor.

Headaches are very common, very painful, and very costly. Each year Americans spend over $1 billion for medical care to treat headaches, plus the cost of time missed from work and school. Although adults in their thirties and forties are the most likely persons to have headaches, kids can have them, too; in any given month over 40% of teenagers report having had a headache. An estimated 4 to 11 percent of teenagers have migraine headaches.

Children with migraines miss more than twice as many school days each year as other kids. Mondays are the most common day for migraines in school-age kids, with 50% more migraines reported on Mondays than on Tuesdays and twice as many on Mondays as on Saturdays.

Headaches run in families.[1] For example, chronic tension headaches are three times more common among those who have a close relative with frequent tension headaches than for kids who don't have headaches in the family.

Apparently no age is completely immune to having headaches. Babies get them, too. Recurrent vomiting may be the only signal that toddlers and preschoolers are having migraine headaches. Even infants as young as twelve months old have been diagnosed as having migraines.

Like Michael Fahnestock, many parents worry when their child has recurrent headaches that there is a brain tumor, but tumors are incredibly rare. About half of all headaches in children are due to muscle tension. About 25% are due to migraine, and the rest are due to fever, head injuries, sinus infections, dental problems, jaw problems, uncorrected vision problems, and ear infections. Less common causes of headache include high blood pressure, meningitis, lead poisoning, carbon monoxide poisoning, eating very cold foods, altitude sickness, and overdoses of vitamins or medications. Withdrawing from certain foods, drinks, and herbs can also cause headaches.

### TENSION HEADACHE TRIGGERS

- Emotional stress
- Physical stress, lack of sleep, fatigue, heat, noise
- Poor posture
- Pain, pinched nerves
- Eyestrain, poor lighting
- Other illnesses, colds, flu

*Muscular tension headaches* are typically caused by emotional stress, anger, and depression. They can also be caused by physical stress (e.g., fatigue, cold, heat, irregular meals, noisy environment), poor posture, pain, pinched nerves, grinding teeth, eyestrain, poor circulation, and illnesses elsewhere in the body. Whew! Given this long list, it's surprising

that not *all* kids get tension headaches. Tension headaches are usually most painful in the forehead or the back of the head. They feel like a band tightening around the head or a sense of pressure all over. They seldom throb, and are not aggravated by motion, light, or sound.

*Migraine headaches* can provoke pain, clenched muscles, and thus tension headaches. Often the two go together. Although migraine headaches and tension headaches can occur simultaneously, migraines have their own painfully unique characteristics. People who have migraine headaches are called *migraineurs*.

### CHARACTERISTICS OF MIGRAINE HEADACHES

- Run in families
- Recurrent headaches; pain-free between episodes
- Aura: symptoms preceding the headache
- Typically last two to seventy-two hours
- Pounding or throbbing on one side of head; can hurt all over
- Often sensitive to light or sound
- Often have upset stomach, nausea, or vomiting
- Prefer to remain lying down in quiet, dark room
- Improved with sleeping

*Mike was really on the ball in putting together his daughter's symptoms with his wife's history of headaches. Migraine headaches are also more common in women, adding more weight to the possibility that Kim was having migraines.*

Like Kim, some migraneurs experience symptoms such as flashing lights or other images *just before* the headache starts. These symptoms are known as the headache's *aura*. Less often, migraneurs have other symptoms such as temporary blindness, tingling, or severe weakness in the arms or legs on one side of the body. Usually these symptoms last for a few minutes and go away when the actual headache begins, which is usually within an hour. Some people are so troubled by the aura symptoms that they actually look forward to the headache itself. For example, one of my colleagues has aura symptoms which include temporary blindness; when the headache starts, he can finally see again.

A migraine headache is typically a moderate to severe throbbing or pounding headache on one side of the head. However, many children experience migraine headaches as a kind of vague pain all over the head. Most migraines are accompanied by nausea or a stomachache, making the sufferers truly miserable. When struck with a headache, most prefer to lie in a very quiet, dark room and to lie very still; moving makes the pain worse. Migraines typically last several hours, but they can last up to three days. Even after the headache is over, many sufferers feel wiped out and achy for a day or so.

Like tension headaches, migraines can be triggered by many different things.

## MIGRAINE HEADACHE TRIGGERS

- Stress, tension, or anxiety
- Being overtired, late nights
- Diet: chocolate, cheese, aspartame, nitrites, MSG, caffeine
- Menstrual period, birth control pills
- Bright light, flashing lights
- Chinook winds

Children who suffer from migraines do not necessarily experience any more *stress* than other children, but they seem to respond differently to stress, often feeling more anxious about challenges than other children. They also appear to be more sensitive to pain and are more excitable and anxious about hurting themselves in sports and games.[2] Magnetic Resonance Imaging (MRI) studies indicate that the brain's cortex tends to be especially active and excitable in migraineurs.[3] Many migraineurs get their migraines after the tension has eased (e.g., after the exam is over) rather than while they are worried about it; thus some folks are most prone to getting a headache on the weekends or as soon as they've unpacked the suitcases on vacation. Super-sensitivity to changes in stress provides the rationale for mind-body therapies such as self-hypnosis, biofeedback, and meditation.

About 25% of families identify *fatigue* as a trigger for migraines. Grandmothers who urge us to eat right, exercise, and get enough sleep have a pretty good strategy for minimizing headaches and a host of other health problems.

*Missing meals* or *eating certain foods* (such as chocolate, cheese, aspartame, nitrites, MSG, caffeine, and red wine) have also been blamed for migraines. Although some children and adults are sensitive to certain foods, foods have taken an unfair rap in many cases. *Chocolate* may indeed be a trigger for some migraine sufferers,[4] but in a randomized, double-blind crossover trial only *two* out of twenty-five adults who initially attributed their symptoms to chocolate had consistently negative reactions to it.[5] These results were duplicated in a more recent study of sixty-three women who had thought their headaches were triggered by chocolate, but when they were actually blind-tested (they didn't know whether or not they were getting chocolate) it turned out that chocolate was not really the culprit.[6] If your child gets headaches after eating chocolate, try going three months without any chocolate and keep track of whether or not she has fewer headaches. Children do not *need* chocolate as part of a healthy diet, but they may not need to live a life of total deprivation to avoid headaches either.

The amino acid, tyramine, found in *cheese*, especially aged cheeses, has also been blamed for migraines. However, the vast majority of people can eat cheese safely. Several studies in children have shown that tyramine does *not* trigger migraines.[7]

The artificial sweetener, *aspartame* (Nutrasweet) triggers some adult migraines, but no studies have yet linked it to headaches in children. Most adult headaches are not triggered by aspartame, but then again, it's not as if we *need* aspartame. If your child has frequent migraines, try omitting aspartame for three months and keep track of her headaches. Careful monitoring may uncover other triggers as well.

*Nitrites* and *nitrates* are used to cure and preserve many meats such as hot dogs, bacon, salami, and dried meat sticks. Nitrites and nitrates trigger migraines in some people. Again, try going several months without these products and monitor your child's headaches carefully.

*MSG* is the key ingredient held responsible for "Chinese restaurant syndrome": headache, dizziness, flushing, sweating, and abdominal cramps. When you eat out, ask to have your child's food prepared without MSG; most restaurants accommodate this request without a fuss. Because many people now steer clear of MSG, manufacturers have started calling it by other names: hydrolyzed vegetable protein (HVP), hydrolyzed plant protein (HPP), and "natural flavor enhancers." Read labels carefully. Sensitive children who consume small amounts of MSG in ordinary foods every day may end up with chronic headaches.[8]

*Caffeine*, found in coffee, tea, cola, and chocolate, is addictive. Quitting coffee cold turkey not only results in more yawns, but in more headaches, irritability, and depression; it actually changes the EEG.[9] Likewise, the most common cause of post-operative headaches in adults is having abstained from coffee (as well as breakfast) prior to the operation! Children who drink two to three cans a day of caffeine-containing sodas are just as susceptible to withdrawal headaches as adult coffee drinkers who try to quit suddenly, who oversleep on the weekend and miss their morning dose, or who undergo surgery.[10] If your child is a regular cola drinker, gradually reduce her intake over two weeks to avoid withdrawal headaches.

Paradoxically, caffeine is a potent pain reliever that effectively combats headache pain. It is so effective, it is included in many headache remedies such as Anacin and Excedrin. People who start taking these medications every day for mild aches and pains may end up addicted to caffeine and suffer severe headaches when they try to stop using them.

*Menstrual periods* and *birth control pills* are common triggers for migraines in teenage girls and adult women. *Bright* or *flashing lights* trigger symptoms for some sufferers. Although some factors seem to trigger migraine headaches directly, others seem to work in combination. A teenager who usually tolerates nitrates without any problem could develop a raging headache if she has a bacon cheeseburger the day after a sleepless slumber party, especially if it's the wrong time of the month.

Many people feel their headaches are related to various *changes in the weather*. A Canadian neurologist listened to his patients complain that the warm westerly Chinook winds in Alberta triggered their migraines; looking back over the headache diaries kept by 75 patients, he found that patients were much more likely to develop a headache in the two days before or during high Chinook winds (wind speeds more than 38 mph) than at other times.[11] No one knows why. But if your child complains that certain kinds of weather trigger her migraines, well, it may not be all in her head.

Migraine sufferers who keep careful track of their headaches using a *headache diary* often find that their headaches occur more often at certain times of the day. In a study of fifteen meticulous migraine sufferers, the headaches occurred most often between 6 A.M. and 10 A.M. and were less likely between 8 P.M. and 4 A.M.[12] This is the same timing as adult heart attacks. It is also the same rhythm of the rising and falling of several stress hormones, suggesting a complex interaction between hormones, blood vessels, inflammation, and pain.

So what actually causes a migraine? Sophisticated imaging and biochemical studies are getting us much closer to answering that question. So far it looks like all the various migraine triggers focus in on the brainstem, the part of the brain closest to the spinal cord. Chemical imbalances in certain centers there, triggered by factors in the environment, start a wave of chaotic neural discharges firing across the brain, flooding the brain with serotonin and other hormones, leading to leaky blood vessels, pain, and swelling.

Have you ever had an *ice-cream headache?* Many people have. The problem is not the ice cream per se but the temperature. The headache occurs when cold food hits the nerves on the roof of the mouth, triggering a pain sensation that feels as if it comes from the forehead or behind the eyes. This type of headache may have a strikingly sudden onset, but it usually resolves within a minute. Your child can still eat ice cream and popsicles, but she may have to go slowly, allowing the ice cream to melt on her tongue before letting it hit the roof of the mouth.

## DIAGNOSIS

There are no blood tests or X rays that differentiate between tension headaches and migraines. X rays may help make the diagnosis of a sinus headache. Expensive tests such as MRIs (Magnetic Resonance Imaging), CT (Computed Tomography) scans and EEGs are rarely necessary or helpful.[13] The most helpful information is a complete picture of the child's symptoms. If your child has frequent headaches, keep a diary or calendar noting the headaches, when they start, what seems to trigger them, how long they last, what seems to relieve them, and any other symptoms. This kind of record is more useful than a hundred CT scans or MRIs, and it doesn't cost you a penny. The best diagnostic test is keeping track of symptoms and triggers and getting a thorough physical examination by your pediatrician to make sure there aren't any neurological symptoms.

## WHAT IS THE BEST WAY TO TREAT HEADACHES?

The two most important aspects of any headache treatment are:

1. Recognize and address the underlying cause of the headache
2. Prevent it or treat it early rather than wait it out

The treatment for a sinus headache involves treating the sinus infection, while the treatment for a stress headache involves managing the stress. A headache signifying meningitis requires different therapy than a headache from a head injury. No matter what causes the pain, it's better to treat it early rather than wait until the body starts screaming even more loudly with worse symptoms.

This chapter does *not* cover the specific treatments for all causes of headaches. It focuses on treatments for tension headaches and migraine headaches.

## SEE YOUR HEALTH CARE PROFESSIONAL IF YOUR CHILD HAS:

- A very severe headache
- Headache accompanied by fever or stiff neck (possible meningitis)
- Headache and vomiting following a blow to the head (possible brain injury)
- Headache with seizures, dizziness, confusion, double vision, or trouble hearing
- Headache that is worse with "bearing down," coughing, or sneezing
- Headaches that are worse in the morning and get better during the day
- Headache that lasts longer than two days or gets worse over time

Also seek professional care if you suspect that your child might have a sinus infection, a dental problem or jaw problem, lead poisoning, high blood pressure, or some other serious problem underlying her headaches.

Let's tour the Therapeutic Mountain to find out what works for tension and migraine headaches. If you want to skip to my bottom-line recommendations, flip to the end of the chapter.

## BIOCHEMICAL THERAPIES: MEDICATIONS, HERBS, NUTRITIONAL SUPPLEMENTS

### Medications

To treat everyday *tension headaches*, all your child may need is a nonprescription pain reliever and a nap in a dark, quiet room.

## NONPRESCRIPTION PAIN RELIEVERS

- Aspirin
- Acetaminophen (Tylenol, Panadol, and other brands)
- Ibuprofen (Advil, Motrin, and others)
- Naproxen (Aleve; by prescription: Anaprox or Naprosyn)

*Aspirin* is inexpensive and widely available. It has even proven effective in treating some migraine headaches. Aspirin should *not* be taken when your child has influenza or chicken pox because of the risk of developing Reye's syndrome, a potentially deadly disorder of the liver and brain. Because of this risk, many physicians now steer clear of aspirin; most pediatricians also recommend the chicken pox vaccine for your child. Aspirin can cause an upset stomach and bleeding of the stomach lining; frequent or high doses can cause ringing in the ears.

*Acetaminophen* (Tylenol and other brands) is the most widely used nonprescription pain reliever. Generic brands are just as effective as name brands. Acetaminophen is inexpensive and is safe if taken in recommended doses. Acetaminophen starts to work in thirty to forty-five minutes; benefits last for about four hours. Overdoses poison the liver and can be fatal.

*Ibuprofen* (Advil, Motrin, and other brands) is at least as effective as acetaminophen and lasts about two hours longer. Ibuprofen can cause upset stomach. If used as recommended, it is safe, and many kids prefer its flavor to acetaminophen's.

*Naproxen* (Aleve) has made the transition from a prescription to a nonprescription medication. In the process, the price dropped about 75%. Naproxen is a powerful pain reliever that lasts up to twelve hours. It can cause stomach upset and may only be tolerable if taken with food. It is very effective for migraines but is probably overkill for simple tension headaches. I recommend that migraine sufferers keep some on hand to treat severe headaches.

Combining caffeine with any of these non-prescription pain relievers boosts their effectiveness.[14] You can either buy a combination product (such as Extra Strength Excedrin) or have your child take her pain reliever with a cup of coffee or cola.

For *migraine headaches*, additional medications have proven effective in prevention and treatment. If your child has migraines more than once a month, talk with your health care professional about preventive medications.

## PREVENTIVE MEDICATIONS FOR MIGRAINES

- *Beta-blocker medications:* propranolol (Inderal) and others
- *Blood pressure medications:* calcium-channel blockers (Flunarizine and others); ACE inhibitor (Lisinopril and others)
- *Antidepressant medication:* amitryptiline (Elavil) SSRIs
- Methysergide (Sansert)
- *Antihistamines:* cyproheptadine (Periactin)
- *Seizure medications:* phenobarbital, phenytoin (Dilantin), carbamazepine (Tegretol)

*Beta-blocker medications* such as propranolol (Inderal) have been the medication of choice for preventing migraine headaches for over twenty years. In adults, propranolol reduces migraine headaches an average of 43%—about the same reduction achieved with biofeedback training.[15] Propranolol also pre-

vents pediatric migraines. Promising candidates for preventing pediatric migraine include propranolol's relatives, nadolol, timolol, atenolol, and metoprolol. Propranolol should *not* be used in children suffering from asthma, heart failure, or depression, because it can worsen these disorders.

*Calcium-channel blocking drugs* were originally used to treat high blood pressure. Lowering blood pressure does not necessarily prevent migraine headaches, and it looks like calcium-channel blockers affect the balance of different chemicals that contribute to migraine headaches as well as chemicals causing high blood pressure. It may take several months before taking them starts to reduce headache frequency. They are not a perfect cure; even after six months, calcium-channel blockers such as Flunarizine cut headache frequency by only about 50%. Angiotensin-converting enzyme (ACE) inhibitors, such as Lisinopril, are also effective for some patients in cutting the frequency of migraine episodes.[16] Be very careful using these powerful medications in young children.

Certain *antidepressant* drugs called tricyclic antidepressants (such as amitryptiline) and selective serotonin reuptake inhibitors (such as fluoxetine) successfully prevent migraines in adults (even those who were not depressed), but have not been thoroughly tested with controlled trials in children.[17] They may be useful to try in children who have migraines and depression, but I do not recommend them as first-line migraine prevention for children who are not depressed.

*Sansert* is an effective migraine preventer, but because of its severe side effects, it is not much used in the United States.[18] *Periactin,* a widely used prescription *antihistamine,* also prevents migraines; its side effects include drowsiness and increased appetite.[19] Periactin has not yet been compared to other treatments. I do not recommend it for children.

In the past, the seizure medications *phenobarbital* and *Dilantin* were used to prevent migraines, but they have substantial side effects and have not been rigorously tested as migraine treatments for children. *Valproate* prevents migraines in older children and adults, but it is rarely used unless the migraineur also suffers from seizures because of the potential for serious side effects.[20] There is less evidence supporting the use of other seizure medicines such as carbamazepine (Tegretol).

In general, there are a lot of medications that may offer some benefit in terms of *preventing* migraines. None of them offers 100% protection and most can cause serious side effects. I'd reserve prescription medications for those children who have not been sufficiently helped by nonprescription medications, lifestyle changes, massage, acupuncture, and mind-body therapies such as biofeedback.

## TREATMENT MEDICATIONS FOR MIGRAINE (PRESCRIPTION ONLY)

- Ergotamine and dihydroergotamine (DHE)
- Sumatriptan (Imitrex), zolmitriptan (Zomig), and others
- Antihistamines (Benadryl and others)
- *Antinausea medications:* metoclopromide (Reglan), prochlorperazine (Compazine), and chlorpromazine (Thorazine)
- *Topical anesthetics:* intranasal lidocaine
- Sedatives and narcotics (butalbital, Valium, Demerol, morphine)
- Steroids (dexamethasone and prednisone)
- Combinations (Midrin and Fiorinal)

*Ergotamine*, which is derived from the ergot fungus that grows on wheat, is one of the oldest medications used to treat migraines. Ergotamine is better absorbed and more effective when caffeine is added. If it is taken as soon as the child feels the headache coming on, Cafergot (caffeine and ergotamine) frequently minimizes subsequent symptoms. Cafergot has significant side effects including cold hands and feet from blood vessel spasms. Synthetic *dihydroergotamine* (DHE) is available by prescription for injection (in the emergency room, for example) and by nasal spray (Migranal nasal spray) and suppositories. The injection and nasal spray cost about five to ten times as much as ergotamine pills, but if nausea is a big problem with your child's migraines, she may not be able to take a pill in the midst of her headache, and it's good to have some other options. If your child ends up taking this medication frequently, she can grow dependent on it and suddenly stopping it may lead to rebound headaches.

*Sumatriptan* (Imitrex) was the first serotonin 5-HT(1) agonist medication to treat migraine headaches. It is available for use by mouth, by nose spray, and by injection. Newer medications in the same family include zolmitriptan (Zomig), naratriptan (Amerge), and rizatriptan (Maxalt); they are all fairly expensive. Sumatriptan starts to work in minutes, relieving the pain, the oversensitivity to lights and sounds, and the nausea and vomiting of migraine headaches. It works best when given at the beginning of headache symptoms and usually works with just one dose; it is *not* a preventive medication. Sumatriptan causes a brief rise in blood pressure, which is safe for most adolescents but may be hazardous in those with severe heart disease or those with high blood pressure. Other side effects include experiencing an awful taste and tingling in the mouth, flushing, tingling all over the body, warmth, and light-headedness. It has proven useful in teenagers as well as adults, and has become one of the most commonly used migraine medications in emergency rooms.[21] It's definitely better than placebo pills, but it may not be worth the cost over simpler and less expensive medications such as ibuprofen combined with antinausea remedies.[22]

*Antihistamines* (like Benadryl and Periactin) often cause drowsiness and help sufferers sleep.

Nausea and vomiting are among the most troublesome migraine symptoms. *Antinausea medications*, such as metoclopromide, not only treat nausea, but by promoting normal intestinal movement, they aid the absorption of other pain medicines. Two other powerful prescription antinausea medications (prochlorperazine and chlorpromazine) effectively relieve intractable migraine headaches as well as the nausea that accompanies them.[23] They are generally only used in emergency rooms, where they are given by injection to migraine sufferers who have not found relief with typical home treatments.[24] These medications may cause drowsiness, dizziness, and a drop in blood pressure.

Remember the shot of numbing medicine you got last time you went to the dentist? Well, a related numbing medicine or *topical anesthetic,* lidocaine, can help relieve headache pain for over half of adults suffering from migraine if some is squirted up the nose soon after the headache starts.[25] It has been used for a while to treat cluster headaches in adults, but it may not last long enough (not much more than an hour) to help with migraines. There are still no studies evaluating lidocaine as a pediatric headache treatment.

Many of the *sedative* medications used to treat migraine work by promoting sleep, which is the way people historically handled migraines. Sedatives such as butalbital and Valium work solely by putting the patient to sleep; they do not address the underlying cause of the headache, and I do *not* recommend them. *Narcotic* pain relievers (such as Demerol, morphine, and codeine) are widely used in emergency rooms as migraine treatments, but they carry the risk of addiction. Emergency room personnel have become wary of persons showing up in the ER complaining of headaches and demanding narcotic medications. None of these medications actually addresses the cause of headaches, but they have been used for many years when no other effective medication was available.

Midrin is the brand name of a *combination medication:* acetaminophen, isometheptene, and dichloralphenazone. Midrin is effective in adults but has *not* been evaluated in children. Fiorinal is the combination of aspirin, caffeine, and butalbital (a sedative). Midrin and Fiorinal can be addicting and are not any more effective than other headache medications. I do not recommend them.

## Herbs

As there are many kinds of headaches, there are many traditional remedies. Herbal headache remedies include: angelica, balm mint, chamomile, cowslip flowers, ginseng, feverfew, hawthorn, lavender, peppermint, rosemary, skullcap, valerian, violet flowers, and white willow bark. Willow bark is the original source of aspirin (now made synthetically); the bark itself contains very small quantities of the painkiller. Most of the other herbs have not been systematically studied.

Migraine sufferers who eat as little as two to three *feverfew* leaves a day report a dramatic decrease in the frequency and severity of their headaches.[26] Feverfew is a member of the Chrysanthemum family of plants and is easily grown in the home garden. A double-blind study showed that 25 milligrams twice daily of freeze-dried feverfew leaves effectively prevented migraines in adults.[27] Feverfew is used preventively; you cannot wait until your child has a headache and then expect feverfew to relieve it. It must be taken daily to work. Suddenly stopping it or missing several doses can cause rebound headaches. About 10% of those who take feverfew develop sores in their mouths. The amount of active ingredient in different commercial products varies widely, and some contain no active ingredients at all. Herbal products are not well regulated in the United States. Biochemical analysis has shown great variability in the strength, potency, and purity of commercially available feverfew preparations.[28] American-grown feverfew contains hardly any active compounds at all compared with plants grown in England. So, even though it may be helpful theoretically, I do not recommend feverfew to my patients here in the United States.[29]

*Capsaicin* is the spicy ingredient in hot peppers. It appears to decrease the nerve transmitters responsible for pain. Hot peppers have long been a folk remedy for painful conditions. In an experimental trial, capsaicin nasal spray successfully reduced pain in adults suffering from cluster headaches (a type of adult headache related to migraine).[30] Capsaicin has *not* been studied as a treatment of childhood headaches. It can certainly sting and cause severe irritation if it gets in the eyes. Do not spray pepper up your child's nose. If you want to try it, use it in food.

*Ginger* is a traditional remedy for headaches and upset stomachs. It is widely used in East Africa and in Ayurvedic medicine as a headache cure. Certain compounds in ginger appear to work the same way as aspirin does, blocking inflammation and pain. There are several case reports that taking raw ginger or ginger powder daily helped prevent migraines in adults.[31] There are *no* studies evaluating its effectiveness in preventing or treating children's headaches. Nevertheless, ginger is safe, inexpensive, and widely available. If you want to give it a try for your headache-prone child, keep careful track of her headaches for a month before and

for at least three months after boosting her ginger intake.

*Tiger Balm* is a popular nonprescription salve used for all kinds of aches and pains, including headache pain. It contains a number of herbal extracts including menthol, cajuput, camphor, and clove oil. In a randomized, controlled crossover trial among 57 adults who came to clinic suffering from a severe tension headache, Tiger Balm was significantly more effective than placebo rubs in relieving headache pain; in fact, it worked faster and was as strong as acetaminophen (nonaspirin pain reliever) taken by mouth.[32] Although this salve may cause a little tingling and tickle the nose, Tiger Balm is very safe. Massage it into the temples, neck, and shoulders as soon as a headache starts.

*Valerian* and *skullcap* are traditional sedative herbs, but recent reports raise the possibility that chronic use of valerian can cause liver trouble. *Lavender, chamomile,* and *mint* are used in many stress-related conditions because they are so calming. Unfortunately, there are *no* studies evaluating their effectiveness in treating adults or children suffering from headaches.

An *herbal bath* may be soothing. Herbs traditionally added to the headache sufferer's bath include balm mint, chamomile, hops, St. John's wort, lavender, rosemary, peppermint, and rose. Put the dried herbs in an old pillowcase or a stocking to make cleanup easier. Alternatively, you can add a few drops of the essential oils of these herbs to the bathwater. There are no scientific studies evaluating the effectiveness of herbal baths as headache treatments; you can experiment to find out what works best for your child.

Headaches can be a *side effect* of herbs. Ginkgo causes headache and upset stomach even at normal doses. Hops (even in the innocuous sleep pillow—see Chapter 24, Sleep Problems) have also been accused of causing headaches and nausea. Ephedra, commonly used to treat congestion and colds, can cause high blood pressure, rapid heart rate, and headache.

## Nutritional Supplements

### NUTRITIONAL SUPPLEMENTS FOR HEADACHES

*No:* vitamin A, vitamin D, zinc, niacin
*Probably not helpful:* vitamin B6
*Maybe:* magnesium

It is much better for your child to get her vitamins and minerals from foods rather than from pills. Excessive vitamin A causes a buildup of pressure inside the brain that produces such severe symptoms, it has been mistaken for a brain tumor. Overdoses of vitamin D can also cause headaches. Excessive zinc can cause headaches as well as stomachaches, nausea, vomiting, and decreased appetite. Niacin injections were used in the 1940s to treat headache pain, but later studies showed that they were no better than a placebo for curing headache pain. I do *not* recommend them.

For many women, headaches are one of many troublesome symptoms of the premenstrual and early pregnancy periods and are sometimes a side effect of oral contraceptive pills. Vitamin B6 has been suggested as a safe supplement to prevent hormonal headaches, but unfortunately, it turns out to be no better than placebo pills in preventing them.[33]

Children who suffer from migraines have lower levels of magnesium in their blood than healthy children, with even lower magnesium levels during headaches.[34] Platelets, the blood cells that appear to be dysfunctional triggers of migraines, also have lower levels of magnesium in headache sufferers.[35] This has led to a fair amount of speculation as to whether magnesium supplements might be helpful in preventing migraines.[36] So far, the only studies of magnesium supplements have been done in women whose migraines are part of the premenstrual syndrome. In a comparison study, magnesium supplements (360 milligrams taken three times daily) were significantly more effective than placebo pills in reducing premenstrual symptoms including migraine.[37] These results are promising, but we are a long way from completely understanding all of the risks and benefits of supplements with a single mineral and how megadoses might affect the balance of other minerals and functions elsewhere in the body. I recommend that your child eat plenty of magnesium-rich foods such as figs, nuts, seeds, citrus fruits, corn, apples, and dark green vegetables rather than relying on magnesium supplements. If you're going to give supplements, give a balanced multivitamin and mineral product from a reputable manufacturer. If you're giving calcium supplements to a teenage girl to help build up her bones, make sure the supplement also contains magnesium.

## LIFESTYLE THERAPIES: NUTRITION, EXERCISE, ENVIRONMENT, MIND-BODY

### Nutrition

Food allergies and food sensitivities are commonly blamed for migraine headaches. A British study showed that 93% of children suffering from weekly migraines and other allergy symptoms (e.g., skin rashes, diarrhea, wheezing) markedly improved when they consumed a low-allergen diet.[38] This diet (only one type of meat, one fruit, one vegetable, one carbohydrate, water, and vitamins allowed) for three to four weeks is gradually supplemented with one new food each week.[39] Any foods provoking headaches are withdrawn. The foods that provoke symptoms most often are cow's milk, egg, chocolate, orange, wheat, corn, cheese, tomato, cane sugar, benzoic acid, and the yellow dye tartrazine.[40] Other studies have confirmed these findings in adult migraine sufferers.[41] In another study, however, even children with frequent migraines that were thought to be triggered by foods did not have symptoms when given them under double-blind study conditions.[42]

Avoiding allergenic foods is rarely successful because it is difficult to change family eating habits. In a study of adults with chronic headache, 75% identified one or more foods as headache triggers. However, most of them did not act on this knowledge. They ate just like people who didn't suffer from chronic headaches, except they drank a little less red wine.[43] This may be one reason physicians rarely pursue food sensitivities in the treatment of headache; even when extensive tests are done, families rarely follow through on the rigorous diets required.

There are no reliable tests that can tell you in advance which foods will cause problems for a particular child, so if you want to find out whether your child has a true sensitivity, you need to start with the bare bones and gradually add things. An alternative approach is to eliminate those foods most commonly associated with headaches in other children and then slowly add them back, one at a time. Many children who are sensitive to particular foods do eventually "outgrow" their sensitivity and tolerate these foods later without any symptoms. Besides being extremely difficult to institute, these diets run the risk of nutritional deficiencies unless supervised by a pediatric nutrition expert. *See your health care professional before starting any special diet.*

## Exercise

Being overly tired is a setup for developing a headache. Make sure your child gets *plenty of rest*, especially during periods of increased stress. Going to bed in a quiet, dark place is useful even after one feels the aura for a migraine starting. For many people, going to bed is the main treatment for migraines. Usually by the time the sufferer awakens, the headache is gone. Rest is also helpful for many of the illnesses (such as influenza, intestinal flu, strep throats, and sinus infections) that cause headaches.

Vigorous *exercise during the day* (when the child is not having a headache) is one of the best remedies for stress. Aerobic exercise seems to be a natural antidepressant. Exercise programs can be very useful in preventing migraine headaches as well as relieving the stress that triggers tension headaches.[44]

## Environment

Being in a *quiet, dark environment* is soothing for many headache sufferers. Often the stress that precipitates a headache is due to loud noises (e.g., construction noises right outside), bright lights, or overstimulation. Relaxing in bed in a quiet, dark room helps reduce the environmental stress level.

*Pressure, heat,* and *cold* have all been reported to ease headache pain. Some folks feel better if they stand under a hot shower or apply a *heat pack* to their neck and shoulders. Others prefer *ice packs* to the back of the neck or forehead. Nowadays you can purchase a special gel-filled headband that can be tightened around the head with a Velcro strap; the headband can either be heated in the microwave or cooled in the freezer and then strapped around the head, applying pressure and the most favored temperature for the headache sufferer. This device was actually studied in 15 adults with severe headaches and found to be helpful and have fewer side effects than many headache medicines.[45] Other home remedies include a ten- to fifteen-minute *hot foot bath* or *soak*. The heat dilates the blood vessels of the feet and promotes general relaxation.

Exposure to *toxic chemicals, fumes,* and *carbon monoxide* is a hidden cause of many headaches. When I was studying hypnosis, we learned of a girl with severe recurrent headaches who had been evaluated for several serious illnesses. Her headaches responded briefly to hypnotherapy but then recurred. Finally her parents looked for an environmental cause. They found it in their own garage (which was next to the girl's bedroom); a faulty furnace was spewing carbon monoxide into the air and poisoning their daughter. When the furnace problem was corrected, their daughter's headaches disappeared. Carbon monoxide poisoning can occur wherever there is incomplete combustion such as from a leaky car exhaust pipe, smog, and fumes from charcoal being burned indoors during a power outage.

## Mind-Body

Stress is a definite trigger for headaches. Children who report bullying or other distressing events at school are much more likely to suffer from headaches than other kids. If your child suffers from recurrent headaches, keep a diary or log of her symptoms. You can use a regular calendar or make your own. Write down the date and time of the headache (was it a school day? a weekend? first thing in the morning? after school? just before or during a menstrual period?), the events, food, or other factors that seemed to trigger it, what you did to treat it, how long it lasted, and if anything seemed to make it worse or better. By keeping careful track of your child's symptoms, you will be well on the way to determining their cause and the best ways to prevent and treat them.

Mind-body therapies such as *biofeedback, hypnosis*, and *progressive relaxation* effectively prevent headaches for many children and have fewer side effects than most medications.[46] Remember, no method is 100% effective for all children. However, mind-body therapies can help 50 to 75 percent of headache sufferers.[47] The combination of *deep breathing, autogenic training,* and *progressive muscle relaxation* can even ease headaches after they've started as well as reduce the frequency of getting them in the first place. These techniques require training and regular practice. Most adults require about two months of practice before they notice fewer symptoms.

### EFFECTIVE MIND-BODY THERAPIES FOR PREVENTING MIGRAINES

- Hypnosis
- Autogenic training
- Biofeedback: thermal and EMG
- Progressive relaxation

Several studies have demonstrated that the most effective preventive therapy for migraines in children is *relaxation*, whether through self-hypnosis, the relaxation response (meditation), autogenic training, biofeedback, or progressive muscle relaxation.[48] As with other therapies, one type may work better for your child than another. A review of many studies found that relaxation therapy alone improved symptoms for 38% of adults with migraine headaches and 45% of those with tension headaches. Unlike the benefits of medication, which tend to wear off soon after the medication is stopped, the benefits of relaxation training last for several years beyond the initial training period.[49] Some of these therapies can be learned and practiced at home after a few training sessions with a professional—all of which leads to lower cost than continuous treatment with prescription medications.[50]

*Self-hypnosis* is even more effective than the most commonly prescribed medication, propanolol, in preventing migraines in children.[51] Children as young as six years old can learn hypnosis to help them prevent headaches. Hypnosis is simply being in a very relaxed state of mind in which the child's attention is focused on pleasant, healing images.

You can help your child relax through *deep breathing exercises* (in which the child watches her belly rise and fall with each breath), *progressive muscle relaxation,* or repeating a favorite phrase, affirmation, or prayer. Relaxing, pain-reducing images for your child might include the following:

1.  Imagine that the pain is like a bunch of bubbles. Take a deep breath in. Each time you breathe out, blow the bubbles out of your head and watch them disappear as they float up into a soft, blue sky.
2.  Imagine yourself in your favorite place. It may be home in bed with your parent reading you a story. It may be at the beach or in the woods or Disneyland. Imagine yourself there feeling very safe and happy.
3.  Imagine the sun warming your hands and feet.
4.  Imagine the pain as a point on a dial inside your head. Reach over and gradually turn the dial down until it is at zero.
5.  Imagine the pain as a thermometer reading. Watch the thermometer go down and down as the headache disappears. Imagine putting an ice cube at the bottom of the thermometer so it goes down even faster.

I'm sure you and your child can imagine even more ways of blowing away or turning down the pain.

*Autogenic training* is a kind of self-hypnosis in which the person tells herself several relaxing statements over and over. Autogenic training is an effective treatment for chronic tension headaches.[52]

*Biofeedback* is particularly useful in preventing pediatric migraine headaches, and I almost always refer my migraine headache patients to a psychologist who can help train them in biofeedback techniques. The simplest example of thermal biofeedback is the old-fashioned mood ring. More sophisticated devices use more sensitive thermistors to measure temperature and can display the results in colors, lights, or sounds. Children can learn thermal biofeedback readily, and many science museums around the country now contain exhibits using thermal biofeedback devices to teach kids about biofeedback. Electromyographic (EMG) biofeedback provides information about muscle tension to help one learn to relax specific muscles.

Preventing and treating headaches is an area in which biofeedback therapy really shines.[53] Thermal (fingertip temperature) feedback has proved especially helpful in preventing migraines and drastically reducing the need for medication; for many children, biofeedback is even more effective than medication.[54] Benefits persist for at least six years in those who have participated in just eight to ten weeks of biofeedback training.[55] Newer studies suggest that fewer formal training sessions are necessary if children continue to practice relaxation techniques at home; this makes biofeedback a more financially attractive treatment option.[56] By relaxing tense muscles, EMG biofeedback has been especially helpful for those with chronic tension headaches.[57] Controlled studies document the effectiveness of EMG biofeedback training in reducing the pain and frequency of muscle tension headaches in children as young as six years old.[58]

*Progressive relaxation exercise* combined with *diaphragmatic breathing* can help reduce the frequency and intensity of headaches for many children. As preventive therapy for headaches, they can be as effective as biofeedback training and less costly.[59] Relaxation exercises increase the child's sense of mastery, decrease her sense of distress, decrease her muscle tension, and distract her from pain. The benefits of progressive relaxation exercises, self-hypnosis, and autogenic training can persist for years in children with both tension headaches and migraine headaches.

Mind-body techniques are most effective if practiced regularly. Children benefit from home practice and the encouragement of supportive parents.[60] Most successful programs combine biofeedback training with imagery, breathing, or relaxation techniques. I recommend professional relaxation, hypnosis, and/or biofeedback training as first-line treatment for children with frequent or severe headaches. Even those children who end up requiring medications may benefit from these nondrug therapies.

## BIOMECHANICAL THERAPIES: MASSAGE, SPINAL ADJUSTMENTS, SURGERY

### Massage

Massage is one of the most widely used headache remedies. It is a perfectly natural response to headache pain, and it has proven effectiveness. In one study, adult headache sufferers who came to the doctor looking for stronger medication were offered either massage of acupuncture; both massage and acupuncture relieved pain for most patients, but massage appeared to have a slight edge.[61] In a randomized trial of 26 adult migraneurs, those who received 30-minute massages ten times over five weeks had a significant increase in the number of days free of headaches, better sleep, and less distress than those who did not receive massage therapy.[62] Massage is one of the most underutilized therapies in medicine. Just about every child would benefit from having a parent provide massages on a regular basis, and this is particularly true for kids with recurrent headaches.

### RECIPE FOR A HEAVENLY HEADACHE MASSAGE

1. Start by massaging your child's forehead. Put your thumbs together at the center and top of her forehead and slowly stroke away from the center. Repeat this movement, moving gradually down toward the eyebrows with each repetition.
2. Next, massage her temples slowly using tiny circular motions.
3. Move to the back of the skull at the place where the skull meets the spine. Rub from the center away toward the ears and make slow, gentle circles in all the tender spots.
4. Then massage the back of the neck, moving from the back of the skull downward toward the shoulders.
5. Before doing the shoulders themselves, try a brisk scalp rub. Use your fingertips or knuckles to lightly "scrub" your child's scalp as if you were giving her a shampoo, first one side, then the other.
6. Gently knead the muscles of the shoulders and upper back. Experiment with what feels best for your child.
7. Finish the head and neck massage by massaging your child's face. In general, it feels best if you use your thumbs, moving from the center toward the sides of the face. Slide

along the bones that form the rim of the eye socket. Rub from the bridge of the nose down to the tip. Be sure to massage the jaw from the chin up toward the ears. Gently tug and wiggle her earlobes.

8. If your child is too tender to be touched on the head, neck, or shoulders, try giving her a foot rub instead. It may help relax her, and in one study of adults, reflexology (specialized foot rubs) effectively reduced headaches for 81% of patients.[63]

Be very gentle. There are often sore spots where the muscles have been tightly tensed. It is better to massage these spots lightly, focusing on the less painful areas and coming back to the tight spots, gradually increasing pressure as your child tolerates it. If your child's head or neck is tender, you may want to give her a foot massage first to help her relax. You might try adding one or two drops of lavender, peppermint, or eucalyptus oil to one teaspoon of plain vegetable oil as a special headache massage lotion because they are relaxing and help decrease pain.[64] If your child's headaches are particularly severe or recurrent and you want professional assistance, see a massage therapist or physical therapist to learn how to help.[65]

## Spinal Adjustments

Cranial and spinal adjustments or manipulation are widely used to treat headaches and neck aches, and many chiropractors claim that this is the treatment of choice for headaches.[66] If you've found help there, no need to give it up. However, a Danish study reported in the *Journal of the American Medical Association* in 1998 found that there was no benefit to chiropractic therapy beyond that found in a group that received massage.[67] I know the chiroprac-

tors will hate me for saying it, but I think you should stick with massage for your child—at least until better studies prove that chiropractic has more to offer and is a cost-effective alternative to parent-provided massage.

## Surgery

There is no need for surgery to treat most childhood headaches. However, surgery can be lifesaving for severe head trauma.

## BIOENERGETIC THERAPIES: ACUPUNCTURE, THERAPEUTIC TOUCH, HOMEOPATHY

### Acupuncture

Two small studies found that adult migraine sufferers improved just as much when they simply monitored their headaches over time as when they received acupuncture.[68] (Keeping track of your child's headaches can be therapeutic in itself!) On the other hand, several studies show that true acupuncture *is* more effective than sham treatments in reducing migraine frequency and pain as well as the need for pain medications in adults.[69] A study from Germany reported that acupuncture was effective in 80% of adults with migraine headaches.[70] Several other studies also suggest that acupuncture effectively prevents many migraine headaches.[71] Other studies suggest that acupuncture is as effective in preventing migraines as a standard medications.[72] One study looked at acupuncture in pediatric migraine sufferers and found it offered significant benefit.[73] I refer more and more of my migraine patients to my acupuncture colleagues as do my physician colleagues who specialize in pain treatment.

Acupuncture has also been recommended for muscle tension headaches as well as migraines.[74] A Swedish study compared acupuncture to physical therapy (massage, ice massage, progressive relaxation, biofeedback, transcutaneous electrical nerve stimulation, and general relaxation) for adults with chronic tension headache; both treatments improved symptoms, but the combination of physical therapies was better than acupuncture.[75] It is not surprising that a multifaceted approach worked better than a single therapy. In a controlled study, true acupuncture was more effective than sham acupuncture in preventing adults' chronic tension headaches.[76] More studies are needed to examine the role of acupuncture in the treatment of tension headaches in children. So far, it looks promising. If your child's headaches have not responded to other remedies, acupuncture therapy is worth trying.

## Therapeutic Touch

Therapeutic Touch successfully treats tension headaches. In a comparison trial, Therapeutic Touch effectively relieved tension headaches in 90% of recipients, and relief was sustained for over four hours.[77] Therapeutic Touch is safe, and I often use it in my practice for both patients and colleagues who have headaches.

## Homeopathy

A recent study compared homeopathic remedies to placebo pills in 68 adults with migraine headaches; although their daily headache diaries did not show any benefit from homeopathy, those who took the remedies seemed slightly better to their neurologists.[78] In three other studies, homeopathy was no better than placebo pills.[79] The most commonly recommended homeopathic headache remedies are: Belladonna, Bryonia, Gelsemium, and *Nux vomica*. There are no studies evaluating the effectiveness of homeopathic remedies in treating headaches in children. They are certainly safe, but I do not routinely recommend them.

※

# WHAT I RECOMMEND FOR HEADACHES

## PREVENTING HEADACHES

If your child has frequent headaches, keep a diary or log of the headaches, headache triggers, and remedies.

1. *Lifestyle—exercise.* Make sure your child gets plenty of regular sleep at night and vigorous aerobic exercise during the day.

2. *Lifestyle—nutrition.* If your child suffers from other allergy symptoms (runny nose, diarrhea, skin rashes) as well as frequent headaches, see your health care professional or a nutritionist to discuss the possibility of a low-allergenic diet. Try avoiding nitrates, nitrites, aspartame, MSG, chocolate, and aged cheeses and monitor your child's headaches. Avoid sudden changes in caffeine consumption. Give your child calcium and magnesium-rich foods. Also consider including ginger and hot peppers as part of her diet.

3. *Lifestyle—environment.* Avoid known allergens and toxins such as carbon monoxide and lead. Try using a gel pack–filled headband that can be tightened around the head to apply pressure to the painful areas. These headbands can be cooled or heated, as preferred by the child.

4. *Lifestyle—mind-body.* Have your child practice relaxation exercises or meditation regularly to help minimize stress and build a sense of mastery. Consider professional mind-body therapies such as self-hypnosis, guided imagery, or biofeedback training.

5. *Biochemical—medications, herbs, and nutritional supplements.* See your physician about preventive prescription medications such as beta-blockers. Consider giving your child a dietary supplement containing calcium and magnesium (check with your doctor about the proper dose for your child).

6. *Biomechanical—massage.* Try giving your child a massage every night before bed.

7. *Bioenergetic—acupuncture.* If it's acceptable to your child and a pediatric acupuncturist is available, consider acupuncture therapy.

*See your health care professional if your child has a headache and:*

- You are concerned about possible meningitis (fever, stiff neck, spotted rash) or your child is lethargic or irritable

- Your child has recently suffered a head injury *and* vomits more than three times, vomits more than one hour after the injury, has difficulty hearing or seeing properly, has clear or bloody fluid coming out of the nose or ears, has a seizure, or becomes more clumsy, off-balance, or dizzy

- The headache is severe and won't go away with simple home remedies

- You are concerned about a possible sinus or tooth infection: facial pain, runny nose or thick mucus from the nose, fever, or pain in the jaw, teeth, ears, or eyes

- You are concerned that your child has an underlying serious illness: frequent recurring headaches despite home remedies; the child seems unwell, tired, has a poor appetite, is not growing well, has a change in personality, or becomes clumsier

## TREATING HEADACHES

1. *Biochemical—medications.* If your child's migraines are only moderately severe, try a nonprescription pain reliever such as acetaminophen (Tylenol), ibuprofen (Advil or Motrin), or naproxen (Aleve) in combination with caffeine; consider asking your pediatrician for a prescription for metoclopromide (Reglan) to help with the nausea and help the medications actually get into the child's system. For children with more severe migraines, see your physician about sumatriptan or zolmitriptan to have on hand to treat the headache in its early stages.[80] You are much better off starting with something strong than starting weak and working your way up.

2. *Biochemical—herbs.* Try rubbing a little Tiger Balm salve into the temples, the neck, and the upper shoulders at the first sign of a headache.

3. *Lifestyle—environment.* Have your child lie quietly for a few minutes in a dark room; try an ice pack on the back of her neck. Alternatively, try a hot foot bath or warm towels around her feet.

4. *Biomechanical—massage.* Try a head, neck, and shoulder massage. If she is too sore, try a foot massage instead. Consider adding oil of peppermint, lavender, or eucalyptus to the massage oil. Consider seeking professional help from a licensed massage therapist or physical therapist.

## RESOURCES

National Headache Foundation
5252 N. Western Ave.
Chicago, IL 60625
(800) 843-2256
http://www.headaches.org/

American Council for Headache Education
875 Kings Highway, Suite 200
West Depford, NJ 08096
(800) 255-ACHE
http://www.achenet.org/

American Massage Therapy Association
820 Davis St.
Evanston, IL 60201-4444
(847) 864-0123;
Fax (847) 864-1178
http://www.amtamassage.org/

### Books

Lipton, Richard; Newman, Lawrence; MacLean, Helene. *Migraine: Beating the Odds: The Doctor's Guide to Reducing Your Risk.* Addison Wesley, 1992.

Solomon, Seymour. *The Headache Book.* Consumer Reports Books, 1991.

Saper, Joel R.; Magge, Kenneth. *Freedom from Headaches.* Fireside Books, 1986.

Sinclair, Marybetts. *Massage for Healthier Children.* Wingbow Press, 1992.

Thomas, Sara. *Massage for Common Ailments.* Fireside Books, 1988.

*To find a biofeedback therapist in your area, contact:*

Biofeedback Certification Institute of America
10200 West 44th Ave., Suite 304
Wheatridge, CO 80033
(303) 420-2902

*To find a pediatrician skilled in hypnosis, contact:*

Society for Developmental and Behavioral Pediatrics
19 Station Lane
Philadelphia, PA 19118
(215) 248-9168
http://www.sdbp.org/default.html

American Society of Clinical Hypnosis
33 W. Grand Ave., Suite 402
Chicago, IL 60610
(312) 645-9810
http://www.asch.net/

# 21
# HYPERACTIVITY (ATTENTION DEFICIT HYPERACTIVITY DISORDER)

Sandra Vincent called me in late September about her first-grader, Brian. She had always known Brian was active, but his teacher had called her in to discuss the possibility that Brian was hyperactive. His teacher said that Brian had a hard time sitting still and was usually out of his chair even before she'd finished calling attendance. He frequently shouted out answers impulsively, even if another child had been called on. Sandra wanted to bring him in for an evaluation and to discuss different treatments. She didn't like the idea of Brian having to take medicine every day just to be able to go to school, and she wanted to know if there were any other options.

Hyperactivity is shorthand for the diagnosis of *attention deficit hyperactivity disorder* (ADHD or ADD). ADHD is divided into three subtypes: one in which the primary problem is inattention; a second in which the primary problem is hyperactivity; and a third, mixed type. ADHD is the most commonly diagnosed behavioral disorder in children, and the number of kids diagnosed as ADHD skyrocketed in the 1980s and 1990s.[1] A study reviewing the medical records of over 20,000 school-age children in 44 different states found that 9% of children had been diagnosed with attention or hyperactivity problems.[2] In the 1990s approximately 5 to 10 percent of elementary school children were on medications for hyperactivity; the medication rates were highest for boys (two to four times more commonly than girls) and for Caucasian children (at least twice as common as for African American children).[3]

ADHD is not just a problem for kids in grade school. Increasing numbers of preschool kids are also being diagnosed as ADHD and being treated with stimulant medications.[4] In the early 1990s, nearly 1% of Baltimore County high school students were taking medications for hyperactivity. Prescriptions for hyperactivity medications increased more than tenfold between the 1970s and the 1990s.

There has been a national uproar and a great deal of concern about these high rates of diagnosis and drug treatment. Are we labeling normal behavior as a medical problem (over-diagnosis)? Are parents failing to teach discipline? Are teachers failing to enforce it? Are we creating a nation of addicts? What is going on? It's become such a hot topic that the American Academy of Pediatrics and the National Institutes of Health convened special task forces to look into the issue and to make standardized recommendations about evaluation, diagnosis, and treatment.[5]

Many speculate that ADHD simply reflects a poor fit between children's temperaments and current cultural and social expectations. Rather than be confined to crowded classrooms year after year, children used to stay at home and learn from their parents by active example. Although most children seem to have adapted to the demands of modern society, some simply don't have the disposition to sit still, pay attention, and wait their turn without one-to-one supervision. It doesn't take long before these children are labeled as trouble-makers; the label often becomes a self-fulfilling prophecy.

To some degree, impulsiveness, short attention span, and high activity levels are normal. Normal toddlers are messy, impatient, distractible, and very active. But things that are normal for two-year-olds are not necessarily normal for ten- or sixteen-year-olds. Before diagnosing ADHD, one has to be sure that the child is not simply acting his age. It's also important to rule out learning disabilities that impair a child's school performance. About one-third of children with ADHD also have another learning disability.

## SYMPTOMS OF ADHD

AT LEAST SIX SYMPTOMS OF SEVERE *IMPULSIVENESS:*

- Often acts before thinking
- Has difficulty organizing work
- Often blurts out answers, interrupts others' activities
- Has difficulty waiting his turn in group games or activities
- Shifts excessively from one activity to another
- Needs a lot of supervision
- Often engages in physically dangerous activities, e.g., runs into the street without looking

AT LEAST SIX SYMPTOMS OF *SHORT ATTENTION* AND/OR *HYPERACTIVITY:*

- Shorter than average attention span; distractibility; inattention
- Often fails to finish things he starts
- Has difficulty sustaining attention in tasks or activities
- Has difficulty following through on instructions
- Is easily distracted
- Does not seem to listen to what is being said to him
- Runs about or climbs things excessively
- Difficulty sitting still, fidgets with hands or squirms in seat
- Has difficulty staying seated
- Moves about excessively during sleep
- Is always on the go or acts as if "driven by a motor"

Symptoms of ADHD appear *before the child is seven years old*, but often the diagnosis is not made until the child's behavior starts causing problems in the classroom. Children don't have to have all of the above symptoms to be diagnosed as having ADHD. However, they do need to exhibit at least several of these characteristics more than is normal for their age *for at least six months*. One also needs to account for other causes of disruptive behavior (such as the acute stress of a death in the family, schizophrenia, depression, mental retardation, or petit mal seizures). Certain illnesses, such as itchy skin rashes and pinworms, can also make children irritable, distracted, and squirmy. ADHD may also be the first sign of thyroid problems. These conditions must be addressed before diagnosing ADHD.

*Sandra was curious about what actually causes ADHD—is it a genetic disease? Too much sugar? Bad parenting? Or what?*

## POSSIBLE CAUSES OF HYPERACTIVE BEHAVIOR

- Other medical problems
- Genetic factors or congenital problems
- Learning problems and other mental health issues
- Dietary problems
- Problems of arousal and low self-esteem

*Physical problems* such as impaired *hearing* and *vision* can cause problem behavior that is easily mistaken for hyperactivity. If your child can't hear the teacher, he can't very well pay attention to what she says. If your child can't see the blackboard, he's likely to pay more attention to what's on his neighbor's desk.

Another physical problem that can cause daytime hyperactivity is *poor sleeping* at night. Among the many causes of sleep problems, one of the biggest culprits is partially blocked breathing, called obstructive sleep apnea. Sometimes breathing is temporarily blocked during a cold or sinus infection. In these cases, breathing, sleep, and behavior return to normal when the infection clears. Chronic blockages are usually due to large adenoids or tonsils. Nighttime breathing blockages result in loud snoring and frequent stops and starts in breathing, daytime sleepiness, and poor growth. These obstructions can be easily corrected with surgery, which often results in dramatic improvements in behavior and growth. Sometimes it's a simple case of allergies causing the obstruction; treating the allergy can dramatically improve sleep at night and behavior during the day.

Brain damage due to *lead* poisoning has long-term effects on language and concentration skills. Lead levels are often elevated in hyperactive children. The higher the lead level, the more hyperactive symptoms. *Chelation therapy* (which removes lead from the system) helps improve hyperactive behavior in children with elevated lead levels. Thanks to stricter environmental regulations, the average blood lead level has dropped over the last twenty years, and lead poisoning accounts for very little of the ADHD seen nowadays.

*Brain damage* from any cause can result in problems in thinking, memory, and attention. Even minor damage from *head injury* can cause learning and behavior problems.

*Cigarette smoke* adversely affects many aspects of a child's health, including behavior. Maternal *smoking during pregnancy* subtly limits the oxygen supply to the baby's brain, and can contribute to hyperactivity.[6] In studies of children whose mothers used moderate amounts of alcohol, marijuana, and cigarettes during pregnancy, cigarettes had even more impact on intelligence and behavior than alcohol or drugs.[7] Maternal *smoking after pregnancy* also affects children's behavior; the more she smokes, the worse the child's behavior.[8] Exposure to smoke at home is a bigger risk factor for school failure than are recurrent ear infections.[9] Children of *alcoholic fathers* are also at increased risk of behavioral problems such as hyperactivity.[10]

*Pinworms* are a common childhood infection. The worms live in the large intestine and crawl out at night to lay their eggs on the skin. The worms' lifestyle leads to several symptoms in the child: an itchy bottom at night and irritability and distractibility throughout the day. Pinworms can be easily eradicated with medication, dramatically improving a child's disposition and behavior.

## DIAGNOSIS

The diagnosis of ADHD or hyperactivity is based on the child's symptoms. There are no blood tests, urine tests, X rays, or other laboratory tests that prove ADHD. Parents and teachers may be asked to complete questionnaires or daily diaries of the child's behavior to help confirm the diagnosis. The most widely used daily behavior diaries are the *Conners Parent Rating Scale* and the *Conners Teacher Rating Scale*. Other questionnaires include the *Child Behavior Checklist*, the *Yale Children's Inventory*, the *Behavior Rating Profile*, and the *ADD-H Comprehensive Teacher Rating Scale*, (ACTeRS). There is also a questionnaire specifically for adolescents who might have ADHD called the *ADD/H Adolescent Self-Report Scale*. If your child's symptoms and tests are *not* suggestive of any of other physical, emotional, or learning problems and they *are* consistent with ADHD, the diagnosis is made.

*I gave Sandra copies of the Conners parent and teacher rating scales for her and Brian's teacher to fill out over the next two weeks.*

Hyperactivity *runs in families*. Many parents whose children are diagnosed with hyperactivity report that they, too, have attention problems or *learning disabilities;* they also have an increased risk of substance abuse, depression,

and having been delinquent as children.[11] Between 30 and 70 percent of children who meet the criteria for ADHD also have learning disabilities, language problems, or slow learning. Learning problems such as dyslexia can also lead to distractibility. Language problems can be addressed by proper school evaluations. It's hard to pay attention if you can't understand or remember the directions. Improved language skills can dramatically improve academic and social performance.

*Sandra said that Brian's father had also had problems in school and wanted to make sure that Brian didn't have a specific learning disability. She scheduled an appointment for him to be tested by the school psychologist.*

Children who are *grieving* for a significant loss, such as the loss of a parent through death or divorce, are often inattentive to their school environment, may act out their sadness through aggression, or act impulsively in dangerous situations out of despair and hopelessness. Anxiety and depression can also mimic attention deficit disorder. Before a child is diagnosed with attention deficit disorder, consider whether the child has a long-term behavioral disorder or a reaction to an upsetting situation.

*Brian didn't seem to be suffering from any particular stresses this year and didn't appear to be anxious or depressed except about his school performance. While she was filling out the Conners scale and waiting for the results of the school psychologist's tests, Sandra wanted to do something to help Brian. She wondered if his problems weren't just caused by his grandparents' frequent indulgence of Brian's sweet tooth.*

The anti-*sugar* mania of the 1970s and 1980s was taken to its illogical extreme by the famous Twinkie defense. In 1978, a gunman named Dan White shot San Francisco's mayor and city supervisor. In his defense, White pleaded that his criminal behavior was due to his steady diet of Twinkies! Excellent scientific studies since then have proven that hyperactive children, even those whose parents swore the problem was sugar before the studies, were not made hyperactive by eating large amounts of sugar.[12] Sugar is not the culprit; sugar does not make kids or adults crazy, criminals, delinquents, or aggressive.[13] This is fortunate because almost all healthy fresh and dried fruits, starches, and grains are broken down into sugar during digestion.

On the contrary, sugar and other carbohydrates may exert a calming effect.[14] Have you ever indulged in "comfort foods"? Rice pudding, oatmeal, mashed potatoes, and other high-carbohydrate foods actually seem to calm the brain, reducing aggressive behavior.[15] Sucrose (plain table sugar) given before painful procedures such as blood drawing or circumcision helps calm infants and reduces pain.[16] Hyperactive children may unconsciously be trying to treat their symptoms by eating sweets.

After sugar was off the hyperactivity hook, another dietary villain was sought. Despite much concern about artificial sweeteners, *aspartame* has been exonerated from blame for hyperactivity.[17] Even in amounts ten times higher than that consumed by the average child, aspartame has no adverse effects on the behavior of hyperactive children.[18]

The same thing may be true of *caffeine*. More than 75% of all children regularly consume caffeine from soft drinks or chocolate.[19] On a weight basis, children typically consume more caffeine than adults. For example, a twenty-five-pound toddler who drinks a can of cola consumes about *twice* as much caffeine (for his size) as a 120-pound woman who drinks one strong cup of coffee a day. Caffeine improves attention in normal children and adults.[20] Hyperactive children tend to drink more caffeine-containing sodas than their unaffected peers. Again, hyperactive kids may be unconsciously treating their symptoms with caffeine.

Dr. Ben Feingold, a San Francisco allergist, developed his theory about hyperactivity from his observation that hyperactivity increased as Americans increased their intake of *artificial colorings and flavorings*. He was also alarmed at the increasing use of children's aspirin in the 1960s and 1970s, knowing that its active ingredient, salicylate, could trigger asthma symptoms in some patients. He became convinced that subtle allergic reactions to artificial colorings, flavorings, and salicylate were the basis for about 50% of cases of hyperactivity.

Based on this belief, he began treating hundreds of children with the Feingold diet, which excluded numerous processed and natural foods. Although he did not perform any controlled scientific studies, enthusiasm for his approach infected millions of frustrated families with hope that radically restricting their child's diet would improve intolerable behavior.

## FEINGOLD DIET AVOIDS

- Artificial colors and flavors, especially yellow dyes (tartrazine)
- Medicinal salicylate compounds such as aspirin, Pepto-Bismol, and oil of wintergreen
- Foods containing natural salicylates such as almonds, apples, apricots, berries, cherries, citrus, cloves, cucumbers, currants, grapes, raisins, nectarines, peaches, plums, prunes, strawberries, tea, and tomatoes

There has been a great deal of confusion about what items are actually excluded from this diet. For example, artificial preservatives, stabilizers, and other chemical ingredients, shunned by many parents, were not excluded from the original Feingold diet.

In the best study of the Feingold diet, three

dozen hyperactive children and their families were placed on experimental diets for up to two months.[21] The participating families were told only that the study was evaluating the effect of different foods on behavior. For this reason, every week during the study, all of the food in the study households was removed and replaced with free food, prepared and delivered by study personnel. The families did not know when they were on the Feingold diet and when they were on a similar diet that contained hidden artificial flavors and colors and natural salicylates. The children's behavior was closely monitored at home, at school, and in behavior/learning laboratories by parents, teachers, and trained observers, none of whom knew which diet the children were eating during any given week. Among school-age children, the Feingold diet did *not* improve attention, hyperactivity, or disruptive behavior. Among preschool children, parents reported modest improvements during the Feingold diet weeks, but these improvements were not discernible in the lab by objective observers and were nowhere near as dramatic as Feingold had originally claimed. The researchers concluded that there may be some preschool children whose behavior is improved by the Feingold diet, but there was no benefit for school-age children.

In a somewhat similar study in Pittsburgh, a nutritionist gave families advice about two different diets, each of which was to be followed for a month: the Feingold diet (though it was not named as such) and a comparison diet. The families in the study bought and prepared their own food based on the nutritionist's recommendations.[22] The children's teachers noted somewhat improved behavior on the Feingold diet, but parents did not.

In three later studies, children were knowingly placed on the Feingold diet. Those who seemed to improve were kept on the diet, and later tested the forbidden foods. Those who seemed to react to the foods were instructed to adhere strictly to the diet. Later, they were tested in double-blind studies comparing capsules or foods containing artificial colors versus placebos. Their behavior was closely monitored by parents and others who did not know when the child was given the real test substance and when the placebo was given. Under these conditions (in which parents had been strongly convinced of the efficacy of the Feingold diet before the study), fewer than 5% of children had consistently negative reactions to the artificial colors. The negative reactions included irritability, restless sleep, and other allergic reactions, not just hyperactivity. Similarly, double-blind challenges of yellow dye demonstrated that the majority of children were not adversely affected by it.

Numerous studies have also evaluated the possibility that hyperactivity is due to *food allergies*.[23] For the most part, these studies are not very convincing that food allergies play a significant role in hyperactive behavior in most children. When allergies do play a part, the child often has other symptoms, such as eczema or hay fever that make him uncomfortable and irritated.

The bottom line about food sensitivities is that the vast majority of hyperactivity is *not* due to food sensitivity of any kind. The main benefit of restrictive diets seems to be in the powerful placebo effect of making an entire family change its eating habits. There are rare children who experience behavioral as well as physical changes because of food allergies (see Chapter 4).[24] If you suspect your child has a food allergy, please have him evaluated by a health care professional who is experienced in pediatric nutrition.

*Sandra asked, "If it's not sugar or food allergies, then what is it? And is there any possibility that this is just a phase he's going through and that he'll outgrow it?"*

The real situation underlying ADHD seems

to be a *problem with arousal*. Arousal or vigilance is the state of being watchful, awake, and alert. Hyperactive children actually seem to be less aroused (less alert or vigilant) than other children. Have you ever noticed that when you are very tired it is difficult to concentrate, and that the only way to stay awake (if you must stay awake) is to move about or fidget? In addition to fidgeting, you might daydream or complain of being bored. Medications that increase arousal allow the child to stop fidgeting and to pay attention more easily. It takes a certain amount of alertness to inhibit impulsive behaviors; when watchfulness is decreased, there is more impulsive behavior and less thought about the consequences of that behavior.

An emerging scientific theory implicates different parts of the brain in the arousal/self-control/planning dysfunction found in ADHD. Scientific interest is currently focused on the frontal lobes, the basal ganglia (specifically the caudate nucleus and the globus pallidus) and the nerves in the brain that rely on the neurotransmitter dopamine.[25] Sophisticated imaging techniques such as functional Magnetic Resonance Imaging (fMRI) and PET scans are being used to try to pinpoint the various areas of the brain involved. But it will be awhile before all this basic science translates into new and effective treatments for ADHD.

Kids with ADHD also often suffer from poor sleep.[26] So there may be problems overall with arousal, sleeping, and wakefulness. In any event, if your child is diagnosed as having ADHD, be sure you talk with your pediatrician about sleep issues as well.

Without help, hyperactive children frequently become disruptive in a regular classroom and are soon labeled as the "bad kids." Children whose behavior frequently meets with disapproval often end up with poor self-images. This is certainly true of hyperactive children who frequently suffer from *low self-esteem*. Low self-esteem exacerbates feelings of hopelessness and aggressiveness. This is the basis for mind-body therapies that are essential to the treatment for hyperactivity.

Some children outgrow their hyperactivity, but may remain distractible and impulsive throughout adolescence and young adulthood. Some learn to compensate for their disability, developing different strategies for staying focused and attentive. When followed over four years, only 15% in one group studied had a complete remission of symptoms, and these tended to be the kids who had fewer problems initially.[27] Even those without hyperactivity continue to have problems with distractibility and impulsiveness, impaired schoolwork and social interactions. Children who suffer from hyperactivity during school years remain more accident-prone and have higher rates of car crashes than other teenagers and young adults.[28] They have much higher rates of serious injuries, hospitalizations, visits to emergency rooms and clinics, and a much higher overall cost of health care.[29] They are about twice as likely as other teenagers to smoke cigarettes. Without ongoing treatment, they are also at much higher risk of developing substance abuse problems, unintended pregnancy, and antisocial behavior, resulting in rates of unemployment and imprisonment that are five to ten times higher than in the general population.[30]

## WHAT IS THE BEST WAY TO TREAT HYPERACTIVITY?

Now let's talk about what you really want to know: how to treat ADHD. Many parents are cautious about agreeing to put their child on a lengthy course of stimulant medications; in a survey of 381 Australian children with ADHD seen in a pediatric clinic, 69% of parents were giving stimulant medications and 64% were giving or had recently given some kind of complementary or alternative medical therapy such as the Feingold diet, restricting sugar, avoiding allergens, or taking vitamins or herbs.[31] Let's tour the Therapeutic Mountain to find out what works. If you want to skip to my bottom-line recommendations, flip to the end of the chapter.

## BIOCHEMICAL THERAPIES: MEDICATIONS, HERBS, NUTRITIONAL SUPPLEMENTS

### Medications

Stimulant medications have been the mainstay of medical treatment for hyperactive children for over twenty years. They have proven effectiveness helping children improve classroom behavior and academic performance.[32] Although stimulant medications are effective, the American Academy of Pediatrics recommends that they never be used as the only treatment for hyperactivity. Lifestyle, especially mind-body therapies, are integral to the success of a comprehensive treatment program.[33] Medications help with symptoms of inattention, impulsiveness, distractibility, memory, and hyperactivity, but they do not correct the underlying disorder or other learning disabilities such as dyslexia.

### PRESCRIPTION MEDICATIONS TO TREAT HYPERACTIVITY

- Methylphenidate (Ritalin, Ritalin SR— sustained release)
- Dextroamphetamine (Dexedrine, Dextrostat, Adderall)
- Pemoline (Cylert)
- Tomoxetine
- Clonidine

It may seem paradoxical that the medications which are most effective in treating hyperactivity are stimulants, but it is true. This is probably because ADHD is primarily a problem of low arousal. By increasing arousal, stimulants decrease symptoms. Tranquilizers and sedatives are not helpful for hyperactive children. Interestingly, only about half of children who are diagnosed as having ADHD end up with a prescription for a stimulant medication.[34] So, drug therapy is not necessarily inevitable even if your child is diagnosed as having ADHD.

*Ritalin* is the most widely prescribed medication used to treat hyperactivity, accounting for 93% of all stimulant medications prescribed for children. Ritalin benefits attention, impulsiveness and activity, but it has little effect on aggressive behaviors or poor social skills. Ritalin is helpful for adolescents suffering from attention deficits and impulsiveness as well for younger children who are hyperactive. Ritalin is significantly more effective than intensive behavioral management alone.[35] Overall, stimulant medications are more effective than any other kind of psychiatric medication or behavioral therapy alone for most kids with ADHD. But it's not for everyone.

The best way to tell if your child will benefit from Ritalin is the double-blind, placebo controlled crossover trial.[36] This means that you, your child, and your health care provider together conduct a brief (three-week) study. The physician talks with the pharmacist who will make up three different preparations:

1. A dummy or placebo pill
2. A low dose of Ritalin
3. A higher dose of Ritalin

Your child will take each of the medicines for one week. Neither you, your child, nor your child's physician will know the order of the medications. During each week, you and the child's teacher or day care provider will keep careful track of your child's symptoms on a symptom diary (such as the Conners parent and teacher rating scales).

At the end of the three weeks, you return to

your doctor with the symptom diaries for each of the three treatment periods and your best guess about when your child was taking the real medication. After reviewing the records, the physician contacts the pharmacist to find out when the child was taking placebo, low dose, and higher dose of Ritalin. This may sound like a complicated process, but it is the easiest and most objective way to determine if your child will really benefit from taking Ritalin. Most parents would rather go through a three-week trial and know for sure rather than having their child on months and years of medication without really knowing if that's what he needs.[37] I do not prescribe Ritalin to any of my patients until we have gone through this process. Not all pharmacies are geared to do this kind of study. Your physician may need to contact a pharmacy at the closest university or hospital to prepare the trial medications; it's definitely worth the effort.

Children can continue taking Ritalin for years and still receive the same benefits without increasing the dose.[38] Side effects include decreased appetite, stunted growth, insomnia, dizziness, stomachaches, tics, and headaches. On the other hand, Ritalin results in less daydreaming, staring, irritability, and nailbiting.[39] Despite older warnings against epileptic children using Ritalin, studies show it does not provoke seizures.[40] The regular form must be given at least twice daily (at breakfast and lunch time) in order for effects to last throughout the school day; some kids who engage in after-school sports activities may need up to three doses to get through the day.[41] The sustained-release preparation (Ritalin-SR) can be given just once a day, which is far more convenient.

*Dexedrine* and *Adderall* are chemically related to Ritalin. Dexedrine has been used for over fifty years to treat school children with behavior problems.[42] It is an effective stimulant medication that starts acting within an hour. Dexedrine is as effective as Ritalin; Adderall requires dosing only once a day; for some children, one or the other of these medications is more effective than Ritalin.[43] Their side effects are similar to Ritalin and include decreased appetite, insomnia, irritability, tics, and stomachaches; these side effects seem to be more common with Dexedrine than with Ritalin.[44]

Please treat these medications with care; lock them up at home, and deliver them to the school nurse yourself if doses must be given at school. A lot of prescription stimulant medication is finding its way to the street these days, and a fair number of cases of Ritalin poisoning have been reported to Poison Control Centers.[45]

Many parents are worried that giving their kids these powerful stimulant medications (formerly referred to as "speed") may lead them to become drug addicts. This is an understandable concern, especially since kids with ADHD have an increased risk of alcohol and drug problems. However, a study showed that kids with ADHD who were treated with stimulants (such as Ritalin or Adderall) had a *lower* risk of substance abuse problems than those kids who didn't receive stimulant medications;[46] in fact, the kids who received stimulant medications had about the same risk as kids who didn't have any ADHD—terrific news!

Several studies have shown *pemoline (Cylert)* is as effective as Ritalin and Dexedrine in improving attention and learning. It is long-acting and can be given just once a day, but your child may need to take it for several days before improvements become apparent. Cylert may cause serious liver problems; several cases have resulted in death or the need for a liver transplant. If your child takes Cylert, he needs regular tests to monitor liver function. Because of its side effects, it is never the first medication I choose when treating a child with ADHD.

A new medication, *tomoxetine*, is an antidepressant medication that works about as well as Ritalin—at least in one study conducted so far; it's given twice daily and doesn't decrease appetites as much as Ritalin.[47] Other medications used to treat hyperactive children include antidepressants and the blood pressure medicine *clonidine*. Some children are given Ritalin during the day and clonidine in the evening. Clonidine can make kids sedated and worsen depression and lower blood pressure. I am hesitant to prescribe it, especially because clonidine overdoses reported to Poison Control Centers have skyrocketed over the last ten years; most prescriptions that resulted in overdoses were for ADHD.[48] *Antidepressant medications* such as desipramine are effective, but can result in serious side effects. Five children have died as a result of cardiac side effects when taking antidepressant medication for hyperactivity. All of these prescription medications should be taken only under the close supervision of a qualified health care professional. They are never my first choice of treatments for ADHD.

## Herbs

Traditional herbal medicine has remarkably little to say about hyperactivity, probably because it is largely a twentieth-century diagnosis. The German Commission E (which is roughly equivalent to the U.S. Food and Drug Administration) recommends *valerian* to treat states of restlessness, which has been interpreted to mean that it is approved for treating ADHD. However, sedative medications are *not* helpful for children with ADHD (remember, it is more than simple restlessness!), and there is little reason to think that sedative herbs would be helpful. In fact, sedatives may make children drowsy, confused, and even more likely to be erratic and impulsive. Valerian can definitely help with sleep, and for the child who is occasionally restless after a poor night's sleep, valerian may be a reasonable remedy. But there are no data suggesting it is an effective treatment for ADHD.

In addition to valerian, hops, passion-flower, chamomile, kava kava, and lemon balm have been recommended as calming herbs for hyperactive children. There are no studies suggesting that any of these herbs alone or in combination are effective treatments for ADHD. I do not routinely recommend sedative herbs to treat ADHD.

### HERBS POPULARLY USED TO TREAT ADHD

- *Sedative herbs:* valerian, chamomile, hops, passionflower
- *Memory-enhancing herbs:* ginkgo
- *Antioxidants and others:* pycnogenol, ginkgo, spirulina, evening primrose oil, detoxifiers, coffee

Once *ginkgo* became a popular remedy for adults concerned with memory problems, it wasn't long before it was marketed for children. There are no studies showing that ginkgo helps with pediatric learning problems. Its main benefit is improving sluggish circulation in older adults who have atherosclerosis. There's no reason to think it will help kids with ADHD. It can cause bleeding problems in children who already take anticoagulants or aspirin regularly, and it can interfere with some antidepressant medications. I do not recommend it for children.

Pine bark extract contains *antioxidant chemicals* known as pycnogenols or oligomeric proanthocyanidins (OPCs). These compounds are also found in grapeseed extract, apples, grapes, raspberries, and blackberries in lower concentrations, and are among the large family of flavonoids. They are potent antioxidants. Pycnogenols became widely marketed as ADHD remedies in the mid-1990s. There are numerous testimonials about their efficacy in treating ADHD.[49] It's not clear exactly how they might improve brain function. They are safe, but until there are studies evaluating their benefits compared with other treatments for ADHD, I do not routinely recommend them for this condition.

Another widely marketed natural product is *spirulina*, also known as blue-green algae, and affectionately called "pond scum" by those familiar with its source. Spirulina actually is made up of several thousand different species of blue-green algae, the microscopic growth in water that turns it greenish. Spirulina contains about 65% protein, a variety of B-complex vitamins, and several trace minerals. However, it can also contain pesticides, animal feces, bacteria, fungi, fertilizer, heavy metals, and other contaminants from the water in which it grows. There are several reports of patients becoming very ill after taking it. There are no studies showing that it is helpful for kids with ADHD. I do not recommend it.

*Evening primrose oil* contains gamma linoleic acid (GLA), which has potent antioxidant and anti-inflammatory properties. It's helpful for some kids with eczema. Two trials have evaluated its effectiveness in treating kids with ADHD, but neither showed that it had any significant benefit. I do not routinely recommend it for ADHD, but I do occasionally recommend it for other conditions.

Because heavy metals (such as lead) have been blamed for problem behavior in some children, a few herbalists recommend *detoxifying teas* such as red clover lemon grass, and milk thistle. There are no scientific studies showing that these herbs help alleviate symptoms.

Supplementing your child with America's favorite herb, *coffee*, makes more sense than using just about any other herb to treat ADHD. Caffeine has been evaluated in numerous studies as an alternative treatment that is fairly safe, inexpensive, and readily available. However, caffeine is not nearly as effective as the prescription stimulants.[50] Low doses of caffeine may benefit children who are already taking Ritalin, boosting the benefits without substantially increasing side effects.[51] Caffeine's well-known side effects include feeling jittery, nervous, anxious, and eventually tired when the effects wear off.

## Nutritional Supplements

Deficiencies of zinc, magnesium, iron, pyridoxine (vitamin B6), and vitamin C have been suspected of causing hyperactivity in some children. Hyperactive children who have low zinc levels may be less likely to respond to stimulant medications than children with normal zinc levels.[52] On the other hand, a New Zealand study showed no association between children's zinc levels and their behavior as rated by parents and teachers. A double-blind controlled study of hyperactive children given megadoses of vitamin C, B-vitamins, and calcium (vs. placebo) showed no behavioral improvements with the supplement. If anything, children treated with megavitamins tended to have worse behavior, and over 40% developed signs of liver toxicity. Iron supplements may cause problems unless the child is iron deficient to begin with. There are few data supporting the use of magnesium or pyridoxine supplements to treat ADHD.[53] I do not recommend megavitamins as routine treatments for children with ADHD.

Fish oil—today's version of cod liver oil, is being used to treat just about every ailment under the sun—from asthma to arthritis to ADHD. Fish oil contains a special kind of fatty acid known as omega-3 fatty acids or docosahexanoic acid (DHA), which is an important part of cell membranes. There are no studies suggesting that it is useful in treatment ADHD. I do not routinely recommend it in this condition.

Melatonin is an antioxidant hormone produced by the pineal gland. Unlike most other hormones such as insulin, it is sold over the counter without a prescription. Melatonin helps regulate normal sleep and wakefulness cycles and other biological biorhythms such as temperature fluctuations over the day. Two studies have shown that it can improve sleep for kids with ADHD (in doses of 0.5 to 3 milligrams nightly), but it is contraindicated for children with epilepsy because it may increase the frequency of seizures in these children.[54] Even though it improved nighttime sleep, it had no impact on daytime ADHD symptoms; I do not routinely recommend it.

It's not that I'm generically opposed to dietary supplements. But I think that kids with ADHD, like all kids, should receive a high-quality multivitamin/multimineral and a healthy diet rich in fruits, vegetables, whole grains, and organic proteins, and not rely on single nutrient supplements.

## LIFESTYLE THERAPIES: NUTRITION, EXERCISE, ENVIRONMENT, MIND-BODY

### Nutrition

Just because there is compelling evidence *against* the "sugar causes hyperactivity" hypothesis does not mean your child should subsist on cookies, cola, and candy bars. Sugar is bad for your child's teeth, and it replaces many more healthy foods needed for a balanced diet. If you are convinced that sugar makes your child's symptoms worse, temporarily eliminate all sweets from his diet (without telling anyone else), and then ask his teachers or other adults how they think he's doing. Check it yourself several times. If you remain convinced that sugar is the culprit, your child can live without cakes, cookies, and candy, but don't expect it to be easy.[55]

The latest dietary interest is in foods with a low glycemic index. The glycemic index reflects how quickly the body absorbs the energy in foods and how quickly those foods lead to a leap and then fall in blood sugar levels. The theory is that high-glycemic foods result in a roller coaster for blood sugar and a number of hormones, causing fluctuations in the ability to concentrate. Raw sugar, fruit juices, plain bagels, plain toast, doughnuts, and candy have high-glycemic indexes. Whole fruits, whole grain cereals and breads, vegetables, and dairy products have low glycemic indexes. Low-glycemic foods may help prevent obesity and diabetes as well as reduce mood and attention swings; they also tend to be richer in fiber, minerals, and vitamins than high-glycemic foods. I think that a diet emphasizing low-glycemic foods makes sense for just about everybody.

Avoiding artificial dyes may be helpful in a small minority of hyperactive children.[56] Rare children do have reproducible reactions (including irritability, restlessness, and sleep disturbances) when challenged with the yellow dye tartrazine.

Despite vivid testimonials to the contrary, there have been numerous studies demonstrating the ineffectiveness of the Feingold diet.[57] The diet is so restrictive, it's quite possible that children who adhere to it will end up with more nutritional deficiencies than those who eat a normal diet. On the basis of all existing evidence to date, I do not recommend the Feingold diet.

Others who believe that hyperactivity is a symptom of food allergy suggest that hyperactive children might benefit from a "few foods diet."[58] This diet includes only lamb and turkey, rice and potato, bananas and pears, root vegetables, green vegetables, sunflower oil, milk-free margarine, and bottled water. It avoids the most common food allergens: cow's milk, soy, corn, wheat, citrus, tomatoes, eggs, peanuts, and artificial preservatives and colors. If children improve after two weeks on this diet, one new food per week is gradually added. A few allergic children do improve on this kind of regimen (see Chapter 4, Allergies), and it may result in improved sleep and irritability as well as improved attention. This restrictive diet is extremely difficult for most families to maintain and only a minority of children seem to benefit from it. Avoiding food allergens and food sensitivity probably helps only a small minority of children. I do not typically recommend restrictive diets unless all other measures have failed to help or the child has other allergic symptoms. If you decide to pursue dietary therapy, make sure you seek the help of a trained nutritionist so your child does not develop any preventable nutritional deficiencies.

## Exercise

Exercise is great for hyperactive kids. Kids with ADHD are often a bit clumsy, struggling with eye-hand coordination. Go for large muscle exercises such as running, soccer, and swimming. If your child is involved in team sports, let the coach know that extra directions may be needed. Keep the child close to the coach or team leader so his attention is less likely to wander. Teams and activities with close adult supervision (such as scouting) are better bets than unorganized, after-school pick-up games.

Martial arts training in small groups may be helpful in promoting discipline, coordination, and self-esteem. Relaxing exercise such as yoga, *Qi Gong,* and *Tai Chi* may have special benefits for the hyperactive child. A comparison study showed that hyperactive children who were taught simple yogic breathing exercises, slowly moving stretches, and relaxing postures had improved self-esteem.[59] Teaching a child how to relax through movement is a perfect therapy for hyperactive children, who are on the move and need to develop relaxation skills.

Because hyperactive kids tend to have a lot of injuries, they often end up in the emergency room for stitches and casts. Make sure your youngster wears proper protective gear whenever he goes out to Rollerblade, scooter, ride a bike, or engage in contact sports.

## Environment

### ENVIRONMENTAL STRATEGIES

- Reduce lead exposure
- Organize home environment
- Music
- Limit television-watching time

Help prevent your child from developing *lead poisoning* by keeping your home free of paint chips and dust. Dry dusting and sweeping just stir up the dust, so use a wet mop and a damp duster. High phosphate cleaners are especially effective at removing lead dust. Wet-mop hard floors at least twice a month, vacuum and dust window ledges weekly, and have toddlers wash their hands several times daily (at least before all meals and bedtime). Do not store your child's juice in glazed pottery or pewter containers, because both may contain lead that can leach into your child's juice. Keep lead-containing objects, such as watch batteries, fishing weights, and old, soldered toy soldiers away from toddlers. If you or your spouse work in a high-lead occupation (foundries, firing ranges, etc.) change your clothes as soon as you get home so you don't spread lead dust from your clothes to your house. Removal of lead-based paint should always be done by professionals who are trained and have the proper equipment to get rid of the lead without astronomically increasing airborne lead levels.

Your health care practitioner can test your child for lead poisoning. Most pediatricians test at least once during infancy and toddlerhood if lead poisoning is a problem in your area. If levels are high, treatment can help your child excrete the lead.

Help your child create an *organized environment* at home. Minimize clutter to minimize distractions. Calm colors and simple lines help reduce overstimulation.

## OPTIMAL EDUCATIONAL ENVIRONMENT FOR KIDS WITH ADHD

- Structured learning environment (order and predictability)
- Simple instructions, repeated frequently about work assignments
- Visual as well as verbal instructions
- Use tape recorders, computer-assisted instruction, and other audiovisual equipment to reinforce assignments
- Frequent feedback, e.g., daily checklists or report cards
- Tests given with extended time, quiet setting with few distractions
- One-to-one tutorials or very small groups
- Attend to other learning problems such as memory and language-processing problems

Can *music therapy* help? An interesting Israeli study compared normal and hyperactive boys' work performances while they listened to different kinds of music: fast-paced vs. slower tempo vs. no music.[60] As expected, the hyperactive boys tended to make more mistakes than the normal boys. Their performance plunged even more while listening to fast-paced music. While listening to calmer, slow tempo music, however, they did nearly as well as the normal boys. These intriguing results bear repetition in a variety of classroom settings. Pending such studies, it makes sense to keep all environmental cues (musical and otherwise) as orderly as possible to help hyperactive children maintain a steady pace.

OK, I know this will make me unpopular, but I firmly believe that one of the most helpful things parents can do is to turn off the *television*.

Several studies suggest that more television viewing is linked to a higher risk of developing ADHD. Instead, spend some time in one-to-one activities with your child. Do *not* allow the child to have a television in his room; it is far too distracting and is linked to obesity and violence as well as reduced attention spans.

Environmental and mind-body approaches overlap when it comes to optimizing the educational setting for children.

## Mind-Body

Mind-body or behavioral therapy is the cornerstone of treatment for hyperactive children. Parents must learn to express disapproval of a child's unwanted behavior while still expressing love for the child himself. Take every opportunity to praise your child whenever he behaves as you would like, even if it is only for a few minutes. Over the long term of months and years, appropriate treatment can eventually rebuild self-esteem, but it is far easier to maintain and improve self-esteem from the time your child is young rather than waiting until it is already severely impaired.

## MIND-BODY THERAPIES

- Structured schedule
- Step-by-step instructions
- Positive reward for desired behavior
- Tutoring
- Biofeedback and relaxation training
- Professional counseling

First, review your child's *daily schedule*. Make sure there *is* a schedule. Everything should be as routine and predictable as possible—mealtimes, nap time, and bedtime, exercise time, story time, day care or school time, bath time, cleanup time, relaxing time, chore time, and so on. It may help for you and your child to sit down and make a poster or chart together, listing all the day's activities and the times and places they occur. Try to stick as much as possible to the schedule, even on weekends and vacation time. Organization and structure are very important for hyperactive children.

*Break every activity down into smaller steps.* Hyperactive children need specific, detailed, step-by-step instructions. You can't just say, "Get ready for dinner." You have to first tell them to wrap up the game, then put it away, then go wash their hands and face, and finally, come to the table and sit down. You may have to go through this exact same routine a thousand times before they get it. If you vary it, your child may not get it right, even though he's done the same thing a hundred times before.

*Reward your child* for getting things right. He should get at least four compliments for every correction! Many families find a chart and sticker system helpful. Put all your child's daily activities on a chart hung on his bedroom door. He gets a regular star (or ordinary sticker) for doing each activity when you remind him and a gold star (or special sticker) for doing each activity without needing to be reminded. Some parents use vouchers instead of stickers. When he has earned a certain number of vouchers, he can trade them in for a special reward.

*Tutoring* can be extremely helpful. It provides one-to-one attention and addresses other learning disabilities better than a single teacher in a crowded classroom can. Tutoring also provides an opportunity for immediate feedback. Private tutoring can be expensive, but volunteer tutors are often available at community centers and literacy programs. Also, call your school to arrange an Individual Educational Assessment and Plan so your child gets all the school services to which he is entitled by law.

*Biofeedback* that focuses on reducing mus-cle tension in the forehead (EMG biofeedback) not only reduces muscle tension, but seems to result in more relaxed behavior. EMG biofeedback also seems to improve language skills and helps children feel more in control of their behavior.[61] One study showed that EMG biofeedback works as well as Ritalin in improving behavior.[62] Biofeedback is especially helpful when used along with other behavioral therapies such as structured scheduling and rewards for relaxed behavior.[63] Don't expect results overnight. Biofeedback training takes at least six to eight weeks and possibly as long as six months with regular practice at home to achieve maximal effectiveness.

In the 1990s EEG biofeedback became a popular alternative treatment for ADHD. In this form of biofeedback, the child receives real-time information about his current brainwave or EEG activity.[64] Children with ADHD often produce too much slow wave activity (theta) in certain parts of the brain (which is consistent with being underaroused), and the theory is that by learning to regulate their brainwave activity through biofeedback, these kids can improve their behavior. There are many case reports about how helpful this approach is.[65] It's fairly time-consuming, requiring two to three sessions weekly for at least eight weeks and is often combined with tutoring and coaching for specific learning problems. A typical course of treatment involves 35 to 50 sessions. That much one-to-one attention could be beneficial in itself. Most insurance won't pay for EEG biofeedback because it's still considered experimental. I do not routinely recommend it, yet.

*Relaxation training* can be very helpful in teaching a hyperactive child how to relax. It can be done in groups or with an individual therapist. There are several types of relaxation training: progressive muscle relaxation, deep breathing, autogenic training (similar to self-hypnosis), and even yoga exercises. Relaxation training of any sort works best if the parents are involved and the child continues to practice regularly at home. Learning the relaxation skills can help improve the hyperactive child's self-esteem as well.

*Professional counseling* by a psychologist or psychiatrist can be helpful for a number of reasons. First, a mental health professional can help insure an accurate diagnosis and can reassure you that your child is not suffering from another problem such as depression or anxiety, both of which are difficult to diagnose in young children. Second, a professional can provide more in-depth education about attention deficit disorder. Professionals can also provide additional behavioral, communication, and problem-solving strategies for dealing with the child's hyperactivity and self-esteem. They can also help families deal with the stresses inherent in having a child labeled difficult, different, bad, or handicapped.

Last, but not least, seek the support of other parents and families with hyperactive children. You are not alone and you don't need to feel alone. National support groups, local support groups, and even Internet support groups are available.

Neurophysiological retraining therapies, which have not been proven effective in comparison studies, include patterning, visual retraining, and vestibular stimulation.

## BIOMECHANICAL THERAPIES: MASSAGE, CHIROPRACTIC

### Massage

Although it makes sense that *massage* would help children learn to relax, there is only one study so far evaluating it for ADHD. This study evaluated the benefits of daily massage among 28 boys with ADHD; they reported less fidgeting and greater happiness in the group who received massage.[66] While this is very nice, we need longer-term studies and more objective outcome measures before insurance companies are likely to pay for this sort of thing. I don't routinely recommend massage for ADHD on the basis of existing evidence, but I'll keep my eyes open to look for future studies.

### Chiropractic and Surgery

Some chiropractors and cranio-sacral therapists also claim to improve ADHD symptoms by adjusting the bones and soft tissues in the neck and skull. There are no studies evaluating these claims, and I don't routinely recommend chiropractic as a therapy for children or adolescents with ADHD.

*Surgery* has no place in the treatment of ADHD.

## BIOENERGETIC THERAPIES: ACUPUNCTURE, HOMEOPATHY

### Acupuncture

ADHD is not a diagnosis made in Traditional Chinese Medicine. Although there are case reports of dramatic improvement in ADHD with acupuncture treatments, acupuncture has not been evaluated in a comparison study for ADHD.[67] I do not routinely recommend acupuncture therapy for ADHD.

### Homeopathy

Homeopathy is another route that many parents have explored while looking for non-drug treatments of their child's ADHD. Again, a few cases appear to have responded dramatically, but few studies have compared homeopathy with placebo remedies or with standard medications.[68] The homeopathic remedies that appear to be most helpful are Stramonium,

Cina, *Hyoscyamus niger, Veratrum album,* and *Tarentula hispanica.* Until there are larger studies comparing homeopathic treatments with other standard therapies (such as stimulant medications or herbs and mind-body therapies), I do not recommend them routinely. On the other hand, homeopathy is safe and may be worth exploring.

## WHAT I RECOMMEND FOR HYPERACTIVITY (ADHD)

### PREVENTING HYPERACTIVITY

1. *Lifestyle—environment.* Do not smoke, drink, or use recreational drugs during pregnancy. Do not smoke around your child.

Keep your child's environment free of lead. Get professional help in removing lead paint. Keep your dust levels down with weekly damp-mopping and dusting.

Do not put a television set in a child's bedroom, and limit all television and video games to less than two hours daily.

2. *Lifestyle—exercise.* Protect your child from damaging head injuries by insisting he use proper protective equipment while bicycling, Rollerblading, and engaging in contact sports. Always use seatbelts and child restraint devices when riding in a car.

---

*Take your child to your health care provider to be evaluated for:*

- Hearing problems, vision problems, thyroid problems, sleep problems, lead poisoning, pinworms, allergies, eczema, and other health problems that may interfere with learning and behavior

*Take your child to a clinical psychologist or educational specialist for:*

- Intelligence testing and testing for special learning problems, additional testing for emotional problems or stresses that may trigger problem behavior, advice about behavioral management, information about hyperactivity and support

- Fill out formal behavior rating scales such as the Conners parent and teacher scales—these will help you determine objectively how serious your child's symptoms are and how much he improves with various treatments

---

## TREATING HYPERACTIVITY

1. *Lifestyle—mind-body.* Accept your child as he is. Avoid blaming him or yourself. Remember that he is not trying to misbehave. Be patient and persistent in reminding him of your expectations about his behavior.

Give your child clear structure. Make his routine consistent, orderly, low-key, and predictable. A wall chart of his daily activities may be helpful. Have consistent mealtimes, bedtimes, chore times, study times, play times, etc. Also be consistent in terms of your expectations.

Break down tasks into smaller steps and make sure they're clear to him.

Reward him regularly for desired behavior. Lavishly praise positive behavior; he should get at least four compliments for each correction. Give feedback immediately. Use time-out rather than physical punishment for discipline. Focus on building self-esteem.

Consider having him tutored in his most challenging subjects. Get as much academic help and help for any learning disabilities that the school provides.

Teach your child relaxation skills. These can be breathing exercises, progressive muscle relaxation, yoga, or other methods. Reward your child for his efforts to practice relaxation skills.

Consider taking your child to a professional counselor for training in relaxation skills or biofeedback. Support and encourage your child's practice at home.

Recognize that having a child with ADHD is stressful for most parents. Recognize your own needs for time out and breaks. Seek support. Regularly talk with your child's teachers and other parents whose children are hyperactive.

2. *Lifestyle—exercise.* Regular vigorous exercises and stretching relaxing exercise such as yoga or *Tai Chi* may be helpful. Focus on sports with close interaction between child and coach (such as martial arts training or small teams).

3. *Lifestyle—environment.* Reduce excessive stimulation in your child's environment. Consider playing slow tempo rather than fast-paced background music. Reduce the amount of time he spends in front of a television, and do not allow one in his room.

4. *Biochemical—medications.* In conjunction with your health care provider and your child's teacher, do a double-blind crossover of stimulant medication (such as Ritalin) vs. placebo to determine whether or not your child will benefit from medical treatment. If he does, make sure he gets it regularly and recheck his need for the same dose every year. Do not rely on sedative medications.

5. *Biochemical—nutritional supplements.* If you are interested in milder, natural stimulants, consider giving your child extra caffeine in the form of coffee, tea, or cola beverages. Remember that even natural stimulants can have side effects such as decreased appetite, feeling jittery, and insomnia. Give him a high-quality multivitamin/multimineral daily.

## RESOURCES

### Support Groups

CHADD: Children and Adults with
  Attention Deficit Disorder
8181 Professional Place, Suite 201
Landover, MD 20785
(800) 233-4050; (301) 306-7070;
  Fax: (301) 306-7090
http://www.chadd.org/

National Attention Deficit Disorder
  Association
1788 Second Street, Suite 200
Highland Park, IL 60035
(847) 432-ADDA; Fax: (847) 432-5874
http://www.add.org/
mail@add.org

Learning Disabilities Association
4156 Library Road
Pittsburgh, PA 15234
(412) 350-0223
http://www.ldanatl.org

National Center for Learning Disabilities
(212) 545-7510
http://www.ncld.org/

ADD Warehouse (offers books, videos,
  and tapes about ADHD)
(800) 233-9273
http://addwarehouse.com/

ERIC Clearinghouse on Disabilities and
  Gifted Education
Council for Exceptional Children
1920 Association Drive
Reston, VA 22091-1589
(800) 328-0272

Association for Applied
  Psychophysiology and Biofeedback
10200 W. 44th Ave.
Wheat Ridge, CO 80033
(888) 830-2272
http://www.npginc.com/aapb/

### Books

Barkley, R. *Taking Charge of ADHD: The Complete, Authoritative Guide for Parents.* Guilford Press, 1995.

Garber, S.; Spizman, R. F. *Beyond Ritalin: Facts About Medication and Other Strategies for Helping Children, Adolescents and Adults with Attention Deficit Disorders.* HarperCollins, 1997.

Gordon, Michael. *Jumpin' Johnny Get Back to Work!* GSI Publications, 1991.

Grad, L.; Flick; Parker, Harvey C. *Power Parenting for Children with ADD/ADHD: A Practical Parent's Guide for Managing Difficult Behaviors.* Center for Applied Research in Education, 1996.

Hallowell, E. M.; Ratey, J. J. *Driven to Distraction: Recognizing and Coping with Attention Deficit Disorder from Childhood Through Adulthood.* Simon and Schuster, 1995.

Ingersoll, B. *Daredevils and Daydreamers: New Perspectives on Attention-Deficit/Hyperactivity Disorder.* Doubleday, 1997.

Kurcinka, Mary. *Raising Your Spirited Child: A Guide for Parents Whose Child Is More Intense, Sensitive, Perceptive, Persistent, Energetic.* HarperCollins, 1992.

Moss, Robert A. *Why Johnny Can't Concentrate: Coping with Attention Deficit Problems.* Bantam Books, 1990.

Parker, Harvey C. *The ADD Hyperactivity Handbook for Schools: Effective Strategies of Identifying and Teaching ADD Students in Elementary and Secondary Schools.* Specialty Press, 1992.

Silver, L. B. *The Misunderstood Child: A Guide for Parents of Learning Disabled Children.* 2nd ed. McGraw-Hill, 1992.

Wodrich, D. *Attention Deficit Hyperactivity Disorder: What Every Parent Wants to Know.* Paul H. Brookes Publishing, 1994.

Zeigler, Dendy C. A. *Teenagers with ADD: A Parent's Guide.* Woodbine House, 1995.

# 22

# JAUNDICE

Steven Chen called me just as the office opened one morning about his newborn daughter, May. Steven's mother, Rose, was in town helping with the new baby and had noticed May was becoming jaundiced. May was a little yellow in the face the previous evening, but now the jaundice was noticeable on her chest as well. Rose told Steven that when he was a baby, he had jaundice and underwent many blood tests. She had been told to stop nursing him and he had to stay three extra days in the hospital under special lights. Rose had continued to be extra cautious with his health throughout his infancy. She wanted him to make sure that his bad luck wasn't starting in his daughter.

Steven's wife, Bonnie, was much less concerned. Her pregnancy and delivery had been completely normal. May had weighed 7 pounds, 6 ounces at birth, and had gone home twenty hours after her delivery. After a day or so, Bonnie's milk supply had come in, and now she was nursing six or seven times a day. A public health nurse was coming to visit them later that afternoon for a routine checkup following the early discharge, but Rose was urging him to come in right away to get May started on therapy. He felt trapped between his mother's concern and his wife's confidence, and he wanted some professional advice about what to do.

## WHAT IS JAUNDICE?

Jaundice is a yellow color of the skin and the whites of the eyes. It is caused by a buildup of the yellow pigment *bilirubin* in the blood. Bilirubin is a normal breakdown product of the hemoglobin in red blood cells. Every day about 1% of our red blood cells die and are replaced with new cells. Red blood cells contain iron and hemoglobin. Rather than waste the useful iron in the dead red blood cells, the body saves and recycles it. Hemoglobin, the molecule that carries the iron, is easily replaced, so while the iron is saved, the old hemoglobin is broken down and metabolized in the liver.

The first by-product of hemoglobin breakdown is biliverdin which is a green pigment. Biliverdin is transformed into bilirubin, which is yellow (see chart). This is why bruises change color over several days from reddish purple (fresh blood) to green (biliverdin) to yellow (bilirubin). The liver processes bilirubin to prepare it for excretion. If the liver gets backlogged, some of the bilirubin spills over into the bloodstream, turning the skin and the whites of the eyes yellow. Once the liver has finished with the bilirubin, it passes it on to the gallbladder (which functions as a kind of holding tank), which in turn passes it on to the intestines for excretion. Before it passes out of the body, it faces another hurdle. An enzyme in the intestines can free the bilirubin to be reabsorbed into the blood. The longer it takes for the intestinal contents to be excreted, the more chance there is for bilirubin to be reabsorbed into the blood. It then has to return to the liver to be reprocessed and then on to the gallbladder and intestines.

Where Bilirubin Comes From and Where It Goes

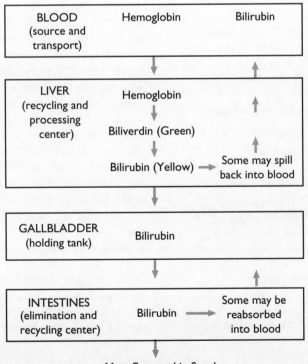

Most Excreted in Stool

Jaundice is not an illness; it is simply a sign that bilirubin has built up in the blood. For reasons that no one quite understands, levels tend to be higher in the morning than in the evening—just the opposite of temperatures, which tend to be highest in the afternoon and evening and lowest in the morning. Babies tend to have higher bilirubin levels than adults.

## WHY DO BABIES HAVE HIGHER BILIRUBIN LEVELS THAN ADULTS?

Now that you know where bilirubin comes from, you can easily see the different factors that can cause it to build up in babies.

### WHY BABIES HAVE HIGH BILIRUBIN LEVELS

*Higher turnover of red blood cells*

- Fewer red blood cells needed after birth
- Bruising during birth (forceps or vacuum-assisted deliveries)
- Diseases such as Rh, ABO, genetically fragile blood cells

*Slower liver metabolism or excretion*

- Babies are slower than adults; genetic differences in metabolism
- Diseases slow down liver metabolism
- Diseases block secretion from the liver to the gallbladder

*Slower movement through the intestines, allowing time for reabsorption*

First, babies *have more red blood cells* for their size than adults. They need more red

blood cells to help carry oxygen before they are born. Once they are breathing on their own, babies do not need so many red blood cells. The extra blood is broken down and recycled to supply future needs. The extra work of breaking down blood cells creates a backlog for the liver, and some bilirubin tends to spill over into the blood.

To compensate for thinner air (less oxygen), babies born at high altitudes have higher hemoglobin levels than their sea-level counterparts; babies born at high altitudes are also more likely to be jaundiced than babies born at sea level. Babies who get bruises on their head from pushing during delivery (or from the forceps or vacuum extractors used to assist delivery) are also more likely to become jaundiced because of the extra work for the liver in breaking down the blood in the bruises.

Certain *diseases* can also cause a higher turnover of red blood cells. In the bad old days, the most feared cause of jaundice was *Rh disease*. Rh disease occurs when the mother has Rh-negative blood and the baby has Rh-positive blood. Rh-negative mothers make antibodies to the Rh factor in their baby's blood cells, breaking them down rapidly, leading to anemia, high bilirubin levels, and sometimes death or permanent disability, called kernicterus. Fortunately, scientists found a way to block this reaction: Rhogam. Rhogam derails the destructive reaction against babies' blood so Rh-negative mothers can have normal, healthy Rh-positive babies without breaking down their red blood cells.

Rh disease was terrible and frightening. High bilirubin levels meant the possibility of kernicterus, which was to be avoided at all costs. The memory of kernicterus has been linked to jaundice in the minds of older parents and physicians alike. The fear of kernicterus is why many people fear jaundice. The good news is that kernicterus has virtually disappeared in full-term babies with the advent of Rhogam, so younger parents and physicians are less likely to panic at the first tinges of yellow skin.

Other blood group differences (such as A, B, O, AB blood types) between mother and baby can also lead to breakdown of the baby's red blood cells. These differences are rarely as severe as Rh disease. Mothers with type O blood are the most likely to have an immune reaction to their babies' blood. A mother who has O-positive blood makes antibodies to blood types A, B, and AB. If the mother has blood type O and the baby has one of the other types, it is called an ABO set-up or ABO incompatibility. This is why physicians check mothers' blood types during pregnancy. If the mother is type O, her baby's blood type is checked soon after delivery. Careful monitoring and early treatment can prevent damage from ABO incompatibility.

Some genetic diseases of the blood result in fragile blood cells which are easily destroyed. These diseases have long names such as glucose-6-phosphate dehydrogenase (G6PD) deficiency and hereditary spherocytosis. G6PD is common in certain racial groups such as Sephardic Jews, Greeks, and Nigerians, but it is rare in most other peoples. Genetic diseases causing fragile blood cells can be diagnosed with simple blood tests.

Even under normal circumstances, the newborn's liver has a lot of work to do metabolizing broken down blood cells. However, babies' livers, like the rest of them, are not as speedy or developed as adults'. They just aren't as adept at the hemoglobin recycling program. Bilirubin builds up as it waits for the liver to metabolize and excrete it. Excessive bilirubin spills into the bloodstream and appears as yellow in the skin and eyes. Low birth weight and premature babies are more likely to become jaundiced because their livers are even less fully developed and ready to metabolize bilirubin than full-term babies.

The rate at which the liver gets up to full speed varies slightly from baby to baby and in different ethnic groups. Asian babies have a higher rate of jaundice than other races. Hispanic babies are more prone to jaundice than Caucasians, and African-American babies are least likely to be jaundiced. These differences are not just because it's easier to see jaundice in certain racial groups; the bilirubin levels really differ in different races. The differences are probably due to differences in liver metabolism in different races. For unknown reasons, boys are more likely to become jaundiced than are girls.

If there are *liver diseases* such as hepatitis or other illnesses that slow down the liver, a backlog of bilirubin accumulates, spills into the blood, and causes jaundice. Hypothyroidism slows metabolism throughout the body, including the liver. Any other major illness, such as sepsis or meningitis, can also slow liver metabolism. Blockages in the pathway from the liver to the intestines by way of the gallbladder can also lead to bilirubin buildup.

Once bilirubin has made it to the *intestines*, you'd think the way would be clear to excretion in the stool, but there is another hurdle before bilirubin's final exit. The longer the bilirubin stays in the intestines, the more chance it will be reabsorbed into the blood. From there it has to go back to the liver to be remetabolized and reexcreted. This process is known as the *entero* (intestinal) *hepatic* (liver) *circulation*.

Anything that slows down the intestines can slow the excretion of bilirubin and increase its enterohepatic circulation. Everyone who has changed a newborn baby's diaper knows that newborn stool is dark, thick, and sticky. This thick, sticky stool, known as *meco-*

*nium*, builds up before the baby is born. It needs to be cleared out before normal stool can pass. Every time a baby drinks milk (Mom's or formula), the intestines contract, moving the meconium and stool along on their way out. The less often the intestines contract, the more slowly meconium is excreted. Babies who are constipated or who don't pass a stool within the first day of life are more likely to develop jaundice than those who pass a stool in the first twenty-four hours.

The most common cause of slowed excretion is not consuming calories frequently. Formula-fed babies get a full complement of calories at every meal from day one. Breast-fed babies have smaller meals until their mother's milk supply comes in. The less frequently breast-fed babies nurse (for example, if the baby is fed only every four hours or if water is substituted for a feeding), the less the intestines are stimulated and the more slowly the mother's milk supply comes in. Overall, breast-fed babies are about twice as likely to be jaundiced as formula-fed babies. In the first few days of life, they tend to take in fewer calories, have less stimulation to move their bowels, and have fewer bowel movements.

For reasons no one quite understands, there is an enzyme in some women's breast milk that enhances bilirubin's reabsorption from the intestines. Families that have this particular enzyme tend to have babies who become mildly jaundiced after they're a week old and they tend to stay mildly jaundiced for about a month. But they don't seem to be at higher risk of developing kernicterus or any other problem—except for being slightly less photogenic for the first few weeks!

In light of all the factors that can cause increased bilirubin, it's not surprising that so many babies become jaundiced. Jaundice is common even among perfectly normal healthy babies with perfectly normal deliveries. About 35% of babies have visible jaundice (bilirubin levels of 7.0 or higher), but only about one to two per hundred have bilirubin levels above 15, (the old treatment level), and only about one to two per 1,000 babies reach bilirubin levels of 18 to 20 or more, the current treatment level for most babies.

Jaundice typically becomes noticeable around the third day of life as the red blood cells break down and the liver falls behind on metabolizing it. Bilirubin levels are highest on the fourth or fifth day of life. They gradually decline over the next several days as the liver gets into gear and the mother's milk supply comes in. Breast-fed babies who carry the enzyme that makes it easy to break down and reabsorb bilirubin in their intestines can be jaundiced for several weeks.

Because newborn jaundice doesn't show up right away, pediatricians recommend that babies who are discharged within 24 hours of birth should be seen be a doctor or nurse within the first three to five days of life. This is the reason so many hospitals and health plans are moving toward having nurses visit new babies at home. In most cases, if the nurse thinks the baby is jaundiced, but otherwise healthy, there is usually a quick call to the doctor to get approval to check the bilirubin, and then the nurse can draw the blood right at home. The blood test can be run at the lab without the baby having to make the trip to the hospital. Even if phototherapy is needed, it can be set up at home as well. This home-based approach to care is much more convenient for everyone while still making sure that babies get the therapy they need.

*May had typical newborn jaundice. Because she was breast-feeding, Asian, and jaundice ran in her family, she was at higher risk than the average baby of being visibly jaundiced, but she was not necessarily in any danger.*

---

**TAKE YOUR CHILD TO A HEALTH CARE PROFESSIONAL FOR AN EVALUATION IF:**

- The mother is Rh-negative or blood type O
- Abnormal or fragile blood types or severe jaundice run in your family
- Jaundice is visible within the first 48 hours of life
- The jaundice lasts longer than ten days
- The jaundice extends all the way down to the chest or the belly button
- The baby is more than three weeks premature
- The baby develops dark urine or pale stools
- The baby acts sick, is very sleepy, or is not interested in nursing
- The baby has trouble breathing or is breathing very fast
- You are concerned about the baby in any way

---

These could be signs that your baby has a serious problem as a cause for the jaundice or that your child needs additional treatment.

*May first became visibly jaundiced when she was three days old. She had no signs of serious illness; it was safe for her to be evaluated and treated at home.*

## DOES JAUNDICE CAUSE BRAIN DAMAGE?

In the days when Rh disease caused devastating red blood cell destruction, anemia, and even death, autopsies showed bilirubin deposits (or staining) in the brain. This brain staining accompanied by either death or permanent disability was attributed to bilirubin. Many studies over the past forty years have looked at whether bilirubin causes brain damage in babies who are not affected by Rh disease.

Bilirubin does affect hearing. However, these hearing deficits resolve as soon as the bilirubin levels drop to normal. Many babies also become sleepier when they are jaundiced, but when the jaundice resolves, their sleepiness disappears. Long-term follow-up studies of thousands of otherwise healthy, full-term babies have failed to demonstrate *any* long-term adverse effect of typical newborn jaundice on IQ, development, or behavior.[1] These studies do not necessarily apply to very premature babies or babies whose jaundice is due to other serious problems such as hypothyroidism. Sick babies tend to have persistent problems following high bilirubin levels, but among healthy premature babies, the long-term effects are not serious if the jaundice is monitored and treated. Some researchers have even suggested that bilirubin itself is not toxic to the brain; in fact, it may be a protective antioxidant that simply marks injured areas.[2] For the vast majority of babies, jaundice is not dangerous, not brain damaging, and not life-threatening. On the other hand, for a few, it can be a sign of a serious problem that requires prompt medical attention. So how do you know whether or not to be worried?

## DIAGNOSIS

Talking to parents about family history of jaundice, liver disease, blood problems, and how the baby is currently doing (feeding, sleeping, peeing, and pooping) can uncover other clues to the diagnosis. A physical examination can point the way to other conditions contributing to jaundice. The bilirubin level in the blood can be determined easily by a blood test. Along with a bilirubin level, your health care professional will check the baby's and mother's blood type and may test the blood cells themselves. Depending on the results of the initial discussions, examination and blood tests, other laboratory studies may be helpful.[3]

Because so many babies are out of the hospital in less than one day, some doctors recommend that bilirubin levels be checked before they go. It turns out that babies who have bilirubin levels less than 6 mg/dL on the first day of life have a very, very low risk (about 2%) of developing significant jaundice later on.[4] Checking a blood test early may be reassuring for some families.

*I reassured Steven that based on what I had observed while they were in the hospital, May was probably fine, but I'd have the public health nurse check her and draw a blood sample that afternoon to measure her bilirubin level.*

## What Is the Best Way to Prevent and Treat Jaundice?

The best way to prevent jaundice is to feed your baby early and often—at least eight to ten times daily during the first week of life. Also make sure your baby is exposed to some sunlight every day. Let's consider all your options to find out what works best in treating jaundice; if you want to skip to my bottom-line recommendations, flip to the end of the chapter.

### Biochemical Therapies: Medications, Herbs, Nutritional Supplements

#### Medications

Although a number of medications have been tested over the years, none has caught on as the mainstay of treatment for newborn jaundice.

*Activated charcoal* binds bilirubin. It is not absorbed into the bloodstream, so it passes through the intestines, absorbing toxins on the way out. It helps and prevents bilirubin's reabsorption from the intestines. A Minneapolis

### MEDICATIONS TO PREVENT OR TREAT JAUNDICE

- Activated charcoal (no longer used)
- Agar (rarely used as an adjunctive treatment)
- Phenobarbital (effective, but has side effects)
- Protoporphyrin (experimental; high-risk groups only)

study from the 1960s showed that feeding babies activated charcoal from the time they were four hours old decreased their bilirubin levels somewhat. However, the charcoal was not very helpful if it was started later when the babies were actually jaundiced. Activated charcoal never really caught on as a jaundice treatment, but it is used to treat some cases of poisoning.

*Agar*, an extract of seaweed, also absorbs bilirubin in the intestines and helps prevent its reabsorption. Different kinds of agar have varying abilities to absorb bilirubin. Most absorb far too little to affect newborn jaundice. Even the highest medical grade agar is not very potent. In a study my colleagues and I did at Yale in the 1980s, the most absorbent agar lowered bilirubin levels only a couple of points.[5] This difference was statistically significant, but it probably had little real impact on the health of the babies over the long run. High-grade agar is used in some medical centers as an adjunctive treatment to light therapy, but in most medical centers, it's never used and is not even available.

*Phenobarbital*, the well-known seizure medication, lowers bilirubin levels by reviving liver metabolism. Because of its sedative effects, it is rarely used nowadays to treat typical newborn jaundice.

*Protoporphyrins* are chemicals that look enough like hemoglobin to fool the enzymes that usually break it down, thereby decreasing bilirubin levels. Giving an injection of protoporphyrin within the first day of life lowers bilirubin levels throughout the first weeks of life (when they are typically highest). The trouble is that you have to know in advance which babies are going to have jaundice or a lot of babies end up being treated unnecessarily. Protoporphyrins also have side effects such as skin irritation. They have not caught on as primary therapy for jaundice except in countries where there are many babies with fragile blood cells and high rates of jaundice.

Several medications increase bilirubin levels. They are contraindicated in newborns because of the risk of shifting jaundice from a benign condition to a worrisome problem. For this reason, medications such as sulfa drugs and ceftriaxone are not used in babies less than two weeks old.

## Herbs

No herbs have proven safe and effective in treating newborn jaundice. Herbal remedies traditionally used for adults with liver disease or jaundice (such as aloe vera gel, cascara bark, dandelion root, parsley, and milk thistle) have not been evaluated in babies and may not be safe. Several herbal remedies can actually cause liver damage and jaundice. For example, the Chinese herbs *yin-chen* and *cheun-lin*, which are traditionally used to treat jaundice, displace bilirubin from the blood to other tissues, such as the brain![6] Other herbs, such as chaparral and *Jin Bu Haan (Lycopodium serratum)* actually cause liver toxicity and jaundice. Other herbs used to treat liver problems in Traditional Chinese Medicine, such as licorice root, may cause problems with the salt balance in the blood and lead to puffiness and high blood pressure. Goldenseal, which is sometimes recommended as an herbal antibiotic, can bump bilirubin off its carrier protein, making it easier for the bilirubin to pass into the brain. It should never be used in babies less than three months old. I do not recommend any herbal remedies to treat newborn jaundice.

## Nutritional Supplements

Fearing that the baby might be dehydrated, many mothers give water supplements. Jaundice is not caused by dehydration. Water supplements do not improve jaundice.[7]

Megadoses of niacin can actually cause jaundice in older children. No vitamins or minerals have proven helpful in treating newborn jaundice. I do not recommend any dietary supplements as treatments for newborn jaundice.

## LIFESTYLE THERAPIES: NUTRITION, ENVIRONMENT

### Nutrition

#### Feeding frequency

As they say about Chicago voting, do it early and often. Frequent feeding, especially for breast-fed babies, results in lower bilirubin levels and less jaundice.[8] Nursing mothers should breast-feed their newborn babies at least eight to ten times daily. Jaundiced babies may be a little sleepy, but wake them up to nurse every two to three hours. Frequent nursing in the first week of life helps mothers produce more milk more quickly, stimulates the babies' intestines to move things along, and helps babies eliminate bilirubin.[9] Breast milk also helps protect babies against infectious diseases, allergic diseases, colds, and asthma. Keep on nursing!

#### Formula supplements

Supplementing with formula seriously sabotages the eventual success of breast-feeding.[10] Because jaundice is generally so benign and breast-feeding is so beneficial, most pediatricians do not recommend formula supplements for jaundiced breast-fed babies. Rather than stopping or interrupting breast-feeding, I recommend that you nurse your baby more often, at least eight times daily. If your baby is very jaundiced and seems to be hungry even after she nurses, please discuss the situation with your health care professional or a lactation (breast-feeding) specialist.

If you are already feeding your baby formula, you may want to choose a special casein-hydrolysate formula rather than a standard cow's milk formula. At least one study suggests that babies who drink these special formulas have a significantly lower risk of developing jaundice than babies who drink regular formula.[11] If you are on WIC (Women, Infants & Children supplemental food program), you may need a prescription from your pediatrician for this special formula.

## Environment

Light therapy (phototherapy) is the mainstay of jaundice therapy. Phototherapy was discovered years ago by a nurse and physician who observed that infants who were taken outside on bright, warm days or whose cribs were near the window were much less likely to be jaundiced than babies whose cribs were away from the window.[12] Astute pediatricians since then have noted that jaundice occurs more commonly during the fall and winter months when babies are exposed to less sunlight.

In the presence of sunlight, our skin changes bilirubin to another form which is much more easily excreted by the kidneys. This change allows bilirubin to bypass the liver and intestines to be excreted directly by the kidneys without the possibility for reabsorption.

Phototherapy is recommended at different bilirubin levels depending on the baby's age.[13] These levels are now a few points higher than they were in the 1970s and 1980s; this means that fewer babies need to be treated. The changes in pediatric practice were based on evidence that most jaundice is not harmful and many treatments are costly and distressing.[14] The changes mean that many parents can be

spared the costs and concerns of repeated tests and hospitalization.

---

### BILIRUBIN LEVELS LEADING TO PHOTOTHERAPY AT DIFFERENT AGES

| BABY'S AGE | BILIRUBIN LEVEL FOR PHOTOTHERAPY |
|---|---|
| Less than 24 hours old | Any jaundice |
| 25 to 48 hours old | 12 to 15 or higher |
| 49 to 72 hours old | 15 to 18 or higher |
| 73 or more hours old | 17 to 20 or higher |

---

*May's bilirubin level was 15 at four days of age, and both she and her mother had type A (Rh-positive) blood. The nurse encouraged more frequent breast-feeding and two outdoor strolls per day to help bring down the bilirubin. However, it was overcast and rainy, and May never made it outside. When the nurse returned the following day, May's bilirubin had climbed to 18 so she was started on home phototherapy.*

Phototherapy can be provided by standard fluorescent lights, special blue-green spectrum fluorescent lights, halogen lights, or special blankets containing fiber-optic lights ("bili blankets"). These phototherapy products are available only by prescription. The most potent type of light therapy is the combination of placing a baby on top of a bili blanket while shining standard fluorescent lights from above.[15] Sandwiching the baby between lights is called double phototherapy. Single phototherapy, such as the bili blanket alone, is also effective, particularly with the newer high-intensity products. Bili blankets have two main advantages over conventional light therapy: 1) the baby's eyes do not need to be covered; and 2) the baby can be snuggled by the parents rather than being confined to an incubator. I generally recommend the "sandwich" approach for when the baby is sleeping, and the bili blanket for the times the baby is being fed, cuddled, or played with.

Phototherapy has few side effects. Because of the light intensity with overhead light therapy, the baby's eyes need to be protected to prevent eye damage. Recent studies have suggested that it's better to cover the baby's head with a box made of light-proof plastic than to cover the eyes with cloth or gauze eye patches; this is because the eye patches increase the risk of the baby developing conjunctivitis. Despite this small increase in risk, most babies still get the eye patches because they are far more convenient for all concerned. The room temperature may need to be turned up if the baby is lying naked on top of a bili blanket. The baby may also need some extra milk to compensate for the increased evaporation of fluid from the skin during phototherapy. Long-term follow-up studies have not indicated any increased risk of skin cancer or other skin diseases in children who received phototherapy as infants.

*By the time May was a week old, her bilirubin level was down to 13; she was nursing well and her mother's milk was in. She had a total of three blood tests, four nurse visits, five calls to the physician (me), two days of home phototherapy, and had avoided extra trips to the office and an expensive hospital stay. Her grandmother, Rose, was very impressed at the changes in health care in the twenty-three years since Steven was born. Bonnie was confident that May was basically a healthy baby and was glad not to have had to make repeated trips to the clinic in the first week after her delivery.*

## BIOMECHANICAL THERAPIES: SURGERY

### Surgery (Transfusions)

If a baby's bilirubin level climbs into potentially dangerous levels despite changes in feeding and despite light therapy (phototherapy), *blood transfusions* can be helpful. This is called an *exchange transfusion* because some of the baby's blood (containing high bilirubin levels) is removed and exchanged for low-bilirubin blood. This procedure must be done in the hospital by physicians who are experienced in the care of newborn infants. It rapidly reduces bilirubin levels, but the procedure itself causes significant side effects in over 10% of babies.[16] Because of the risks of this potentially lifesaving procedure, most physicians prefer to use it as a last resort, relying on frequent feeding and phototherapy as the mainstays of treatment.

The American Academy of Pediatrics recommends that exchange transfusion be performed for babies whose bilirubin levels have climbed to 20 mg/dL by the time they are 48 hours old. It also recommends exchange transfusion for babies who reach bilirubin levels of 25 mg/dL if they are 49 hours or older. It's an arbitrary cutoff, but the line has to be drawn somewhere. Even though this is the official guideline, your pediatrician may recommend an exchange transfusion at slightly higher or lower bilirubin levels, depending on your baby's individual situation.

## BIOENERGETIC THERAPIES: ACUPUNCTURE, THERAPEUTIC TOUCH/PRAYER, HOMEOPATHY

### Acupuncture

There is no role for acupuncture or related therapies in treating newborn jaundice.

### Therapeutic Touch/Prayer

Prayer-healing has been shown to prevent red blood cells from breaking down in test tubes.[17] Other studies have shown that prayer healing and Therapeutic Touch can increase hemoglobin levels in normal adults.[18] There are no studies specifically evaluating the effectiveness of prayer or Therapeutic Touch in treating jaundiced newborns, but because both therapies are safe, I encourage you to try them along with other therapies if they are consistent with your family's beliefs.

*Homeopathy*

There are no scientific studies evaluating the risks or benefits of homeopathy in treating newborn jaundice.

## WHAT I RECOMMEND FOR JAUNDICE

*Take your baby to your health care professional if:*

- The mother is Rh-negative or blood type O

- Abnormal or fragile blood types or severe juandice run in your family

- The baby becomes excessively sleepy or unresponsive (sleeping for more than four or five hours in a row in the first week of life)

- The baby develops a fever or acts sick

- Jaundice is visible within the first 48 hours of life

- The jaundice extends all the way down your child's chest to the belly button

- The jaundice lasts longer than ten days

- You are concerned about her in any way

1. *Lifestyle—nutrition.* Feed your baby at least eight to ten times daily.

2. *Lifestyle—environment.* Take your baby outside to get some sunlight every day. Avoid the high-intensity hours between 10 A.M. and 2 P.M. If your baby develops higher bilirubin levels, use professional phototherapy.

3. *Bioenergetic—prayer.* If they are consistent with your family beliefs, try prayer and Therapeutic Touch to help stabilize hemoglobin and reduce bilirubin levels.

4. *Biomechanical—surgery.* If your baby develops very high bilirubin levels despite other therapies, she may need an exchange transfusion, exchanging her high-bilirubin blood for lower bilirubin blood.

RESOURCES

*Internet*

America Academy of Pediatrics
http://www.medem.com/default.cfm

General Pediatrics
http://www.generalpediatrics.com/
CommonProbProf.html

# 23

# RINGWORM AND OTHER FUNGAL INFECTIONS

Marie Washington brought in her sons, Irving and Michael, to be treated for ringworm and athlete's foot, which they'd picked up at school. Eight-year-old Irving had silver-dollar size scaly patches on his arms and legs. Michael, the sixteen-year-old star of his basketball team, was complaining of itching and burning on his feet. He had cracked, peeling skin around his toes. Marie wanted to know:

- If ringworm was really caused by worms
- If only athletes could get athlete's foot
- What was the best way to treat both boys?

Despite its name, ringworm is caused by a fungus, not worms. Ringworm (*tinea corporis*) is the most common fungal infection in children over a year old. The same types of fungus that cause ringworm also cause infections on the feet (athlete's foot, or *tinea pedis*), in the groin (jock itch, or *tinea cruris*), and in the scalp (*tinea capitis*). *Tinea* simply means fungal infection. The second part of each medical name refers to the body part affected (*capitis* = head, *corporis* = body, *pedis* = feet). Several types of fungus cause infec-

tions in humans. They have long, poetic names such as *Trichophyton, Microsporum,* and *Epidermophyton.* And they are causing problems at epidemic levels while becoming more resistant to older, widely used medications.

*Tinea corporis* is one of the most common skin conditions of childhood. It is passed from person to person. Outbreaks occur among participants in contact sports. When this happens to wrestlers, it's called *trichophytosis gladiatorum.* Kids can also pick up these infections from dogs and cats or from the clothing or equipment of infected persons.

*Tinea capitis* (ringworm of the scalp) is usually caused by *Trichophyton tonsurans* and less commonly by *Microsporum canis*. Although most fungal infections are passed from person to person, scalp ringworm can be caught from dogs or cats. These fungi can cause big pimple-like swellings, mushy areas, and crusting on the scalp, called a *kerion*. Kerions can look so serious they have fooled experienced doctors into thinking that something other than a simple fungal infection was responsible, leading to costly treatment errors and even hospitalization. The infection can also look like plain old ringworm or it might cause patchy bald areas on the head and swollen lymph nodes in the neck. When the fungi cause the scalp hairs to break off, the resulting bald patches with dots of broken hairs are called *black dot ringworm*. Tinea capitis is common in school-age kids, but becomes much less of a problem once kids enter puberty and their scalps become oilier and less hospitable to fungus.

Unlike tinea capitis, which fades as adolescence begins, *tinea pedis*, athlete's foot, is unusual before adolescence but becomes more common as hormones (and high-top sneakers) kick in. In one study of marathon runners, about 11% had symptoms, and twice that many carried the ringworm fungus. This finding points out the need for careful hygiene in the locker room. Even if your buddy doesn't have any symptoms, he could still be carrying the fungus that will make you miserable. Athlete's foot occurs even among those whose only exertion is Monday morning quarterbacking. Once the fungus has set in and the skin starts to scale, itch, and break down, the scene is set for bacterial infections to move in, creating an even bigger problem.

Fungal infections of the fingernails and toe-nails is known as *onychomycosis*. These are much less common in children than in older adults, but they can occur. And they are difficult to treat. The nail may become thick and yellow, with ridges or curls. Treatment nearly always requires antifungal medications taken by mouth.

Fungal infections can mimic several other skin conditions such as eczema, impetigo, insect bites, psoriasis, plain old dandruff, and allergic reactions. Special tests may be needed to make the right diagnosis. Some fungi glow under black lights; your doctor may use a special light (known as a Wood's lamp) to see if the infected skin glows in the dark. Alternatively, she may scrape a tiny bit of skin onto a slide and examine it under a microscope to be sure it's a fungus and not an imitator. Sometimes a culture is necessary to be certain. Culture results can take several weeks. Most folks are eager to take action much sooner, so you may start therapy even without these diagnostic tests.

## WHAT'S THE BEST WAY TO TREAT FUNGAL INFECTIONS?

All therapies take several weeks to eradicate fungus; there are no quick cures. Let's tour the Therapeutic Mountain to find out what works best. If you want to skip to my bottom-line recommendations, flip to the end of the chapter.

### BIOCHEMICAL THERAPIES: MEDICATIONS, HERBS, NUTRITIONAL SUPPLEMENTS

#### *Medications*

Medical treatments are similar for most fungal infections except for those affecting the scalp. Scalp infections require medication that reaches beneath the skin surface because they usually involve the deep hair shafts. Most other fungal infections on the skin respond to medicated creams.

the more expensive 2.5% prescription formulations.[1]

## NONPRESCRIPTION MEDICATIONS FOR FUNGAL INFECTIONS

- Undecylenic acid (Desenex, Pedi-Dri, Cruex)
- Miconazole (Micatin, Monistat)
- Clotrimazole (Lotrimin, Mycelex)
- Tolnaftate (Tinactin, Desenex, and others)
- Selenium sulfide shampoo (Selsun and others)

*Undecylenic acid* (Desenex and other brands) has been used to treat athlete's foot for over thirty years. The most commonly recommended antifungal agents in our clinic are undecylenic acid, clotrimazole, and miconazole because they have proven safety and effectiveness and are inexpensive. They are applied twice daily until after the rash has been gone for at least one week to ensure that all the fungi have been eliminated. I prefer creams and lotions to powders and sprays because they tend to stay on better, but you can experiment to find out what works best for your child.

*Tolnaftate* (Tinactin) is another effective antifungal medication. It is traditionally used to treat athlete's foot and jock itch, and it is effective against ringworm, too. Tolnaftate is also applied twice daily. Improvement is usually apparent within ten days, although complete cure may take a month or more.

*Selenium sulfide shampoo* (Selsun, Exsel) is an adjunctive therapy to treat fungal infections in the scalp. It does not eradicate the infection, but it helps prevent it from spreading to others. Nonprescription strength (1%) selenium sulfide shampoo appears to be as effective as

## PRESCRIPTION MEDICATIONS FOR FUNGAL INFECTIONS

- Griseofulvin (Fulvicin, Grisactin, Grifulvin V)
- Imidazoles: ketoconazole (Nizoral), oxiconazole (Oxistat), econazole (Spectazole), itraconazole (Sporanox), fluconazole (Diflucan), sulconazole 1% (Exelderm), butenafine 1% (Mentax)
- Allylamines: terbinafine (Lamisil), naftifine (Naftin)
- Others: halprogin (Halotex), ciclopirox (Loprox)

A wide variety of prescription medications have been developed to fight fungal infections. Some are taken by mouth while others are applied directly to the rash. Mild infections typically respond to topical application, but deep-seated or widespread infections require a systemic approach that includes oral medication. Many of these medications have not been thoroughly tested or approved for use in children, but that hasn't stopped doctors from recommending them when a stubborn fungal infection fails to capitulate to older, approved drugs.

For fungal infections in the scalp *(tinea capitis),* the oral medicine *griseofulvin* is the treatment of choice because of its low toxicity and low cost; it has been around since 1958, so we know a lot about how safe it is. Like penicillin, griseofulvin is derived from our old friend, the *Penicillium* mold. It must be taken daily for at least six to eight weeks to eradicate fungal infections. Because fungi, like bacteria, have gradually adapted to medications, the dose required to knock them out has gradually increased over the last ten years. It is one of the rare medicines that actually works better if it is taken with food, especially fatty foods. Try giving it to your child with a glass of whole milk. It can interfere with the effectiveness of birth control pills; children taking seizure medications may need to take higher than usual doses of griseofulvin to achieve the same effect as children who are not taking other medications.

*Ketoconazole* and *itraconazole* are prescription antifungal medications that kill yeast and fungus throughout the body; they can eradicate symptoms and even prevent outbreaks in kids who are frequently exposed to fungi, such as wrestlers. Itraconazole has become the treatment of choice for fungal infections affecting the fingernails or toenails—sites that are notoriously difficult to treat. *Econazole* works quickly; it is effective within two weeks against ringworm and within one month against athlete's foot. *Fluconazole* has been heavily marketed as a treatment for yeast infections; it is also effective against ringworm on the scalp. It is available in a liquid form that can be taken by mouth. All of the prescription imidazole medications are effective, but they are significantly more expensive than their nonprescription relatives. Imidazoles can also cause an upset stomach and markedly interfere other medications, including allergy medicines, seizure medicines, asthma medicines, heart medicines, and others.

The *allylamines,* terbinafine and naftifine, are the newest and most effective antifungal medications. *Terbinafine* (Lamisil) is effective in treating even difficult cases of athlete's foot and tinea capitis within 2 to 4 weeks.[2] However, terbinafine in large doses has been blamed for causing cancer in laboratory animals and it may cause side effects when given to patients who are already taking other medications such as cimetidine, rifampin, or phenobarbital. The usual tablets contain too much medication for

children, so you may ask your physician or pharmacist for help cutting the tablets into the right-sized doses for your child; liquid suspensions are not yet available. *Naftifine* is another powerful antifungal medication for treating athlete's foot.[3] Like all fungal medicines, it can cause burning and stinging when applied to already irritated skin.

The most cost-effective medical approach to the typical fungal infection of the skin is to start with an inexpensive but effective nonprescription medication (such as miconazole); if there is no improvement after a month of twice daily use, see your physician about a more expensive and powerful prescription medication.[4]

## Herbs

*Tea tree oil* has antibacterial and antifungal properties and has been recommended as a treatment for fungal infections. In an Australian study it was compared to tolnaftate for the treatment of athlete's foot. Although patients reported improved symptoms with both preparations, tea tree oil failed to kill the fungi.[5] Tea tree oil is safe when applied to nonirritated skin. You can try it if you are reluctant to use medication. As with any treatment, if the skin becomes more irritated, stop using it.

*Garlic* extracts have proven antifungal effects in test-tube studies and have been tried in field experiments in army recruits with mixed success.[6] They have not yet been tested against fungal skin infections in children. Garlic poultices can cause burns and severe skin irritation if left on too long.

Plants have evolved many tricks over the ages to ward off fungal infections. Several essential oils have shown effectiveness against fungal infections in guinea pigs and test-tube studies: *Artemisia nelagrica, Artemisia afra, Caesulia axillaris, Chenopodium ambrosioides*, *Cymbopogon citratus* (lemongrass), and *Mentha arvensis.*[7] For mild fungal infections such as one patch of simple ringworm, you may want to try a massage with an oil containing lemongrass, mint, oregano, marjoram, sage, lavender, or rosemary oil.[8] Or add a few drops of these oils to the rinse cycle in your laundry to help kill the fungal spores lingering on clothes. However, these oils should not be used as the sole treatment for serious or widespread fungal infections or those affecting the scalp or nails.

Ringworm of the scalp is rare on the Indian subcontinent, where many people use hair dressings containing vegetable oil. A recent test-tube study showed that the most popular Indian hair oils (mustard oil, coconut oil, and Amla oil) had antifungal properties.[9] Although these results are preliminary, they are intriguing. These vegetable oils are safe and inexpensive and may be worth trying as preventive or adjunctive therapy, but do *not* forsake medications that have proven effectiveness for treating fungal infections that have already taken hold in the scalp.

Some herbalists recommend teas to help the immune system fight fungal infections. Teas reputed to have this effect are burdock, cleavers, dandelion root, echinacea, nettles, peppermint, and red clover. Teas used as washes for fungal infections are agrimony, burdock, and marigold. There are no studies evaluating the effectiveness of any of these teas or tinctures as treatments for fungal infections. I do *not* recommend them as primary treatments.

Lemon juice and cider vinegar have both been recommended as ways to make the skin more acid (lower pH) and less hospitable for fungi. There are no scientific studies documenting their effectiveness in treating children with fungal infections, but they are inexpensive and safe. They may be worth trying as preventive or adjunctive therapies for fungal infections.

## Nutritional Supplements

Vitamin C in powder or crystal form has been recommended as topical treatment for fungal infections of the skin, but there are no studies evaluating its use.

## LIFESTYLE THERAPIES: NUTRITION, EXERCISE, ENVIRONMENT

### Nutrition

There are no studies suggesting that any particular dietary supplement eradicates fungal infections. I try yogurt with just about everything, but there are no studies showing it works for serious fungal infections. There's a lot of anecdotal experience suggesting it's helpful for diaper rashes caused by yeast (see Chapter 15, Diaper Rash).

### Exercise

Exercise common sense. If your child is in gym class at school and takes showers in a common area, make sure he has shower sandals to keep his feet out of direct contact with the inevitable fungus on the floor. If your child has an infection, it's even more important to wear shower shoes to prevent the infection from spreading to others. Have him dry his feet well after a shower to make them less hospitable for fungi. After showering is the perfect time to apply antifungal medication. Even if your child doesn't have athlete's foot, he may want to dust his feet with antifungal powder several times a week in the locker room to prevent picking up a case.

### Environment

Fungi love to live in warm, damp environments. High-top sneakers are perfect breeding grounds for athlete's foot fungus. If your child is prone to athlete's foot, have him forget the high-tops for a while and go with more breathable shoes such as sandals or thongs when he's not playing basketball. It takes a day or so for regular shoes to dry out from normal sweat. Changing shoes and socks twice daily helps reduce moisture; try not to wear the same shoes two days in a row, and look for cotton socks. Also, put those sneakers in the washing machine with the white clothes, detergent, and bleach. You may find that as the shoes are cleaned and dried and the rash clears, there is a remarkable improvement in foot odor.

Children *can* catch fungal infections from pets and farm animals. If your pets or livestock have skin problems, have them checked by your veterinarian and treated promptly to reduce your child's chances of catching a fungal infection.

## BIOMECHANICAL THERAPIES

None of these therapies has scientifically proven benefits in treating children with ringworm or other fungal infections. I do *not* recommend them.

## BIOENERGETIC THERAPIES: ACUPUNCTURE, REIKI/THERAPEUTIC TOUCH, HOMEOPATHY

### Accupuncture

I don't know of any acupuncturists who treat fungal infections with acupuncture.

### Reiki/Therapeutic Touch

I have never treated anyone with a fungal infection with Reiki or Therapeutic Touch, but I suspect that these therapies may be helpful in reducing the annoying itch and redness that often accompany fungal infections. I would not rely on these therapies alone to treat fungal infections, but I'm curious to see studies evaluating their effectiveness as adjunctive treatments.

### Homeopathy

Commonly used homeopathic remedies for fungal infections include Calcarea, Dulcamara, Graphites, Sepia, Sulfur, and Tellurium. None has proven effectiveness, but they are safe when used as recommended.

# WHAT I RECOMMEND FOR RINGWORM AND OTHER FUNGAL INFECTIONS

## PREVENTING FUNGAL INFECTIONS

1. *Lifestyle—environment.* Use good hygiene. Prevent athlete's foot by using shower shoes, sandals, or flip-flops in the gym showers and locker room. Keep the feet clean and dry. Avoid high-top sneakers. Change socks and shoes frequently. Wash sneakers in the washing machine and dry them thoroughly. If your pets or livestock develop skin problems, have them evaluated and treated promptly to prevent possible spread to your children.

2. *Biochemical—herbs*. Consider rinsing your child's feet in lemon juice or vinegar after showering in public places to make the skin more acidic and less hospitable to fungi. Or consider a mini-massage with essential oils of sage, lavender, lemongrass, rosemary, or a poultice with crushed garlic.

---

*See your health care provider if:*

- You suspect a fungal infection of the scalp (this requires prescription medication); it may also benefit from regular shampooing with selenium sulfide shampoo

- The rash is not improving after ten days of therapy or is getting worse with home treatment

- The rash is spreading

- The rash involves the toenails or fingernails

---

## TREATING FUNGAL INFECTIONS

1. *Biochemical—medications*. Treat twice daily with nonprescription antifungal medications containing clotrimazole (Lotrimin, Mycelex), miconazole (Monistat), tolnaftate (Tinactin), or undecylenic acid (Desenex, Cruex, Caldesene) for at least four weeks. Continue treatment for at least one week after all symptoms have resolved to make sure the fungi have been eradicated.

2. *Biochemical—herbs*. Consider tea tree oil or other essential oils applied to the rash twice daily for four weeks. Or try a garlic poultice twice daily for no more than twenty minutes at a time.

If the rash is not gone within a month with nonprescription treatments, see your health care provider to evaluate the need for prescription medication.

RESOURCES

*Internet*

American Academy of Dermatology
http://www.aad.org/pamphlets/tineav.html

American Academy of Family Practice
http://familydoctor.org/handouts/316.html

National Center for Emergency Medicine Informatics
http://www.ncemi.org/cse/cse1117.htm

University of Iowa Virtual Hospital
http://www.vh.org/Patients/IHB/Peds/Infectious/ScalpFungus.html

# 24
# SLEEP PROBLEMS

- GETTING YOUR INFANT TO SLEEP THROUGH THE NIGHT
- GETTING YOUR TODDLER TO BED
- NIGHTMARES AND NIGHT TERRORS
- INSOMNIA

"Our baby is four months old and still waking up to nurse at 2 A.M. and 5 A.M. When will he outgrow the need for middle-of-the-night feeds so we can get some sleep? He still sleeps with us. Is that OK? Will giving him rice cereal at bedtime help him sleep better?"

"Our three-year-old is driving us nuts. Every night it's the same thing. We put her to bed, and then she wants a glass of water; next it's a story; by that time she has to go to the bathroom again. We get her in bed and five minutes later she's up again; if we don't read her another story, she starts crying. Bedtime started out as a fifteen minute process, and now it takes an hour. How can we get back to a reasonable routine?"

"Our four-year-old has been waking up a few hours after we put him to bed, screaming like someone is killing him. We rush into the room to find him sitting up in bed, staring blankly. He doesn't seem to know we're there and won't talk about the bad dream. In the morning, he doesn't even seem to remember it. This has happened several times. Should we take him to a psychiatrist?"

One of the most common and frustrating problems parents face is getting their children to sleep through the night. Babies' sleep patterns differ from adults' sleep. They learn sleep and wakefulness cycles just as they learn hunger cycles, bladder control, language, and walking—over time. Children's sleeping patterns change throughout infancy and early childhood, from initially waking every few hours to nurse, to sleeping several hours at a time, to intermittently waking again in later infancy, to full night's sleep plus naps at toddler age, to school-age regular nighttime sleep, to adolescents who may require more sleep as they go through growth spurts. It takes the average two-month-old over 25 minutes to fall asleep, while the average nine-month-old needs just over 15 minutes to drift off. Most infants awaken every few hours to nurse until they are three to four months old, and some continue to do so for the first year and a half. By six months of age, over 80% of infants sleep at least five hours in a row. Believe it or not, in pediatric circles five to six straight hours of sleep is considered "sleeping through the night."

### TYPICAL SLEEP PATTERNS

| AGE | TOTAL SLEEP | NAPS |
| --- | --- | --- |
| Newborn | 16 to 17 hours | A.M. and P.M. |
| 6 to 12 months | 14 to 15 hours | A.M. and P.M. |
| Toddlers | 12 hours | P.M. |
| School age | 10 hours | None |
| Older school age | 8 hours | None |
| Teenagers | 8 to 10 hours | None |

Almost all children give up naps by first grade; some outgrow naps by the time they are three years old. School-age children typically need fewer than ten hours of sleep, but should get at least eight hours a night. Adolescents often sleep more during periods of intense growth and maturation. During illnesses and recovery from injury, children sleep more. Each child is different.

The two main phases of sleep are rapid-eye-movement, REM (dream) sleep and non-REM sleep. Non-REM sleep is quiet sleep during which the child moves from wakefulness into deeper sleep with slower brain waves. During deepest sleep the brain waves are very slow and the child is very still. This is when growth hormone secretion reaches its peak. REM sleep is fairly light and physically active sleep. Following REM sleep the child may briefly waken before returning to quiet sleep and repeating the cycle. Like cats, infants can enter REM sleep almost immediately. Older children and adults sleep quietly (non-REM) for about 70 to 90 minutes before REM sleep starts. A teenager who sleeps eight hours goes through about four or five repetitions of this cycle every night.

If you think your child has sleep difficulties, you are not alone. Neither is your child. In national surveys of thousands of children, almost half were reported to have some kind of sleep difficulty. The most common problem (27%) was getting toddlers to go to bed; 10 to 15 percent of kids had a hard time falling asleep or awoke in the middle of the night at least once a week.[1] Fifteen to 20 percent had troubles waking up in the morning or felt fatigued during the day from inadequate sleep.[2] Fifteen percent had frequent nightmares or night terrors; 5% walked in their sleep.[3] Other problems included bed-wetting and teeth grinding during sleep. Children's sleep problems frequently disrupt parents' sleep, resulting in fatigue, frustration, anger, and guilt.

Parents aren't the only ones who are stressed,

exhausted, and depressed when their children have trouble sleeping.[4] The kids suffer, too. Children and adolescents who don't get enough sleep are less able to pay attention in school, more irritable, more unhappy, and less likely to comply with parental or teacher requests.[5] Many kids who are inattentive or impulsive are actually sleepy; they tend to fall asleep more during the day and to fall asleep more quickly at night than their better rested peers. Any time a child is being evaluated for attention deficit hyperactivity disorder, depression, or oppositional behavior, the clinician and parent should pay close attention to the child's sleep.[6] And any time a parent is concerned about a child's behavior, they should reflect on the child's sleep patterns—regular bedtime, regular place to sleep, and having a bedtime similar to their peers rather than their parents. Poor sleep may be a precursor to depression and other psychiatric and behavioral problems.[7]

## FACTORS THAT INTERFERE WITH NORMAL SLEEP

- Illness, pain, allergies
- Anxiety, depression, tension, or stress
- Change in routine, travel
- Being overtired
- Too much TV
- Caffeine-containing beverages or foods
- Medications and alcohol
- Difficult temperament

Ear infections are perhaps the best example of a *painful illness* that awakens children in the middle of the night. Teething and itchy rashes can also keep a child from a sound sleep as can breathing problems from congestion or asthma. Diabetes and bladder infections increase urination and thereby increase nighttime awakening. Strangely enough, cow's milk *allergies* can interfere with sleeping as well.[8] There is at least one study showing that sleep dramatically improves when allergic children stop drinking milk.[9] (See Chapter 4, Allergies.)

Like adults, children can suffer from *stress, anxiety, depression,* or *tension* that keeps them awake. Preschool-age children may be concerned about parental disputes or disruptions in normal routines. School-age children and adolescents may worry about upcoming tests, peer pressure, dates, or scary movies. Major catastrophes and natural disasters often trigger nightmares. Following the 1989 San Francisco earthquake nightmares were eight times more frequent in Bay Area students than among students living in Tucson, Arizona.[10] Try to keep evening time quiet and relaxed. Discuss family disagreements during the day when coping and communication are at their best rather than before bed when they tend to be strained.

Paradoxically, being *overtired* is a common cause of sleep problems. When a child becomes overtired, he compensates for his fatigue by increasing levels of stress hormones (such as epinephrine) that keep him awake. It takes a certain calm focus to allow the events of the day to slide away and allow sleep to set in.

School-age children who watch more *television,* especially those who watch violent shows, are much more likely to have sleep problems than children who watch less.[11] Nowadays somewhere between 25 and 50 percent of kids have televisions in their rooms, making it far too easy to overindulge in TV. If your child has trouble sleeping, remove the TV from his room and limit him to less than 90 minutes daily of television, preferably nonviolent shows. When he watches, stay with him; you might be surprised how much violence there is in kids' shows, and how much it helps your child to talk with you about what he's viewing.

Adults are not the only ones who are kept awake by *caffeine*. Its stimulant effects are found in tea, cola, and chocolate as well as coffee. I saw a teenager who complained of being unable to fall asleep before 11:30 P.M. and then having trouble getting up for his 6 A.M. alarm. It turned out he was drinking massive quantities of cola after supper while doing his homework. His ability to fall asleep dramatically improved when he decided not to drink any cola after 4 P.M.

Common cold *medications* and herbal remedies also contain potent stimulants: ephedrine, pseudoephedrine, phenylpropanolamine, ephedra, *Ma Huang,* and ginseng.[12] If you are nursing your baby, check with your health care professional before taking nonprescription cold medications because some of them end up in breast milk and may keep your baby awake. *Alcohol* is another common ingredient in many nonprescription cold remedies. While alcohol may initially seem to knock your child out, it actually induces a relatively light sleep, a full bladder, and a rebound awakening after a few hours—not good therapy for a child suffering from a cold—or any child for that matter.

Infants who have trouble falling asleep or who waken frequently in the middle of the night are more likely to be viewed as having *difficult temperaments* than children who sleep soundly. Children with persistent sleep problems are also more likely to have temper tantrums and other behavior problems.[13] It is difficult to sort out whether less adaptable children are more likely to have sleep problems or whether children who awaken their parents in the middle of the night are labeled as troublesome. Children with attention deficit disorder awaken frequently in the middle of the night and also suffer more commonly than other children from night sweats and bed-wetting.[14] Behavior problems don't necessarily stop the minute a child gets in bed.

Sleep patterns can be substantially improved with a few straightforward measures. In a study of breast-fed infants and their parents, one group was taught how to train their infant to sleep through the night; the other group was put on a waiting list and not given any special instructions on infant sleep until the baby was eight weeks old. Those who were taught the techniques were able to train their infants to sleep better through the night (100% were sleeping at least five consecutive hours by the time they were eight weeks old compared to only 23% of control group infants). The trained group also rated their babies temperaments as significantly easier than the untrained group whose babies were still waking frequently.[15] Parents who are taught to train their infants to sleep through the night also report an increased sense of competence as parents.[16] This study raises the possibility that the advantages of early sleep training may extend beyond peaceful parental slumber to benefit infant temperament and parental confidence.

Infants who are *put into bed after they have fallen asleep* or *who fall asleep in the presence of a parent* are more likely to awaken in the middle of the night (and wake their parents) than infants who fall asleep by themselves in their crib. This is a strong argument for putting your child down to sleep while he is still awake. If your child is already used to falling asleep while you are holding him or rocking him, try making the change first at nap time. When he learns to fall asleep on his own at nap time, try putting him down at night while he is still awake. By learning to fall asleep on his own, he can later put himself to sleep when he awakens in the middle of the night without waking you.

*Nightmares* are most common between the ages of three and six years old. Children who awaken with nightmares are generally fully awake, can be comforted by parents, and can tell their parents details about the bad dream.

Children who suffer from nightmares are not maladjusted, more anxious, or under more stress than other children. Nightmares are not due to behavior problems, seizures, or brain wave abnormalities. They are simply bad dreams. Adults who suffer from nightmares tend to be more sensitive and creative than those who aren't beset by troubling images at night.[17] Children, of course, have more vivid imaginations than adults, and have active fantasies about imaginary friends, ghosts, monsters, and all kinds of creatures. It's no surprise that many of them turn up in dreams. Nightmares can be inspired by anything from television violence to shadows cast by a night light to actual scary experiences.

### FREQUENT NIGHTMARE TOPICS

- Scary animals
- Monsters
- Strangers attacking or chasing them
- Being abandoned or helpless in a strange place
- Being shot (more common with increasing media violence)

*Night terrors* occur most commonly in children between the ages of one and four years old. Unlike dreams or nightmares, they do not occur during REM sleep. Rather, they occur in the deepest stages of sleep. Night terrors tend to occur within the first two hours of sleep whereas nightmares occur during dream sleep in the later part of the night (between 3 A.M. and 6 A.M.). During a night terror episode, the child utters terrifying screams, sits bolt upright and stares ahead with a glassy gaze. His eyes are open and he appears to be awake, but he does not notice or respond to his parents. This is very unnerving for the parent who is trying to comfort an obviously distraught child who is so soundly asleep that he really doesn't hear anything. Often, the child doesn't even recall the incident the following morning. The episodes typically last fewer than fifteen minutes. Children who start having night terrors before the age of four tend to have more frequent episodes than children who start having them later. No one knows why some children have night terrors and why they usually outgrow them by school age. They tend to run in families and they are *not* signs of a psychiatric problem. However, if your child has frequent night terrors (more than twice a week), see your health care professional for advice. Some prescription medications are helpful for this condition.

## WHAT IS THE BEST WAY TO TREAT SLEEP PROBLEMS?

The best treatments for all children's sleep problems are to:

- Prevent them in the first place
- Treat the underlying problem if there is one
- Reassure yourself and your child that good sleep is attainable
- Use proper sleep habits, such as bedtime routines

Lifestyle therapies are the best bet. Let's tour the Therapeutic Mountain to make sure we cover all the bases. If you want to skip to my bottom-line recommendations, flip to the end of the chapter.

## BIOCHEMICAL THERAPIES: MEDICATIONS, HERBS, NUTRITIONAL SUPPLEMENTS

I do not recommend biochemical therapies for children who simply don't want to go to bed when their parents want them to sleep. Nor are they appropriate therapy for infants who still waken in the middle of the night to nurse or feed. The only time I recommend such therapies is for children who have undergone a significant life change or disruption in their sleep-wake cycle, such as those who have been in a natural disaster, witnessed a death, traveled across three or more time zones, or are hospitalized. Even under these circumstances, biochemical remedies should supplement, not replace, parental reassurance and lifestyle therapies. Do not use any medication, herbal remedy, or nutritional supplement daily for more than five days without consulting your health care professional. Tolerance to sleeping medications begins to develop within a week, and higher doses may be needed to achieve the same effect.

## Medications

The medication most commonly recommended for children suffering from temporary sleep disruption is diphenhydramine (Benadryl). Benadryl is an inexpensive *antihistamine* whose main side effect is drowsiness and may help your child sleep after a long flight across several time zones. Benadryl is very safe when taken as recommended. However, some who take Benadryl become more aroused and excitable. It's impossible to predict in advance if your child is will react this way. Benadryl given thirty minutes before bedtime to children with troubled sleep significantly reduces the time it takes to fall asleep and decreases episodes of awakening in the middle of the night, but some children who take it feel drowsy and "out of it" the next day. These hangover effects typically disappear within a few days of regular use—not a habit I'd encourage.

## MEDICATIONS USED FOR CHILDREN'S SLEEP

- *Antihistamines:* diphenhydramine (Benadryl), hydroxyzine (Vistaril), trimeprazine (Temaril)
- *Benzodiazepines:* diazepam (Valium), lorazepam (Ativan), alprazolam (Xanax)
- *Sedatives/barbiturates:* phenobarbital, secobarbital, chloral hydrate, and others

Hydroxyzine (Vistaril) is a prescription antihistamine similar to Benadryl. It is frequently used to help hospitalized patients fall asleep. Another prescription antihistamine, trimeprazine (Temaril), was studied in three-year-old children with sleep problems. The usual doses were not very helpful, but higher doses (three times the normal antihistamine dose) knocked the toddlers out and kept them out throughout the night. The medication is not a long-term cure, but it has few side effects. Most physicians prefer behavioral (lifestyle) changes rather than relying on antihistamines for typical toddler sleep problems.

Stronger sleeping medications are available with a prescription from your health care professional. I do *not* recommend sleeping pills for children unless you have tried safe home remedies without success and you have your child thoroughly evaluated by a professional. Many sleeping pills make children feel groggy or hungover the next day. Some can lead to addiction. A few can be fatal if an overdose is taken.

The most commonly prescribed sleep medications for adults are *benzodiazepines* such as Valium, Ativan, and Xanax and *sedatives* such as phenobarbital and secobarbital. The benzodiazepines help reset the biological clock for those suffering from jet lag. Benzodiazepines also suppress deep sleep, the time when sleep terrors are most likely to occur. Valium and imipramine have been useful in treating children suffering from sleep terrors. I do not routinely recommend them because of the risk of serious side effects, because safe alternatives (such as hypnosis) are available, and because most children outgrow night terrors without any treatment.

## Herbs

Traditional folk medicine has long relied on herbs as sleep aids. Most, such as *chamomile*, are given as tea; some, such as *valerian*, are taken in the form of tablets and capsules. Still others, such as *lavender,* may be included in bathwater, massage oil, or as a few drops of essential oil on a favorite pillow or blanket. In Europe, a small fancy pillow known as a "sleep pillow" is tucked under a sleepless child's regular pillow. A sleep pillow filled with a combination of dried sedative herbs makes a lovely, aromatic gift.

### HERBS TRADITIONALLY USED
### FOR INSOMNIA

- Chamomile
- Balm mint (also known as lemon balm) and catnip
- Hops
- Kava kava
- Lavender
- Passionflower, skullcap, and valerian
- St. John's wort

*Chamomile* flowers are among the safest and most widely used herbal remedies for children. I often recommend chamomile tea as a nighttime sleep aid. Chamomile is calming and soothing (and was given to Peter Rabbit fol-

lowing a harrowing escapade in Mr. MacGregor's garden). It is said to help prevent nightmares. Chamomile is widely available in commercial herbal teas in your local grocery store. It has a pleasant aroma and taste. It is easily grown in the garden and often can be found growing wild along roadsides.

*Balm*, also known as *lemon balm* because of its refreshing fragrance, is included in herbal tea blends used to treat insomnia, anxiety, and "nerves." It is also commonly used to calm an upset stomach. Balm is often cultivated in household gardens because it attracts bees. Balm leaves are also tasty additions to summer salads. *Catnip* is from the same family of plants. Not only is it attractive to cats, it is also said to be soothing and sedating, allaying anxiety and preventing nightmares.

*Hops* are proven sedatives that have been traditional herbal remedies as least as far back as Roman times. They are genetically related to the *Cannabis* (marijuana) family of plants. Hops are traditional ingredients in European "sleep pillows," having been used by King George III to cure his insomnia. Tea made from hops can also be added to bathwater for a relaxing soak. Hops are best used soon after they are picked. Within a year after drying, they lose 90% of their effectiveness.

*Kava kava* is a traditional beverage in the Pacific Islands, where it has been used historically on social occasions to induce a carefree state of conviviality and lack of anxiety. It has become more popular in the United States as an anti-anxiety herb and to help adults with a lot on their minds to relax and fall asleep. There are no studies evaluating it in children, and there is some potential for misuse by teens who may make the mistake of driving while under the influence of kava (yes, it can impair driving performance).

*Lavender* flowers are often included in bedtime herbal tea blends. A few drops of essential oil of lavender can also be added to the child's evening bath or to a massage oil to help him relax. Lavender has a pleasant, soothing scent. *Passionflower* is a common herbal sleep remedy that is included in several herbal tea blends. Its name is not derived from its use as an aphrodisiac, but from the flower's imagined resemblance to the crucifixion scene (the passion of Christ). There are no studies evaluating its safety or effectiveness in children.

Despite its creepy name, *skullcap* is a common ingredient in herbal bedtime teas. It is a traditional sedative that was initially used to treat rabies! A potential problem with skullcap is liver toxicity. I do not recommend it, although you often find it in commercially available teas marketed to improve sleep.

The name *valerian* comes from the Latin, *valere*, to be strong or well. Valerian root was used as a sedative in ancient Greece, Rome, China, and Persia and was also used by American Indians. Valerian decreases the length of time it takes to fall asleep and improves the quality of sleep without leaving that drowsy morning-after feeling that is common with many sleep medications.[18] In adults suffering from insomnia, it improves the quality of sleep and reduces nighttime awakening as effectively as several prescription sleep medicines.[19] Because it improves nighttime sleep, it may reduce daytime drowsiness.[20] One drawback of valerian is its unpleasant scent, which can be described as musky, stale, sweaty gym socks. Phew! A more serious drawback is valerian's toxic effect on the liver.[21] There is substantial variation in the amount of the sedative compounds in different varieties and preparations of valerian.[22] However, I have used valerian myself when I've had to deal with jet lag, and I've recommended it to adolescents having trouble falling asleep in the hospital. The combination of valerian and lemon balm is widely used in Europe where herbal products are more commonly used and better regulated.

The leaves and flowers of *St. John's wort*

have been used since ancient Greece, and they remain one of the most commonly recommended herbal remedies for a variety of sleep disturbances, including nightmares. St. John's wort is also believed to balance the central nervous system in cases of depression and is an excellent choice for children whose sleep is disturbed due to a recent loss, such as the death of a grandparent or pet. One potential side effect of St. John's wort is photosensitivity; that is, when a child takes tea made from this plant, his skin may become extra sensitive and he may be easily sunburned. Another problem is that St. John's wort may cause the body to metabolize other drugs more quickly so they are less likely to benefit the child. If your child takes any other medication, be sure to talk with your doctor before starting St. John's wort.

*Combinations* of the above herbs are widely available in commercial teas such as Nighty Night, Sleepy Time, Surrender to Sleep, Tension Tamer, Calming Tea, and others. This is certainly a convenient way to go because the herbs have been selected, combined, and are available in easy-to-use teabags. No matter what blend you choose, *avoid herbal teas before bed if your child is prone to bed-wetting!* Also, *avoid stimulating herbs:* coffee, tea (with caffeine), cocoa, chocolate, cola, ephedra *(Ma Huang)*, guarana, ginseng, and mate! They can all keep your child awake long after he should be finished counting sheep.

*Warning:* Herbal products are not regulated by the federal government with the same degree of safety considerations as drugs are. Herbal products may not contain any of the active ingredients we associate with the herb on the label; or herbal products may be contaminated with heavy metals (such as lead, cadmium, and mercury), pesticides, herbicides, etc.; or they may be "spiked" with drugs. So, herbs may cause some toxicity themselves, and commercially marketed products may present additional hazards. The most commonly reported problems involve liver damage; if your child develops diarrhea, dark urine, or pale stools while taking an herbal remedy, stop the herbs and see your doctor immediately.

## Nutritional Supplements

The amino acid *L-tryptophan* is an effective sleep promoter in both adults and children.[23] It was one of the most popular supplements sold until it was banned in 1989 due to its reported association with the deadly disease eosinophilia myalgia syndrome, EMS. Before it was banned, L-tryptophan was linked to over 5,000 cases of EMS, including twenty-seven deaths. Because all of the EMS cases could be traced to the L-tryptophan from a single manufacturer, a search was made for possible contaminants. It turns out that the problem was probably not due to L-tryptophan, but to a contaminant introduced in the manufacturing process. Nevertheless, since the EMS outbreak, L-tryptophan supplements are no longer available in the United States.

L-tryptophan is a precursor to the brain chemical serotonin, which plays an important role in regulating sleep and minimizing depression. L-tryptophan effectively reduces the time it takes for adults to fall asleep. In a controlled study, supplemental L-tryptophan also helped infants fall asleep faster.[24] Breast milk contains substantially more L-tryptophan than formula. Cow's milk contains minute amounts of L-tryptophan as well as other compounds believed to promote sleep. Rather than taking supplements, I recommend that you breast-feed or give your child a glass of milk thirty to sixty minutes before bedtime. Be sure your child brushes his teeth after the milk to reduce the risk of cavities!

Calcium and magnesium supplements are frequently recommended to adult sufferers of insomnia. However, there are no scientific studies evaluating the usefulness of such supplements in children. Children generally get all the calcium they need from milk. If your child does not nurse or drink milk, make sure he gets plenty of calcium from other foods such as yogurt, tofu, fish, and calcium-supplemented soy milk, rice milk, or orange juice.

Vitamin B12 supplements have been reported to be useful in a few adults and teenagers suffering from sleep problems, but vitamin supplements have not been compared with other therapies as sleep aids for children.[25] I do not recommend them.

Melatonin is a hormone produced by the pineal gland, deep in the brain. People with insomnia generally produce less melatonin than those who sleep well.[26] Melatonin supplements have become a popular over-the-counter sleep remedy, used especially by adults who have to work the night shift and by airline personnel who have to combat jet lag. Several studies have shown that it can improve sleep for children with attention deficit hyperactivity disorder or insomnia using doses of 2 to 5 milligrams before bed. However, I don't think it's wise for most children to try melatonin until more research has been done. For one thing, I'm always leery about giving people extra hormones when they haven't been proved to have a deficiency. There's also data suggesting that melatonin supplements may increase the frequency of seizures in some kids who already have a seizure problem.

## LIFESTYLE THERAPIES: NUTRITION, EXERCISE, ENVIRONMENT, MIND-BODY

The primary treatment for childhood sleep problems is creating a healthy lifestyle. Paying attention to your child's diet, exercise patterns, and sleep environment are key to improving sleeping patterns.

## Nutrition

### FOODS TO HELP WITH SLEEP

*Yes:* Milk and high-protein foods
*No:* Rice cereal
*Yes:* Sweets, followed by brushing teeth

Formula-fed babies generally fall asleep faster and sleep longer between feedings than breast-fed babies. This is because the fat in formula takes longer to digest and longer to empty from the stomach than the fat in human milk. Mother's milk completely empties from the stomach within two hours, while formula may take three to four hours to make the same transition. This means that nursing babies' stomachs empty sooner, and they are hungry sooner than formula-fed babies. Children who breast-feed through the second year of life may awaken in the middle of the night to nurse, especially if they sleep with their parents; this is not a problem for the child unless it is a problem for you. It is the norm in many parts of the world. You need to decide if this is what you want for your family.

*Protein-rich foods* contain a rich mixture of amino acids, including tryptophan. Tryptophan is an important precursor to hormones that affect sleep and mood. Dieters who cut back on protein may find themselves having trouble sleeping at night or focusing during the day. A wide body of research (and my grandmother) suggests that eating a protein-rich meal late in the day helps you sleep better at night. While no one has specifically evaluated the impact of turkey sandwiches on sleep latency in teenagers, I often recommend such a late-night snack for kids who have trouble falling asleep.

*Hot beverages* are traditionally used before bedtime to induce a state of relaxed drowsiness in older children and adults. You might try a cup of warm (caffeine-free) herbal tea or a glass of *warm milk*. There are many other compounds as well as L-tryptophan in milk that may contribute to sleepiness. Unless your child is allergic to milk or has problems with bed-wetting, it's worth a try.

Despite common myths to the contrary, adding *rice cereal* to your babies' evening bottle does not help him sleep better through the night. A randomized, controlled trial done at the Cleveland Clinic clearly demonstrated that adding rice cereal to the evening feeding did not improve infants' sleep.[27] A similar study done at Johns Hopkins had identical results.[28] It turns out that many parents become frustrated with night wakenings and add cereal just about the time the baby is learning to sleep through the night on his own anyway. The cereal erroneously receives the credit for the baby's accomplishment in learning to fall asleep and stay asleep.

*Sweets* have long been known to induce a pleasant torpor and are often called "comfort foods." Honey is a traditional ingredient in home sleep remedies. Try adding a teaspoon of honey to a cup of hot tea before bed or give your child a cup of hot cocoa. To avoid the risk of botulism, do *not* give honey to infants under a year of age. If you give your child something sweet to help him sleep, do so *before* he brushes his teeth!

*Do not put your child to bed with a bottle* in his mouth. Falling asleep with a bottle of milk or juice will rot your baby's teeth. Decay can start as soon as the teeth begin to emerge (usually between five and seven months of age). If your child is already in the habit of going to bed with a bottle and can't seem to fall asleep without one, here's a trick that will eliminate that habit within a week. The first night, dilute the milk or juice (whatever the child has been taking to bed) with ⅛ water. The next night, go to ¼ water; the third night, half water; the fourth night, ¾ water. The fifth night, nothing but water in the bottle. Most children don't like the taste of water as much as whatever they were drinking before. Some may protest at the watering down, but many will not even be aware of the gradual change. By the time you've reached pure water, most children willingly release the bottle altogether. If not, you can at least be assured that the water will not harm your child's teeth.

## Exercise

Many physicians (and grandmothers) recommend that vigorous exercise be avoided in the hour just before bedtime. Regular daytime exercise can certainly contribute to sound sleep, but avoid running, dancing, spinning, and other frenetic exercises in the hour before bed.[29] Elite athletes may get away with a good night's sleep after an evening run, but don't bet on it for your youngster.[30] Better bets are reading stories, listening to quiet music, and taking a hot bath.

## Environment

Bed and bedtime should be as pleasant as possible. Do not send your child to bed during the day as a punishment. Associating bedtime with punishment will only make him want to avoid it.

### SLEEPING ENVIRONMENT

- Light (dark), sound (quiet), temperature (cool)
- With parents vs. alone
- Hot bath before bed
- Music: Bach vs. Barney
- Favorite stuffed animal, blanket, pacifier
- Sleep position (face up vs. face down)

Emphasize the day-night differences in the environment. Pay attention to light, sounds, and temperature. Most children sleep better in a *cool* environment. *Quiet* and *dark* are conducive to sleep, but are not essential. Many children feel more comfortable with a night-light or having their bedroom door open so they feel safe.

*Should a baby sleep with his parents or not?* This question must be answered by parents according their own values and beliefs.[31]

### CO-SLEEPING BENEFITS

- Lower risk of Sudden Infant Death Syndrome (SIDS)
- Cultural norm
- Easier breast-feeding

The risk of Sudden Infant Death Syndrome (SIDS) is actually lower in the those cultures in which infants routinely sleep with their parents for the first year of life. Co-sleeping results in lighter sleep from which it is easier to awaken; while this may hamper parental sleep, it may protect the baby from SIDS.[32] Parents rarely roll over on their babies and crush them or smother them unless the parent is very drunk or takes a strong sedative drug or they are sleeping right next to a wall or with too many blankets. In many cultures it is unthinkable for a baby *not* to sleep with his parents; in those cultures in which co-sleeping is the norm, it does not seem to be associated with any increased risk of behavioral problems.[33] Most nursing mothers find it convenient to have the baby in bed with them so when the child awakens to feed there is no need to get up. I'm strongly in favor of co-sleeping. On the other hand, there are some drawbacks.

One of the drawbacks of letting the baby sleep with you is that the baby learns to fall asleep only with you present, and doesn't learn to fall asleep by himself; later on when you want the privacy of your own bed back it is harder to get the baby to fall asleep by him-

## CO-SLEEPING DRAWBACKS

- Baby learns to depend on parental presence to fall asleep
- Parents awaken when baby awakens
- More sleep problems reported by parents
- Challenges to parental intimacy

self in his own bed. Some parents are light sleepers who awaken every time the baby moves or awakens. For these parents, it may be preferable to have the baby in a crib nearby for the first few months when the baby requires a nighttime feed, and then move the baby's crib to another room when a night feeding is no longer needed. *Parents must be attuned to and honor their own needs as well as the baby's needs.* Parents who are exhausted and irritable from insufficient sleep are prone to making poorer parenting decisions than parents who are well rested.

Flexibility is important when the toddler or infant is acutely ill. Children with chronic conditions such as asthma don't necessarily have more sleep problems than other children. However, children with acute illnesses such as colds, sore throats, and ear infections often feel more comfortable with a parent nearby. Many parents choose to allow the child back in bed with them for a few nights. Children often want to continue this pattern after the illness has resolved. In these cases, the parents need to help the child reestablish a bedtime routine for falling asleep in their own beds and staying there. Some parents bring a large mattress into the child's room when the child is ill so the parents can sleep on the floor near the child without having the child come into the parents' room.

A *hot bath* before bed is a time-honored way of relaxing for sleep. Again, make sure the bath time is relatively quiet and calm. Too much excitement can rev up a child just when you want him drowsy.

*Music* is a key component of many families' bedtime routine. Some families start with soothing classical music or lullabies when the child is still an infant. Keeping to a routine of the same music every night helps the child use it as a stimulus to sleep. One of the advantages of using the same taped music is that it can be brought along in the car or on trips so that at least that aspect of the bedtime routine can be maintained no matter where the family is. *What music works best?* Common sense says that if the music is calming for parents, it will contribute to a calm, relaxing atmosphere for the child. One of my physician colleagues swears that Gregorian chants have miraculous sleep-inducing effects on her infant daughter. Other children prefer Bach and some like Barney. You'll have to experiment to find out what works best for your family.

Many children grow attached to *certain objects* such as a favorite blanket, stuffed animal, pacifier or pillow. In a survey of toddlers' parents in a Cleveland area clinic, over half reported that their child needed a transitional object (blanket, pacifier, toy, thumb-sucking) to help them fall asleep. Having this object along can help ease the way to sleep when the family is in the car, at the grandparents', or otherwise outside of the usual sleep environment.

Sudden Infant Death Syndrome (SIDS) is the sudden, unexpected death during sleep of a baby, usually between one and five months old. It is the second leading cause of death among infants. The number of SIDS deaths could be cut in half if all babies were put to sleep on their backs (supine) rather than on their tummies (prone). *Lay your baby down to sleep on his back, not facedown.* SIDS deaths have declined dramatically since widespread publicity has changed sleep habits from tummy sleeping to back or side sleeping.[34] The

American Academy of Pediatrics, the National Institute of Child Health and Human Development, the Indian Health Service, the Consumer Product Safety Commission, and the Bureau of Maternal and Child Health all recommend that you put your baby to sleep on his back or side to reduce the risk of SIDS. This is one time you should pay attention to medical authorities; rarely are we in such strong agreement![35]

### TO REDUCE THE RISK OF SUDDEN DEATH DURING SLEEP, DO *NOT*:

- Put your infant to sleep on his stomach
- Smoke cigarettes or use heroin, crack, or cocaine
- Overheat or overbundle your baby
- Put your infant to sleep on a sheepskin, water bed, or a natural fiber mattress

Parental *smoking* and *drug use* markedly increase the risk of SIDS. Several studies have shown an increased risk of SIDS among babies who are *overbundled* or who sleep in *overly warm* rooms.[36] Although *sheepskin* and *lambskin* are soft and cuddly, they may increase your child's risk of suffocation. Studies also show an increased risk of SIDS among infants who sleep on *natural fiber mattresses*. *Waterbeds* may also be problematic. Unlike firmer foam bedding, natural fibers and water beds tend to conform to the baby, making it difficult for the baby to turn his head away from possible suffocation if he lies on his tummy with his nose facing into the mattress.

## Mind-Body

The most important thing you can do to help your child learn to fall asleep at night is to establish a bedtime routine or ritual. The routine should suit your needs as a parent and be consistent with your family beliefs.

### COMMON ELEMENTS OF A BEDTIME ROUTINE

- Same bedtime every night
- Going through the same routine of bathing, brushing teeth, toileting, putting on pajamas, stories, songs, lights out, shades drawn every night
- Wearing special clothes (pajamas) to bed; bed clothes should not be the same as day clothes; warm the sleep clothes (but not daytime clothes) on the radiator or the dryer so they are warm and snugly
- Special bedtime stories or prayers
- Special bedtime lullabies or other music
- Bedtime massage—back rubs, stroking the forehead, foot rubs, etc.
- Favorite blanket, stuffed animal, pacifier, or pillow in bed
- Same words for good night
- A hug and "I love you" from parents

By establishing the *same bedtime* and *same routine* every day, you help your child establish a regular sleep-wake cycle. Our innate circadian rhythms are actually slightly longer than twenty-four hours, so it is natural for all of us to stay up a bit later each night and wake a bit later each morning. If you allow your child to stay up later on weekends and sleep in the next morning, you may have a real struggle on Mondays when you try to revert to the old schedule and your child's body wants to continue the later pattern. The same thing can happen during vacations.

Children who go to sleep early tend to awaken early, and those who stay up later tend to sleep later. You may need to adjust your child's bedtime to reflect your family's needs. If you are a night owl and like to sleep late in the morning, you may want to establish a late bedtime for your child. On the other hand, if you have to be up early for work, you may want your child asleep earlier. Children who have long afternoon naps are less sleepy for early bedtimes than those whose afternoon naps are cut shorter. Adjust bedtimes and nap times to find the schedule that works best for you. Try to follow the same pattern at least three days in a row. If you switch sleep patterns every day, your child will just be confused and irritable.

It is very important to *put the child down to sleep while he or she is still awake*. Studies using all-night time-lapse photography show that children as young as three weeks old who are put to bed while they are still awake can learn to put themselves to sleep. In fact, infants who learn to put themselves to sleep in their crib learn to fall asleep more easily on their own when they waken in the middle of the night.

If you allow the child to fall asleep in your arms, he will learn that he can *only* fall asleep in your arms. He will then fuss and cry until you come pick him up and he will not fall asleep until you are holding him. Babies are often drowsiest right after a meal. Try putting your infant down as soon as you've finished the last nursing of the evening. Falling asleep is a skill and a habit. Teach your child early on that he or she can fall asleep on his own and you will save yourself many later struggles.

Try to put your child to sleep in the *same place* every night. If you are out visiting friends or family for the evening when your child's bedtime comes, try to put your child to sleep using as many of the same routines as possible—pajamas, story, song, favorite blanket, or stuffed animal, etc.

## WHAT TO DO WHEN YOUR BABY WAKES UP IN THE MIDDLE OF THE NIGHT

- Check the baby: Does he need to be fed? Does the diaper need changing? Is he in pain (e.g., an open diaper pin, a hair wrapped around a finger or toe, ill)?
- Attend to his needs for nourishment, hygiene, or pain relief
- Reassure him that you love him and are nearby with a few brief words, a pat on the tummy, stroking his head or patting his hand
- When you finish, leave the room
- If he keeps crying, recheck him in 5 minutes; repeat the above, then leave the room
- If the baby keeps crying, recheck him in 10 minutes; repeat the above, then leave the room
- If the baby keeps crying, recheck him in 15 minutes; repeat the above, then leave the room, etc.
- Reward your self for hanging in there and teaching your child a new skill!

Make your middle-of-the-night visits as *brief* and *boring* as possible so your baby isn't interested or stimulated by them. Make sure his basic needs are met. Reassure him by speaking a few loving words and patting him on the tummy or stroking his head. If you have a music tape that helps him fall asleep, turn it on. Make sure he has his favorite blanket or toy nearby where he can see and touch it. Do not get your baby out of bed except to change diapers or feed him. Do not rock, cuddle, and walk your baby back to sleep or he will grow dependent on your ministrations. If you teach him to need this kind of attention in the middle of the night he will continue to demand it long after you want to go to sleep. If this is OK with you, offer him all the cuddling and entertainment you want.

If your baby is used to you getting up and playing with him or holding him and rocking him back to sleep and you stop doing those things, *he will probably cry* so you will do them again. This is the most difficult part for parents, and the part requiring the most self-control. If you want him to fall asleep on his own, leave the room even though he cries for you to return. It seems cruel to leave the baby alone and crying, but remind yourself of your long-term goal. If he's still crying after five minutes (he probably will be), go back and recheck him. It may help for you to set a small timer so you know when five minutes are up. Go through the same routine of checking and brief reassurance. Then leave. Next time wait ten minutes. Repeat this procedure, waiting an extra five minutes each time before going back to recheck, so that the intervals between rechecking lengthen to 15 minutes, then 20 minutes, then 25 minutes, etc. You don't need to recheck him if he's not crying. This technique is called "Ferberizing" in honor of Dr. Richard Ferber, the Boston pediatrician who developed it. Ferberizing has been successfully used by thousands of American parents.

The first few nights this process may take longer than it would have taken simply to go in, pick him up and rock him or cuddle him until he falls back asleep. That's OK. Within a week, there will be much less protest, and fewer night wakenings because your child will have learned to put himself back to sleep. Even after your child has learned this skill, things may briefly fall apart the next time he becomes ill. Children who are ill often have legitimate needs for their parents in the middle of the night, so feel free to go comfort your child as needed during illnesses. After your child has recovered, he may want to continue the habit of extra attention. Then you may be called upon to repeat this routine until he has

relearned to put himself back to sleep.

Acknowledge yourself for having the discipline to teach your child to put himself to sleep. This is one of the most difficult parenting tasks; many parents give in night after night rather than listen to their child cry. Give yourself some small reward for hanging in there for the first five minutes, then ten minutes, and so forth. Go ahead and brag to your friends, family, and colleagues. You've earned it!

Many parents just can't stand to hear their baby cry, even for five or ten minutes at a stretch. There is an alternative to help your infant learn to sleep through the night called *scheduled waking*.

## SCHEDULED WAKING

- Keep a diary of your child's night wakenings
- Note what time your child usually wakes up
- Set the timer for 10 minutes before your child usually wakes
- Awaken your child *before* he wakes himself
- Feed or soothe him
- Repeat for each of the usual night wakening times
- Every few days, reduce the number of times you waken your child

Scheduled wakenings may seem bizarre, but they work. It takes a bit longer than Ferberizing, but it generally works within six weeks.[37] It may be worth trying for parents who don't want to ignore their child's cries, but who do want to eliminate the nighttime wakenings. This strategy has also proven successful in reducing night terrors in children who tend to have them at the same time each night.[38]

Truthfully, I could neither Ferberize my child nor do scheduled wakenings. When he awoke and wanted me, I was there. I cuddled him; I rocked him; I nursed him; I sang to him. I got less sleep, but I didn't feel guilty, either. Managing your child's sleep is an individual choice every family must make (and live with!).

Interestingly, although my son awoke frequently in the night until he was two (and I soothed him back to sleep), once he started sleeping through the night, he rarely protested bedtime, did not get out of bed, and almost never reported nightmares or night terrors. Perhaps he knew deep down that being in bed was safe, and that comfort was available if necessary.

## WHAT TO DO IF YOUR TODDLER KEEPS GETTING OUT OF BED

- Follow bedtime ritual (be firm about good night)
- Explain consequences of getting out of bed
- Follow through with consequences

For parents of many toddlers, the most difficult part of getting them to bed is the seemingly endless requests for more water, another story, another back rub, etc. What starts out as a fifteen-minute routine turns into a nightly hour and a half battle. The parents wearily give in to each request, not wanting to be cruel and hoping that this is the last thing the child wants. Parents may warn the child, "This is the last . . . ," but give in to one more thing to avoid a tantrum or crying. This is a tough situation. Fortunately, it responds well to tough love. Tough love in this situation means setting limits, establishing clear consequences, and then sticking to them. It sounds easy, but it is challenging. If it was easy, you wouldn't be facing the problem now. Be firm, be consistent, and be willing to put up with (and ignore) some serious crying for the first few days.

First, establish a *bedtime routine* that all adults in the house can live with. Make sure all adults know what's going on and agree with the plan so the child can't play one against another. Decide in advance how long the routine will take. Plan ahead. If you want the real bedtime to be 9 P.M. and the routine involves a bath, brushing teeth, a story, and a prayer, you'll need to start the routine by 8:15. Warn the child at 8 P.M. that it's time to start wrapping up the evening's activities and get ready for bed. Go through the bedtime routine you have agreed on in advance. Praise your child for cooperating with each phase of the routine (bath, tooth-brushing, picking the bedtime story, lying quietly while the story is read, prayer, etc.). Positive reinforcement for following each part of the bedtime routine is very effective in getting children to cooperate with bedtime, reducing tantrums and staying in bed once lights are out.

Decide in advance what the *consequences* of getting out of bed will be. For most parents, the consequence is simply leading the child back to bed, having him get into bed, and repeating that it is now bedtime and the child is expected to remain in bed. The consequence must be immediate (not after five more minutes of TV or cuddling), loving, and firm. You may decide that the consequence for getting out of bed a second time is that the child's bedroom door is closed or the music is turned off. You can anticipate that the child will get out of bed to test these limits, and most likely he will cry. This is normal. Your child is not being bad; he is simply testing the rule to see if it's a real rule or not. It's up to you to make clear that it is a real rule and you will enforce it by an immediate return to bed. The consequence must be immediate to be effective. Telling a three-year-old that the consequence is no TV the following day is nearly meaningless; many adults can't remember a consequence for that long!

There are numerous studies showing that

this technique is effective. Most children get the idea within a week. Be prepared to be firm for five to seven days in a row and be prepared for a temporary escalation in whining, complaining, and crying. Don't try to start this rule/consequences routine when you are dealing with another major stressor or disruption in routines such as a new baby in the house or you will doom yourself to frustration and failure. By and large, the only times this technique does not work is when parents are unable to *follow through with enforcing the limits* they wanted to set.

There is an alternative for getting your toddler to bed. This is a sneakier way of introducing limits. Instead of forcing your child to go to bed at your preset time immediately, let him stay up as late as he wants. Go through your bedtime routine in a calm, relaxed fashion. The next night, start the routine 15 minutes earlier. Be sure to give your child 15 to 20 minutes of warning so that he can wrap up his activities and be ready for bedtime routines. Every few days, push the routine back 15 minutes earlier so that your child's biological clock is gradually reset to your desired bedtime. This technique takes a bit longer, but it may save you a few tantrums, and it does have proven effectiveness.[39]

### Nightmares and Night Terrors

*Do not talk about your child's fears or anxieties right before bed.* Talking about the monsters in the closet or anxieties about an upcoming test may temporarily comfort your child, but it may also keep the anxieties spinning in his mind as he tries to fall asleep. Instead, reassure your child that everything is all right and that you can talk about such issues in the morning. If you postpone talking about your child's concerns, make sure that you really do set aside time the following morning to discuss them. Alternatively, you can talk about them early in the evening, well before bedtime so that fears are resolved before the child gets in bed.

Being wakened by a terrified screaming child is a frightening event for most parents. First reassure yourself that the house is not on fire and there is no immediate emergency. *Remain calm* as you enter your child's room. Ask to hear about the scary dream. Listen and be sympathetic, letting your child know you hear him and understand his fears. While you listen, calmly stroke his back, forehead, or hand; then reassure him that you are there and he is loved. Many children are comforted by hearing that parents, too, have frightening dreams sometimes, but that everything is really OK. Reassure the child that you can talk more about the dream in the morning if he would like to discuss it further.

*Hypnosis* can help reduce the frequency of insomnia, nightmares, and night terrors.[40] The noted child hypnotherapist, Dr. G. Gail Gardner, describes a simple technique that parents can use to help children reduce the frequency of nightmares and improve self-esteem.[41] During the daytime when your child feels relaxed and comfortable, begin to discuss the nightmare. Have the child tell you the story of the bad dream from beginning to end. When he has finished, ask him to pretend that the nightmare is a scary story that you read together and that he can make up a new, happy ending. Have him start at the beginning of the dream again, and this time, when the scary part comes (e.g., big animals chase him), instead of feeling frightened and running, he can be brave (e.g., turn around and ask the animals why they chase him) or ask for help from a superhero or fairy godmother or see the situation transformed (the monsters turn into soft butterflies) and see how things turn out differently (e.g., the monster becomes his friend, he is a hero, or the butterflies fly away). When he has completed the story to his satisfaction, tell him that he can do the same thing with his dreams at night *while he is dreaming them*. It is true. Becoming involved with dreams and changing them at the time one is dreaming is called *lucid dreaming*. Children who learn to become involved in their dreams in this way develop a powerful sense of self-esteem. This technique of rewriting the nightmare is also known as *rehearsal*, and it has proven effective in adult sufferers of severe nightmares.[42]

Professional *hypnotherapy* has also been used to help children with night terrors. After getting the night terrors under control with medication, school-age children trained in self-hypnosis gradually learn to control their night wakening with hypnosis alone, eliminating the need for medication.[43]

Another therapy, *recording*, developed at the University of New Mexico, has proven effective in adults suffering from severe, recurrent nightmares.[44] In recording therapy, the child recalls the nightmare while he is relaxed and comfortable in a safe place. He then writes down the nightmare or draws it in great detail. Although this technique is very simple, it has proven very helpful.

Several of these techniques can be combined for children who suffer from severe nightmares. One ten-year-old boy who suffered from recurrent nightmares after a car ran into his house benefited from such a combined program: progressive relaxation, reminding himself that "it is only a dream," and reconstructing positive endings for his nightmares. Within weeks he was able to sleep through the night.[45]

## Insomnia

For insomnia in older children and teenagers, the problem is likely to be *anxiety* about upcoming events or *overstimulation* from activities or caffeine. Make sure the child uses his bed only for sleeping. Have him listen to music, talk on the phone, do his homework, and other activities somewhere else. Have him engage in relaxing activities such as reading or listening to quiet music for the hour before he goes to bed.

*Meditation* has proven helpful for adults suffering from insomnia.[46] So has hypnosis.[47] An easy technique is to use a tape recording that includes calming sounds and music as well as a monotone voice and a repetitive, relaxing message that emphasizes the child's ability to fall asleep and stay asleep. This kind of tape can be used either for problems falling asleep or for problems of waking up in the middle of the night and not being able to fall asleep again.

*Progressive relaxation* is an easy technique for most older children and teenagers to learn and it is remarkably effective in allowing a child to relax so he can fall asleep. With this technique, the child focuses on one part of the body at a time, starting with the feet. As he focuses on that part of the body, he intentionally tightens the muscles there as tight as he can, holds it for a few seconds, and then releases. Attention moves from the feet to the lower legs, upper legs, hips, belly, chest, lower back, upper back, hands, arms, neck, and head. By the time the child tightens and relaxes the facial muscles, the whole body is generally quite relaxed and ready to fall asleep.

Progressive relaxation and pleasant imagery have also proven useful in children who are afraid of the dark or who are reluctant to go to bed.[48] Confronting oneself with potentially scary thoughts (such as fear of the dark, monsters, or tests) while one is very relaxed gradually drains the fear from the scary thought. This technique is called *desensitization* when used by professional therapists. It effectively reduces fears of the dark and nightmares.[49]

*Biofeedback* training can help insomniacs learn to affect their brain wave activity. By giving patients information about their brain waves and muscle tension, biofeedback devices help patients progress from normal waking rhythms (beta activity), through light relaxation (alpha rhythm), into the deep theta and delta states normally achieved only with deep sleep or meditation. Even young children can learn to use biofeedback to improve their sleep.[50] Biofeedback is taught initially in an office or institution, but devices are available for home use so the child can continue to practice at home in his own bed.

## BIOMECHANICAL THERAPIES: MASSAGE, SURGERY

### Massage

Many parents and children enjoy a relaxing massage before falling asleep. In a study of adolescent psychiatric patients, a nightly back rub was more effective than watching relaxing videotapes in helping the children fall asleep. The positive effects of massage carried over into the day, helping the children manage their anxiety and depression and decreasing their levels of stress hormones.[51] Massage can be as simple as a back rub, stroking a child's forehead or gently rubbing his hands or feet. Elaborate rituals are unnecessary. Scented oils containing one or more of the essential oils described in the herbs section (e.g., lavender) may also help the child relax and feel drowsy. If you feel uncertain about the best way to massage your child, check out one of the many books or videos on massage from your local library, or schedule a visit with a local massage therapist who treats children, and ask her to show you effective strategies.

### Surgery

If your child suffers from *severe snoring* consider taking him to an ear/nose/throat (ENT) doctor for an evaluation for *sleep apnea*. Sleep apnea or severe breathing obstruction is a chronic condition that affects about 10% of children with severe snoring. In this condition the child's adenoids and tongue block airflow during sleep, resulting in loud snoring, long, frequent pauses in breathing, and increased work to breathe that results in poor growth, daytime sleepiness, and hyperactivity;[52] it can also lead to high blood pressure.[53] After removing the obstruction, the child's sleep returns to normal, resulting in improved wakefulness during the day and an improved appetite, growth and general disposition.[54]

## BIOENERGETIC THERAPIES: THERAPEUTIC TOUCH, PRAYER, HOMEOPATHY

### Therapeutic Touch

Therapeutic touch has proven benefits in helping patients relax, and in decreasing anxiety.[55] Case reports (anecdotes) in adults suggest that it helps patients fall asleep and rest easily.[56] A study in nursing home patients showed that Therapeutic Touch significantly improved sleep in elderly residents.[57] I regularly use Therapeutic Touch and Reiki to treat hospitalized children. Many fall asleep during the treatment. They all become very relaxed, and several older children have been able to stop using sleeping pills.

### Prayer

This chapter would not be complete without including my grandmother's favorite advice about falling asleep: *Count your blessings.* I know that the standard advice is to count sheep, and that counting sheep has worked for thousands of people. It is boring and therefore effective. However, counting your blessings, enumerating all the things for which you are grateful, has the added benefit of generating feelings of gratitude. This is one of the most potent anti-anxiety and antidepressant techniques I know. Since we know that anxiety is a major contributor to sleep problems, I think my grandmother was really on to something.

## Homeopathy

There are no scientific studies evaluating the effectiveness of homeopathic remedies as sleep aids in children. Traditional homeopathic remedies for sleep problems include: Arsenicum (nightmares or other symptoms worse after midnight), Belladonna (for sudden frights), *Calcarea carbonica* and *phosphorica,* Chamomile (for teething or irritable infants), *Coffea cruda* (treating sleeplessness with extremely dilute concentrations of coffee is another perfect example of the homeopathic principle of like cures like), Ignatia (for insomnia due to grief), *Kali phosphoricum* (for night terrors), Lycopodium, *Natrum muriaticum* (nightmares), *Nux vomica* (for insomnia due to overindulgence in caffeine or overstimulation), Passiflora (for insomnia due to an overactive mind in older children and teenagers), Pulsatilla, *Rhus toxicum* (for restless sleep), Silica, and Sulfur. I do not recommend homeopathic remedies, but they are certainly safe and most are inexpensive. If they've worked for you, keep using them.

# WHAT I RECOMMEND FOR SLEEP PROBLEMS

*Take your child to a health care professional if:*

- Your child's sleep does not improve with lifestyle changes or home remedies

- Your child's nightmares interfere with daytime activities or his ability to sleep by himself

- Your child has other symptoms and you are concerned that something more serious is going on (such as an ear infection, diabetes, a bladder infection)

- You think your child may need medication (long travel, severe stress)

- You think your child may need surgery (sleep apnea)

- You are becoming increasingly frustrated by your child's wakefulness

1. To help an infant learn to go to sleep:
- Feed thirty minutes before bed, do not put to bed while nursing
- Put him to sleep in the same place every night while still awake
- Create a consistent bedtime routine; put him to sleep on his back to minimize the risk of SIDS

2. To help decrease awakenings in the middle of the night:
- Check on your child to make sure he's not hungry or in pain
- Leave the room; if he still cries, recheck him at longer and longer intervals

3. For children who won't go to bed on time:
- Establish a brief, consistent bedtime routine
- Set firm limits, state consequences, and stick to them *or* let the child stay up as late as he wants, gradually move bedtime earlier by 15 minutes every few nights
- Do not let him watch more than ninety minutes of television daily; bedtime should not be delayed to watch "special" programs

4. For children with nightmares:
- Prevent nightmares by minimizing your child's exposure to scary or violent movies, television, and news before bedtime
- Reassure your child at the time he awakens
- Briefly listen to him if he wants to describe the nightmare; discuss the nightmare with him the next day; have him record the details of the nightmare by keeping a dream journal or drawing a picture of the scary dream; give him the opportunity to rewrite the nightmare with a different ending

5. For a child who has night terrors:
- Reassure yourself that your child is normal; most children outgrow them
- Do not try to waken your child or to soothe him unless he wakens; do stay in the room with him in case he wakes up and wants you

6. For school-age children or teenagers with insomnia:
- Encourage vigorous exercise during the day, not before bed
- Remove the television from the bedroom
- Try a warm bath before bed; relaxing music or activity before bed; using the bed only for sleep (not for homework, TV, telephone); counting blessings; practicing meditation; progressive muscle relaxation, or other relaxation technique
- Avoid caffeinated beverages and food; consider a glass of warm milk
- Discuss stresses during the day when coping skills are highest rather than the evening when coping skills ebb
- *Biochemical*—Consider a hot cup of chamomile tea with honey before bed
- *Biomechanical*—Consider a back rub before bedtime to help him relax
- *Bioenergetic*—Consider a Therapeutic Touch or Reiki treatment to help him relax; have him count his blessings

## RESOURCES

### Internet

American Sleep Apnea Association
http://www.sleepapnea.org/awake.html

American Academy of Sleep Medicine
http://www.aasmnet.org/

Longwood Herbal Task Force (information on sedative herbs)
http://www.mcp.edu/herbal/

National Institutes of Health: National Center on Sleep Disorders Research
http://rover.nhlbi.nih.gov/about/ncsdr/

National Sleep Foundation
http://www.sleepfoundation.org/about.html

Sleep Disorders Center
http://www.sleepscene.com/index.htm

### Books

Ferber, Richard. *Solve Your Child's Sleep Problems*. Simon and Schuster, 1986.

Huntley, Rebecca. *The Sleep Book for Tired Parents: A Practical Guide to Solving Children's Sleep Problems*. Parenting Press, 1991.

LaBerge, Stephen. *Lucid Dreaming*. Ballantine, 1985.

Wiseman, Anne Sayre. *Nightmare Help*. Ten Speed Press, 1989.

# 25
# SORE
# THROATS

Peter Phillips brought in his daughter, Angela, first thing one cold winter morning for a shot of penicillin. Six-year-old Angela had been ill for a day with a very sore throat, swollen, tender glands in her neck, and a fever. Her throat was so sore she couldn't even drink orange juice. Peter had been suffering from laryngitis himself; his voice was raspy and faint. He had heard there was a flesh-eating strain of Strep that could kill you, so he wanted Angela treated as rapidly as possible. He also didn't want to miss a day of work, so he wanted to take her directly from the office to school.

## WHAT CAUSES SORE THROATS?

Sore throats are the third most common cause for doctor visits in the United States. There are different kinds of sore throats and different causes for each kind. Viruses cause most of the problems, but overuse, irritants, bacterial infections, and a variety of other things can all make for a painful throat.

*It sounded as though Peter had laryngitis and Angela had tonsillitis or pharyngitis.*

*Pharyngitis* can be caused by viruses, bacteria, allergies, irritants, overuse, or emotions. In only a minority of cases—about 15 to 20 percent—does the bacteria, group A beta-hemolytic *Streptococcus* cause the pharyngitis; another 45% of cases are caused by viruses and the rest are a mixed bag.[1] *Tonsillitis* is usually caused by a viral or bacterial infection. Viruses, irritants, and overuse can also cause *laryngitis*.

| TYPE OF SORE THROAT | BODY PART AFFECTED | SYMPTOMS |
|---|---|---|
| Pharyngitis | Pharynx, back of throat | Pain, fever, redness, sometimes ulcers or red spots on palate or back of throat |
| Tonsillitis | Tonsils | Pain, fever; red, swollen tonsils, sometimes with pus or white spots |
| Laryngitis | Larynx, voice-box, lower throat, and upper windpipe | Hoarseness, whisper-voice, cough, sometimes pain; usually sound worse than they feel |

## CAUSES OF SORE THROATS

- *Viruses:* Epstein-Barr virus (infectious mononucleosis), adenovirus, cocksackievirus (hand-foot-mouth disease), herpes virus (cold sores), canker sores, others
- *Bacteria:* various kinds of Streptococcus, Staphylococcus, Mycoplasma, Diphtheria (rare in vaccinated people), and other bacteria
- *Allergies:* to dust, pollen, animals, pollutants
- *Irritants:* tobacco smoke, air pollution
- *Miscellaneous:* overuse, grief, anger, and other strong emotions

The most famous sore throat *virus* is the *Epstein-Barr virus* (EBV), the cause of infectious mononucleosis, or "mono." Teenagers with mono typically suffer from sore throats, swollen lymph glands, a swollen spleen (a giant waystation for lymph cells in the upper left side of the belly), and fatigue. Mono usually lasts for two weeks. Unfortunately, the fatigue can last weeks or even months, causing kids to miss major amounts of school. The sore throat can be so severe and the tonsils so swollen that it is hard to swallow anything. This makes it easy for mono sufferers to become dehydrated. Dehydration makes them feel worse and even less like drinking, a downward spiral of symptoms that is best avoided by drinking plenty of fluids throughout the illness. Mono is uncommon before school age. Despite its reputation, the "kissing disease" is rarely caught from affectionate family members kissing each other.

*It didn't sound as if anyone in the Phillips family was suffering from mono.*

Preschoolers' and summertime sore throats are usually caused by *adenovirus*. Adenovirus sore throats are often very painful and may be accompanied by conjunctivitis or pinkeye (see Chapter 11).

*Adenovirus was not a likely cause for either of the Phillips's symptoms.*

*Enteroviruses* causes about 10% of sore throats in children.[2] *Coxsackievirus* (hand-foot-mouth disease), *Type I Herpes virus* (cold sores), and *chancre sores* can all cause red spots or blisters in the mouth and throat. Coxsackievirus also causes tiny blisters or red spots on the palms of the hands and the soles of the feet. Children typically feel ill and complain of pain a day or two before the blisters appear and for several days afterward. *Herpes virus II* can cause sore throats in teenagers experimenting with oral sex. And the new scourge, *AIDS*, can also cause a sore throat and other flulike symptoms soon after infection occurs.

*Group A beta-hemolytic Streptococcal pneumoniae* bacteria *(Strep)* are responsible for only 5% of pharyngitis cases in adults, but up to one-third of sore throats in children, especially in the winter and early spring. True Strep throat is rare in children under three years old outside of crowded day care settings. Infections are spread from one person to another by mucus from the nose and mouth. Symptoms appear within a week after exposure. About 2 to 5 percent of children carry Strep bacteria without having any symptoms.[3] Strep carriers are *not* at risk of developing the most feared consequences of Strep infection—rheumatic fever and kidney disease—but they can infect others. Strep's symptoms typically last about three days, but can go on for a week. Strep infections are easily treated with antibiotics. Because antibiotics prevent Strep's serious consequences, they are important to diagnose and treat. Once a child has had a bout with rheumatic fever, it is strongly recommended that antibiotics be taken regularly to prevent recurrences.[4]

Other kinds of Strep *(Group C* and *Group G beta-hemolytic Streptococcus)* cause sore throats that look just like Group A Strep. Infections caused by these kinds of Strep also yield to antibiotics. Group C and Group G Strep do not lead to rheumatic fever or kidney disease.

*Mycoplasma pneumonia* bacteria cause sore throat and "walking pneumonia" in school-age children. The symptoms caused by *Mycoplasma* look just like those caused by Strep except that Mycoplasma also causes coughing, while Strep rarely does. A few other bacteria can also cause sore throat symptoms; these included gonorrhea, diphtheria, plague, syphilis, tularemia, and other nasty bugs.

*Allergies* (see Chapter 4) cause sore throats as well as itchy eyes and watery noses. The most common and easily avoided throat irritant is tobacco smoke. Ironically, in the 1950s menthol cigarettes were advertised as medically approved sore throat remedies. Now we know that nothing could be further from the truth. The menthol may be soothing, but the tobacco smoke makes things much worse. Children whose mothers smoke have more frequent and more severe sore throats. Other irritants include air pollution, fumes, smoke from woodstoves, dry air, mouth-breathing, and the nasal drainage that drips down the back of the throat from colds or allergies.

A sore throat due to *overuse* is a common affliction of cheerleaders, singers, and sports enthusiasts. Although adults may recognize that a "lump in the throat" is due to *grief, anxiety, anger, or other strong emotions*, children may not be able to interpret this feeling except to say they have a sore throat.

*Peter admitted that he smoked about a pack a day. His wife had quit smoking about a month earlier and was trying to get him to quit, but he said he just didn't have time, and there was no lung cancer in his family anyway. Peter also reported that since the furnace had been on this winter, the air in the house was very dry. They had a humidifier, but it was up in the attic, gathering dust. I advised him to stop smoking now and to get the humidifier up and running.*

Even experienced clinicians are accurate only about 50% of the time when they guess whether or not Strep is the culprit behind a sore throat based on symptoms and physical exam alone.[5]

## DIAGNOSIS

Most children who have other symptoms such as a runny nose or a cough do *not* have Strep or mono and do *not* need any diagnostic tests. Although many doctors have tried to develop scoring tests to predict which patients need antibiotics and which ones don't, none of these clinical scoring systems is as good as some simple lab tests.

## LABORATORY TESTS FOR SORE THROATS

- Infectious Mononucleosis—blood tests
- Strep throat—throat swab for rapid test and/or culture

Blood tests are useful for diagnosing *infectious mononucleosis*. The test doesn't become positive until the disease has been present at least four or five days. A negative test in the first day or two of illness could be wrong. Children who have mono can also have a Strep infection.

## HOW CAN YOU TELL A STREP THROAT FROM OTHER TYPES OF SORE THROATS?

| *Symptoms* | *Strep* | *Viruses* | *Irritants* | *Allergies* |
|---|---|---|---|---|
| Rapid onset of symptoms | √ | | | |
| Fever | √ | √ | | |
| Red throat | √ | √ | √ | √ |
| Pus or white patches on tonsils | √ | √ | | |
| Swollen glands in neck | √ | √ | | |
| Trouble swallowing | √ | √ | √ | √ |
| Headache | √ | | | √ |
| Nausea, vomiting | √ | | | |
| Bad breath | √ | | | |
| Red, sandpapery skin rash | √ | | | |
| Hoarse voice | | √ | √ | √ |
| Cough | | √ | √ | √ |
| Watery or red eyes | | √ | | √ |
| Runny nose | | √ | | √ |
| Fatigue | √ | √ | | √ |
| Under three years old | | √ | √ | √ |

The only way to be absolutely sure an infection is caused by Strep is with a laboratory test. This means your child will need a swab of the back of the throat. The swab is tested either with a rapid test that checks for signs of Strep (like a tracker following an animal's footprints) or a throat culture that checks for the presence of the bacteria themselves (like seeing the animal directly).

A rapid Strep test can be ready within minutes. If the test is positive (meaning Strep is present), you can start antibiotics the same day. The bad thing about rapid tests is that a negative result doesn't necessarily mean that your child doesn't have Strep. If a tracker doesn't see footprints, it doesn't mean there is no animal—just that the signs weren't visible. Rapid tests miss up to 10 to 30 percent of cases. If the rapid test is negative, many physicians perform a throat culture to make sure an infection isn't missed; others, who are more confident of their rapid strep tests, don't bother with the culture.[6]

On the other hand, some doctors just go ahead and get a throat culture and don't bother with rapid tests at all.[7] Throat cultures are the gold standard for diagnosing Strep throats. They are very reliable. But it takes at least twenty-four to forty-eight hours for the results to come back.

If you want to minimize your child's chances of being over-treated with antibiotics, insist that a throat culture be performed *before* filling a prescription for antibiotics. Do *not* treat your child with leftover antibiotics before getting a throat culture. You *can* treat your child's discomfort with analgesics or other home remedies.

I prefer to do a rapid test, and process the test while the patient is still in the office. If the test is positive, we start antibiotics that day. If the test is negative, we do a throat culture and wait for the results before starting antibiotics.

With this approach, most patients who need antibiotics get them right away. Those who don't need them avoid unnecessary antibiotics (allergic reactions, upset stomachs, medication costs). My only exceptions to this approach are children who:

- Have symptoms of scarlet fever as well as sore throat
- Have the classic symptoms of a Strep infection during a Strep outbreak
- Have had rheumatic fever

These children all get a throat culture to confirm the diagnosis *and* antibiotics even before the culture results are back because of their high risk of serious disease. Early treatment (within the first two days of symptoms) helps children feel better significantly faster than delaying treatment for a day or two while waiting for the cultures to come back.

*The rapid Strep test for Angela was positive, so no culture was needed. Peter's rapid test and his throat culture were negative for Strep.*

## WHY IS A STREP THROAT WORSE THAN ANY OTHER KIND OF SORE THROAT?

The two reasons Strep throat is more serious than other kinds of sore throat are: *rheumatic fever* and *glomerulonephritis* (kidney disease). Rheumatic fever follows strep infections about two to three weeks after the sore throat is gone. Just after World War II, before antibiotics were widely available, strep throat was followed by rheumatic fever in 2 to 3 percent of soldiers. Treatment with ten days of antibiotics reduces this risk tenfold. Treatment can be delayed as long as nine days after the first sore throat symptoms appear and still effectively prevent rheumatic fever.

Many people think rheumatic fever is a disease of the past, but outbreaks still occur. In the 1980s, outbreaks were reported in Ohio, Pennsylvania, Salt Lake City, San Diego, New York, and Nashville. Most of the recent outbreaks have been in suburban or rural middle-class neighborhoods, and the initial illnesses were so mild that many people had not even visited their doctors. It turns out that Strep bacteria come in different varieties—some of which cause very nasty infections and others of which are more benign—and these varieties shift and change in subtle patterns year to year, leading to differences in disease severity over time.[8]

One to three weeks after some strains of Strep infection, the immune reaction between the Strep bacteria and the child's antibodies (immune molecules) can settle in the kidneys, resulting in a serious kidney disease known as *post-Streptococcal glomerulonephritis*.

If not treated, the bacteria from a Strep throat sometimes spread, leading to ear infections, lymph node infections, and abscesses in the tonsils and throat. Strep bacteria can also cause serious, life-threatening infections such as shock, septicemia, and infections of the skin, connective tissues, and muscles. These complications, though well publicized, are extremely rare. Some strains of Strep are more aggressive than others. Some are also more contagious (easier to spread) than others. It is impossible to sort out all of these strains of Strep without special laboratory tests.

## WHAT'S THE BEST WAY TO TREAT A SORE THROAT?

The best treatment depends on what's causing the sore throat. Let's tour the Therapeutic Mountain to find out what works. If you want to skip to my bottom-line recommendations, flip to the end of the chapter.

## BIOCHEMICAL THERAPIES: MEDICATIONS, HERBS, NUTRITIONAL SUPPLEMENTS

### *Medications*

#### MEDICATIONS USED TO TREAT SORE THROAT SYMPTOMS

- Analgesics: acetaminophen, ibuprofen (nonprescription)
- Throat lozenges (nonprescription), antacid gargles (nonprescription)
- Antibiotics (prescription only): penicillin, erythromycin, others

Some medications just help you live with the uncomfortable symptoms while the body does the healing work. *Analgesics*, for example, soothe sore throat pain, but they don't wipe out viruses or bacteria. The most widely used analgesics are *acetaminophen* (Tylenol and other aspirin-free pain relievers) and *ibuprofen* (Advil or Motrin). Aspirin is not recommended because of its association with the sometimes fatal Reye's syndrome. Acetaminophen and ibuprofen are both effective pain remedies. Ibuprofen works a bit sooner and lasts a bit longer than acetaminophen and may be slightly more effective against pain.[9] That's what I take and that's what I give my son when he has pain.

Similarly, *throat lozenges* containing benzocaine (such as Cepastat) help numb sore throat pain, but they don't do anything to treat an underlying infection. Some children have had serious side effects from benzocaine. I do not recommend lozenges for children under four years old because of the risk that they will choke on them. Chloraseptic throat spray significantly reduces sore throat symptoms compared with a placebo. I use throat sprays when I have a severe sore throat, but young children who hate the taste and temporary stinging, may be difficult to convince that they're worth it.

*Antacids* (such as Maalox) coat and soothe not only the stomach lining but also the throat. For children with frequent mouth and throat irritation from cancer chemotherapy, canker sores, or fever blisters, I often recommend Magic Mouthwash—a combination of Tylenol, Maalox, and Benadryl. This is a soothing combination of safe ingredients that can be repeated several times daily. Ask your physician to help you calculate the right dose for your child.

*Antibiotic* treatment reduces Strep throat symptoms, consequences, and the chance that the sufferer will pass the illness on to someone else. Antibiotics are *not* useful for treating sore throats caused by viruses, allergies, irritants, overuse, or emotions.

### ANTIBIOTICS TO TREAT STREP THROAT (ALL REQUIRE A PRESCRIPTION)

- Penicillin, amoxicillin (Amoxil)
- Erythromycin, azithromycin (Zithromax), clarithromycin (Biaxin)
- Combinations: amoxicillin-clavulanic acid (Augmentin) and erythromycin-sulfisoxazole (Pediazole)
- Cephalosporins: cefadroxil (Duricef), cefaclor (Ceclor), cefuroxime (Ceftin), cephalexin (Keflex), cefpodoxime (Vantin), and others
- Clindamycin (Cleocin)

Our good old friend *penicillin* (which is actually derived from the *Penicillium* mold—does that make it a natural remedy?) remains the official treatment of choice for children with true Strep throats. Penicillin decreases the length of symptoms by about a day. More important, it dramatically reduces the subsequent risk of developing rheumatic fever. Penicillin can be given as an injection, pills, or syrups. If taken by mouth, it must be given at least twice daily for at least ten days to eradicate Strep bacteria.[10] Most parents quit giving medication by the sixth day because the child is better and the need for medication seems less pressing, but penicillin is markedly less effective when taken less than ten full days. It also requires refrigeration, which is a drawback for families who are about to go on camping trips. For maximal absorption and effectiveness, penicillin should *not* be given within an hour before or two hours after mealtime—pretty inconvenient for today's busy families. I give parents the choice of whether they want their child to receive an injection or oral medication. As much as most people hate needles, I'm surprised how often families choose to "take the shot and get it over with."

*Amoxicillin* is a derivative of penicillin that is also inexpensive and effective. It tastes better than penicillin, and it can be given as little as once a day and still work.[11] Like penicillin, it requires refrigeration. If amoxicillin is given to patients with mononucleosis (mono), they break out in a rash. This is one of the reasons physicians don't just give antibiotics to everyone who has a sore throat.

For children who are allergic to penicillin, the antibiotic of choice has been *erythromycin*. However, more and more strains of Strep have become resistant to erythromycin. It has to be given three or four times daily, and it often causes an upset stomach. About a third of patients stop taking it because of side effects. New antibiotic relatives of erythromycin, *azithromycin* (Zithromax) and *clarithromycin* (Biaxin), are more effective treatments for Strep throat. Azithromycin is even effective with only five days of treatment. Both of these new antibiotics cost more ($30 to $50) than penicillin (about $5 to $10) or erythromycin (about $15).

The *combination antibiotics* and the *cephalosporins* (such as Duricef and Vantin) are more effective and more expensive than penicillin, amoxicillin, or erythromycin. Some are more convenient because they only require dosing once or twice a day and they do not require refrigeration. Cefpodixime (Vantin) taken twice daily for five days or cefuroxime (Ceftin) taken twice daily for four days are as effective as penicillin taken three times daily for ten days. Most combination medications or cephalosporins cost three to four times as much as penicillin or erythromycin. They can also cause upset stomach and diarrhea and wipe out the "good" bacteria in the bowels, leading to yeast infections.

*Clindamycin* is a powerful antibiotic that effectively eradicates Strep. Based on Swedish studies, it is my choice for Strep throats that are resistant to penicillin and cephalosporins. Clindamycin also does an excellent job of clearing Strep from carriers who keep reinfecting family members. Unfortunately, it also kills many of the "good" bacteria in the bowels, leading to diarrhea. If clindamycin is recommended for your child, be sure to stock up on extra yogurt and supplemental *Lactobacillus* to replace the healthy bacteria in the intestines that have been wiped out by antibiotics.

*Trimethoprim-sulfamethoxazole* (Bactrim or Septra), *tetracycline*, and *sulfa* drugs are *not* effective in eradicating Strep from the throat. They are *not* recommended for Strep throat, though they can be very helpful in other infectious illnesses.

It doesn't hurt to wait a day or two to start antibiotics, but the sooner treatment starts, the sooner the child will feel better. Delaying treatment for twenty-four to forty-eight hours may allow the body to build up its own antibodies (immune defenses against this and future attacks) and prevent subsequent infections.[12] One study found that children who were treated immediately had an eight times higher risk of developing another Strep infection within the next four months than children whose treatment was delayed for two days.[13] Other studies have found *no* difference in recurrence risks between those treated immediately and those whose treatment is delayed by forty-eight hours.[14] I do *not* withhold antibiotic therapy from a child who is sick with a Strep throat. I also don't rush to treat a child who has a sore throat before appropriate laboratory tests have established a diagnosis.

Pretty much whenever I recommend antibiotics, I also recommend that the child gets extra helpings of yogurt or kefir containing active cultures; also, there are a number of products containing the healthy bacteria (*Lactobacillus* and *Bifidobacterium*) that normally live in the intestines. Providing these supplements helps reduce the diarrhea that often accompanies administration of potent antibiotics. They are safe and they're natural. There's even a name for this class of bacteria: PRO-biotics. A good balance for "anti-biotics."

*After weighing all the options (and at Peter's urging), Angela reluctantly agreed that the best choice for her was a shot of penicillin. This way they didn't need to remember all the doses of medicine for the next ten days. They also decided to stop at the grocery store on the way home to stock up on Stonyfield Farms organic yogurt.*

### When can your child return to school or day care?

Children are no longer contagious to others when they have completed twenty-four hours of antibiotic therapy. Even children who have received an injection should wait twenty-four hours before returning to school or day care to make sure the medicine has had a chance to begin eradicating the Strep bacteria and reducing the risk of spreading the infection.

No antibiotic is 100% effective.

## REASONS FOR ANTIBIOTIC FAILURE

- Failure to take medication
- Reinfection from other family members or peers
- Not a bacterial infection
- Resistant bacteria, requiring different antibiotic
- Weak immune system

The main reason antibiotics fail is that people fail to take them often enough and long enough. Even if the child takes all of her doses, if someone else in the family is infected and not treated, that person can reinfect the child. Infection can go back and forth between family members like a Ping-Pong ball. For repeated, recalcitrant infections, it's worth testing and treating every infected person in the household. Children can also get reinfected by close peers in school and day care. In some cases, a second, more powerful antibiotic is needed. Antibiotics are *not* effective against viruses; if your child's sore throat is not due to bacteria, antibiotics won't help. Some children's throats are just more susceptible to the Strep bacteria. Antibiotics can't do the job alone; they require a healthy immune system to wipe out bacteria and keep them out. If antibiotics haven't worked for your child, see your health care provider to discuss alternative antibiotics or other measures to support the immune system.

Lest you think that modern medicine can only treat bacterial sore throats, here's some reassuring news. The antiviral medication *acyclovir* is effective in reducing children's mouth and throat pain caused by cold sores (which are caused by Herpes viruses).[15] It only benefits patients who get started on it within the first three days of symptoms. If your child suffers from severe cold sores that also cause sore throats, don't just wait around hoping it will get better. Help is a prescription pad page away.

## Herbs

There are no scientific studies specifically evaluating the effectiveness of any herbal remedy in treating sore throats. No herbal remedy replaces antibiotics for treating Strep throat. However, herbal remedies have a long history of soothing irritated sore throats. The table lists some of the most commonly used herbal treatments that can help your child deal with the discomfort:

## HERBAL REMEDIES TO SOOTHE SORE THROATS

- *Demulcents (throat soothers):* horehound, licorice, mullein, slippery elm bark
- *Immune boosters:* echinacea
- *Inflammation easing:* chamomile, licorice
- *Bacteria fighters:* goldenseal
- *Astringent:* gum myrrh, mullein
- *Miscellaneous:* honey, sage, thyme, oil of eucalyptus, mustard, essential oils of chamomile, lavender, and lemon

*Horehound* is a demulcent and expectorant (loosens mucus) ingredient in many cough drops and candies. I recommend horehound cough drops or hard candies for children over four (who are unlikely to choke on hard drops) to help soothe their sore throats, and I use them myself. Horehound is an ingredient in Ricola Natural Herb Cough Drops.

*Licorice root* is a demulcent, soothing sore throats; it also eases inflammation by blocking the breakdown of the body's own steroids. Licorice tea may be especially useful in treating sore throats due to cold sores or chancre sores.[16] Be careful not to overdo it with licorice. Taking too much on a long-term basis can cause problems with the balance of blood salts, blood pressure, and heart function.

*Chamomile* is one of my favorite home remedies. It helps reduce inflammation—that's the body's reaction to a problem, and it leads to pain, redness, and swelling. A bit of chamomile tea or a gargle made from a strong cup of chamomile tea may help ease the inflammation of a painful sore throat. It has few side effects; it's readily available, inexpensive, and very few people are allergic to it.

*Mullein* leaves and flowers are boiled into tea as a demulcent and astringent useful against coughs, colds, and sore throats. It is used on the Indian subcontinent and by American Indians for sore throats and respiratory problems because it is so soothing. *Slippery elm bark* is another of my favorite remedies because it is so soothing to mucous membranes. It is the main ingredient in Throat Coat tea available in grocery stores. Slippery elm bark lozenges are also available as sore throat soothers.

*Comfrey* tea is a demulcent (throat soother), but contains dangerous pyrollizidine alkaloids which can cause serious liver problems; I do not recommend comfrey tea. *Red clover* blossoms and leaves are traditionally brewed into a strong tea, used as a gargle for an inflamed throat. Red clover can also cause bleeding problems, so I suggest you use it cautiously, if at all.

*Echinacea (purple coneflower):* A Nebraska farmer stole the idea for this remedy from local Indians who had long used it as an anti-infective agent. It is now widely used in Germany as a stimulant for the immune system, especially in treating the common cold and sore throats. It stimulates several components of the immune system, and if taken during the first twenty-four hours of having common cold symptoms, it does speed recovery from the cold. However, it does not kill Strep effectively or help prevent rheumatic fever. Echinacea is very safe, but most herbalists recommend that it be used on a short-term basis (less than six weeks at time) only.

*Goldenseal* root contains the active ingredient berberine. Berberine kills many bacteria (including strep) in test-tube studies.[17] It was used by the Cherokee Indians to treat ulcers and arrow wounds. Goldenseal also stimulates the immune system. There are *no* studies evaluating its effectiveness in treating people with Strep throat, and it is close to extinct from overharvesting; I do not recommend it.

*Gum myrrh* is the gum resin of trees indigenous to East Africa and Arabia. It has been used since ancient times as a perfume and incense. It is also an ingredient in mouthwashes and gargles for its fragrance and its mildly astringent properties.

Though not technically an herb, *honey* is traditionally added to tea or lemonade to help soothe sore throats. To avoid the risk of botulism, do not give honey to infants under one year of age.

Other traditional herbal remedies: compresses of *sage* and *thyme*, flannel mufflers of *eucalyptus oil*, and *mustard* poultices. Some families add *chamomile, lavender,* and *thyme* to steam baths to soothe the mucous membranes of the nose and throat. Others massage the child's neck and throat with massage oil and add essential oils of *chamomile, lemon,* and *thyme*. There are no scientific studies evaluating the effectiveness of these remedies, but I encourage parents to follow their families' safe healing traditions.

*Peter decided he would get some slippery elm bark lozenges for Angela and make some hot licorice and slippery elm bark tea for both of them. He wanted to talk to his wife about echinacea and goldenseal extracts before purchasing them.*

## Nutritional Supplements

Sugar-free *vitamin C* lozenges or *zinc* lozenges may be helpful in relieving sore throat pain, but there are no studies comparing their effectiveness to other throat lozenges, horehound candy, or other hard candy. Both seem to reduce symptoms of the common cold in adults, so if sore throat is just one of several cold symptoms, vitamin C and zinc lozenges may be worth a try for older children and adolescents.

*Raw garlic* and *onions* have antibacterial properties, though they have never been specifically tested as treatments for sore throats.[18] You might try giving your child raw garlic blended with mashed potatoes or in a blender with vegetable juices. Some of my European colleagues swear by this remedy. Having tried it once, I cannot in good conscience recommend that you try to force onion juice down the throat of any child who is already unhappy. It tastes terrible.

*Peter decided that extra orange juice would be good for everyone in the family, and that pesto (made with raw garlic and basil) would make a great dinner. He decided to stop at the grocery store on his way home and pick up a gallon of orange juice, spaghetti noodles, and pesto ingredients along with the yogurt and kefir. I reminded him that to get the amount of vitamin C that helps reduce cold symptoms, he'd have to drink at least five glasses of OJ a day. That's one way to make sure everyone is getting plenty of fluids! But for someone with a really sore throat, capsules or crystalline vitamin C sprinkled in applesauce might be easier to swallow.*

## LIFESTYLE THERAPIES: NUTRITION, EXERCISE, ENVIRONMENT, MIND-BODY

### Nutrition

As with other infectious diseases, drinking *plenty of fluids* is the order of the day. Your child's fluid intake is sufficient if it necessitates diaper changes or visits to the bathroom every two to three hours.

One of the most time-honored sore throat remedies is the saltwater gargle:

- ½ teaspoon of salt (or ¼ teaspoon of salt plus ¼ teaspoon baking soda)
- 8–16 ounces of warm water

Other home remedies are:

- Hot tea with honey
- Honey mixed with roasted onion
- Honey and lemon juice (or cider vinegar) in 6–8 ounces of hot water
- Apple juice and clove tea (spiced apple cider)

There are no scientific studies evaluating the effectiveness of any of these home remedies, but I encourage families to use home remedies that are safe, don't cost much, and seem to make everyone feel better. Remember warm chicken soup, too!

### Exercise

*Rest* is indicated for every infectious disease. Rest allows the body to concentrate its energy on healing rather than exercise. Teenagers suffering from mono may be fatigued for months after the acute infection has resolved. They should *not* participate in contact sports such as football or soccer for at least a month to protect their spleens. There's no point in forcing a fatigued teenager out onto the football field or gym floor. Continue mild, regular exercise such as yoga, *Tai Chi,* or walking to keep the muscles from becoming weak and wasted. This is not the time for wind sprints.

Rest and patience are the mainstay of therapy for children whose throats are sore from too much talking, shouting, or singing.

*Peter realized that Angela needed her rest. He decided that he would take the day off to stay home with her, rent comedy movies, drink tea, and take naps.*

## Environment

For sore throats due to allergens and irritants, the best treatment is environmental: avoid the irritant. Do *not* smoke and do not allow others to smoke around your child. Avoid other sources of smoke, exhaust, and chemical fumes.

*Humidity* is the mainstay of treatment for laryngitis. Humidity also reduces throat irritation caused by dry winter air.

*I suggested Peter get the humidifier out of the attic, clean it off, and get it going.*

*Cold* foods and drinks are also soothing to sore throats. Even kids who won't eat their normal food when they are sick can often be coaxed to try ice cream, lemon sorbet, popsicles or even plain ice cubes.

## Mind-Body

There are no studies evaluating the effectiveness of mind-body techniques such as hypnosis, biofeedback, or meditation in treating children with sore throats.

## BIOMECHANICAL THERAPIES: MASSAGE, SPINAL MANIPULATION, SURGERY

### Massage, Spinal Manipulation

There are no studies evaluating the effectiveness of either massage or spinal manipulation in treating children with sore throats. Massage can be very soothing and, if done by parents, inexpensive.

### Surgery

At one time, tonsillectomy was the most common operation performed on children. Thankfully those days are long gone. However, there still are times when tonsillectomy is beneficial. Carefully performed studies in Pittsburgh have shown that some children with recurrent infections do benefit from surgery. Those who had seven or more culture-proven infections with Strep and underwent a tonsillectomy had only half the number of infections in the next year compared with similar children who did not have surgery. The benefits only lasted a year or two. Three years later, the number of infections was identical in both groups.[19] Tonsillectomy is a safe procedure for children between the ages of two and twelve years; it can often be done on an outpatient basis without the need for overnight hospitalization.

*This was Angela's first Strep throat, so there was no need to discuss surgery.*

## BIOENERGETIC THERAPIES: ACUPUNCTURE THERAPEUTIC TOUCH/PRAYER, HOMEOPATHY

### Acupuncture

There are no studies comparing acupuncture to other therapies for sore throats. I do not recommend acupuncture for the treatment of acute infectious diseases such as Strep throat. There is a point between the base of the thumb and first finger (known as LI4) that is effective in reducing all kinds of pain in the head, mouth, and neck. You can find it on yourself by massaging the area deeply. It is the point where deep massage feels a bit uncomfortable or odd. You can try massaging this point on both of your child's hands for several minutes as an experiment to see if it helps decrease his pain.

### Therapeutic Touch/Prayer

There are no scientific studies evaluating the effectiveness of Therapeutic Touch or prayer in treating children with sore throats. Because both are so safe, they are certainly worth trying if they are consistent with your beliefs.

## Homeopathy

There are no scientific studies evaluating the effectiveness of homeopathic remedies in treating sore throats. I do not recommend homeopathic treatment of Strep throats. For sore throats due to allergies, viruses, or irritants, you may wish to try a homeopathic remedy. Bear in mind that many homeopaths caution that effective therapies often make the patient feel worse before they feel better and that most sore throats are better in a day or two anyway. Homeopaths recommend that if you are going to use a homeopathic remedy, avoid giving your child cough drops or other remedies that contain eucalyptus, menthol, camphor, or other strongly aromatic substances.

The most commonly recommended homeopathic remedies for sore throats are: Aconitum, Apis, *Baryta carbonica,* Belladonna, Bryonia, *Hepar sulph,* Ignatia, Lachesis, Lycopodium, *Mercurius vivus, Nux vomica,* Phytolacca, Pulsatilla, *Rhus toxicum,* Silica, and Sulfur.

✳

## WHAT I RECOMMEND FOR SORE THROATS

### PREVENTING SORE THROATS

1. *Lifestyle—environment.* Minimize throat irritants. Do not smoke and do not allow others to smoke around your child. Avoid allergens. Minimize your child's exposure to other children with sore throats.

2. *Lifestyle—exercise.* Avoid overusing the throat.

3. *Biochemical—medications.* Have your child immunized against diphtheria.

---

*See your health care professional if you suspect Strep or if your child:*

- Is not better within forty-eight hours of starting treatment

- Has trouble swallowing her own saliva or starts drooling

- Develops signs of dehydration (such as fewer than four wet diapers within twenty-four hours or no tears when crying)

- Has severe pain

- Has trouble breathing

---

## TREATING SORE THROATS

1. *Biochemical—medications.* For sore throat pain, try analgesics (such as Tylenol, Advil, or Motrin), gargles with antacids (such as Maalox), anesthetic throat sprays or lozenges for children over four years old. If your child has a Strep infection, I recommend a full course of antibiotics.

2. *Lifestyle—nutrition.* Encourage your child to drink plenty of fluids. Saltwater gargles may be helpful for children who are old enough to gargle. Yogurt and kefir may help replace healthy bacteria that have been wiped out by antibiotics.

3. *Biochemical—herbs.* Try sucking on horehound drops for children over four years old or sipping hot tea with lemon and honey (slippery elm bark, licorice, or comfrey tea). No honey for infants less than one year of age.

4. *Lifestyle—environment.* Offer cold noncarbonated drinks, popsicles, sorbet, ice cream, ice cubes, or frozen yogurt. Humidifiers may help those with laryngitis.

5. *Lifestyle—exercise.* Rest.

6. *Biochemical—nutritional supplements.* Consider vitamin C and zinc lozenges if your child's sore throat is one of many cold symptoms.

7. *Biomechanical—surgery.* If your child has had many recurrent Strep throats, having her tonsils out may be helpful.

RESOURCES

*Internet*

Boston Medical Center
http://www.bostonchildhealth.org/
Health_Ed/Handouts/sorethroat.html

Iowa Virtual Children's Hospital
http://www.vh.org/Patients/IHB/Peds/
Infectious/Strep.html

Lucile Packard Children's Hospital
http://www.packardchildrenshospital.org/
health/respire/pharton.htm

National Institute of Health Center for
Complementary and Alternative Medicine
(list of alternative therapies)
http://nccam.nih.gov/cam/diseases/
Pharyngitis.html

# 26

# VOMITING AND NAUSEA

Jack Burnside called me about his eighteen-month-old daughter, Patrice, who had started vomiting the day before. She had thrown up about three times, most recently in the car on the way to the grocery store to get some cola and chicken soup to settle her stomach. Jack had stopped giving her milk, and started giving her clear liquids such as flat soda. His wife was concerned that their baby, Anna, was also spitting up after nursing. He had several questions:

- What caused the girls' vomiting?
- Should he bring in Patrice, Anna, or both for evaluations and treatment?
- What were the safest and most effective remedies for vomiting?

## WHAT CAUSES VOMITING?

Vomiting is a distinctly uncomfortable experience, but it can also help eliminate toxins from the body before they do serious damage. Vomiting is generally preceded by nausea, the feeling that one is about to vomit. Children who are nauseated generally avoid food, although most will still sip liquids if they are offered. Children vomit more easily than adults.

*Gastroenteritis* (also known as the intestinal flu) is the most common cause of nausea, vomiting, diarrhea, and abdominal pain in children. Technically, this illness is not a "flu" because it is not caused by the influenza virus, but this doesn't stop health care practitioners and parents alike from calling it the "flu bug." Gastroenteritis is normally caused by a viral infection and is over within forty-eight hours.

*Patrice's symptoms sounded as if they were due to plain old gastroenteritis. We agreed that Jack would try some simple home remedies and would bring her in the next day if she was still vomiting or developed any signs of dehydration.*

## CAUSES OF VOMITING

- Gastroenteritis (intestinal flu)
- Spitting up (gastroesophageal reflux)
- Food poisoning
- Swallowed phlegm dripping into the throat from the nose or sinuses
- Overeating, food intolerance, or food allergies
- Side effect of severe coughing
- Side effect of other treatments (medications, herbs, vitamins, anesthesia)
- Motion sickness
- Pregnancy
- Symptom of other illnesses (e.g., appendicitis, Strep throat, bladder infection, migraine headache)

All babies *spit up* milk from time to time. Spitting up is common in babies who are fed too much too quickly. It usually looks like a lot more is coming up than there is. If you are concerned about how much milk is being regurgitated, try this simple test. Take a measuring tablespoon of milk and spill it on the floor, an old rag, or a towel. You'll probably be as surprised as I was the first time I tried this experiment at how much milk it looks like, even when you know perfectly well that it's only a tablespoon.

*Gastroesophageal reflux* is when the stomach (gastric) contents move backwards up into the swallowing tube (esophagus). Refluxing stomach acid can cause heartburn pain. Severe, persistent reflux leads to inadequate nutrition and poor growth. In a Chicago area study of nearly 1,000 babies, reflux was reported in 50% of infants less than three months old, but climbed to 67% (two-thirds) at four months. Most babies had outgrown the problem by the time they were seven to eight months old. Severe reflux not only causes a mess, it can also lead to severe heartburn, nausea, irritability, poor growth, and breathing problems such as

coughing or turning blue. If severe vomiting occurs in the first few days of life, it may be due to *intestinal obstruction* which requires immediate professional evaluation and treatment.

*Anna had been drinking avidly. She was gaining weight normally and had no other symptoms. She was so eager to eat that she seldom paused to burp. She was so tired by her vigorous feeding that she often fell asleep immediately after eating; when she was laid down, she spit up undigested milk. When Jack and his wife actually measured the amount she was spitting up, it was only about one and a half teaspoons.*

Vomiting can be a useful reaction for *eliminating tainted food* (food poisoning) before it is absorbed into the system. If your child is vomiting because of food poisoning, it is better not to suppress the symptoms, but to allow Nature to rid the body of the poisons.

Children also vomit if they *swallow a lot of phlegm*. Children suffering from colds, ear infections, bronchitis, and particularly Strep throat and sinus infections are prone to vomiting because the excessive phlegm irritates the stomach. The best way to reduce this kind of vomiting is to treat the underlying condition and to remove extra phlegm with frequent nose blowing, a bulb syringe, or nasal aspirator.

*Overeating* frequently causes indigestion, heartburn, and nausea, but it rarely causes vomiting in adults. Children seem to be more sensitive than adults to this manifestation of overindulgence. A trip to the ballpark or circus, complete with hot dogs, candy, soda pop, etc., sometimes ends unpleasantly in a rushed trip to the bathroom. *Certain foods*, such as green apples, have a well-deserved reputation for causing nausea and stomachaches. *Food allergies,* such as cow's milk and egg allergy can also manifest as vomiting. However, vomiting is seldom the only sign of a food intolerance (see Chapter 4, Allergies).

*Severe coughing* can trigger vomiting. Vomiting triggers a reflex that actually relieves the coughing spasm. In the old days, ipecac (the medicine used to induce vomiting in case of accidental poisoning) was used to treat children with asthmatic coughs. Nowadays effective asthma medicines don't necessarily cause vomiting.

Speaking of ipecac, many common *medications, herbs, and vitamins* and even the *anesthetics* used during surgery induce nausea and vomiting. Aspirin and ibuprofen commonly cause a queasy stomach. The antibiotic erythryromycin frequently causes nausea and vomiting, although smaller doses are sometimes used to help speed stomach emptying. Chemotherapy for cancer is notorious for causing nausea and vomiting that is so severe that some patients refuse continued treatment. Several Chinese herbs, notably *chuanwu* and *caowu* (the roots of aconitum), used as anti-inflammatory therapy, and *bajiaolian* (used to treat snake bite, tumors, and swollen lymph glands) have caused serious nausea and vomiting.[1] African herbal remedies have also been reported to have serious side effects, including vomiting and dehydration.[2] Herbs high in tannins (such as uva ursi) can also cause nausea. Vitamin A overdoses (doses of at least 300,000 international units or 60 milligrams) and excessive vitamin D can cause vomiting, headaches, and other serious neurologic problems. Zinc can also cause nausea and overdoses can lead to vomiting. Anyone who has had major surgery can tell you that one of the worst parts of an operation is feeling sick to your stomach right after you wake up from the anesthesia. Depending on the type of operation, anywhere from 30 to 80 percent of children experience nausea and vomiting within twenty-four hours of general anesthesia.

Children are also more susceptible than adults to *motion sickness*. Motion sickness can be brought on by the motion of a car, boat, airplane, or amusement park ride. Exhaust fumes and overexcitement make motion sickness worse.

Other conditions also include vomiting and nausea as key symptoms. Morning sickness is a classic early sign of *pregnancy*—an all too common condition in American teenagers. If *constipation* continues long enough, the child may become nauseated and may even vomit. Children suffering from *migraines* often experience nausea, and vomiting as cardinal symptoms of their "sick headaches." Abdominal pain, nausea, and vomiting are also symptoms of severe *lead poisoning*.

---

### TAKE YOUR BABY OR CHILD TO BE EVALUATED IF SHE:

- Spits up more than a tablespoon of milk with each feeding
- Is losing weight or not gaining weight as well as predicted
- Is less than ten weeks old and has very forceful (projectile) vomiting
- Is vomiting even small amounts (less than a tablespoon) of water
- Has violent retching
- Vomits up bile (greenish fluid) or blood or coffee grounds–like material
- Has a temperature over 100.5°F if she is less than two months old
- Has a temperature over 103.9°F at any age
- Has severe abdominal pain, especially the lower right side (could be appendicitis)
- Vomits more than three times or more than an hour following a head injury
- Vomits continuously for more than 24 hours
- Seems uninterested in drinking or appears to be dehydrated
- Or if you are concerned about her symptoms or appearance

---

Other serious causes of vomiting include appendicitis, bladder or kidney infections, and meningitis. Rare genetic diseases such as hereditary fructose intolerance or severe vitamin B12 deficiency can also cause vomiting. Vomiting is also one of the signs of hepatitis (liver disease). Children who have suffered a head injury often vomit once or twice within the first hour following the injury.

If your child is having one of these symptoms, she may have something more complicated than simple gastroenteritis or spitting up and may need more therapy than you can provide at home.

Dehydration can occur within a day, especially if your child has diarrhea as well as vomiting. If your child has any of these signs, she needs to be evaluated by a health care professional to determine the cause of the vomiting and the potential need for fluids by vein (intravenous).

### SIGNS OF DEHYDRATION

IF YOUR CHILD:

- Voids (pees/urinates) less than four times per day or less than half of what is normal for her
- Doesn't have tears when she cries
- Loses weight
- Has sunken eyes or a sunken fontanel (soft spot on baby's head)
- Has dry lips and tongue, or stringy saliva
- Hands and feet are much cooler than her arms and legs

## WHAT CAN BE DONE TO PREVENT VOMITING?

Prevent food poisoning by keeping hot foods hot and cold foods cold. Cook all meat, poultry, and eggs thoroughly to kill bacteria that cause vomiting and diarrhea. Wash all poultry products well before cooking. Wash the cutting board, knives, and other utensils and your hands after preparing poultry. Do not leave foods prepared with mayonnaise (such as chicken salad or tuna salad) out of the refrigerator for more than an hour before eating them. Do not let your child eat raw dough made with eggs that have not been cooked.

Avoid motion sickness by having the child sit in the front seat, keeping a window open, and encouraging her to look out at the horizon rather than reading.

Avoid spreading infectious gastroenteritis by frequently washing your hands and your child's hands. Treat underlying illnesses promptly. Keep your child's nose cleaned out when she has a cold or sinus infection to prevent her from swallowing lots of phlegm.

Prevent spitting up by slowing feedings, frequent burping, thickening feedings with rice cereal, or keeping your child upright for twenty to thirty minutes after feeding.

*I suggested that Jack and his wife try slowing down Anna's feedings, having her burp at least twice each feeding and once afterward. I also suggested that they keep her upright for half an hour after she had been fed to give the milk a chance to pass through the stomach, making it less likely that it would come back up when she lay down. Anna continued to grow well and stopped spitting up when she was about five months old.*

## WHAT IS THE BEST WAY TO TREAT VOMITING?

The best way to treat vomiting depends on what is causing it. The treatments for motion sickness are not necessarily the same as for food poisoning or chemotherapy-induced vomiting. Let's tour the Therapeutic Mountain to find out what works for different kinds of vomiting. If you want to skip to my bottom-line recommendations, flip to the end of the chapter.

## BIOCHEMICAL THERAPIES: MEDICATIONS, HERBS, NUTRITIONAL SUPPLEMENTS

### Medications

Because vomiting is often the body's way of eliminating toxins from the system, and because young children are more prone to suffering side effects, medications to suppress nausea and vomiting are *not* recommended for children under two years old. If your young child is undergoing chemotherapy or requires some other therapy that causes nausea, ask your health care provider about safe treatments to minimize symptoms.

### NONPRESCRIPTION ANTINAUSEA MEDICATIONS

- Meclizine (Antivert)
- Diphenhydramine (Benadryl)
- Dimenhydrinate (Dramamine)
- Cyclizine (Marezine)
- Emetrol; Coca-Cola syrup
- Pepto Bismol

*Antivert* is commonly used to prevent and treat motion sickness. It starts working within one hour and lasts for 12 to 24 hours. It is not recommended for children younger than twelve. It can cause drowsiness, restlessness, blurred vision, and a drop in blood pressure. It should not be taken if the teenager is planning to drive or operate dangerous equipment. Overdoses can cause seizures. Although it sounds scary, Antivert is actually safe enough to be used during pregnancy to treat morning sickness.

*Benadryl* is one of the most commonly used medications for motion sickness, nausea, and vomiting. It is often used in combination with more powerful drugs to prevent nausea due to chemotherapy. Benadryl is fairly safe even for young children. It causes drowsiness, increased thirst, and dry mouth in most children, irritability and excitement in a few.

*Dramamine* is the classic medication used to prevent motion sickness. It is chemically similar to Benadryl and has similar side effects: drowsiness or irritability, confusion and dry mouth. It is not approved for use in children less than two years old, but it is the number-one choice for treating motion sickness in children between 2 and 12 years old.

*Cyclizine* is approved for children of all ages. It starts working within 30 to 60 minutes. However, after the death of an Alaskan teenager was attributed to Cyclizine abuse, enthusiasm for this drug has waned.

*Emetrol, Nausetrol,* and *Naus-A-Way* are all carbohydrate (sugar) solutions with phosphoric acid. Although they are marketed as antinausea medications, they are actually pretty similar to *Coca-Cola syrup*. There is no scientific evidence that any of these medications are any more effective than flat soft drinks in reducing nausea and vomiting.

### PRESCRIPTION MEDICATIONS FOR VOMITING

- Prochlorperazine (Compazine), promethazine (Phenergan), chlorpromazine (Thorazine)
- Metoclopramide (Reglan)
- Trimethobenzamide (Tigan), hydroxyzine (Vistaril)
- Ondansetron (Zofran)
- Scopolamine (Transderm Scop)
- Others

*Compazine, Phenergan,* and *Thorazine* are chemically related, powerful treatments for vomiting due to other medications and surgery. They can be very sedating. Phenergan helps prevent motion sickness. They are not typically used for children less than two years old.

*Reglan* is used to treat infant's gastro-esophageal reflux and, in combination with other medications, to prevent chemotherapy-induced vomiting. It should *not* be used in babies who simply spit up a bit after feeding if they are growing well and do not have other problems.

*Tigan* and *Vistaril* are sedating medications related to nonprescription Benadryl and Dramamine. Tigan is commonly used in hospitalized adults and is approved for use in children as young as two years old. Vistaril is often given in combination with other antinausea medications and is safe for young children.

*Ondansetron* (Zofran) is a powerful medicine used to help prevent nausea and vomiting in patients undergoing chemotherapy.

*Transdermal scopolamine* is chemically related to poisonous belladonna and is available as an adhesive patch to prevent motion sickness. Because younger children are more susceptible to its side effects (dry mouth, drowsiness, blurred vision), it is not recommended for children under twelve years old.

*Other effective medications* that treat the serious nausea and vomiting accompanying cancer chemotherapy are steroids, sedatives, and droperidol.[3] These medicines are sometimes combined with Reglan and Benadryl to enhance their antiemetic (antivomiting) effect. These combinations have the risk of severe sedation and other side effects. They should only be used under the supervision of a physician with extensive experience in treating children with chemotherapy.

*Medications are not indicated for the vast majority of children suffering from gastroenteritis, spitting up, or food poisoning. Neither Patrice nor Anna needed medication for their symptoms.*

## Herbs

*Ginger* is my favorite home remedy to prevent and treat nausea. I recommend it regularly to patients who require chemotherapy or those recovering from surgery. In fact, recent studies have shown it to be helpful in treating the morning sickness of pregnancy, sea sickness, and nausea caused by chemotherapy.[4] In a study of postoperative nausea, ginger was as effective as the powerful medicine Reglan.[5] Ginger is very safe. The total dose of powdered ginger root is typically divided into four doses over the course of a day. The tea can be sipped throughout the day. I usually combine ginger and peppermint tea, sometimes adding a little chamomile as well to the recipe. If your child would rather take pills or capsules, you can put powdered ginger into empty gelatin capsules.

### GINGER ROOT (TAKE FOUR DOSES DAILY)

- *Over twelve years old:*
  250 milligrams per dose
- *Six to twelve years old:*
  125 milligrams per dose
- *Three to six years old:*
  50 to 75 milligrams per dose
- *Under three years old:*
  25 milligrams per dose

You can also prepare homemade ginger tea:

### GINGER TEA

1 quart of water, plus
3–5 slices (about 2 inches chopped)
    ginger root

Simmer together for 10 to 20 minutes. Tea can be poured over peppermint leaves or chamomile flowers and allowed to steep for another 10 minutes. Sweeten as desired and sip as needed.

You can also try ginger soda, but check to make sure the ginger ale you buy contains real ginger and not just ginger flavoring. You can also add freshly grated ginger (⅛ teaspoon at a time) to your child's juice, applesauce, or hot cereal. Some teenagers prefer to chew on candied ginger or candies with ginger flavoring. Younger children sometimes complain that ginger is too spicy, so I usually don't recommend it for kids less than six years old.

Other traditional tummy-settling teas contain *chamomile* and *peppermint*. You can find this combination ready made at your grocery store under several brand names (such as Celestial Seasonings' Grandma's Tummy Mint tea). Sometimes *catnip* and other members of the *mint* family are added or substituted for peppermint. Common additions include anise, dill, fennel, lemon balm, lime flowers, and meadowsweet. Some herbalists recommend bitter herbs (such as gentian) to treat stomach upsets and stimulate appetites. These herbs don't taste very good and may not be helpful if the child is also having diarrhea. The combination of chamomile, vervain, licorice, lemon balm, and mint has proven useful in treating infants suffering from colic (see Chapter 10, Colic), a common newborn condition often thought to be due in part to an upset stomach.[6]

*Jack chose to try ginger, mint, chamomile, and lemon balm for Patrice. He also decided to change from root beer to real ginger ale for Patrice; this is the remedy his mother had used when he was ill as a child. We agreed that he would alternate ginger ale with chicken broth so that Patrice would get the balance of salt (from chicken broth) and sugar (from ginger ale) that her body needed.*

Clove tea (10 cloves in 12 ounces of boiling water, steeped ten minutes and strained) and cinnamon tea (1 to 2 sticks of cinnamon to 1 cup of boiling water, steeped 10 minutes and drained) are also traditional, tasty remedies for nausea. You can experiment and combine different ratios of ginger, clove, and cinnamon. Basil tea (½ ounce of dry basil, plus one cup of boiling water, steeped for 5 minutes and strained) is an old English remedy for nausea.

Goldenseal *(Hydrastis canadensis)* and barberry *(Berberis vulgaris)* tinctures are frequently recommend for diarrhea and may be helpful if the child is suffering from gastroenteritis—both vomiting and diarrhea. The dose of either tincture is two to three drops diluted in four ounces of water, sipped slowly over an hour. However, because goldenseal is close to extinct from overharvesting, herbalists seldom recommend it anymore.

## Nutritional Supplements

Vitamin B6 (pyridoxine) has proven effective in reducing the nausea and vomiting of pregnancy.[7] The dose is 10 to 25 milligrams every eight hours until symptoms are controlled. Although it is not clear exactly how pyridoxine works, it is an ingredient in a European medication used to treat morning sickness, Debendox.[8] Pyridoxine has also been used to treat the nausea caused by radiation therapy.[9] There are no studies evaluating the effectiveness of B6 in treating gastroenteritis, reflux, or other causes of nausea and vomiting in children. Because pyridoxine is generally safe, you can try giving your child 10 milligrams of vitamin B6 an hour before traveling to help minimize motion sickness.

There are no other nutritional supplements which have proven effective in treating childhood nausea or vomiting.

## LIFESTYLE THERAPIES: NUTRITION, EXERCISE, ENVIRONMENT, MIND-BODY

### Nutrition

Giving *small amounts of clear fluids frequently* is the mainstay of treatment for vomiting. Small amounts means 1 to 2 tablespoons at a time. Frequently means every 5 to 15 minutes. To give your child's stomach a chance to settle, wait for 15 to 30 minutes after a vomiting spell before trying again. Avoid large volumes at one time. Often a child who vomits after four ounces of soda guzzled in two minutes can easily tolerate a tablespoon repeated every five minutes over an hour—which is equivalent to the same four ounces.

To replace fluid losses, especially if your child has diarrhea as well as vomiting, use a commercially prepared rehydration fluids (such as Pedialyte) or make your own.

## HOMEMADE REHYDRATION SOLUTION

1 quart clean water
½ teaspoon salt or ¼ tsp salt + ¼ tsp salt
    substitute (potassium)
8 teaspoons of sugar *or* 1 cup of infant
    rice cereal

Use measuring spoons to measure precisely. Mix thoroughly. If you prefer to avoid straight sugar, you can substitute rice cereal.

A traditional Japanese home remedy for upset stomach is miso soup. Some children love it, but others really don't care for the flavor. You can find miso soup in most health food stores. This is one of my favorite home remedies for an upset stomach. A more American version is chicken bouillon or chicken broth.

If your baby is breast-feeding, continue to do so, even if the baby spits up every time she nurses. If she becomes uninterested in breast-feeding or has fewer wet diapers than usual, she needs to be evaluated professionally for dehydration and possible additional therapy.

*Avoid solid food* until the vomiting has stopped for at least two to four hours. Most children won't be hungry for solids until their stomachs have settled a bit anyway. Start cautiously with small amounts. Resume with bland foods such as rice, bananas, dry toast, Cheerios, teething biscuits, and crackers. Start with small amounts given frequently rather than one large meal. For at least a day or two, avoid greasy foods such as meats, fried eggs, or anything else that is fried. If your child is prone to motion sickness, give her a few crackers or some toast before leaving on a trip. An empty stomach can actually make her nausea worse than having a little something on board.

*Avoid very cold* foods and beverages as these can be hard on the stomach.

*Avoid very sweet beverages.* Studies in cyclists showed that lower sugar solutions (6% glucose) were better absorbed and caused less nausea than higher sugar beverages (12% glucose).[10]

*Thickening feedings* may help minimize spitting up in babies with mild to moderate reflux.[11] You can thicken feedings by adding one to two tablespoons of infant rice cereal to each ounce of formula. Thickened feedings are most effective in combination with keeping the baby upright for 20 to 30 minutes following a feeding.

If your child has chronic problems with vomiting or serious spitting up, consider having her evaluated for a possible allergy to cow's milk. In one study of children who had been referred to gastroenterology specialists for reflux, 41% turned out to be allergic to cow's milk, which is the main ingredient in most formulas.[12] Some children will improve markedly when they are switched to soy, and some will require a more elemental formula. See your doctor if you think this is the problem.

## Exercise

Although exercise helps build strong muscles, lungs, and heart, it has some side effects on the intestines. Most long distance runners are familiar with runner's diarrhea. Vomiting is also common after long runs or intense bicycle rides, possibly because the blood that normally supplies the stomach and intestines is diverted away to supply the muscles, interfering with normal gut function. Exercise also sometimes induces gastroesophageal reflux, resulting in heartburn and nausea.[13] Your child is not likely to suffer these symptoms unless she is exercising vigorously as part of a track or cross-country team. If your child does have heartburn with exercise, consider cutting back on the intensity of her workout.[14] Light exercise actually encourages the stomach to empty promptly. Adequate training minimizes diarrhea, cramping, and nausea associated with intense exercise.[15]

Interestingly, in a study of airline pilots-in-training, a program of endurance training actually increased their symptoms of air sickness.[16] Despite the fact that they were in better condition with respect to their heart, lung, and muscles, they were more susceptible to motion sickness after training—an interesting trade-off. I wouldn't let this study deter me from recommending aerobic exercise to any but the most motion sickness–prone child.

As with most illnesses, rest is beneficial. If your child is tired, encourage her to rest. Try lying down with her to read a story or listening to quiet, soothing music.

### Environment

Avoid stale, stuffy air. Do not let your child become chilled, but do keep fresh cool air flowing around your child's face.

Keep an empty receptacle (a pot, bowl, or basin) near your child's bed or wherever she is resting so that if the urge strikes, she does not need to run all the way to the bathroom and worry about losing it on the way.

Some children are soothed by a cool, damp cloth placed on the forehead and over the eyes or the back of the neck. Gently clean your child's face after she vomits. If she is old enough, have her swish some water in her mouth and spit it out afterward to clean the taste of vomit out of her mouth.

Keep your baby upright after eating for at least thirty minutes. Sleeping on her tummy (prone) may result in less spitting up than sleeping on her back (spine). If she has serious problems with spitting up or reflux, you can consult a physical therapist about making a special foam wedge or sling to keep your baby's head and chest elevated while she sleeps, or you can buy one ready-made (Infant Reflux Wedge, available from Pedicraft, 4134 St. Augustine Road, Jacksonville, FL 32207; 800-223-7649).

### Mind-Body

Several studies have shown that *hypnosis* can be helpful in reducing intractable vomiting,[17] for children struggling with the severe nausea and vomiting due to cancer chemotherapy,[18] for cutting back on the gagging children sometimes have when trying to swallow pills,[19] and for eliminating habitual vomiting.[20] Desensitization therapy, relaxation therapy, and biofeedback have also proven useful in treating air sickness in pilots and nausea in patients undergoing chemotherapy.[21] If your child has recurrent vomiting from chemotherapy or motion sickness, it is probably worthwhile to consult a hypnotherapist. If your child has a simple case of food poisoning or gastroenteritis, the vomiting will probably be over by the time you get an appointment to see a psychologist anyway.

For most people, there is something vaguely shameful about vomiting. It is important to reassure your child that you love her and will stay with her, that it's OK to vomit if she needs to, and that vomiting will help clear the toxins from her system.

## BIOMECHANICAL THERAPIES: MASSAGE, SPINAL MANIPULATION, SURGERY

### Massage

Massaging the belly could trigger more nausea in sensitive children. Rather than massage the abdomen directly, you might try an old folk remedy frequently recommended by Edgar Cayce: Soak a cotton flannel cloth in castor oil and lay the cloth over your child's abdomen. Cover with a towel, and let the child rest for an hour or so before gently rinsing off with a baking soda and water solution. There are no scientific studies evaluating this remedy, but it is safe and inexpensive.

### Spinal Manipulation

There are no scientific studies evaluating the effectiveness of chiropractic or osteopathic adjustment in treating children with nausea or vomiting. I do not recommend spinal manipulation as a treatment for children with these primary symptoms.

### Surgery

Surgery is unnecessary to treat the flu, but it can be lifesaving if the vomiting is due to appendicitis. If your child has severe abdominal pain, especially if it localizes on the right, lower side where the appendix is located, please seek medical care immediately. Surgeons are probably the most skilled physicians around when it comes to figuring out belly pain and vomiting.

## BIOENERGETIC THERAPIES: ACUPUNCTURE, THERAPEUTIC TOUCH/REIKI, HOMEOPATHY

### Acupuncture

There are numerous studies evaluating the effectiveness of acupuncture and acupressure in treating nausea and vomiting. The point most often used is Pericardium 6 (P6), located about one inch above the wrist crease, between the two tendons leading to the palm. This is about where your watch clasp falls on your wrist.

In several comparison studies, acupuncture therapy given before surgery significantly reduced *postoperative nausea* and vomiting in adults for up to six hours after surgery.[22] Real acupuncture or acupressure is more effective than sham (placebo) acupuncture in preventing postsurgical nausea and reducing the need for antinausea medication in adults.[23] In fact, acupuncture stimulation is as effective as an antiemetic medication.[24] Applying pressure to the P6 point intermittently following the initial acupuncture treatment prolongs its antiemetic effect for up to 24 hours.[25]

Acupuncture treatment at the P6 point has also proved useful in treating *morning sickness*. Comparison studies have shown that daily pressure (using wrist bands) at the P6 point was more effective than sham or placebo acupressure (pressure at another point) in reducing nausea.[26] Acupressure wrist bands reduce not just the nausea, but also the anxiety, depression, and other emotional discomforts that accompany morning sickness.[27] While acupressure therapy is effective, it may need to be repeated as often as every two hours to achieve consistent control of symptoms.[28]

Stimulation of the P6 point has even proved effective in treating nausea due to *cancer chemotherapy*.[29] Like medications, acupuncture improves symptoms, but does not cure the underlying cause. Treatment may need to be repeated every few hours.

Unfortunately, there have been few studies of acupuncture in children. The studies that have been done have had mixed results, but more recent studies confirm accupuncture's effectiveness and acceptability in children as well as adults. When it is provided by a well-trained, licensed health professional, acupuncture is extremely safe and low in side effects compared with antiemetic medications.[30] I recommend acupressure with Sea-Bands for most patients I see with ongoing nausea or vomiting such as children with cancer who need ongoing chemotherapy.

## Therapeutic Touch/Reiki

There are no studies specifically evaluating the effects of hands-on healing practices for patients with nausea. I have used Reiki and Therapeutic Touch several times with patients with severe nausea, and they told me it was very helpful; a few of them actually turned down their powerful nausea medicines, saying they were no longer necessary. Similarly, although there are no studies specifically eval-

uating the benefits of prayer in treating nausea, I wouldn't hesitate to recommend prayer if consistent with your family values and beliefs.

## Homeopathy

As expected from the homeopathic principle of "like cures like," all of these remedies actually *cause* vomiting if taken in higher, nonhomeopathic doses: *Aconitum* (aconite), *Antimonium tartaricum* (tartar emetic), *Arsenicum album* (arsenic), *Bryonia alba* (white bryony), *Cinchona officianalis* (China officianalis), *Ferrum metallicum* (iron), Ipecac, *Nux vomica* (poison nut), Phosphorus, and Pulsatilla. There are no scientific studies evaluating the effectiveness of homeopathy in treating children with nausea or vomiting. I do not recommend them.

## WHAT I RECOMMEND FOR VOMITING

*Take your baby or child to be evaluated if she:*

- Spits up more than a tablespoon of milk with each feeding

- Is losing weight or not gaining weight as well as predicted

- Is less than ten weeks old and has forceful (projectile) vomiting

- Is vomiting when she drinks even small amounts (less than a tablespoon) of water

- Has violent retching

- Has a yellowish tinge to her skin or eyes (jaundice)

- Vomits up bile (greenish fluid) or blood or coffee grounds–like material

- Has a temperature over 100.5°F if she is less than two months old

- Has a temperature of over 103.9°F at any age

- Has severe abdominal pain, especially in the lower right side (could be appendicitis)

- Vomits more than three times or more than an hour following a head injury

- Vomits continuously for more than twenty-four hours

- Seems uninterested in drinking or appears to be dehydrated

- Or see a health professional if you are concerned about her symptoms or appearance

## FOR BABIES WHO SPIT UP (OR HAVE REFLUX)

1. *Lifestyle—nutrition.* Small, frequent feedings, frequent burping, consider thickening feedings by adding 1 to 2 tablespoons of dry rice cereal to each ounce of formula.

2. *Lifestyle—environment.* Keep the baby's head elevated during sleep; keep the baby's head elevated while feeding and for at least thirty minutes afterward.

## FOR GASTROENTERITIS

1. *Lifestyle—nutrition.* Small amounts of rehydration fluid (Pedialyte), ginger soda, miso soup, broth, rice water, or herbal tea containing ginger, chamomile, lemon balm, and mint sipped frequently; avoid solid foods and milk until the child has had at least two to four consecutive hours without vomiting; start with bananas, crackers, toast, and rice. Avoid very cold or very sweet foods.

2. *Biochemical—medications.* Avoid them unless you have consulted a health care professional.

## FOR MOTION SICKNESS

1. *Lifestyle—environment.* Fresh air (keep the window open or stay on deck); ride in the front seat; focus on the horizon (count telephone poles or other distant objects); don't let the child read or focus on objects close up inside the car or boat.

2. *Biochemical—herbs.* Consider ginger supplements (can chew on ginger root or candied ginger or sip ginger soda).

3. *Biochemical—nutritional supplements.* Consider pyridoxine (vitamin B6) supplements—10 milligrams an hour or two before the ride.

4. *Lifestyle—nutrition.* Eat a light snack before traveling so the stomach isn't completely empty.

5. *Bioenergetic—acupuncture.* Consider acupressure or massage to the P6 point on the inside of the wrist. Elastic bands that rub this point are widely available under the trade name, Sea Bands. I frequently recommend them.

6. *Biochemical—medications.* Consider medications such as Benadryl or Dramamine before the trip. If home remedies are unsuccessful, see your physician for stronger prescription medications.

7. *Lifestyle—mind-body.* If home remedies have not worked, consider professional hypnotherapy to prevent severe, recurrent motion sickness.

## FOR MORNING SICKNESS

1. *Biochemical—nutritional supplements.* Vitamin B6 (pyridoxine): 10 to 25 milligrams one to three times daily.

2. *Biochemical—herbs.* Ginger: tablets, soda, or freshly grated.

3. *Bioenergetic—acupuncture.* Acupuncture or acupressure at the P6 point (one inch above the wrist crease between the tendons leading to the palm of the hand). Try Sea Bands.

4. *Lifestyle—mind-body.* If home remedies have not worked, consider professional hypnotherapy, relaxation therapy, or biofeedback.

*For vomiting due to other causes, treat the underlying problem.*

## RESOURCES

### Internet

American Academy of Family Practice
http://www.aafp.org/afp/981115ap/eliason.html

American Society of Health Systems Pharmacists
http://www.ashp.org/bestpractices/tg/nausea.pdf

U.S. Centers for Disease Control and Prevention (food safety)
http://www.cdc.gov/foodsafety/

Longwood Herbal Task Force (information on ginger)
http://www.mcp.edu/herbal/ginger/ginger.htm

Motion Sickness Information
http://www.choc.com/pediatric_adv/hhg/motionsi.htm

NASA (motion sickness in space)
http://ccf.arc.nasa.gov/dx/basket/factsheets/sms.html

National Cancer Institute (chemotherapy-associated nausea)
http://rex.nci.nih.gov/PATIENTS/aboutbc/treatment-chemo.html#nausea

National Food Safety Database
http://www.foodsafety.ufl.edu/index.html

# 27
# WARTS

Nick Evans brought his six-year-old daughter, Amy, to be treated for warts. Amy had had a few warts on her knees for the last two months, but over the last week she had developed four new warts on her hands. The warts didn't hurt, but Amy kept picking at them and biting them, making them bleed. Nick had heard about having warts burned or frozen off, but he wondered if there wasn't some less drastic but still effective treatment.

## WHAT CAUSES WARTS?

Frogs and toads don't! There are several kinds of warts, and all are caused by human papilloma viruses (HPV). This chapter covers the two kinds of warts that most often affect kids: common warts (usually found on the hands, face, knees, or elbows) and plantar warts (painful warts on the soles of the feet). Over the course of a lifetime, 75% of us develop warts. Warts are second to acne as the leading reason for visits to dermatologists. For reasons no one quite understands, common warts seldom appear before the age of two or after the age of forty. People with serious problems with their immune system can develop extensive warts.

Common warts are dry, bumpy, and firm. Plantar warts grow into the skin on the soles of the feet and look flat. Warts can be skin color, pink, tan, yellow, gray, black, or brown. Warts often contain brown dots and do not contain the whorls and ridges of fingerprints. If the top is cut off, warts bleed because tiny blood vessels grow into their center.

Warts are spread from person to person, but they are not highly contagious. However, athletes who use communal showers or go barefoot in the locker room are slightly more likely to catch plantar warts. If your child takes a gym class or plays a team sport that involves locker rooms and showers, have her wear flip-flops, sandals, or other shower shoes to prevent direct contact between her feet and the floor, which may be harboring wart viruses.

## What Is the Best Way to Treat Warts?

Most warts go away without any therapy other than patience. Interestingly, kids with eczema have fewer warts than other kids. A person with a healthy immune system gets rid of 80% of warts within two to three years.

Big warts and those that have persisted for at least twelve months are unlikely to go away by themselves. They might need treatment. Even when warts do go away, they often recur. With apologies to Tom Sawyer fans, spunk water (from an old tree stump) and dead cats have no proven efficacy in treating warts. Let's tour the Therapeutic Mountain to find out what does work; if you want to skip to my bottom-line recommendations, flip to the end of the chapter.

## Biochemical Therapies: Medications, Herbs, Nutritional Supplements

### Medications

The British call topical wart remedies (those applied directly to the skin) "wart paint." The most commonly used topical medication to treat warts is *salicylic acid* (the active ingredient in Compound W and Duofilm). It is available as a liquid, gel, or in "plasters" that can be placed directly on the wart. Plasters contain higher concentrations of medication and are the least messy to apply. For best results with topical wart medicine:

1. Soak the wart in warm water to soften it.
2. Peel away loose skin on top of the wart or pare down plantar warts until you get to the tender part; you don't need to make it bleed!
3. Apply the wart medicine. Don't let it get on healthy skin.
4. Cover the medication with a dressing such as a Band-Aid or piece of tape.
5. Repeat daily until the wart is gone—up to three months.

These medications may cause some burning or blistering on healthy skin. Be careful. You may want to apply a protective emollient, such as Vaseline, to the healthy skin around the wart to prevent the wart paint from irritating the healthy skin.

Professionally applied medications may include other acids, bleomycin, cantharidin (an irritating chemical extracted from the blister beetle known as "Spanish fly"), podophyllum, tretinoin, liquid nitrogen (to freeze the wart), or silver nitrate. Silver nitrate doesn't burn and is safe even on babies' tender skin. Most of the others on this list are pretty caustic and should only be applied by an experienced professional who is used to working with squirming children.

Some families and physicians have been trying *acne remedies* on warts—benzoyl peroxide, retinoic acid, and other agents. These medications typically cause some irritation, which may help recruit the body's own immune system to eliminate the wart. You might try some nonprescription benzoyl peroxide on your own warts as a home remedy before seeing the doctor for a more costly and potentially irritating treatment.

Because our own immune system rids us of wart viruses all the time, a few clever immunologists are trying to boost the immune response to warts with a variety of medications. The most common immunologic approach to treat stubborn warts is injecting the wart with *interferon*. Others have tried applying agents that cause severe irritating allergies reactions, such as *squaric acid dibutylester (SADBE)* or *dinitrochlorobenzene (DBCB)* on the wart itself, which seems to help in about 67% of kids with resistant warts. The wart sufferer or the parent who applies the remedy may develop widespread allergic reactions if the application is not precise, so it is definitely not a first-line therapy.

There are a lot of weird wart remedies, and not all of them come from fictional characters. Believe it or not, a few years ago someone noticed that patients who suffered from both peptic ulcers and warts who started taking *cimetidine* for their ulcers soon saw their warts melt away. A few brave dermatologists started recommending cimetidine (which is taken by mouth) to patients who had a variety of different kinds of warts all over their skin. Based on several case reports of remarkable success with cimetidine,[1] a few comparison studies have been done, but the results have not been conclusive—some studies say it works (usually within four to six weeks) and others say it's no better than placebo pills.[2] I do not recommend cimetidine as a first-line approach to treatment, but since cimetidine is unlikely to cause side effects, you might ask your doctor about trying cimetidine for four to eight weeks if the warts have resisted other remedies.

*Nick decided to treat Amy's warts with Compound W every day.*

## Herbs

Common herbal remedies applied to warts include the juice of dandelion stalks, tincture of thuja (white cedar), milk of bitterroot herbs, milkweed juice, tea tree oil, and fresh elderberry juice. None of these remedies has undergone scientific study, but because so many warts go away with the mere suggestion that they will, I support families' choices to use safe home remedies, including herbal salves.

If you want to take the physicians' immunological approach to the next level, you might try applying something to your child's wart that you already know will cause a rash, but beware of potential side effects. Some doctors apply *Candida* (a well-known yeast/fungus) and a few brave parents have tried rubbing a bit of poison ivy leaf on the skin. I'd like to know how the parents do this without getting poison ivy themselves—gloves? I think this is a risky practice and I do not recommend it.

## Nutritional Supplements

Some folks advocate the application of vitamin A, vitamin E oil, or a paste of baking soda and castor oil to the wart several times daily until the wart is gone. Some crush a vitamin C tablet or an aspirin, mix it with water to make a paste, and apply it to the wart. Others advise rubbing the wart with a cut raw potato and burying the potato under a tree in the backyard under a full moon. Vitamins A, C, and E, castor oil, crushed aspirin, and raw potatoes have not been scientifically studied as wart treatments, but they are inexpensive and safe. Cover the wart with a Band-Aid after any treatment to minimize messiness.

## LIFESTYLE THERAPIES: ENVIRONMENT, MIND-BODY

### Environment

Keep warts in the *dark*. Cover the wart tightly with a piece of adhesive tape or a Band-Aid. Some people use duct tape; use whatever is handy. Keep the wart covered for a week. Take the tape off to check the wart, wash it well, and let it air out. Re-cover it for another week and take another peek. Many warts disappear in six weeks with this simple cover-up treatment. This technique seems to prompt the immune system to attack the wart, perhaps by increasing the temperature or humidity at the site. I could not find any scientific studies evaluating this technique, but several pediatricians I know say that this is their favorite wart remedy because it is so inexpensive and free of side effects.

A recent study showed that by *heating* warts to 45 to 50 degrees Centigrade for thirty to sixty seconds, warts disappeared twice as well as in an untreated group.[3] You can try soaking warts in hot water (careful not to scald the child!) for five to thirty minutes, three times a week; warts that respond to this treatment usually begin to melt within three weeks of the hot treatment. Now if I had warts, I think I'd volunteer for hot tub therapy!

Several severe environmental strategies are used as surgical approaches to eliminating warts—freezing, burning, zapping, etc. (See the Surgery section below.)

## Mind-Body

Hypnosis can be effective in getting rid of warts. In one study ten patients with warts on both the right and left sides of their body were given the hypnotic suggestion that the warts would disappear from just one side. Nine out of ten patients had warts disappear just on that one side (without any other treatment); the tenth lost warts on both sides.[4] Children have especially good imaginations, and hypnosis or suggestion can work well in removing warts for them. Hypnosis can sometimes cure warts that have failed to respond to caustic conventional medical therapies. Involving the child in making the wart go away is more effective than simply telling him that a placebo will work.[5] Hypnosis is even effective in children whose immune systems are suppressed by illness or chemotherapy.[6]

I often use the technique my childhood doctor used with me: I tell the child that she can tell her warts to go away and that when she comes back in a month, I will give her a quarter for every wart she has made disappear. You can help your child imagine the wart disappearing, feeling the warmth or tingling as the blood carries it away. The more vivid the imagery, the more effective the treatment. Hypnotherapy or suggestion works best if the child is *convinced* that the wart will go away, *involved* in the cure, and something is *done* to the wart.

No one knows whether hypnosis works by shrinking the blood vessels supplying the wart or by stimulating the immune system to fight the wart-causing virus. This would be a fascinating area for additional research because, either way, there are important implications for other, more serious illnesses such as cancer.

*Before applying the Compound W to Amy's warts, Nick planned to have her soak them in hot water for five minutes. After applying the Compound W, they covered each wart with a Band-Aid. Amy received a sticker each day she soaked, put the medicine on, and covered it with a Band-Aid. If she accumulated five stickers in a week, she could pick out her own video to rent on the weekend. I asked Amy to return to the clinic in a month so we could count the warts. For every wart she got rid of, I'd pay her a quarter. We repeated this routine once. Within three months all of Amy's warts had disappeared, without a single scar, and she was very proud of herself.*

## BIOMECHANICAL THERAPIES: SURGERY

### Surgery

The most common surgical wart treatment is freezing the wart with liquid nitrogen. The treatment consists of soaking the wart (to soften it), paring it down (especially for warts on the feet), and then applying liquid nitrogen until the wart freezes. The liquid nitrogen is applied with a cotton swab or sprayed directly on the wart. Treatments are repeated every one to three weeks until the wart is gone. This works well for warts on the hand but is often painful and ineffective for warts on the sole of the foot.

Most of the time when parents come to me asking to have the wart frozen, they have tried a nonprescription treatment for a week or so, and the wart is still there. Usually it takes at least a month for a home remedy to work. I generally reserve liquid nitrogen or other surgical treatments for children who have already tried a mind-body technique (suggestion or hypnosis), home therapy with wart paint, and covering the wart with a Band-Aid or tape. If the warts survive three to six months of this treatment, I'll go ahead and use liquid nitrogen. It is inexpensive and has few side effects, but liquid nitrogen on normal skin (if the child moves during the application) can be quite painful.

Warts can also be electrically cauterized (zapped), lasered, or cut off. I don't recommend these treatments unless all else has failed, because they are painful and can leave scars.

## BIOENERGETIC THERAPIES

I'm not aware of any studies suggesting that acupuncture is useful in treating warts. I haven't tried treating warts with Therapeutic Touch or Reiki, and I'm not aware of any reports that they help. These kind of healing therapies are unlikely to be harmful, and it might be worthwhile to combine them with guided imagery and a few simple home remedies.

In a controlled trial in Canada, a combination homeopathic remedy was no more effective than a placebo in treating plantar warts. In both the treatment and the comparison placebo group, about 25% of patients were cured eighteen weeks after starting treatment.[7] Another randomized, controlled trial also failed to show any benefit from homeopathic remedies in treating warts.[8] On the other hand, homeopathy is safe. I have no objection to trying homeopathy along with home remedies to treat warts, but I don't suggest you rush out and buy new remedies unless you are already a believer in homeopathy or you're a scientist interested in a safe experiment.

# WHAT I RECOMMEND FOR WARTS

*Be patient. Most warts go away by themselves within 24 months.*

---

*Seek professional help if:*

- The wart becomes infected (red, painful, swollen)

- The wart is on the face

- The wart doesn't disappear within six months with home therapy

- You are concerned about the wart

---

1. *Lifestyle—environment.* Make the wart warm and keep it in the dark. Soak it in warm water several times a week. Cover it with a Band-Aid or piece of adhesive tape for a week at a time. Many warts go away in six to eight weeks with this remedy alone.

2. *Lifestyle—mind-body.* Give your child the suggestion that she can make the warts go away. Help her develop vivid imagery about her immune system fighting the warts, the warts melting away, and how the skin might feel tingly or warm as it's working. Consider an incentive for her success (a quarter, a sticker, or a book for every wart she eliminates).

3. *Biochemical—medications.* If suggestion and darkness don't work, try a nonprescription salicylic acid preparation such as Compound W or Duofilm. Apply the medication daily, and keep it covered with a Band-Aid or adhesive tape. If this doesn't work, your doctor may suggest other topical medicines, such as cantharidin or injecting interferon or other immune stimulating medicines into the wart or taking oral medicines such as cimetidine.

4. *Biomechanical—surgery.* If warts have not disappeared with three months of home therapy, see your doctor about zapping the wart with liquid nitrogen or laser treatment.

RESOURCES

*Internet*

American Academy of Dermatology
   http://www.aad.org/pamphlets/warts.html

American Academy of Family Medicine
   http://familydoctor.org/handouts/
   209.html

# REFERENCES

## Chapter 3: Acne

1. Shaw, J. C. Spironolactone in dermatologic therapy. *Journal of the American Academy of Dermatology* 24(1991):236–43.
2. Tucker, S. B., Tausend, R., Cochran, R., et al. Comparison of topical clindamycin phosphate, benzoyl peroxide, and a combination of the two for the treatment of acne vulgaris. *British Journal of Dermatology* 110(1984):487–92.
3. Katsambas, A., Towarky, A. A., Stratigos, J. Topical clindamycin phosphate compared with oral tetracycline in the treatment of acne vulgaris. Ibid. 116(1987):387–91; Norris, J. F. B., Hughes, B. R., Basey, A. J., et al. A comparison of the effectiveness of topical tetracycline, benzoyl-peroxide gel, and oral oxytetracycline in the treatment of acne. *Clinical and Experimental Dermatology* 16(1991):31–3.
4. Bassett, I. B., Pannowitz, D. L., Barnetson, R. A comparative study of tea tree oil versus benzoyl peroxide in the treatment of acne. *Medical Journal of Australia* 153(1990):455–8.
5. Snider, B. L., Dieteman, D. F. Pyridoxine therapy for premenstrual acne flare. *Archives of Dermatology* 110(1974):130–1.
6. Kligman, A. M., Mills, O. H., Leyden, J. J., et al. Oral vitamin A in acne vulgaris: preliminary report. *International Journal of Dermatology* 20(1981):278–85.
7. Labadarios, D., Cilliers, J., Visser, L., et al. Vitamin A and acne vulgaris. *Clinical and Experimental Dermatology* 12(1987):432–6.
8. Michaelsson, G., Juhlin, L., Vahlquist, A. Effect of oral zinc and vitamin A in acne. *Archives of Dermatology* 31(1977):31–6.
9. Weimar, V. M., Puhl, S. C., Smith, W. H., et al. Zinc sulfate in acne vulgaris. Ibid. 114(1978): 1776–8; Michaelsson, op. cit., 31–6; Weimar, op. cit., 1776–8.
10. Michaelsson, G., Edqvist, L. E. Erythrocyte glutathione peroxidase activity in acne vulgaris and the effect of selenium and vitamin E treatment. *Acta Dermato-Venereologica* 64(1984):9–14.
11. Dupre, A., Albarel, N., Bonafe, J. L., et al. Vitamin B12 induced acnes. *Cutis* 24(1979): 210–11.
12. Fulton, J. E., Plewig, G., Kligman, A. M. Effect of chocolate on acne vulgaris. *JAMA* 210(1969): 2071–4.
13. Hoehn, G. H., Acne and diet. *Cutis* 2(1966): 389–94.
14. Wortis, J. Common acne and insulin hypoglycemia. *JAMA* 108(1937):971.
15. McCarty, M. High-chromium yeast for acne? *Medical Hypothesis* 14(1984):307–10.
16. Minkin, W., Cohen, H. J. Effect of chocolate on acne vulgaris [letter]. *JAMA* 211(1970):1856.
17. Feldman, W., Hodgson, C., Corber, S., et al. Health concerns and health-related behaviors of adolescents. *Canadian Medical Association Journal* 134(1986):489–93.
18. Motley, R. J., Finlay, A. Y. How much disability is caused by acne? *Clinical Experimental Dermatology* 14(1989):194–8.
19. Yihou, X. Treatment of acne with ear acupuncture—a clinical observation of 80 cases. *Journal of Traditional Chinese Medicine* 9(1989):238–9; Yihou, X. Treatment of facial skin diseases with acupuncture—a report of 129 cases. Ibid. 10(1990):22–5; Guoqing, D. Advances in the acupuncture treatment of acne. *Journal of Traditional Chinese Medicine* 17(1997):65–72.

## Chapter 4: Allergies

1. Egger, J., Graham, P. J., Carter, C. M., et al. Controlled trial of oligoantigenic treatment in the hyperkinetic syndrome. *Lancet* 1(1985): 540–5.

2. Kahn, A., Mozin, M. J., Rebuffat, E., et al. Milk intolerance in children with persistent sleeplessness: a prospective double-blind crossover evaluation. *Pediatrics* 84(1989):595–603.

3. Niggerman, B., Breiteneder, H. Latex allergy in children. *International Archives of Allergy and Immunology* 121(2000):98–107.

4. Sampson, H. A., Ho, D. G. Relationship between food-specific IgE concentrations and the risk of positive food challenges in children and adolescents. *Journal of Allergy and Clinical Immunology* 100(1997):444–51.

5. Panush, R. S. Food induced ("allergic") arthritis: clinical and seriologic studies. *Journal of Rheumatology* 17(1990):291–4.

6. Bruckner, A. L., Weston, W. L., Morelli J. G. Does sensitization to contact allergens begin in infancy? *Pediatrics* 105(2000):e3.

7. Bindslev-Jensen, C. ABC of Allergies: Food allergies. *British Medical Journal* 7140(1998): 1299–1302; Sampson, H. A. Food allergy. *JAMA* 278(1997):1888–94.

8. Nimmagadda, S. R., Evans, R. Allergy: etiology and epidemiology. *Pediatrics in Review* 20(1999):111–5.

9. Strachan, D. P., Taylor, E. M., Carpenter, R. G. Family structure, neonatal infection and hay fever in adolescence. *Archives of Diseases in Childhood* 74(1996):422–6; Kramer, U., Heinrich, J., Wjst, M., et al. Age of entry to day nursery and allergy in later childhood. *Lancet* 353(1999): 450–4.

10. Gern, J. E., Weiss, S. T. Protection against atopic diseases by measles—a rash conclusion? *JAMA* 283(2000):394–5.

11. Van den Biggelaar, A. H. J., Van Ree, R., Rodrigues, L. C., et al. Decreased atopy in children infected with *Schistosoma haematobium:* a role for parasite-induced interleukin-10. *Lancet* 356(2000):1723–7.

12. Jalonen, T. Identical intestinal permeability changes in children with different clinical manifestations of cow's milk allergy. *Journal of Allergy and Clinical Immunology* 88(1991): 737–42.

13. Sampson, H. A., Scanlon, S. M. Natural history of food hypersensitivity in children with atopic dermatitis. *Journal of Pediatrics* 115(1989):23–7; Bock, S. A. Prospective appraisal of complaints of adverse reactions to foods in children during the first three years of life. *Pediatrics* 79(1987):683–8.

14. Hill, D. J., Firer, M. A., Ball, G., et al. Recovery from milk allergy in early childhood: antibody studies. *Journal of Pediatrics* 114(1989):761–6.

15. Steinman, H. A. "Hidden" allergens in foods. *Journal of Allergy and Clinical Immunology* 98(1996):241–50.

16. Tariq, S. M., Stevens, M., Matthews, S., et al. Cohort study of peanut and tree nut sensitization by age of 4 years. *British Medical Journal* 313(1996):514–7.

17. Hourihane, J. O., Roberts, S. A., Warner, J. O. Resolution of peanut allergy: case-control study. Ibid. 316(1998):1271–5.

18. Shapiro, G. G., Anderson, J. A. Controversial techniques in allergy. *Pediatrics* 82(1988):935–7.

19. King, H. C., King, W. P. Alternatives in the diagnosis and treatment of food allergies. *Otolaryngologic Clinics of North America* 31(1998):141–56.

20. Bock, S. A. Evaluation of IgE-mediated food hypersensitivities. *Journal of Pediatric Gastroenterology* 30(2000):S20–S27.

21. Lewith, G. T., Kenyon, J. N., Broomfield, J., et al. Is electrodermal testing as effective as skin prick tests for diagnosing allergies? A double-blind, randomized block design study. *British Medical Journal* 322(2001):131–4.

22. Meltzer, E. O., Granat, J. A. Impact of cetirizine on the burden of allergic rhinitis. *Annals of Allergy, Asthma, and Immunology* 83(1999): 455–63.

23. Adelsberg, B., R. Sedation and performance issues in the treatment of allergic conditions. *Archives of Internal Medicine* 157(1997): 494–500.

24. Weiner, J. M., Abramson, M. J., Puy, R. M. Intranasal corticosteroids versus oral H1 receptor antagonists in allergic rhinitis:

systemic review of randomized controlled trials. *British Medical Journal* 317(1998):1624–9.

25. Freier, S., Berger, H. Disodium cromoglycate in gastrointestinal protein intolerance. *Lancet* 1(1973):913–15.

26. Grossman, J., Banov, C., Bronsky, E. A., et al. Fluticasone propionate aqueous nasal spray is safe and effective for children with seasonal allergic rhinitis. *Pediatrics* 92(1993):594–9.

27. Busse, W. W. Action and effects of corticosteroids in allergic rhinitis. *Journal of Respiratory Diseases* 12(1991)(S36–S38):3.

28. Valentine, M. D., Schuberth, K. C., Kagey-Sobotka, A., et al. The value of immunotherapy with venom in children with allergy to insect stings. *New England Journal of Medicine* 323(1990):1601–3.

29. Wood, R. A., Eggleston, P. A. Management of allergy to animal danders. *Pediatric Asthma, Allergy, and Immunology* 7(1993):13–21.

30. Rooklin, A. R., Gawchik, S. M. Allergic rhinitis—it's that time again! *Contemporary Pediatrics* 11(1994):19–41.

31. Vinuya, R. Z. Specific allergen immunotherapy for allergic rhinitis and asthma. *Pediatric Annals* 29(2000):425–32.

32. Durham, S. R., Walker, S. M., Varga, E. M., et al. Long-term clinical efficacy of grass-pollen immunotherapy. *New England Journal of Medicine* 341(1999):468–75; Golden, D. B. K., Kwiterovich, K. A., Kagey-Sobotka, A., et al. Discontinuing venom immunotherapy: outcome after five years. *Journal of Allergy and Clinical Immunology* 97(1996):579–87.

33. Passalacqua, G., Albano, M., Fregonese, L., et al. Randomized controlled trial of local allergoid immunotherapy on allergic inflammation in mite-induced rhinoconjunctivitis. *Lancet* 351(1998):629–32; Mungan, D., Misirligil, Z., Gurbuz, L. Comparison of the efficacy of subcutaneous and sublingual immunotherapy of mite-sensitive patients with rhinitis and asthma—a placebo controlled study. *Annals of Allergy, Asthma, and Immunology* 82(1999):485–90.

34. Simons, F. E. R., Gu, X., Johnston, L. M., Simons, K. J. Can epinephrine inhalations be substituted for epinephrine injection in children at risk for systemic anaphylaxis? *Pediatrics* 106(2000):1040–4.

35. Meltzer, E. O. Intranasal anticholinergic therapy of rhinorrhea. *Journal of Allergy and Clinical Immunology* 90(1992):1055–64.

36. Kasahara, Y., Hikino, H., Tsurufuji, S., et al. Anti-inflammatory actions of ephedrines in acute inflammations. *Planta Medica* (1985): 325–31.

37. Sung, C. P., Baker, A. P., Holden, D. A., et al. Effect of extracts of *Angelica polymorpha* on reaginic antibody production. *Journal of Natural Products* 45(1982):398–406; Hikino, H. Recent research on Oriental medicinal plants. *Economic Medicinal Plant Research* 1(1985):53–85.

38. Cyong, J., Otsuka, Y. A pharmacological study of the anti-inflammatory activity of Chinese herbs. A review. *Acupuncture and Electro-Therapeutics* 7(1982):173–202; Kumagai, A., Nanaboshi, M., Asanuma, Y., et al. Effects of glycyrrhizin on thymolytic and immunosuppressive action of cortisone. *Endocrinologica Japononica* 14(1967):39–42; Armanini, D., Karbowiak, I., Funder, J. W. Affinity of liquorice derivatives for mineralocorticoid and glucocorticoid receptors. *Clinical Endocrinology* 19(1983):609–12.

39. Tsuruga, T., Ebizuka, Y., Nakajima, J., et al. Biologically active constituents of *Magnolia salicifolia:* inhibitors of induced histamine release from rat mast cells. *Chemical and Pharmacological Bulletin of Tokyo* 39(1991): 3265–71.

40. Mittman, P. Randomized, double-blind study of freeze-dried *Urtica dioica* in the treatment of allergic rhinitis. *Planta Medica* 56(1990):44–7.

41. Mullins, R. J. Echinacea-induced anaphylaxis. *Medical Journal of Australia* 168(1998):170–1.

42. Bucca, C., Rolla, G., Oliva, A., et al. Effect of vitamin C on histamine bronchial responsiveness of patients with allergic rhinitis. *Annals Allergy* 65(1990):311–4.

43. Duchen, K., Casas, R., et al. Human milk polyunsaturated long-chain fatty acids and secretory immunoglobulin A antibodies and early childhood allergy. *Pediatric Allergy and Immunology* 11(2000):29–39.

44. Lundberg, J. M., Saria, A. Capsaicin-induced desensitization of airway mucosa to cigarette

smoke, mechanical and chemical irritants. *Nature* 302(1983):251–3.

45. Andre, C., Andre, F., Colin, L., et al. Measurement of intestinal premeability to mannitol and lactulose as a means of diagnosing food allergy and evaluating therapeutic effectiveness of disodium cromoglycate. *Annals of Allergy* 59(1987):127–30.

46. Pastorello, E. A., Pravettoni, V., Incorvaia, C., Bellanti, J. A. Food allergy: an update. *Allergy* 54(1999):S43–S45.

47. Cavataio, F., Carroccio, A., Montalto, G., et al. Isolated rice intolerance: clinical and immunologic characteristics in four infants. *Journal of Pediatrics* 128(1996):558–60.

48. Hourihane, J. O., Dean, T. P., Warner, J. O. Peanut allergy in relation to heredity, maternal diet and other atopic diseases: results of a questionnaire survey, skin prick testing and food challenges. *British Medical Journal* 313(1996):518–21.

49. Marini, A., Agosti, M., Motta, G., Mosca, F. Effects of a dietary and environmental prevention programme on the incidence of allergic symptoms in high atopic risk infants: three year follow-up. *Acta Paediatrica Scandinavica* 414(1996)Suppl:1–22; Vadas, P., Wai, Y., Burks, W., et al. Detection of peanut allergens in breast milk of lactating women. *JAMA* 285(2001):1746–48.

50. Saarinen, U. M., Kajosaaari, M. Breast-feeding as prophylaxis against atopic disease: prospective follow-up study until 17 years old. *Lancet* 346(1995):1065–9.

51. Jarvinen, K. M., Makinen-Kiljunen, S., Suomalainen, H. Cow's milk challenge through human milk evokes immune response in infants with cow's milk allergy. *Journal of Pediatrics* 125(1999):506–12.

52. Lovegrove, J. A., Morgan, J. B., Hampton, S. M. Dietary factors influencing levels of food antibodies and antigens in breast milk. *Acta Paediatrica* 85(1996):778–84.

53. Hide, D. W., Matthews, S., Tariq, S., Arshad, S. H. Allergen avoidance in infancy and allergy at 4 years of age. *Allergy* 51(1996):80–93.

54. deBoisseau, D., Matarazzo, P., Rocchiccioli, F., et al. Multiple food allergy: a possible diagnosis in breast-fed infants. *Acta Paediatrica* 86(1997):1042–6.

55. Businco, L., Giampietro, P. G. Lucentim, P., et al. Allergenicity of mare's milk in children with cow's milk allergy. *Journal of Allergy and Clinical Immunology* 105(2000):1031–4.

56. Meydani, W. N., Ha, W. K. Immunologic effects of yogurt. *American Journal of Clinical Nutrition* 71(2000):861–72.

57. Fergusson, D. M., Horwood, L. J., Shannon, F. T. Early solid feeding and recurrent childhood eczema: a 10-year longitudinal study. *Pediatrics* 86(1990):541–6.

58. Paganus, A., Juntunen-Backman, K., Savilahti, E. Follow-up of nutritional status and dietary survey in children with cow's milk allergy. *Acta Paediatrica* 81(1992):518–21.

59. Heiner, D. C., Sears, J. N., Kniker, W. T. Multiple precipitins to cow's milk in chronic respiratory disease. *American Journal of Diseases of Children* 103(1962):40–60.

60. Zeiger, R. S. Dietary aspects of food allergy prevention in infants and children. *Journal of Pediatrics Gastroenterology and Nutrition* 30(2000): S77–S86.

61. Sicherer, S. H. Food allergy: when and how to perform oral food challenges. *Pediatric Allergy and Immunology* 10(1999):226–34.

62. Caffarelli, C., Terzi, V., Perrone, F., Cavagni, G. Food related, exercise induced anaphylaxis. *Archives of Diseases in Childhood* 75(1996):141–4.

63. Tilles, S., Schocket, A., Milgram, H. Exercise-induced anaphylaxis related to specific foods. *Journal of Pediatrics* 127(1995):587–9.

64. Hide, D. W., Matthews, S., Tariq, S., Arshad, S. H. Allergen avoidance in infancy and allergy at 4 years of age. *Allergy* 51(1996):89–93.

65. Platts-Mills, T., Vaughan, J., Squillace, S., et al. Sensitization, asthma and a modified Th2 response in children exposed to cat allergen: a population-based cross-sectional study. *Lancet* 357(2001):752–6.

66. Avner, D. B., Perzanowski, M. S., Platts-Mills, T. A. E., et al. Evaluation of different techniques for washing cats: quantitation of allergen removed from the cat and the effect on airborne Fel D 1. *Journal of Allergy and Clinical Immunology* 100(1997):307–12.

67. McDonald, L. G., Tovey, E. The role of water temperature and laundry procedures in reducing house dust mite populations and allergen content of bedding. Ibid. 90(1992):599–608.

68. Huang, S. W. The effects of an air cleaner in the homes of children with perennial allergic rhinitis. *Pediatric Asthma, Allergy, and Immunology* 7(1993):111–7.

69. Tovey, E. R., McDonald, L. G. A simple washing procedure with eucalyptus oil for controlling house dust mites and their allergens in clothing and bedding. *Journal of Allergy and Clinical Immunology* 100(1997):464–6.

70. Kemp, T. J., Siebers, R. W., Fishwick, D., et al. House dust mite allergen in pillows. *British Medical Journal* 313(1996):916.

71. Huang, S. W., Kimbrough, J. W. Effect of air cleaners on mold count in the air and on the symptoms of perennial rhinitis. *Pediatric Asthma, Allergy, and Immunology* 9(1995): 205–11.

72. Georgitis, J. W. Local hyperthermia and nasal irrigation for perennial allergic rhinitis: effect on symptoms and nasal airflow. *Annals of Allergy* 71(1993):385–9.

73. Zachariae, R., Bjerring, P. Increase and decrease of delayed cutaneous reactions obtained by hypnotic suggestions during sensitization. Studies on dinitrochlorobenzene and diphenylcyclopropenone. *Allergy* 48(1993):6–11.

74. Perloff, M. M., Spiegelman, J. Hypnosis in the treatment of a child's allergy to dogs. *American Journal of Clinical Hypnosis* 15(1973):269–72.

75. Anbar, R. D. Self-hypnosis for management of chronic dyspnea in pediatric patients. *Pediatrics* 107(2001):e21.

76. Locke, S. E., Ransil, B. J., Zachariae, R., et al. Effect of hypnotic suggestion on the delayed-type hypersensitivity response. *JAMA* 272(1994):47–52.

77. Joos, S., Schott, C., Zou, H., et al. Immunomodulatory effects of acupuncture in the treatment of allergic asthma: a randomized controlled study. *Journal of Alternative and Complementary Medicine* 6(2000):519–25.

78. Chari, P., Biwas, S., Mann, S. B. S., et al. Acupuncture therapy in allergic rhinitis. *American Journal of Acupuncture* 16(1988):143–7.

79. Xinsheng, L., Ling, S., Re, J., et al. Acupuncture treatment of Type 1 allergic diseases: a clinical observation. *International Journal of Clinical Acupuncture* 3(1992):109–15.

80. Knipschild, P., Kleijnen, J., Ter Riet, G. Belief in the efficacy of alternative medicine among general practitioners in the Netherlands. *Social Science and Medicine* 31(1990):625–6.

81. Reilly, D. T., Taylor, M. A., McSharry, C., et al. Is homeopathy a placebo response? Controlled trial of homeopathic potency, with pollen in hay fever as a model. *Lancet* 2(1986):881–6; Wiesenauer, M., Ludtke, R. A meta-analysis of the homeopathic treatment of pollinosis with *Galphimia glauca. Forsch Komplementarmed* 3(1996):230–4; Taylor, M. A., Reilly, D., Llewellyn-Jones, R. H., et al. Randomized controlled trial of homeopathy vs. placebo in perennial allergic rhinitis with overview of four trial series. *British Medical Journal* 321(2000):471–6; Weiser, M., Gegenheimer, L. H., Klein, P. A randomized equivalence trial comparing the efficacy and safety of Luffa comp.-Heel nasal spray compared with cromolyn sodium spray in the treatment of seasonal allergic rhinitis. *Forsch Komplementarmed* 6(1999):142–8.

82. Kleijnen, J., Knipschild, P., Ter Riet, G. Clinical trials of homeopathy. *British Medical Journal* 302(1991):316–23.

83. Gennuso, J., Epstein, L. H., Paluch, R. A., et al. The relationship between asthma and obesity in urban minority children and adolescents. *Archives of Pediatrics and Adolescent Medicine* 152(1998):1197–1200.

## Chapter 5: Asthma

1. Centers for Disease Control. Asthma-United States, 1982–1992. *Morbidity and Mortality Weekly Report* 51(1995):952–5.

2. Upton, M. N., McConnachie, A., McSharry, C., et al. Intergenerational 20-year trends in the prevalence of asthma and hay fever in adults: the Midspan family study surveys of parents

and offspring. *British Medical Journal.* 321(2000): 88–92; Sears, M. R. Epidemiology of childhood asthma. *Lancet* 350(1997):1015–20; ISAAC Steering Committee. Worldwide variation in prevalence of symptoms of asthma, allergic rhinoconjunctivitis and atopic eczema. Ibid. 351(1998):1225–32.

3. Crain, E. F., Weiss, K. B., Bijur, P. E., et al. An estimate of the prevalence of asthma and wheezing among inner city children. *Pediatrics* 94(1994):356–62; Joseph, C. L., Foxman, B., Leickly, F. E., et al. Prevalence of possible undiagnosed asthma and associated morbidity among urban schoolchildren. *Journal of Pediatrics* 129(1996):735–42.

4. Brooks, A. M., Byrd, R. S., Weitzman, M., et al. Impact of low birth weight on early childhood asthma in the United States. *Archives of Pediatrics and Adolescent Medicine* 155(2001): 401–6; Clark, C. E., Coote, J. M., Silver, D. A. T., et al. Asthma after childhood pneumonia: six year follow up study. *British Medical Journal* 320(2000):1514–6; Dodge, R., Martinez, D. M., Cline, M. G., et al. Early childhood respiratory symptoms and the subsequent diagnosis of asthma. *Journal of Allergy and Clinical Immunology* 98(1996):48–54.

5. Liu, L. L., Stout, J. W., Sullivan, M., et al. Asthma and bronchiolitis hospitalizations among American Indian children. *Archives of Pediatrics and Adolescent Medicine* 154(2000):991–6; Taylor, W. R., Newacheck, P. W. Impact of childhood asthma on health. *Pediatrics* 90(1992):657–62; Yunginger, J. W., Reed, C. E., O'Connell, E. J., et al. A community-based study of the epidemiology of asthma: incidence rates, 1964–1983. *American Review of Respiratory Disease* 146(1992):888–94; Weitzman, M., Gortmaker, S., Sobol, A. Racial, social, and environmental risks for childhood asthma. *American Journal of Diseases of Children* 144(1990):1189–94.

6. Gennuso, J., Epstein, L. H., Paluch, T. A., et al. The relationship between asthma and obesity in urban minority children and adolescents. *Archives of Pediatrics and Adolescent Medicine* 152(1998):1197–1200.

7. Skobeloff, E. M., Spivey, W. H., Silverman, R.,

et al. The effect of the menstrual cycle on asthma presentations in the emergency department. *Archives of Internal Medicine* 156(1996):1837–40.

8. Glauber, J. H., Farber, H. J., Homer, C. J. Asthma clinical pathways: toward what end? *Pediatrics* 106(2000):590–2.

9. Kwong, K. Y. C., Jones, C. A. Chronic asthma therapy. *Pediatrics in Review* 20(1999):327–34.

10. Strachan, D. P., Butland, B. K., Anderson, H. R. Incidence and prognosis of asthma and wheezing illness from early childhood to age 33 in a national British cohort. *British Medical Journal* 312(1996):1195–9.

11. McConnochie, K. M., Russo, M. J., McBride, J. T., et al. Socioeconomic variation in asthma hospitalization: excess utilization or greater need? *Pediatrics* 103(1999):e75.

12. Steinman, H. A., Weinberg, E. G. The effects of soft-drink preservatives on asthmatic children. *South African Medical Journal* 70(1986):404–6; Freedman, B. J. Asthma induced by sulphur dioxide, benzoate and tartrazine contained in orange drinks. *Clinical Allergy* 7(1977):407–15.

13. Mannix, E. T., Farber, M. O., Palange, P., et al. Exercise-induced asthma in figure skaters. *Chest* 109(1996):312–5.

14. Gustafsson, P. A., Bjorksten, B., Kjellman, N. I. Family dysfunction in asthma: a prospective study of illness development. *Journal of Pediatrics* 125(1994):493–8.

15. Partridge, M. R. Dishing the dirt. *British Medical Journal* 321(2000):58.

16. Harding, S. M., Richter, J. E., Guzzo, M. R., et al. Asthma and gastroesophageal reflux: acid suppressive therapy improves asthma outcome. *American Journal of Medicine* 100(1996):395–405.

17. Schuh, S., Johnson D. W., Stephens, D., et al. Comparison of albuterol delivered by metered dose inhaler with spacer versus a nebulizer in children with mild acute asthma. *Journal of Pediatrics* 135(1999):22–7; Chou, K. J., Cunningham, S. J., Crain, E. F. Metered-dose inhalers with spacers vs. nebulizers for pediatric asthma. *Archives of Pediatrics and Adolescent Medicine* 149(1995):201–5; Parkin,

P. C., Saunders, N. R., Diamond, S. A., et al. Randomised trial spacer vs. nebuliser for acute asthma. *Archives of Diseases in Childhood* 72(1995):239–40.

18. Croft, R. D. Two-year-old asthmatics can learn to operate a tube spacer by copying their mother. Ibid. 64(1989):742–3; Wildhaber, J. H., Dore, N. D., Wilson, J. M., et al. Inhalation therapy in asthma: nebulizer or pressurized metered-dose inhaler with holding chamber? In vivo comparison of lung deposition in children. *Journal of Pediatrics* 135(1999):28–33.

19. Kramarz, P., DeStefano, F., Gargiullo, P. M., et al. Does influenza vaccination prevent asthma exacerbations in children? Ibid. 138(2001):306–10.

20. Fairchok, M. P., Trementozzi, D. P., Carter, P. S., et al. Effect of prednisone on response to influenza virus vaccine in asthmatic children. *Archives of Pediatrics and Adolescent Medicine* 152(1998):1191–5.

21. Rowe, B. H., Bota, G. W., Fabris, L., et al. Inhaled budesonide in addition to oral corticosteroids to prevent asthma relapse following discharge from the emergency department. *JAMA* 281(1999):2119–26.

22. Perera, B. J. C. Efficacy and cost-effectiveness of inhaled steroids in asthma in a developing country. *Archives of Diseases in Childhood* 72(1995):312–6.

23. Matthews, E. E., Curtis, P. D., McLain, B. I., et al. Nebulized budesonide versus oral steroid in severe exacerbations of childhood asthma. *Acta Paediatrica* 88(1999):841–3.

24. Baker, J. W., Mellon, M., Wald, J., et al. A multiple-dosing, placebo-controlled study of budesonide inhalation suspension given once or twice daily for treatment of persistent asthma in young children and infants. *Pediatrics* 103(1999):414–21.

25. Ferguson, A. C., Spier, S., Manjra, A., et al. Efficacy and safety of high-dose inhaled steroids in children with asthma: a comparison of fluticasone proprionate with budesonide. *Journal of Pediatrics* 134(1999):422–7; Moller, C., Stromberg, L., Oldaeus, G., et al. Efficacy of once daily versus twice daily administration of budesonide by turbohaler in children with stable asthma. *Pediatric Pulmonology* 28(1999):337–43.

26. Lipworth, B., J. Systemic adverse effects of inhaled corticosteroid therapy: a systematic review and meta-analysis. *Archives of Internal Medicine* 159(1999):941–55.

27. Sharek, P. J., Bergman, D. A. The effect of inhaled steroids on the linear growth of children with asthma: a meta-analysis. *Pediatrics* 106(2000):e8.

28. Heuck, C., Wolthers, O. D., Kollerup, G., et al. Adverse effects of inhaled budesonide on growth and collagen turnover in children with asthma. *Journal of Pediatrics* 133(1998):608–12.

29. Donahue, J. G., Weiss, S. T., Livingston, J. M., et al. Inhaled steroids and the risk of hospitalization for asthma. *JAMA* 277(1997):887–91.

30. Connett, G. J., Warde, C., Wooler, E., et al. Prednisolone and salbutamol in the hospital treatment of acute asthma. *Archives of Diseases in Childhood* 70(1994):170–3.

31. Grant, G. C., Duggan, A. K., Santosham, M., DeAngelis, C. Oral prednisone as a risk factor for infections in children with asthma. *Archives of Pediatrics and Adolescent Medicine* 150(1996):58–63.

32. Schuckman, H., DeJulius, D. P., Blanda, M., et al. Comparison of intramuscular triamcinolone and oral prednisone in the outpatient treatment of acute asthma: a randomized controlled trial. *Annals of Emergency Medicine* 31(1998):333–5.

33. Shrewsbury, S., Pyke, S., Britton, M. Meta-analysis of increased dose of inhaled steroid or addition of salmeterol in symptomatic asthma. *British Medical Journal* 320(2000): 1368–73.

34. Wilding, P., Clark, M., Coon, J. T., et al. Effect of long-term treatment with salmeterol on asthma control: a double-blind, randomized crossover study. Ibid. 314(1997):1441–6; Condemi, J., Goldstein, S., Kalberg, C., et al. The addition of salmeterol to fluticasone propionate versus increasing the dose of fluticasone in patients with persistent asthma. *Annals of Allergy, Asthma, and Immunology* 82(1999):383–9.

35. Simons, F. E. R., Gerstner, T. V., Cheang, M. S.,

et al. Tolerance to the bronchoprotective effect of salmeterol in adolescents with exercise-induced asthma using concurrent inhaled glucocorticoid treatment. *Pediatrics* 99(1997): 655–9.

36. Ploid, D., Chapuis, F. R., Stamm, D., et al. High-dose albuterol by metered-dose inhaler plus a spacer device versus nebulization in preschool children with recurrent wheezing: a double-blind, randomized equivalence trial. Ibid. 106(2000):311–7.

37. Weinberger, M., Hendeles, L. Theophylline in asthma. *New England Journal of Medicine* 334(1996):1380–8.

38. Stein, M. A., Krasowski, M., Leventhal, B. L., et al. Behavioral and cognitive effects of methylxanthines. *Archives of Pediatrics and Adolescent Medicine* 150(1996):284–8; Bender, B. G., Ikle, D. N., DuHamel, T., et al. Neuropsychological and behavioral changes in asthmatic children treated with beclomethasone diproprionate versus thephylline. *Pediatrics* 101(1998):355–60.

39. Evans, D. J., Taylor, D. A., Zetterstrom, O., et al. A comparison of low-dose inhaled budesonide plus theophylline and high-dose inhaled budesonide for moderate asthma. *New England Journal of Medicine* 337(1997):1412–8.

40. Yung, M., South, M. Randomized controlled trial of aminophylline for severe, acute asthma. *Archives of Disease in Childhood* 79(1998):405–10.

41. Lord, J., Ducharme, M. D., Stamp, R. J., et al. Cost effectiveness analysis of inhaled cholinergics for acute childhood and adolescent asthma. *British Medical Journal* 319(1999): 1470–1; Rodrigo, G., Rodrigo, C., Burschtin, O. A meta-analysis of the effects of ipratropium bromide in adults with acute asthma. *American Journal of Medicine* 107(1999):363–70; Zorc, J. J., Pusic, M. V., Ogborn, J., et al. Ipratropium bromide added to asthma treatment in the pediatric emergency department. *Pediatrics* 103(1999): 748–52.

42. Lin, R. Y., Pesola, G. E., Bakalchuk, L., et al. Superiority of ipratropium plus albuterol over albuterol alone in the emergency department management of adult asthma: a randomized clinical trial. *Annals of Emergency Medicine* 31(1998):208–13.

43. Qureshi, F., Pestian, J., Davis, P., et al. Effect of nebulized ipratropium on the hospitalization rates of children with asthma. *New England Journal of Medicine* 339(1998):1030–5; Plotnick, L. H., Ducharme, F. M. Should inhaled anticholinergics be added to beta agonists for treating acute childhood and adolescent asthma? A Systematic review. *British Medical Journal* 317(1998):971–7.

44. Fost, D. A., Spahn, J. D. The leukotriene modifiers: a new class of asthma medication. *Contemporary Pediatrics* 15(1998):95–108.

45. Bisgaard, H. Leukotriene modifiers in pediatric asthma management. *Pediatrics* 107(2001):381–90.

46. Israel, E., Cohn, J., Dube, L., et al. Effect of treatment with zileuton, a 5-lipoxygenase inhibitor, in patients with asthma. *JAMA* 275(1996):931–6.

47. Pearlman, D. S., Ostrom, N. K., Bronsky, E. A., et al. The leukotriene D4-receptor antagonist zafirlukast attenuates exercise-induced bronchoconstriction in children. *Journal of Pediatrics* 134(1999):273–9.

48. Leff, J. A., Busse, W. W., Pearlman, D., et al. Montelukast, a leukotriene-receptor antagonist, for the treatment of mild asthma and exercise-induced bronchoconstriction. *New England Journal of Medicine* 339(1998):147–52; Kemp, J. P., Dockhorn, R. J., Shapiro, G. G., et al. Montelukast once daily inhibits exercise-induced bronchoconstriction in 6- to 14-year-old children with asthma. *Journal of Pediatrics* 133(1998):424–8.

49. Knorr, B., Matz, J., Bernstein, J. A., et al. Montelukast for chronic asthma in 6- to 14-year-old children. *JAMA* 279(1998):1181–6; Lofdahl, C. G., Reiss, T. F., Leff, J. A., et al. Randomized, placebo controlled trial of effect of a leukotriene receptor antagonist, Montelukast, on tapering inhaled corticosteroids in asthmatic patients. *British Medical Journal* 319(1999):87–90; Malmstrom, K., Rodriguez-Gomez, G., Guerra, J., et al. Oral montelukast, inhaled betamethasone and

placebo for chronic asthma. *Annals of Internal Medicine* 130(1999):487–95.

50. Vinuya, R. Z. Specific allergen immunotherapy for allergic rhinitis and asthma. *Pediatric Annals* 29(2000):425–32; Hedlin, G., Wille, S., Browaldh, L., et al. Immunotherapy in children with allergic asthma: effect on bronchial hyperreactivity and pharmacotherapy. *Journal of Allergy and Clinical Immunology* 103(1999): 609–14.

51. Carter, E. R., Webb, C. R., Moffitt, D. R. Evaluation of heliox in children hospitalized with acute severe asthma. *Chest* 109(1996):1256–61; Kudukis, T. M., Manthous, C. A., Schmidt, G. A., et al. Inhaled helium-oxygen revisited: Effect of inhaled helium-oxygen during the treatment of status asthmatics in children. *Journal of Pediatrics* 130(1997):217–24.

52. Kuo, Y. C., Tsai, W. J., Wang, J. Y., et al. Regulation of broncho-alveolar lavage fluids cell function by the immunoregulatory agents from *Cordyceps sinensis*. *Life Sciences* 68(2001):1067–82.

53. Ghosh, D., Wawrzak, V., Pletnev, M., et al. Molecular mechanism of inhibition of steroid dehydrogenases by licorice-derived steroid analogs in modulation of steroid receptor function. *Annals of the New York Academy of Sciences* 761(1995):341–3.

54. Epstein, M. T., Espiner, E. A., Donald, R. A., Hughes, H. Effect of eating liquorice on the renin-angiotensin aldosterone axis in normal subjects. *British Medical Journal* 1(1977): 488–90.

55. Hamasaki, Y., Kobayashi, I., Hayasaki, R., et al. The Chinese herbal medicine, Shinpi-To, inhibits EgE mediated leukotriene synthesis in rat basophilic leukemia-2H3 cells. *Journal of Ethnopharmacology* 56(1997):123–31; Kobayashi, I., Hamasaki, Y., Sato, R., et al. Saiboku-To, an herbal extract mixture, selectively inhibits 5-lipoxygenase activity in leukotriene synthesis in rat basophilic leukemia-1 cells. Ibid. 48(1995):33–41.

56. Nakajima, S., Tohda, Y., Ohkawa, K., et al. Effects of Saiboku-To (TJ-96) on bronchial asthma. *Annals of the New York Academy of Sciences* 685(1993):549–60.

57. Bielory, L., Lupoli, K. Herbal interventions in asthma and allergy. *Journal of Asthma* 36(1999):1–65.

58. Schwarz, J. Caffeine intake and asthma symptoms. *Annals of Epidemiology* 2(1992):627–35.

59. Dorsch, W., Wagner, H., Bayer, T., et al. Antiasthmatic effects of onions: alk(en)ylsulfiniothioic acid alk(en)yl-esters inhibit histamine release, leukotriene and thromboxane biosynthesis in vitro and counteract PAF and allergen-induced bronchial constriciton in vivo. *Biochemical Pharmacology* 37(1988):4479–86.

60. Dorsch, W., Weber, J. Prevention of allergen-induced bronchial obstruction in sensitized guinea pigs by crude alcoholic onion extract. *Agents and Actions* 14(1984):626–9.

61. Geyman, J. P. Anaphylactic reaction after ingestion of bee pollen. *Journal of the American Board of Family Practice* 7(1994):250–2.

62. Smith, P. F., MacLennan, K., Darlington, C. L. The neuroprotective properties of the *Ginkgo biloba* leaf: a review of the possible relationship to platelet-activating factor (PAF). *Journal of Ethnopharmacology* 50(1996):131–9.

63. Kose, K., Dogan, P. Lipoperoxidation induced by hydrogen peroxide in human erythrocyte membranes. 2. Comparison of the antioxidant effect of *Ginkgo biloba* extract (EGb 761) with those of water-soluble and lipid soluble antioxidants. *Journal of International Medical Research* 23(1995):9–18.

64. Guinot, P., Brambilla, C., Duchier, J., et al. Effect of BN-52063, a specific PAF-acether antagonist, on bronchial provocation test to allergens in asthmatic patients: a preliminary study. *Prostaglandins* 34(1987):723–31.

65. Bauer, K. Pharmacodynamic effects of inhaled dry powder formulations of fenoterol and colforsin in asthma. *Clinical Pharmacology and Therapeutics* 53(1993):76–83.

66. Gupta, S. *Tylophora indica* in bronchial asthma—a double-blind study. *Indian Journal of Medicine* 69(1979):981–9; Thiruvengadam, K. V., Haranath, K., Sudarsan, S., et al. Tylophora indica in bronchial asthma. A controlled comparison with a stand ard anti-asthmatic drug. *Journal of the Indian Medical Association* 71(1978):172–6.

67. Gupta, I., Gupta, V., Parihar, A., et al. Effects of *Boswellia serrata* gum resin in patients with bronchial asthma: results of a double-blind placebo-controlled, 6-week clinical study. *European Journal of Medical Research* 3(1998):511–4.

68. Govindan, S., Viswanathan, S., Vijayasekaran, V., et al. A pilot study on the clinical efficacy of *Solanum xanthocarpum* and *Solanum trlobatum* in bronchial asthma. *Journal of Ethnopharmacology* 66(1999):205–10.

69. Pachter, L. M., Cloutier, M. M., Bernstein, B. A. Ethnomedical (folk) remedies for childhood asthma in a mainland Puerto Rican community. *Archives of Pediatrics and Adolescent Medicine* 149(1995):982–9.

70. Reynolds, R. D., Natta, C. L. Depressed plasma pyridoxal phosphate concentrations in adult asthmatics. *American Journal of Clinical Nutrition* 41(1985):684–8.

71. Sur, S., Camara, M., Buchmeier, A., Morgan, S., Nelson, H. S. Double-blind trial of pyridoxine (vitamin B6) in the treatment of steroid-dependent asthma. *Annals of Allergy* 70(1993): 147–52.

72. Collipp, P. J., Goldzier, S., Weiss, N., et al. Pyridoxine treatment of childhood bronchial asthma. Ibid. 35(1975):93–7; Kaslow, J. E. Double-blind trial of pyridoxine (vitamin B6) in the treatment of steroid-dependent asthma. Ibid. 71(1993): 492.

73. Forastiere, F., Pistelli, R., Sestini, P., et al. Consumption of fresh fruit rich in vitamin C and wheezing symptoms in children. *Thorax* 55(2000):283–8.

74. Soutar, A., Seaton, A., Brown, K. Bronchial reactivity and dietary antioxidants. Ibid. 52(1997):166–70.

75. Mohsenin, V., Dubois, A. B., Douglas, J. S. Effect of ascorbic acid on response to methacholine challenge in asthmatic subjects. *American Review of Respiratory Disease* 127(1983):143–7; Mudway, I. S., Krishna, M. T., Frew, A. J., et al. Compromised concentrations of ascorbate in fluid lining the respiratory tract in human subjects after exposure to ozone. *Occupational Environmental Medicine* 56(1999):473–81.

76. Tolbert, P. E., Mulholland, J. A., MacIntosh, D. L., et al. Air quality and pediatric emergency room visits for asthma in Atlanta, Georgia. *American Journal of Epidemiology* 151(2000):798–810.

77. Grievink, L., Zijlstra, A. G., Ke, X., et al. Double-blind intervention trial on modulation of ozone effects on pulmonary function by antioxidant supplements. Ibid. 149(1999): 306–14; Romieu, I., Meneses, F., Ramirez, M., et al. Antioxidant supplementation and respiratory functions among workers exposed to high levels of ozone. *American Journal of Respiratory and Critical Care Medicine* 158(1998):226–32.

78. Cohen, H. A., Neuman, I., Nahum, H. Blocking effect of vitamin C in exercise-induced asthma. *Archives of Pediatrics and Adolescent Medicine* 151(1997):367–70.

79. Anah, C., Jarike, L., Baig, H. High dose ascorbic acid in Nigerian asthmatics. *Tropical and Geographical Medicine* 32(1980):132–7.

80. Britton, J., Pavord, I., Richards, K., et al. Dietary magnesium, lung function, wheezing and airway hyper-reactivity in a random adult population sample. *Lancet* 344(1994):357–62; Soutar, A., Seaton, A., Brown, K. Bronchial reactivity and dietary antioxidants. *Thorax* 52(1997):166–70; Baker, J. C., Tunnicliffe, W. S., Duncanson, R. C., et al. Dietary antioxidants and magnesium in type 1 brittle asthma: a case control study. Ibid. 54(1999):115–8.

81. Rowe, B. H., Bretzlaff, J. A., Bourdon, C., et al. Intravenous magnesium sulfate treatment for acute asthma in the emergency department: a systematic review of the literature. *Annals of Emergency Medicine* 36(2000):181–90; Ciarallo, L., Brousseau, D., Reinert, S. Higher-dose intravenous magnesium therapy for children with moderate to severe acute asthma. *Archives of Pediatrics and Adolescent Medicine* 154(2000):979–83.

82. Hill, J., Micklewright, A., Lewis, S., Britton, J. Investigation of the effect of short-term change in dietary magnesium intake in asthma. *European Respiratory Journal* 10(1997):2225–9.

83. Demissie, K., Ernst, P., Gray, Donald, K., Joseph, L. Usual dietary salt intake and

asthma in children: a case-control study. *Thorax* 51(1996):59–63.

84. Broughton, K. S., Johnson, C. S., Pace, B. K., et al. Reduced asthma symptoms with n-3 fatty acid ingestion are related to 5-series leukotriene production. *American Journal of Clinical Nutrition* 65(1997):1011–7.

85. Hodge, L., Salome, C. M., Peat, J. K., et al. Consumption of oily fish and childhood asthma risk. *Medical Journal Australia* 164(1996): 137–40; Britton, J. Dietary fish oil and airways obstruction. *Thorax* 50(1995):S11–S15; Schwartz, J., Weiss, S. T. The relationship of dietary fish intake to level of pulmonary function in the first National Health and Nutrition Survey (NHANES I). *European Respiratory Journal* 7(1994):1821–4.

86. Nagakura, T., Matsuda, S., Shichijyo, K., et al. Dietary supplementation with fish oil rich in omega-3 polyunsaturated fatty acids in children with bronchial asthma. Ibid. 16(2000):861–5.

87. Villani, F., Comazzi, R., DeMaria, P., et al. Effect of dietary supplementation with polyunsaturated fatty acids on bronchial hyperreactivity in subjects with seasonal asthma. *Respiration* 65(1998):265–9.

88. Hodge, L., Salome, C. M., Hughes, J. M., et al. Effect of dietary intake of omega-3 and omega-6 fatty acids on severity of asthma in children. *European Respiratory Journal* 11(1998):361–5.

89. Dry, J. Effect of a fish oil diet on asthma: results of a one-year double-blind study. *International Archives of Allergy and Applied Immunology* 95(1991):156–7.

90. Gennuso, J., Epstein, L. H., Paluch, R. A., et al. The relationship between asthma and obesity in urban minority children and adolescents. *Archives of Pediatrics and Adolescent Medicine* 152(1998):1197–1200.

91. Woods, R. K., Abramson, M., Raven, J. M., et al. Reported food intolerance and respiratory symptoms in young adults. *European Respiratory Journal* 11(1998):151–5.

92. Unge, G., Grubbstrom, J., Olsson, P., et al. Effects of dietary tryptophan restrictions on clinical symptoms in patients with endogenous asthma. *Allergy* 38(1983):211–2.

93. Carey, O. J., Cookson, J. B., Britton, J.,

Tattersfield, A. E. The effect of lifestyle on wheeze, atopy, and bronchial hyperreactivity in Asian and white children. *American Journal of Respiratory and Critical Care Medicine* 154(1996):537–40.

94. Lindahl, O., Lindwall, L., Spangberg, A., et al. Vegan regimen with reduced medication in the treatment of bronchial asthma. *Journal of Asthma* 22(1985):45–55; Hoj, L., Osterballe, O., Bundgaard, A., Weeke, B., Weiss, M. A double-blind controlled trial of elemental diet in severe, perennial asthma. *Allergy* 36(1981): 257–62; Harsono, A., Partana, J. S., Partana, L. The allergy management of bronchial asthma in children in Surabaya. *Pediatrica Indonesiana* 30(1990):266–9.

95. Woods, R. K., Weiner, J., Abramson, M., Thien, F., Walters, E. H. Patients' perceptions of food-induced asthma. *Australia and New Zealand Journal of Medicine* 26(1996):504–12.

96. Wilson, N. M. Bronchial hyperactivity in food and drink tolerance. *Annals of Allergy* 61(1988): 75–9.

97. Haas, F., Bishop, M. C., Salazar-Schicchi, J., et al. Effect of milk ingestion on pulmonary function in healthy and asthmatic subjects. *Journal of Asthma* 28(1991):349–55.

98. Woods, R. K., Weiner, J. M., Abramson, M., Thien, F., Walters, E. H. Do dairy products induce bronchoconstriction in adults with asthma? *Journal of Allergy and Clinical Immunology* 101(1998):45–50.

99. Gagnon, L., Boulet, L. P., Brown, J., et al. Influence of inhaled corticosteroids and dietary intake on bone density and metabolism in patients with moderate to severe asthma. *Journal of the American Dietetic Association* 97(1997):1401–6.

100. Porro, E., Indinnimeo, L., Antognoni, G., et al. Early wheezing and breast-feeding. *Journal of Asthma* 30(1993):23–8; Wright, A. L., Holberg, C. J., Taussig, L. M., et al. Relationship of infant feeding to recurrent wheezing at age 6 years. *Archives of Pediatrics and Adolescent Medicine* 149(1995):758–63; Saarinene, U. M., Kajosaari, M. Breast-feeding as prophylaxis against atopic disease: prospective follow-up study until 17 years old. *Lancet* 346(1995):

1065–9; Oddy, W. H., Holt, P. G., Sly, P. D., et al. Association between breast-feeding and asthma in 6-year-old children: findings of a prospective birth cohort study. *British Medical Journal* 319(1999):815–9.

101. Dorsch, W., Scharff, J., Bayer, T., et al. Antiasthmatic effects of onions. *International Archives of Allergy and Applied Immunology* 88(1989):228–30; Wagner, H., Dorsch, W., Bayer, T. H., et al. Antiasthmatic effects of onions: inhibition of 5-lipoxygenase and cyclooxygenase in vitro by thiosulfinates and cepaenes. *Prostagland in Leukotriene Essential Fatty Acids* 39(1990):59–62.

102. Birkel, D. A., Edgren, L. Hatha Yoga: improved vital capacity of college students. *Alternative Therapies in Health and Medicine* 6(2000):55–63; Jain, S. C., Talukdar, B. Evaluation of yoga therapy programme for patients of bronchial asthma. *Singapore Medical Journal* 34(1993): 306–8; Nagarathna, R., Nagendra, H. R. Yoga for bronchial asthma: a controlled study. *British Medical Journal* 291(1985):1077–9; Khanam, A. A., Sachdeva, U., Guleria, R., et al. Study of pulmonary and autonomic functions of asthma patients after yoga training. *Indian Journal of Physiology and Pharmacology* 40(1996):318–24.

103. Vedanthan, P. K., Kesavalu, L. N., Murthy, K. C., et al. Clinical study of yoga techniques in university students with asthma: a controlled study. *Allergy Asthma Proceedings* 19(1998):3–9.

104. Singh, V. Effect of respiratory exercises on asthma: the pink city lung exerciser. *Journal of Asthma* 24(1987):355–9.

105. Nagendra, H. R., Nagarantha, R. An integrated approach of yoga therapy for bronchial asthma: a 3–54 month prospective study. Ibid. 23(1986):123–37.

106. Jain, S. C., Rai, L., Valecha, A., et al. Effect of yoga training on exercise tolerance in adolescents with childhood asthma. Ibid. 28(1991): 437–42.

107. Tiep, B. L., Burns, M., Kao, D., et al. Pursed lips breathing training using ear oximetry. *Chest* 90(1986):218–21.

108. Buchholz, I. Breathing, voice and movement therapy: applications to breathing disorders. *Biofeedback Self-Regulation* 19(1994):141–53.

109. Fluge, T., Richter, J., Fabel, H., Zysno, E., Weller, E., Wagner, T. O. Long-term effects of breathing exercises and yoga in patients with bronchial asthma. *Pneumologie* 48(1994): 484–90.

110. Opat, A. J., Cohen, M. M., Bailey, M. J., et al. A clinical trial of the Buteyko breathing technique in asthma as taught by a video. *Journal of Asthma* 37(2000):557–64.

111. Bowler, S. D., Green, A., Mitchell, C. A. Buteyko breathing techniques in asthma: a blinded, randomized controlled trial. *Medical Journal of Australia* 169(1998):575–8.

112. Gras, N. B., Benchetrit, G. Voluntary control of breathing pattern in asthmatic children. *Percept Motor Skills* 83(1996):1384–6.

113. Huang, S. W., Veiga, R., Sila, U., Reed, E., Hines, S. The effect of swimming in asthmatic children—participants in a swimming program in the city of Baltimore. *Journal of Asthma* 26(1989):117–21.

114. Tanizaki, Y., Kitani, H., Okazaki, M., et al. Clinical effects of complex spa therapy on patients with steroid-dependent intractable asthma (SDIA). *Aerugi-Japanese Journal of Allergology* 42(1993):219–27.

115. Lanphear, B. P., Aligne, A., Auinger, P., et al. Residential exposures associated with asthma in U.S. children. *Pediatrics* 107(2001):505–11.

116. Wood, R. A., Johnson, E. F., Van Natta, M. L., et al. A placebo-controlled trial of a HEPA air cleaner in the treatment of cat allergy. *American Journal of Respiratory and Critical Care Medicine* 158(1998):115–20.

117. Hidden life of spider plants. *University of California at Berkeley Wellness Letter* 10(1994): 1–2.

118. Vanlaar, C. H., Peat, J. K., Marks, G. B., et al. Domestic control of house dust mite allergen in children's beds. *Journal of Allergy and Clinical Immunology* 105(2000):1130–3.

119. Harving, H., Korsgaard, J., Dahl, R. Clinical efficacy of reduction in house-dust mite exposure in specially designed, mechanically ventilated "healthy" homes. *Allergy* 49(1994):866–70.

120. Reiser, J., Ingram, D., Mitchell, E. B., et al.

House dust mite allergen levels and an anti-mite mattress spray (natamycin) in the treatment of childhood asthma. *Clinical and Experimental Allergy* 20(1990):561–7.

121. Warner, J. A., Marchant, J. L., Warner, J. O. Double-blind trial of ionisers in children with asthma sensitive to the house dust mite. *Thorax* 48(1993):330–3.

122. Hahn, D. L., Bukstein, D., Luskin, A., Zeitz, H. Evidence for *Chlamydia pneumoniae* infection in steroid-dependent asthma. *Annals Allergy and Asthma Immunology* 80(1998):45–9.

123. Rosenstreich, D. L., Eggleston, P., Kattan, M., et al. The role of cockroach allergy and exposure to cockroach allergen in causing morbidity and mortality among inner-city children with asthma. *New England Journal of Medicine* 336(1997):1356–63.

124. Lehrer, P. M. Emotionally triggered asthma: a review of research literature and some hypotheses for self-regulation therapies. *Applied Psychophysiology Biofeedback* 23(1998):13–41.

125. Bartlett, S. J., Kolodner, K., Butz, A. M., et al. Maternal depressive symptoms and emergency department use among inner-city children with asthma. *Archives of Pediatrics and Adolescent Medicine* 155(2001):346–53; Weil, C. M., Wade, S. L., Bauman, L. J., et al. The relationship between psychosocial factors and asthma morbidity in inner-city children with asthma. *Pediatrics* 104(1999): 1274–80.

126. Alexander, A. B., Miklich, D. R., Hershkoff, H. The immediate effects of systematic relaxation training on peak expiratory flow rates in asthmatic children. *Psychosomatic Medicine* 34(1972):388–94.

127. Kohen, D. P., Wynne, E. Applying hypnosis in a preschool family asthma education program: uses of storytelling, imagery and relaxation. *American Journal of Clinical Hypnosis* 39(1997):169–81; Smith, J. M., Burns, C. L. C. The treatment of asthmatic children by hypnotic suggestion. *British Journal of Diseases of the Chest* 54(1960):78–81.

128. Henry, M., DeRivera, J. L. G., Gonzalez-Martin, I. J., et al. Improvement of respiratory function in chronic asthmatic patients with autogenic therapy. *Journal of Psychosomatic Research* 37(1993):265–70.

129. Wilson, A. R., Honsberger, R., Chiu, T. J., Novey, H. S. Transcendental meditation and asthma. *Respiration* 32(1975):74–80.

130. Mass, R., Richter, R., Dahme, B. Biofeedback-induced voluntary reduction of respiratory resistance in severe bronchial asthma. *Behaviour Research and Therapy* 34(1996): 815–9.

131. Peper, E., Tibbetts, V. Fifteen-month follow-up with asthmatics utilizing EMG/Incentive inspirometer feedback. *Biofeedback and Self-Regulation* 17(1992):143–51.

132. Feldman, G. M. The effect of biofeedback training on respiratory resistance of asthmatic children. *Psychosomatic Medicine* 38(1976):27–34; Coen, B. L., Conran, P. B., McGrady, A., et al. Effects of biofeedback-assisted relaxation on asthma severity and immune function. *Pediatric Asthma, Allergy, and Immunology* 10(1996):71–8; Scherr, M. S., Crawford, P. L. Three-year evaluation of biofeedback techniques in the treatment of children with chronic asthma in a summer camp environment. *Annals of Allergy* 41(1978):288–92.

133. Smyth, J. M., et al. Effects of writing about stressful experiences on symptom reduction in patients with asthma or rheumatoid arthritis: a randomized trial. *JAMA* 281(1999): 1304–9.

134. Asher, M. I., Douglas, C., Airy, M., et al. Effects of chest physical therapy on lung function in children recovering from acute severe asthma. *Pediatric Pulmonology* 9(1990):146–51.

135. Field, T., Henteleff, T., Hernandez-Rief, M., et al. Children with asthma have improved pulmonary functions after massage therapy. *Journal of Pediatrics* 132(1998):854–8.

136. Nielsen, N. H., Bronfort, G., Bendix, M. F., Weeke, B. Chronic asthma and chiropractic manipulation: a randomized clinical trial. *Clinical and Experimental Allergy* 25(1995): 80–8; Balon, J., Aker, P. D., Crowther, E. R., et al. A comparison of active and simulated chiropractic manipulation as adjunctive treat-

ment for childhood asthma. *New England Journal of Medicine* 339(1998):1013–20.

137. Morton, A. R., Fazio, S. M., Miller, D. Efficacy of laser-acupuncture in the prevention of exercise-induced asthma. *Annals of Allergy* 70(1993):295–8; Tashkin, D. P., Kroening, R. J., Bresler, D. E., et al. A controlled trial of real and simulated acupuncture in the management of chronic asthma. *Journal of Allergy and Clinical Immunology* 76(1985):855–64; Tandon, M. K., Soh, P. F., Wood, A. T. Acupuncture for bronchial asthma? A double-blind crossover study. *Medical Journal Australia* 154(1991): 409–12; Biernacki, W., Peake, M. D. Acupuncture in treatment of stable asthma. *Respiratory Medicine* 92(1998):1143–5.

138. Joos, S., Schott, C., Zou, H., et al. Immunomodulatory effects of acupuncture in the treatment of allergic asthma: a randomized controlled study. *Journal of Alternative and Complementary Medicine* 6(2000):519–25; Jobst, K. A. Acupuncture in asthma and pulmonary disease: an analysis of efficacy and safety. Ibid. 2(1996):179–206.

139. Morton, A. R., Fazio, S. M., Miller, D. Efficacy of laser-acupuncture in the prevention of exercise-induced asthma. *Annals of Allergy* 70(1993):295–8; Fung, K. P., Chow, O. K. W., So, S. Y. Attenuation of exercise-induced asthma by acupuncture. *Lancet* 2(1986):1419–22.

140. Kemper, K. J., Sarah, R., Silver-Highfield, E., et al. On pins and needles: Pediatric pain patients' experience with acupuncture. *Pediatrics* 105(2000):941–7.

141. von Wacker, A. Healing in asthma—a pilot study. *Erfahrungsheilkunde,* July(1996):428–33.

142. Koenig, H. G. *The Healing Power of Faith: Science Explores Medicine's Last Great Frontier.* New York: Simon and Schuster, 1999.

143. Reilly, D., Taylor, M. A., Beattie, N. G. M., et al. Is evidence for homeopathy reproducible? *Lancet* 344(1994):1601–6.

## Chapter 6: Bed-Wetting (Enuresis)

1. Lovering, J. S., Tallett, S. E., McKendry, J. B. Oxybutynin efficacy in the treatment of primary enuresis. *Pediatrics* 82(1988):104–6.

2. Egger, J., Carter, C. H., Soothill, J. F., et al. Effect of diet treatment on enuresis in children with migraine or hyperkinetic behavior. *Clinical Pediatrics* 31(1992):302–7.

3. Esperanca, M., Gerrard, J. W. Nocturnal enuresis: Comparison of the effect of imipramine and dietary restriction on bladder capacity. *Canadian Medical Association Journal* 101(1969):65–8.

4. Pace, G., Aceto, G., Cormio, L., et al. Nocturnal enuresis can be caused by absorptive hypercalciuria. *Scandinavian Journal of Urology and Nephrology* 33(1999):111–4.

5. Banerjee, S., Srivastav, A., Palan, B. M. Hypnosis and self-hypnosis in the management of nocturnal enuresis: a comparative study with imipramine therapy. *American Journal of Clinical Hypnosis* 36(1993):113–9.

6. Combs, A. J., Glassberg, A. D., Gerdes, D., Horowitz, M. Biofeedback therapy for children with dysfunctional voiding. *Urology* 52(1998): 312–5.

7. LeBoeuf, C., Brown, P., Herman, A., et al. Chiropractic care of children with nocturnal enuresis: a prospective outcome study. *Journal of Manipulative and Physiological Therapy* 14(1991):110–5.

8. Bjorkstrom, G., Hellstrom, A. L., Andersson, S. Electro-acupuncture in the treatment of children with monosynaptic nocturnal enuresis. *Scandinavican Journal of Urology and Nephrology* 34(2000):21–6; Serel, T. A., Perk, H., Koyuncuoglu, H. R., et al. Acupuncture therapy in the management of persistent primary nocturnal enuresis. Ibid. 35(2001):40–3.

9. Baozhu, S., Xiyou, W. Short-term effect in 135 cases of enuresis treated by wrist-ankle needling. *Journal of Traditional Chinese Medicine* 5(1985):27–8.

10. Minni, B., Capozza, N., Creti, G., et al. Bladder instability and enuresis treated by acupuncture and electro-therapeutics: early urodynamic observations. *Acupuncture and Elctro-Therapeutics Research* 15(1990):19–25.

11. Capozza, N. Treatment of nocturnal enuresis: a comparative study between desmopressin and acupuncture used separately or in association. *JAMA* 267(1992):1741.

## Chapter 7: Burns

1. Korkmaz, A., Sahiner, U., Yurdakok, M. Chemical burn caused by topical vinegar application in a newborn infant. *Pediatric Dermatology* 17(2000):34–6.

2. Montemarano, A. D., Gupta, R. K., Burge, J. R., Klein, K. Insect repellents and the efficacy of sunscreens. *Lancet* 349(1997):1670–1.

3. Smack, D. P., Harrington, A. C., Dunn, C., et al. Infection and allergy incidence in ambulatory surgery patients using white petrolatum vs. bacitracin ointment. *JAMA.* 276(1996):972–7.

4. Kaplan, J. Z. Acceleration of wound healing by a live yeast cell derivative. *Archives of Surgery* 119(1984):1105–8.

5. Rodriguez-Bigas, M., Cruz, N. I., Suarez, A. Comparative evaluation of aloe vera in the management of burn wounds in guinea pigs. *Plastic Reconstructive Surgery* 81(1988):386–9.

6. O'Keefe, P. A trial of asiaticoside on skin graft donor areas. *British Journal of Plastic Surgery* 27(1974):194–5; Bosse, J. P., Papillon, J., Frenette, G., et al. Clinical study of a new antikeloid agent. *Annals of Plastic Surgery* 3(1979):13–21.

7. Maquart, F. X., Bellon, G., Gillery, P., et al. Stimulation of collagen synthesis in fibroblast cultures by a triterpene extracted from *Centella asiatica. Connective Tissue Research* 24(1990):107–20.

8. Izu, R., Aguirre, A., Gil, N., et al. Allergic contact dermatitis from a cream containing *Centella asiatica* extract. *Contact Dermatitis* 26(1992):192–3.

9. Ivancheva, S., Manolova, N., Serkedjieva, J., et al. Polyphenols from Bulgarian medicinal plants with anti-infectious activity. *Basic Life Sciences* 59(1992):717–28; Gegova, G., Manolova, N., Serkedzhieva, I., et al. Combined effect of selected antiviral substances of natural and synthetic origin: II. Anti-influenza activity of a combination of a polyphenolic complex isolated from *Geranium sanguineum L.* and rimantadine in vivo. *Acta Microbiologica Bulgarica* 30(1993):37–40.

10. Phan, T. T., Hughes, M. A., Cherry, G. W. Enhanced proliferation of fibroblasts and endothelial cells treated with an extract of the leaves of *Chromolanea odorata* (Eupolin), an herbal remedy for treating wounds. *Plastic Reconstructive Surgery* 101(1998):756–65.

11. Garty, B. Z. Garlic burns. *Pediatrics* 91(1993):658–9.

12. Berger, M. M., Cavadini, C., Chiolero, R., et al. Influence of large intakes of trace elements on recovery after major burns. *Nutrition* 10(1994):327–34; Berger, M. M., Spertini, F., Shenkin, A., et al. Trace element supplementation modulates pulmonary infection rates after major burns: a double-blind, placebo-controlled trial. *American Journal of Clinical Nutrition* 68(1998):365–71.

13. Klein, G. L., Nicolai, M., Langman, C. B., et al. Dysregulation of calcium homeostasis after severe burn injury in children: possible role of magnesium depletion. *Journal of Pediatrics* 131(1997):246–51.

14. Gottschlich, M. M., Warden, G. D., Michel, M., et al. Diarrhea in tube-fed burn patients: incidence, etiology, nutritional impact, and prevention. *Journal of Parenteral and Enteral Nutrition* 12(1988):338–45.

15. Matsuda, T., Tanaka, H., Hanumadass, M., et al. Effects of high-dose vitamin C administration on post-burn microvascular fluid and protein flux. *Journal of Burn Care and Rehabilitation* 13(1992):560–6.

16. Haberal, M., Hamaloglu, E., Bora, S., et al. The effects of vitamin E on immune regulation after thermal injury. *Burns Including Thermal Injury* 14(1988):388–93.

17. Jenkins, M., Alexander, J. W., MacMillan, B. G., et al. Failure of topical steroids and vitamin E to reduce postoperative scar formation following reconstructive surgery. *Journal of Burn Care and Rehabilitation* 7(1986):309–12.

18. Subrahmanyam, M. Topical application of honey in treatment of burns. *British Journal of Surgery* 78(1991):497–8; Subrahmanyam, M. Honey impregnated gauze versus polyurethane film (OpSite) in the treatment of burns: a prospective randomised study. *British Journal of Plastic Surgery* 46(1993):322–3.

19. Willix, D. J., Molan, P. C., Harfoot, C. G. A comparison of the sensitivity of wound-

infecting species of bacteria to the anti-bacterial activity of manuka honey and other honey. *Journal of Applied Bacteriology* 73(1992):388–94; Allen, K. L., Molan, P. C., Reid, G. M. A survey of the antibacterial activity of some New Zealand honeys. *Journal of Pharmacy and Pharmacology* 43(1991): 817–22.

20. Efem, S. E., Udoh, K. T., Iwara, C. I. The anti-microbial spectrum of honey and its clinical significance. *Infection* 20(1992):227–9.

21. Postmes, T., van den Bogaard, A. E., Hazen, M. Honey for wounds, ulcers and skin graft preservation. *Lancet* 341(1993):756–7.

22. Patterson, D. R., Everett, J. J., Burns, G. L., et al. Hypnosis for the treatment of burn pain. *Journal of Consulting and Clinical Psychology* 60(1992):713–7.

23. Foertsch, C. E., O'Hara, M. W., Stoddard, F. J., Kealey G. P. Treatment-resistant pain and distress during pediatric burn-dressing changes. *Journal of Burn Care and Rehabilitation* 19(1998):219–24.

24. Field, T., Peck, M., Krugman, S., et al. Burn injuries benefit from massage therapy. Ibid. 19(1998):241–4.

25. Field, T., Peck, M., Hernandez-Rief, M., et al. Postburn itching, pain and psychosocial symptoms are reduced with massage therapy. Ibid. 21(2000):189–93.

26. Lewis, S. M., Clelland, J. A., Knowles, C. J., et al. Effects of auricular acupuncture-like transcutaneous electric nerve stimulation on pain levels following wound care in patients with burns: a pilot study. Ibid. 11(1990):322–9.

27. Sumano, H., Mateos, G. The use of acupuncture-like electrical stimulation for wound healing of lesions unresponsive to conventional treatment. *American Journal of Acupuncture* 27(1999):5–14.

28. Wirth, D. P. The effect of noncontact Therapeutic Touch on the healing rate of full thickness dermal wounds. *Subtle Energies* 1(1990):1–20.

29. Turner, J. G., Clark, A. J., Gauthier D. K., Williams, M. The effect of Therapeutic Touch on pain and anxiety in burn patients. *Journal of Advanced Nursing* 28(1998):10–20.

30. Leaman, A. M., Gorman, D. Cantharis in the early treatment of minor burns. *Archives of Emergency Medicine* 6(1989):259–61.

## Chapter 8: Chicken Pox

1. Duckett, S. Plantain leaf for poison ivy. *Lancet* 303(1980):583.

## Chapter 9: Colds

1. Cohen, S., Doyle, W. J., Skoner, D. P., Rabin, B. S., Gwaltney, J. M. Social ties and susceptibility to the common cold. *JAMA* 277(1997):1940–4.

2. Kogan, M. D., Pappas, G., Us, S. M., et al. Over-the-counter medication use among U.S. pre-school-age children. Ibid. 272(1994):1025–30.

3. Gaffey, M. J., Gwaltney, J. M., Jr., Sastre, A., et al. Intranasally and orally administered antihistamine treatment of experimental rhinovirus colds. *American Review of Respiratory Disease* 136(1987):556–60.

4. Taylor, J. A., Novack, A. H., Almquist, J. R., et al. Efficacy of cough suppressants in children. *Journal of Pediatrics* 122(1993):799–802.

5. Kuhn, J. J., Hendley, J. O., Adams, K. F., et al. Antitussive effect of guaifenesin in young adults with natural colds. *Chest* 82(1982): 713–8.

6. Graham, N. M., Burrell, C. J., Douglas, R. M., et al. Adverse effects of aspirin, acetamino-phen and ibuprofen on immune function, viral shedding and clinical status in rhinovirus-infect volunteers. *Journal of Infectious Diseases* 162(1990):1277–82.

7. Eccles, R., Jawad, M. S., Morris, S. The effects of oral administration of menthol on nasal resistance to airflow and nasal sensation of airflow in subjects suffering from nasal congestion associated with the common cold. *Journal of Pharmacy and Pharmacology* 42(1990):652–4.

8. Gadomski, A. M. Potential interventions for preventing pneumonia among young children: lack of effect of antibiotic treatment for upper respiratory infections. *Pediatric Infectious Disease Journal* 12(1993):115–20.

9. Nyquist, A. C., Gonzales, R., Steiner, J. F., Sande, M. A. Antibiotic prescribing for children with colds, upper respiratory tract infections, and bronchitis. *JAMA* 279(1998):875–7.

10. Barrow, G. I., Higgins, P. G., al-Nakib, W., et al. The effect of intranasal nedocromil sodium on viral upper respiratory tract infections in human volunteers. *Clinical and Experimental Allergy* 20(1990):45–51.

11. Dockhorn, R., Grossman, J., Posner, M., et al. A double-blind, placebo-controlled study of the safety and efficacy of ipratropium bromide nasal spray versus placebo in patients with the common cold. *Journal of Allergy and Clinical Immunology* 90(1992):1076–82.

12. Cowan, P. F. Patient satisfaction with an office visit for the common cold. *Journal of Family Practice* 24(1987):412–3.

13. Zhang, J. S., Tian, Z., Lou, Z. C. Quality evaluation of twelve species of Chinese ephedra (Ma Huang). *Yao Hsueh Hsueh Pao* 24(1989):865–71.

14. Abe, N., Ebina, T., Ishida, N. Interferon induction by glycyrrhizin and glycyrrhetinic acid in mice. *Microbiology and Immunology* 26(1982): 535–9.

15. Denyer, C. V., Jackson, P., Loakes, D. M., et al. Isolation of antirhinoviral sesquiterpenes from ginger *(Zingiber officianale)*. *Journal of Natural Products* 57(1994):658–62.

16. Pinnock, C. B., Douglas, R. M., Badcock, N. R. Vitamin A status in children who are prone to respiratory tract infections. *Australian Paediatric Journal* 22(1986):95–9.

17. Stansfield, S. K., Pierre-Louis, M., Lerebours, G., et al. Vitamin A supplementation and increased prevalence of childhood diarrhea and acute respiratory infections. *Lancet* 342(1993):578–2; Kartasasmita, C. B., Rosmayudi, O., Soemantri, E. S., et al. Vitamin A and acute respiratory infections. *Paediatrica Indonesiana* 31(1991):41–9.

18. Chalmers, T. C. Effects of ascorbic acid on the common cold: an evaluation of the evidence. *American Journal of Medicine* 58(1975):532–6.

19. Baird, I. M., Hughes, R. E., Wilson, H. K., et al. The effects of ascorbic acid and flavonoids on the occurrence of symptoms normally associated with the common cold. *American Journal of Clinical Nutrition* 32(1979):1686–90; Hemila, H. Vitamin C and the common cold. *British Journal of Nutrition* 67(1992):3–16.

20. Eby, G. A., Davis, D. R., Halcomb, W. W. Reduction in duration of common colds by zinc gluconate lozenges in a double-blind study. *Antimicrobial Agents and Chemotherapy* 25(1984):20–4; Farr, B. M., Conner, E. M., Betts, R. F., et al. Two randomized controlled trials of zinc gluconate lozenge therapy of experimentally induced rhinovirus colds. Ibid. 31(1987): 1183–7; Godfrey, J. C., Sloane, B. C., Smith, D. S., et al. Zinc gluconate and the common cold; a controlled clinical study. *Journal of International Medical Research* 20(1992):234–46.

21. Macknin, M. L., Piedmonte, M., Calendine, C., Janosky, J., Wald, E. Zinc gluconate lozenges for treating the common cold in children. *JAMA* 279(1998):1962–7.

22. Chandra, R. K. Excessive intake of zinc impairs immune responses. Ibid. 252(1984): 1443–6.

23. Saketkhoo, K., Januszkiewicz, A., Sackner, M. A., et al. Effects of drinking hot water, cold water, and chicken soup on nasal mucus velocity and nasal airflow resistance. *Chest* 74(1978):408–10.

24. Rennard, B. O., Ertl, R. F., Gossman, G. L., et al. Chicken soup inhibits neutrophil chemotaxis in vitro. Ibid. 118(2000):1150–7.

25. Forstall, G. J., Macknin, M. L., Yen-Lieberman, B. R., et al. Effect of inhaling heated vapor on symptoms of the common cold. *JAMA* 271(1994):1109–11.

26. Ophir, D., Elad, Y. Effects of steam inhalation on nasal patency and nasal symptoms in patients with the common cold. *American Journal of Otolaryngology* 3(1987):149–53.

27. Tan, D. Treatment of fever due to exopathic wind-cold by rapid acupuncture. *Journal of Traditional Chinese Medicine* 12(1992):267–71.

28. Vickers, A. J., Smith, C. Homoeopathic Oscillococcinum for preventing and treating influenza and influenza-like syndromes. *Cochrane Database of Systematic Reviews* computer file (2000)(2):CD001957.

## References

### Chapter 10: Colic

1. Canivet, C., Hagander, B., Jakobsson, I., Lanke, J. Infantile colic—less common that previously estimated? *Acta Paediatrica* 85(1996): 454–8.
2. Barr, R. G., Kramer, M. S., Pless, I. B., et al. Feeding and temperament as determinants of early infant crying/fussing behavior. *Pediatrics* 84(1989):514–21.
3. Lothe, L., Ivarsson, S. A., Ekman, R., et al. Motilin and infantile colic. *Acta Paediatrica Scandinavica* 79(1990):410–6.
4. Moore, D. J., Robb, T. A., Davidson, G. P. Breath hydrogen response to milk containing lactose in colicky and noncolicky infants. *Journal of Pediatrics* 113(1988):979–84.
5. Lindberg, T. Infantile colic and small intestinal function: a nutritional problem? *Acta Paediatrica* 88(1999):58–60.
6. Clyne, P. S., Kulczycki, A., Jr. Human breast milk contains bovine IgG. Relationship to infant colic? *Pediatrics* 87(1991):439–44.
7. Hunziker, U. A., Barr, R. G. Increased carrying reduces infant crying: a randomized controlled trial. Ibid. 77(1986):641–8.
8. Rantava, P., Helenius, H., Lehtonen, L. Psychosocial predisposing factors for infantile colic. *British Medical Journal* 307(1993):600–4.
9. Sethi, K. S., Sethi, J. K. Simethicone in the management of infant colic. *The Practitioner* 232(1988):508.
10. Danielsson, B., Hwang, C. P. Treatment of infantile colic with surface active substance (simethicone). *Acta Paediatrica Scandinavica* 74(1985):446–50.
11. Metcalf, T. J., Irons, T. G., Sher, L. D., et al. Simethicone in the treatment of infant colic: a randomized, placebo-controlled, multicenter trial. *Pediatrics* 94(1994):29–34.
12. Miller, J. J., McVeagh, P., Fleet, G. H., et al. Effect of yeast lactase enzyme on "colic" in infants fed human milk. *Journal of Pediatrics* 117(1990):261–3; Stahlberg, M. R., Savilahti, E. Infantile colic and feeding. *Archives of Diseases in Childhood* 61(1986):1232–3.
13. Weissbluth, M., Christoffel, K. K., Davis, T. A. Treatment of infantile colic with dicyclomine hydrochloride. *Journal of Pediatrics* 104(1984):951–5.
14. Hardoin, R. A., Henslee, J. A., Christenson, C. P., et al. Colic medication and apparent life-threatening events. *Clinical Pediatrics* 30(1991):281–5; Randall, B., Gerry, G., Rance, F. Dicyclomine in the sudden infant death syndrome (SIDS)—a cause of death or an incidental finding? *Journal of Forensic Sciences* 31(1986):1470–4.
15. Weizman, Z., Alkrinawi, S., Goldfarb, D., et al. Efficacy of herbal tea preparation in infantile colic. *Journal of Pediatrics* 122(1993):650–2.
16. Forsyth, B. W. Colic and the effect of changing formulas: a double-blind, multiple cross-over study. Ibid.115(1989):521–6; Barr, R. G., Wooldridge, J., Hanley, J. Effects of formula change on intestinal hydrogen production and crying and fussing behavior. *Journal of Developmental and Behavioral Pediatrics* 12(1991):248–53.
17. Keane, V., Charney, E., Straus, J., Roberts, K. Do solids help baby sleep through the night? *American Journal of Diseases of Children* 142(1988):404–5.
18. Treem, W. R., Hyams, J. S., Blankschen, E., et al. Evaluation of the effect of a fiber-enriched formula on infant colic. *Journal of Pediatrics* 119(1991):695–701.
19. Larson, K. Ayllon, T. The effects of contingent music and differential reinforcement on infantile colic. *Behavior Research and Therapy* 28(1990):119–25.
20. Taubman, B. Parental counseling compared with elimination of cow's milk or soy milk protein for the treatment of infant colic syndrome: a randomized trial. *Pediatrics* 81(1988): 756–61.
21. Schmitt, B. D. *Your Child's Health,* rev. ed. New York: Bantam Books, 1991, pp. 239–43.
22. Loadman, W., Arnold, K., Volmer, R., et al. Reducing the behavior symptoms of infant colic by introduction of a vibration/sound based intervention. *Pediatric Research* 21(1987): 182A.
23. Larsen, J. H. Infants' colic and belly massage. *The Practitioner* 234(1990):396–7.
24. McClure V. S. *Infant Massage: A Handbook for Loving Parents.* New York: Bantam Books, 1989, pp. 137–9.
25. Klougart, N., Nilsson, N., Jacobsen, J. Infantile colic treated by chiropractors: a prospective

study of 316 cases. *Journal of Manipululative and Physiological Therapeutics* 12(1989):281–8.

26. Wiberg, J. M., Nordsteen, J., Nilsson, N. The short-term effect of spinal manipulation in the treatment of infantile colic: a randomized controlled clinical trial with a blinded observer. Ibid. 22(1999):517–22.

27. Krieger, D. *The Therapeutic Touch: How to Use Your Hands to Help or Heal.* New York: Prentice Hall Press, 1989, pp. 138–9.

## Chapter 11: Conjuctivitis (Pinkeye)

1. Subiza, J., Subiza, J. L., Alonso, M. Allergic conjunctivitis to chamomile tea. *Annals of Allergy* 65(1990):127–32.

2. Stoss, M., Michels, C., Peter, E., et al. Prospective cohort trial of Euphrasia single-dose eye drops in conjunctivitis. *Journal of Alternative and Complementary Medicine* 6(2000):499–508.

## Chapter 12: Constipation

1. Morais, M. B., Vitolo, M. R., Aguirre, A. N., Fagundes-Neto, U. Measurement of low dietary fiber intake as a risk factor for chronic constipation in children. *Journal of Pediatric Gastroenterology and Nutrition* 29(1999):132–5.

2. Lloyd, B., Halter, R. J., Kuchan, M. J., Baggs, G. E., Ryan, A. S., Masor, M. L. Formula intolerance in post-breast-fed and exclusively formula-fed infants. *Pediatrics* 103(1999):e7.

3. Iacono, G., Cavataio, F., Montalto, G., et al. Chronic constipation as a symptom of cow's milk allergy. *Journal of Pediatrics* 126(1995):34–9.

4. Bloom, D. A., Buonomo, C., Fishman, S. J., Furuta, G., Nurko, S. Allergic colitis: a mimic of Hirschprung disease. *Pediatric Radiology* 29(1999):37–41.

5. Hyams, J. S., Treem, W. R., Etienne, N. L., et al. Effect of infant formula on stool characteristics of young infants. *Pediatrics* 95(1995):50–4.

6. Anti, M., Pignataro, G., Armuzzi, A., et al. Water supplementation enhances the effect of high fiber diet on stool frequency. *Hepato-Gastroenterology* 45(1998):727–32.

7. Meshkinpour, H., Selod, S., Movahedi, H., Nami, N., James, N., Wilson, A. Effects of regular exercise in management of chronic idiopathic constipation. *Digestive Diseases and Sciences* 43(1998):2379–83.

8. Clark, J. H., Russell, G. J., Fitzgerald, J. F., et al. Serum beta-carotene, retinol and alpha-tocopherol levels during mineral oil therapy for constipation. *American Journal of Diseases of Children* 141(1987):1210–2.

9. McGuire, J. K., Kulkarni, M. S., Baden H. P. Fatal hypermagnesemia in a child treated with megavitamin/megamineral therapy. *Pediatrics* 105(2000):E18.

10. McClung, H. J., Boyne, L. J., Linsheid, T., et al. Is combination therapy for encopresis nutritionally safe? Ibid. 91(1993):591–4.

11. Godding, E. W. Laxatives and the special role of senna. *Pharmacology* 36(1988):230–6.

12. Siegers, C. P., von Hertzberg-Lottin, E., Otte, M., et al. Anthranoid laxative abuse: a risk for colorectal cancer? *Gut* 34(1993):1099–101.

13. Minghan, W., Zhu, C. The therapeutic effect of mulberry in the treatment of constipation and insomnia in the elderly. *Journal of Traditional Chinese Medicine* 9(1989):93–4.

14. Egger, G., Wolfenden, K., Pares, J., et al. "Bread: it's a great way to go": increasing bread consumption decreases laxative sales in an elderly community. *Medical Journal of Australia* 155(1991):820–1.

15. Brown, S. R., Cann, P. A., Read, N. W. Effect of coffee on distal colon function. *Gut* 31(1990):450–3.

16. Mykkanen, H. L., Karhunen, L. J., Korpela, R., et al. Effect of cheese on intestinal transit time and other indicators of bowel function in residents of a retirement home. *Scandinavian Journal of Gastroenterology* 29(1994):29–32.

17. Andrews, P. J., Borody, T. J. "Putting back the bugs": bacterial treatment relieves chronic constipation and symptoms of irritable bowel syndrome. *Medical Journal of Australia* 159(1993):633–4.

18. Van der Plas, R. N., Benninga, M. A., Redekop, W. K., et al. Randomised trial of biofeedback training for encopresis. *Archives of Diseases in Childhood* 75(1996):367–74.

19. McKenna, P. H., Herndon, C. D., Connery, S., Ferrer F. A. Pelvic floor muscle retraining for pediatric voiding dysfunction using interactive computer games. *Journal of Urology* 162(1999):1056–62; Griffiths, P., Dunn, S., Evans, A., Smith, D., Bradnam, M. Portable biofeedback apparatus for treatment of anal sphincter dystonia in childhood soiling and constipation. *Journal of Medical Engineering Technology* 23(1999):96–101.

20. Klauser, A. G., Flaschentrager, J., Gehrke, A., et al. Abdominal wall massage: effect on colonic function in healthy volunteers and in patients with chronic constipation. *Zeitschrift fur Gastroenterologie* 30(1992):247–51.

21. Klauser, A. G., Rubach, A., Bertsche, O., et al. Body acupuncture: effect on colonic function in chronic constipation. Ibid. 31(1993):605–8.

22. Diehl D. L. Acupuncture for gastrointestinal and hepatobiliary disorders. *Journal of Alternative and Complementary Medicine* 5(1999):27–45.

23. Felt, B., Wise, C. G., Olson, A., et al. Guideline for the management of pediatric idiopathic constipation and soiling. *Archives of Pediatrics and Adolescent Medicine* 153(1999):380–85.

## Chapter 13: Cough

1. Johnston, E. D., Strachan, D. P., Anderson, H. R. Effect of pneumonia and whooping cough in childhood on adult lung function. *New England Journal of Medicine* 338(1998):581–7.

2. Smith, M. B. H., Feldman, W. Over-the-counter cold medications: a critical review of clinical trials between 1950 and 1991. *JAMA* 269(1993):2258–63.

3. Taylor, J. A., Novack, A. H., Almquist, J. R., Rogers, J. E. Efficacy of cough suppressants in children. *Journal of Pediatrics* 122(1993):799–802.

4. Committee on Drugs, American Academy of Pediatrics. Use of codeine- and dextromethorphan-containing cough syrups in pediatrics. *Pediatrics* 62(1978):119–22.

5. Kuhn, J. J., Hendley, J. O., Adams, K. E., et al. Antitussive effect of guaifenesin in young adults with natural colds. *Chest* 82(1982):713–8; Hirsch, S. R., Viernes, P. F., Kory, R. C., et al. The expectorant effect of glyceryl guaiacolate in patients with chronic bronchitis. Ibid. 63(1973):9–14.

6. Johnson, D. W., Jacobson, S., Edney, P. C., et al. A comparison of nebulized budenoside intramuscular dexamethasone and placebo for moderately severe croup. *New England Journal of Medicine* 339(1998):498–503.

7. Reijonen, T., Korppi, M., Kuikka, L., Remes, K. Anti-inflammatory therapy reduces wheezing after bronchiolitis. *Archives of Pediatrics and Adolescent Medicine* 150(1996):512–7.

8. Stansfield, S. K., Pierre-Louis, M., Lerebours, G., et al. Vitamin A supplementation and increased prevalence of childhood diarrhea and acute respiratory infections. *Lancet* 342(1993):578–82; Bresee, J. S., Fischer, M., Dowell, S. F., et al. Vitamin A therapy for children with respiratory syncytial virus infection: a multicenter trial in the United States. *Pediatric Infectious Disease Journal* 15(1996):777–82.

9. Bucca, C., Rolla, G., Arossa, W., et al. Effect of ascorbic acid on increased bronchial responsiveness during upper airway infection. *Respiration* 55(1989):214–9.

10. Grievink, L., Smit, H. A., Ocke, M. C., et al. Dietary intake of antioxidant (pro)-vitamins, respiratory symptoms and pulmonary function: the MORGEN study. *Thorax* 53(1998):166–71.

11. Pinnock, C. B., Arney, W. K. The milk-mucus belief: sensory analysis comparing cow's milk and a soy placebo. *Appetite* 20(1993):61–70.

12. Pinnock, C. B., Graham, N. M., Mylvaganam, A., et al. Relationship between milk intake and mucus production in adult volunteers challenged with rhinovirus-2. *American Review of Respiratory Diseases* 141(1990):352–6.

13. Fluge, O., Omenaas, E., Eide, G. E., Gulsvik, A. Fish consumption and respiratory symptoms among young adults in a Norwegian community. *European Respiratory Journal* 12(1998):336–40.

14. Mortensen, J., Falk, M., Groth, S., et al. The effects of postural drainage and positive expiratory pressure physiotherapy on tracheo-

bronchial clearance in cystic fibrosis. *Chest* 100(1991):1350–7.

15. Bourchier, D., Dawson, K. P., Fergusson, D. M. Humidification in viral croup: a controlled trial. *Australian Paediatrics Journal* 20(1984):289–91.

16. Mamolen, M., Lewis, D. M., Blanchet, M. A., et al. Investigation of an outbreak of "humidifi-er fever" in a print shop. *American Journal of Industrial Medicine* 23(1993):483–90.

17. Stein, M. T., Harper, G., Chen, J. Persistent cough in an adolescent. *Journal of Developmental and Behavioral Pediatrics* 20(1999):434–6.

18. Elkins, G. R., Carter, B. D. Hypnotherapy in the treatment of childhood psychogenic cough-ing: a case report. *American Journal of Clinical Hypnosis* 29(1986):59–63.

19. Xinlian, L. 41 cases of cough treated with cup-ping. *International Journal of Clinical Acupuncture* 2(1991):319–22.

## Chapter 14: Cradle Cap

1. Hale, E. H., Bystryn, J. C. Relation between skin temperature and location of facial lesions in seborrheic dermatitis. *Archives of Dermatology* 136(2000):559–60.

2. Peter, R. U., Richarz-Barthauer, U. Successful treatment and prophylaxis of scalp seborrheic dermatitis and dandruff with 2% ketoconazole shampoo: results of a multicentre double-blind, placebo-controlled trial. *British Journal of Dermatology* 132(1995):441–5.

3. Tollesson, A. Fithz, A., Stenlund, K. *Malassezia furfur* in infantile seborrheic dermatitis. *Pediatric Dermatology* 14(1997):423–5.

## Chapter 15: Diaper Rash

1. Healy, C. E. Precocious puberty due to a dia-per ointment. *Indiana Medicine* 77(1984):610.

2. Despard, C. Diaper dermatitis: another simple remedy. *Canadian Medical Association Journal* 139(1988):706.

3. Sharma, V. D., Sethi, M. S., Kumar, A., et al. Antibacterial property of *Allium sativum* Linn.: in vivo and in vitro studies. *Indian Journal of Experimental Biology* 15(1977):466–8; Amer, M.,

Taha, M., Tosson, Z. The effect of aqueous garlic extract on the growth of dermato-phytes. *International Journal of Dermatology* 19(1980):285–7; Prasad, G., Sharma, V. D. Efficacy of garlic *(Allium sativum)* treatment against experimental candidiasis in chicks. *British Veterinary Journal* 136(1980):448–51; Barone, F. E., Tansey, M. R. Isolation, purifica-tion, identification, synthesis, and kinetics of activity of the anticandi-dal compounds of *Allium sativum,* and a hypothesis for its mode of action. *Mycologia* 69(1977):793–824.

4. Lee, T. Y., Lam, T., H. Contact dermatitis due to topical treatment with garlic in Hong Kong. *Contact Dermatitis* 24(1991):193–6.

5. Mahajan, V. L., Sharma, A., Rattan, A. Antimycotic activity of berberine sulfate: an alkaloid from an Indian medicinal herb. *Sabouraudia* 20(1982):79–81.

6. Collipp, P. J., Kuo, B., Castro-Magana, M., et al. Hair zinc, scalp hair quantity, and diaper rash in normal infants. *Cutis* 35(1985):66–70.

7. Bosch-Banyeras, J. L., Catala, M., Mas, P., et al. Diaper dermatitis: value of vitamin A topically applied. *Clinical Pediatrics* 27(1988):448–50.

## Chapter 16: Diarrhea

1. Clemens, J., Rao, M., Eng, M., et al. Breast-feeding and the risk of life-threatening rotavirus diarrhea: prevention or postpone-ment. *Pediatrics* 92(1993):680–5.

2. Long, K. Z., Wood, J. W., Gariby, E. V., et al. Proportional hazards analysis of diarrhea due to Enterotoxigenic *Escherichia coli* and breast-feeding in a cohort of urban Mexican children. *American Journal of Epidemiology* 139(1994):193–205; Samra, H. K., Ganguly, N. K., Mahajan, R. C. Human milk containing specific secretory IgA inhibits binding of *Giardia lamblia* to nylon and glass surfaces. *Journal of Diarrhoeal Diseases Research* 9(1991):100–3; Ruiz-Palacios, G. M., Calva, J. J., Pickering, L. K., et al. Protection of breast-fed infants against *Campylobacter* diarrhea by antibodies in human milk. *Journal of Pediatrics* 116(1990):707–13; Walterspiel, J. N., Morrow, A. L., Guerrero, L., Ruiz-Palacios, G. M.,

References

Pickering L. K. Secretory anti-*Giardia lamblia* antibodies in human milk: protective effect against diarrhea. *Pediatrics* 93(1990):28–31; Glass, R. I., Svennerholm, A. M., Stoll, B. J., et al. Protection against cholera in breast-fed children by antibodies in breast milk. *New England Journal of Medicine* 308(1983): 1389–92.

3. Turner, R. B., Kelsey, D. K. Passive immunization for prevention of rotavirus illness in healthy infants. *Pediatric Infectious Disease Journal* 12(1993):718–22.

4. Figueroa-Quintanilla, D., Salazar-Lindo, E., Sack, R. B., et al. A controlled trial of bismuth subsalicylate in infants with acute watery diarrheal disease. *New England Journal of Medicine* 328(1993):1653–8; Soriano-Brucher, H., Avendano, P., O'Ryan, M., et al. Bismuth subsalicylate in the treatment of acute diarrhea in children: a clinical study. *Pediatrics* 87(1991):18–27.

5. Guarino, A., Canani, R. B., Russo, S., et al. Oral immunoglobulins for treatment of acute rotaviral gastroenteritis. Ibid. 93(1994):12–6.

6. Loeb, H., Vandenplas, Y., Wursch, P., Guersy, P. Tannin-rich carob pod for the treatment of acute-onset diarrhea. *Journal of Pediatric Gastroenterology and Nutrition* 8(1989):480–5.

7. Gupte, S. Use of berberine in treatment of giardiasis. *Archives Journal of Diseases of Children* 129(1975):866.

8. Sachdev, H. P. S., Mittal, N. K., Yadav, H. S. Oral zinc supplementation in persistent diarrhea in infants. *Annals of Tropical Pediatrics* 10(1990):63–9; Roy, S. K., Behrens, R. H., Haider, R., et al. Impact of zinc supplementation on intestinal permeability in Bangladeshi children with acute diarrhea and persistent diarrhea syndrome. *Journal of Pediatric Gastroenterology and Nutrition* 15(1992): 289–96; Sazawal, S., Black, R. E., Bhan, M. K., Bhandari, N., Sinha, A., Jalla, S. Zinc supplementation in young children with acute diarrhea in India. *New England Journal of Medicine* 333(1995):839–44; Bhutta, Z. A., Nizami, S. Q., Isani, Z. Zinc supplementation in malnourished children with persistent diarrhea in Pakistan. *Pediatrics* 103(1999):442; Penny, M. E.,

Peerson, J. M., Marin, R. M., Duran, A., Lanata, C. F., Lonnerdal, B., Black, R., Brown K. H. Randomized, community-based trial of the effect of zinc supplementation, with or without other micronutrients, on the duration of persistent childhood diarrhea in Lima, Peru. *Journal of Pediatrics* 135(1999):208–17.

9. Reid, G. Probiotics in the treatment of diarrheal diseases. *Current Science International* 2(2000):78–83.

10. Arvola, T., Laiho, K., Torkkeli, S., et al. Prophylactic *Lactobacillus* GG reduces antibiotic-associated diarrhea in children with respiratory infections: a randomized study. *Pediatrics* 104(1999):64.

11. Szajewska, H., Kotowska, M., Mrukowicz, J. Z., et al. Efficacy of *Lactobacillus* GG in prevention of nosocomial diarrhea in infants. *Journal of Pediatrics* 138(2001):361–5.

12. Barreto, M. L., Santos, L. M., Assis, A. M., et al. Effect of vitamin A supplementation on diarrhea and acute lower respiratory-tract infections in young children in Brazil. *Lancet* 344(1994):228–31.

13. Rahmathullah, L., Underwood, B. A., Thulasiraj, R. D., Milton, R. C. Diarrhea, respiratory infections and growth are not affected by a weekly low-dose vitamin A supplement: a masked, controlled field trial in children in southern India. *American Journal of Clinical Nutrition* 54(1991):568–77.

14. Avery, M. E., Snyder, J. D. Oral therapy for acute diarrhea: the underused simple solution. *New England Journal of Medicine* 323(1990):891–4.

15. CHOICE study Group. Multicenter, randomized, double-blind clinical trial to evaluate the efficacy and safety of a reduced osmolarity oral rehydration salts solution in children with acute watery diarrhea. *Pediatrics* 107(2001):613–8.

16. Gore, S. M., Fontaine, O., Pierce, N. F. Impact of rice-based oral rehydration solution on stool output and duration of diarrhea: meta-analysis of 13 clinical trials. *British Medical Journal* 304(1992):287–91.

17. Chew, F., Penna, F. J., Peret, L. A., et al. Is dilution of cow's milk formula necessary for

dietary management of acute diarrhea in infants aged less than six months? *Lancet* 341(1993):194.

18. Brown, K. H., Peerson, J. M., Fontaine, O. Use of nonhuman milks in the dietary management of young children with acute diarrhea: a meta-analysis of clinical trials. *Pediatrics* 93(1994):17–27.

19. Bhutta, Z. A., Molla, A. M., Issani, Z., et al. Dietary management of persistent diarrhea: comparison of a traditional rice-lentil based diet with soy formula. Ibid. 88(1991):1010–8.

20. Nurko, S., Garcia-Aranda, J. A., Fishbein, E., Perez-Zuniga, M. I. Successful use of a chicken-based diet for the treatment of severely malnourished children with persistent diarrhea: a prospective, randomized study. *Journal of Pediatrics* 131(1997):405–12.

21. Alarcon, P., Montoya, R., Rivera, J., Perez, F., Peerson, J. M., Brown, K. H. Effect of inclusion of beans in a mixed diet for the treatment of Peruvian children with acute watery diarrhea. *Pediatrics* 90(1992):58–65; Schroeder, D. G., Torun, B., Bartlett, A. V., Miracle-McMahill, H. Dietary management of acute diarrhea with local foods in a Guatemalan rural community. *Acta Paediatrica* 86(1997):1155–61.

22. Sullivan, P. B. Nutritional management of acute diarrhea. *Nutrition* 14(1998):758–62; Boehm, P., Nassimbeni, G., Ventura, A. Chronic nonspecific diarrhea in childhood: how often is it iatrogenic? *Acta Paediatrica* 87(1998):268–71.

23. Khin-Maung, U., Greenlough, W. B. Cereal-based oral rehydration therapy., I. Clinical studies. *Journal of Pediatrics* 118(1991): S72–9.

24. Boudra, G., Touhami, M., Pochart, P., et al. Effect of feeding yogurt versus milk in children with persistent diarrhea. *Journal of Pediatric Gastroenterology and Nutrition* 11(1990):509–12.

25. Isolarui, E., Juntunen, M., Rautanen, T., Sillanaukee, P., Koivula, T. Human *Lactobacillus* strain (*Lactobacillus casei* strain GG) promotes recovery from acute diarrhea in children. *Pediatrics* 88(1991):90–7.

26. Pedone, C. A., Bernabeu, A. O., Postaire, E. R., Reinert, P. *Lactobacillus casei*–fortified

yoghurt reduces the severity and duration of diarrhoea in healthy children. *International Journal of Clinical Practice* 53(1999):179–84.

27. Galovsky, T. E., Blanchard, E. B. The treatment of irritable bowel syndrome with hypnotherapy. *Applied Psychophysiology and Biofeedback* 23(1998):219.

28. Yingchun, L. Observation of therapeutic effects of acupuncture treatment in 170 cases of infantile diarrhea. *Journal of Traditional Chinese Medicine* 7(1987):203–4.

29. Jacobs, J., Jimenez, L. M., Gloyd, S. S., Gale, J. L., Crothers, D. Treatment of acute childhood diarrhea with homeopathic medicine: a randomized trial in Nicaragua. *Pediatrics* 93(1994):719–25.

30. Jacobs, J., Jimenez, L. M., Malthouse, S., Chapman, E., Crothers, D., Masuc, M., Jonas, W. B. Homeopathic treatment of acute childhood diarrhea: results from a clinical trial in Nepal. *Journal of Alternative and Complementary Medicine* 6(2000):131–9.

## Chapter 17: Ear Infections

1. Finkelstein, J. A., Metlay, J. P., Davis, R. L., Rifas-Shiman, S. L., Dowell, S. F., Platt, R. Antimicrobial use in defined populations of infants and young children. *Archives of Pediatrics and Adolescent Medicine* 154(2000): 395–400.

2. Duffy, L. C., Faden, H., Wasielewski, R., Wolf, J., Krystofik, D. Exclusive breast-feeding protects against bacterial colonization and day care exposure to otitis media. *Pediatrics* 100(1997):7.

3. Duncan, B., Ey, J., Holberg, C., Wright, A., et al. Breast-feeding and recurrent otitis media in the first year of life. *Archives Journal of Diseases of Children* 146(1992):482.

4. Adair-Bischoff, C. E., Sauve, R. S. Environmental tobacco smoke and middle ear disease in preschool-age children. *Archives of Pediatrics and Adolescent Medicine* 152(1998):127–33.

5. Schuller, D. E. Prophylaxis of otitis media in asthmatic children. *Journal of Pediatric Infectious Diseases* 2(1983):280–3.

6. Jackson, J. M., Mourino, A. P. Pacifier use and otitis media in infants twelve months or

younger. *Pediatric Dentistry* 21(1999):255–60; Niemela, M., Uhari, M., Mottonen, M. A pacifier increases the risk of recurrent otitis media in children in day care centers. *Pediatrics* 96(1995):884–8.

7. Fleming, P. J., Blair, P. S., Pollard, K., et al. Pacifier use and sudden infant death syndrome: results from the CESDI/SUID case control study. *Archives of Disease in Childhood* 81(1999):112–6.

8. Roberts, J. E., Sanyal, M. A., Burchinal, M. R., Collier, A. M., Ramey, C. T., Henderson, F. W. Otitis media in early childhood and its relationship to later verbal and academic performance. *Pediatrics* 78(1986):423–30.

9. Roberts, J. E., Burchinal, M. R., Collier, A. M., Ramey, C. T., Koch, M. A., Henderson, F. W. Otitis media in early childhood and cognitive, academic and classroom performance of the school-aged child. Ibid. 83(1989):477–85.

10. Hoberman, A., Paradise, J. L., Reynolds, E. A., Urkin, J. Efficacy of Auralgan for treating ear pain in children with acute otitis media. *Archives of Pediatrics and Adolescent Medicine* 151(1997):675–8.

11. Sorenson, H. Antibiotics in suppurative otitis media. *Otolaryngologic Clinics of North America* 10(1977):45–50.

12. Froom, J., Culpepper, L., Jacobs, M., DeMelker, R. A., Green, L. A., Van Buchem, L., Grob, P., Heeren, T. Antimicrobials for acute otitis media? A review from the International Primary Care Network. *British Medical Journal* 315(1997):98–102.

13. Van Buchem, F. L., Dunk, J. H. M., van't Hof, M. A. Therapy of acute otitis media: myringotomy, antibiotics, or neither? *Lancet* 2(1981):883–7.

14. Rudberg, R. D. Acute otitis media: comparative therapeutic results of sulphonamide and penicillin administered in various forms. *Acta Oto-laryngologica* 113(1954):1–79.

15. Lahikainen, E. A. Clinico-bacteriologic studies on acute otitis media: aspiration of tympanum as diagnostic and therapeutic method. Ibid. 107(1953):1–82; Van Dishoeck, H. A. E., Derks A. C. W., Voorhorst, R. Bacteriology and treatment of acute otitis media in children. Ibid. 50(1959):250–62.

16. Halstead, C., Lepow, M. L., Balassanian, N., et al. Otitis media: clinical observations, microbiology, and evaluation of therapy. *Archives Journal of Diseases in Childhood* 115(1968):542–51.

17. Del Mar, C., Glaszious, P., Hayem, M. Are antibiotics indicated as initial treatment for children with acute otitis media? A meta-analysis. *British Medical Journal* 314(1997): 1526–9.

18. Damoiseaux, R. A., Van Balen, F. A., Hoes, A. W., Verheij, T. J., de Melker, R. A. Primary care-based randomised, double-blind trial of amoxicillin versus placebo for acute otitis media in children aged under 2 years. Ibid. 320(2000):350–4.

19. Little, P., Gould, C., Williamson, I., et al. Pragmatic randomised controlled trial of two prescribing strategies for childhood otitis media. Ibid. 322(2001):336–42.

20. Berman, S., Byrns, P. J., Bondy, J., Smith, P. J., Lezotte, D. Otitis media–related antibiotic prescribing patterns, outcomes and expenditures in a pediatric Medicaid population. *Pediatrics* 100(1997):585–92.

21. Kozyrskyj, A. L., Hildes-Ripstein, E., Longstaffe A. E. A., Wincott, J. L., Sitar, D. S., Klassen, T. P., Moffatt, M. E. K. Treatment of acute otitis media with a shortened course of antibiotics: a meta-analysis. *JAMA* 279(1998):1736–42.

22. Hoberman, A., Paradise, J. L., Burch, D. J., Valinkski, W. A., Hedrick, J. A., Aronovitz, G. H., Drehobl, M. A., Rogers, J. M. Equivalent efficacy and reduced occurrence of diarrhea from a new formulation of amoxicillin/clavulanate potassium (Augmentin) for treatment of acute otitis media in children. *Pediatrics Infectious Disease Journal* 16(1997):463–70; DeSaintonge, D. M. C., Levine, D. F., Savage, I. T., et al. Trial of three-day and ten-day courses of amoxycillin in otitis media. *British Medical Journal* 284(1982):1078–81.

23. Green, S. M., Rothrock, S. G. Single-dose intramuscular ceftriaxone for acute otitis media in children. *Pediatrics* 91(1993):23–30.

24. Van Buchem, F. L., Peeters, M. F., Van't Hof, M. A. Acute otitis media: a new treatment strategy. *British Medical Journal* 290(1985):1033–7;

Bollag, U., Bollag-Albrecht, E. Recommendations derived from practice audit for the treatment of acute otitis media. *Lancet* 338(1991):96.

25. Reichler, M. R., Allphin, A. A., Breiman, R. F., et al. The spread of multiply resistant *Streptococcus penumoniae* at a day care center in Ohio. *Journal of Infectious Diseases* 166(1992):1346–53.

26. Williams, R. L., Chalmers, T. C., Stange, K. C., Chalmers, F. T., Bowlin, S. J. Use of antibiotics in preventing recurrent acute otitis media and in treating otitis media with effusion. *JAMA* 270(1993):1344–51.

27. Klein, J. O. Preventing recurrent otitis: what role for antibiotics? *Contemporary Pediatrics* 11(1994):44–60.

28. Roark, R., Berman, S. Continuous twice daily or once daily amoxicillin prophylaxis compared with placebo for children with recurrent otitis media. *Pediatric Infectious Disease Journal* 16(1997):376–81.

29. Berman, S., Luckey, D., Roark, R. Cost-effectiveness analysis of the management of persisting middle ear effusions. *Archives Journal of Diseases of Children* 147(1993):461.

30. Lecks, H. I., Kravis, L. P., Wood, D. W. Serous otitis media: reflections on pathogenesis and treatment, with a comment on the use of intranasal dexamthasone. *Clinical Pediatrics* 6(1967):519–23.

31. Podoshin, L., Fradis, M., Ben-David, J. Ototoxicity of ear drops in patients suffering from chronic otitis media. *Journal of Laryngology and Otology* 103(1989):46–50.

32. Cantekin, E. I., Mandel, E. M., Bluestone, C. D., et al. Lack of efficacy of a decongestant-antihistamine combination for otitis media with effusion ("secretory" otitis media) in children: results of a double-blind, randomized trial. *New England Journal of Medicine* 308(1983): 297–301.

33. Makinen, K. K., Hujoel, P. P., Bennett, C. A., et al. Polyol chewing gums and caries rates in primary dentition: a 24-month cohort study. *Caries Research* 30(1996):408–17; Hujoel, P. P., Makinen, K. K., Bennett, C. A., et al. The optimum time to initiate habitual xylitol gum-chewing for obtaining long-term caries prevention. *Journal of Dental Research* 78(1999):797–803.

34. Kontiokari, T., Uhari, M., Koskela, M. Antiadhesive effects of xylitol on otopathogenic bacteria. *Journal of Antimicrobial Chemotherapy* 41(1998):563–5.

35. Uhari, M., Kontiokari, T., Koskela, M., Niemela, M. Xylitol chewing gum in prevention of acute otitis media: Double-blind randomised trial. *British Medical Journal* 313(1996):1180–4; Uhari, M., Kontiokari, T., Niemela, M. A novel use of xylitol sugar in preventing acute otitis media. *Pediatrics* 102(1998):879–84.

36. Nsouli, T. M., Nsouli, S. M., Linde, R. E., O'Mara, F., Scanlon, R. T., Bellanti, J. A. Role of food allergy in serous otitis media. *Annals of Allergy* 73(1994):215–9.

37. Rundcrantz, H. The effects of position change on eustachian tube function. *Otolaryngology Clinics of North America* 3(1970):103–10.

38. Seely, D. R., Quigley, S. M., Langman, A. W. Ear candles—efficacy and safety. *Laryngoscope* 106(1996):1226–9.

39. Sawyer, C. I., Evans, R. L., Boline, P. D., Branson, R., Spicer, A. A feasibility study of chiropractic spinal manipulation versus sham spinal manipulation for chronic otitis media with effusion in children. *Journal of Manipulative Physiological Therapeutics* 22(1999):292–8.

40. Kaleida, P. H., Casselbrant, M. L., Rockette, H. E., et al. Amoxicillin or myringotomy or both for acute otitis media: results of a randomized clinical trial. *Pediatrics* 87(1991):466–74.

41. Myer, C. M., France, A. Ventilation tube placement in a managed care population. *Archives of Otolaryngology—Head and Neck Surgery* 123(1997):226–8.

42. Paradise, J. L., Feldman, H. M., Campbell, T. F., et al. Effect of early or delayed insertion of tympanostomy tubes for persistent otitis media on developmental outcomes at the age of three years. *New England Journal of Medicine* 344(2001):1179–87.

43. Perrin, J. M. Should we operate on children with fluid in the middle ear? Ibid. 344(2001): 1241–3.

44. Bernard, P. A. M., Stenstrom, R. J., Feldman,

W., et al. Randomized, controlled trial comparing long-term sulfonamide therapy to ventilation tubes for otitis media with effusion. *Pediatrics* 88(1991):215–22.

45. Coyte, P. C., Croxford, R., McIsaac, W., et al. The role of adjuvant adenoidectomy and tonsillectomy in the outcome of the insertion of tympanostomy tubes. *New England Journal of Medicine* 344(2001):1188–95.

46. Friese, K. H., Kruse, S., Ludtke, R., Moeller, H. The homeopathic treatment of otitis media in children—comparisons with conventional therapy. *International Journal of Clinical Pharmacological Therapeutics* 35(1997):296–301.

47. Harrison, H., Fixsen, A., Vickers, A. A randomized comparison of homeopathic and standard care for the treatment of glue ear in children. *Complementary Therapies in Medicine* 7(1999):132–5.

48. Barnett, E. D., Levatin, J. L., Chapman, E. H., Floyd, L. A., Eisenberg, D., Kaptchuk, Klein, J. O. Challenges of evaluating homeopathic treatment of acute otitis media. *Pediatric Infectious Disease Journal* 19(2000):273–5.

49. Jacobs, J., Springer, D. A., Crothers, D. Homeopathic treatment of acute otitis media in children: a preliminary randomized, placebo-controlled trial. Ibid. 20(2001):177–83.

## Chapter 18: Eczema

1. Sanda, T., Yasue, T., Oohashi, M., et al. Effectiveness of house dust-mite antigen avoidance through clean room therapy in patients with atopic dermatitis. *Journal of Allergy and Clinical Immunology* 89(1992):653–7.

2. Fergusson, D. L., Horwood, L. J., Shannon, F. T. Early solid feeding and recurrent childhood eczema: a 10-year longitudinal study. *Pediatrics* 86(1990):541–6.

3. Sampson, H. A., McCaskill, C. C. Food hypersensitivity and atopic dermatitis: evaluation of 113 patients. *Journal of Pediatrics* 107(1985):669–75.

4. Sigurs, N., Hattevig, G., Kjellman, B. Maternal avoidance of eggs, cow's milk, and fish during lactation: effect on allergenic manifestations, skin-prick tests, and specific IgE antibodies in children at age 4 years. *Pediatrics* 89(1992): 735–9.

5. Steinman, H. A., Potter, P. C. The precipitation of symptoms by common foods in children with atopic dermatitis. *Allergy Proceedings* 15(1994):203–10.

6. Barthel, H. R., Stuhlmuller, B. Improvement in atopic dermatitis with change to low salt table water. *Lancet* 344(1994):1089.

7. Paunio, M., Heinonen, O. P., Virtanen, M., et al. Measles history and atopic diseases: a population based cross-sectional study. *JAMA* 283(2000):343–6.

8. Fredriksson, T., Gip, L. Urea creams in the treatment of dry skin and hand dermatitis. *International Journal of Dermatology* 14(1975): 442–4.

9. Munkvad, M. A comparative trial of Clinitar versus hydrocortisone cream in the treatment of atopic eczema. *British Journal of Dermatology* 121(1989):763–6.

10. Schwetz BA. New treatment for eczema. *JAMA* 285(2001):724.

11. Atherton, D. J., Sheehan, M. P., Rustin, M. H. A., et al. Treatment of atopic eczema with traditional Chinese medicinal plants. *Pediatric Dermatology* 9(1992):373–5; Fung, A. Y. P., Look, P. C. N., Chong, L. Y., But, P. P. H., Wong, E. A controlled trial of traditional Chinese herbal medicine in Chinese patients with recalcitrant atopic dermatitis. *Internatonal Journal of Dermatology* 38(1999):387–92.

12. Latchman, Y., Banerjee, P., Poulter, L. W., Rustin, M., Brostoff, J. Association of immunological changes with clinical efficacy in atopic eczema patients treated with traditional Chinese herbal therapy (Zemaphyte). *International Archives of Allergy and Immunology* 109(1996): 243–9.

13. Davies, E., Pollock, I., Steel, H. Chinese herbs for eczema. *Lancet* 335(1990):177; Carlsson, C. Herbs and hepatitis (letter). *Lancet* 336(1990): 1068.

14. Ferguson, J. E., Chalmers, R. J., Rowlands, D. J. Reversible dilated cardiomyopathy following treatment of atopic eczema with Chinese herbal medicine. *British Journal of Dermatology* 136(1997):592–3.

15. Colin-Jones, E., Somers, G. F. A nonsteriodal anti-inflammatory agent in dermatology. *Medical Press* 238(1957):206–11.

16. Adamson, A. C., Tillman, W., G. Hydrocortisone [letter]. *British Medical Journal* 2(1955):1501; Annan, W., G. Hydrocortisone and glycyrrhetinic acid. Ibid. 1(1957):1242.

17. McCallum, D. I. Glycyrrhetinic acid. Ibid. 2(1956):1239.

18. Uehara, M., Sugiura, H., Sakurai, K. A trial of oolong tea in the management of recalcitrant atopic dermatitis. *Archives of Dermatology* 137(2001):42–3.

19. Knight, T. E., Hausen, B. L. Melaleuca oil (tea tree oil) dermatitis. *Journal of the American Academy of Dermatology* 30(1994):423–7.

20. Galland, L. Increased requirements for essential fatty acids in atopic individuals: a review with clinical descriptions. *Journal of the American College of Nutrition* 5(1986):213–28.

21. Bordoni, A., Biagi, P. L., Masi, M., et al. Evening primrose oil (Efamol) in the treatment of children with atopic eczema. *Drugs Under Experimental and Clinical Research* 14(1987):291–7.

22. Morse, P. F., Horrobin, D. F., Manku, M. S., et al. Meta-analysis of placebo-controlled studies of the efficacy of Epogram in the treatment of atopic eczema. Relationship between plasma essential fatty acid changes and clinical response. *British Journal of Dermatology* 121(1989):75–90.

23. Berth-Jones, J., Graham-Brown, R. A. C. Placebo-controlled trial of essential fatty acid supplementation in atopic dermatitis. *Lancet* 41(1993):1557–60; Horrobin, D. F., Morse, P. F. Evening primrose oil and atopic eczema. Ibid. 345(1995):260–1; Biagi, P. L., Bordoni, A., Hrelia, S., et al. The effect of gamma-linoleic acid on clinical status, red cell fatty composition and membrane microviscosity in infants with atopic dermatitis. *Drugs Under Experimental and Clinical Research* 20(1994):77–84; Hederos, C., Berg, A. Epogram evening primrose oil treatment in atopic dermatitis and asthma. *Archives of Diseases in Childhood* 75(1996):494–7.

24. Biagi, P. L., Bordoni, A., Masi, M., et al. A long-term study on the use of evening primrose oil (Efamol) in atopic children. *Drugs Under Experimental and Clinical Research* 14(1988): 285–90.

25. Soyland, E., Funk, J., Rajka, G., et al. Dietary supplementation with very long-chain n-3 fatty acids in patients with atopic dermatitis: a double-blind, multicentre study. *British Journal of Dermatology* 130(1994):757–64.

26. Krowchuck, D. P., et al. Ascorbic acid for treatment of atopic dermatitis. *Pediatrics* 86(1990):125–9.

27. Murch, S. H. Toll of allergy reduced by probiotics. *Lancet* 357(2001):1057–9.

28. Isolauri, E., et al. Probiotics in the management of atopic eczema. *Clinical and Experimental Allergy* 30(2000):1604–10.

29. Ewing, G. L., Gibbs, A. C. C., Ashcroft, C., et al. Failure of oral zinc supplementation in atopic eczema. *European Journal of Clinical Nutrition* 45(1991):507–10.

30. Eigenmann, P. A., Sicherer, S. H., Borkowski, T. A., et al. Prevalence of IgE-mediated food allergy among children with atopic dermatitis. *Pediatrics* 101(1998):8.

31. Neild, V. S., Marsden, R. A., Bailes, J. A., et al. Egg and milk exclusion diets in atopic eczema *British Journal of Dermatology* 114(1986):117–23; Sloper, K. S., Wadsworth, J., Brostoff, J. Children with atopic eczema. II: Immunological findings associated with dietary manipulations. *Quarterly Journal of Medicine, New Series* 80(1991):695–705.

32. Devlin, J., David, T. J., Stanton, R. H. J. Elemental diet for refractory atopic eczema. *Archives of Diseases in Childhood* 66(1991): 93–9.

33. Saarinene, U. M., Karjosaari, M. Breast-feeding as prophylaxis against atopic disease: prospective follow-up study until 17 years old. *Lancet* 346(1995):1065–9.

34. Herrman, M. E., Dannermann, A., Gruters, A., et al. Prospective study on the atopy preventive effect of maternal avoidance of milk and eggs during pregnancy and lactation. *European Journal of Pediatrics* 155(1996):770–4.

35. David, T. J., Waddington, E., Stanton, R. H. J. Nutritional hazards of elimination diets in children with atopic eczema. *Archives of Diseases in Childhood* 59(1984):323–5.

36. Devlin, J., Stanton, R. H., David, T. J. Calcium intake and cow's milk–free diets. Ibid. 64(1989):1183–4.

37. Devlin, J., David, T. J., Stanton, R. H. J. Six food diet for childhood atopic dermatitis. *Acta Dermato-Venereologica (Stockholm)* 71(1991):20–4.

38. Hathaway, M. J., Warner, J. O. Compliance problems in the dietary management of eczema. *Archives of Diseases in Childhood* 58(1983):463–4.

39. Casimir, G. J. A., Duchateau, J., Gossart, B., et al. Atopic dermatitis: role of food and house dust mite allergens. *Pediatrics* 92(1993):252–6.

40. Tan, B. B., Weald, D., Strickland, I., Friedmann P. S. Double-blind controlled trial of effect of house dust mite allergen avoidance on atopic dermatitis. *Lancet* 347(1996):15–8.

41. Von Ehrenstein, O. S., Von Mutius, E., Illi, S., et al. Reduced risk of hay fever and asthma among children of farmers. *Clinical and Experimental Allergy* 30(2000):187–93.

42. Rothenborg, H. W., Menne, T., Sjolin, K. E. Temperature dependent primary irritant dermatitis from lemon perfume. *Contact Dermatitis* 3(1977):37–48.

43. Bruno, G., Milita, O., Ferrara, M., et al. Prevention of atopic diseases in high risk babies (long-term follow-up). *Allergy Proceedings* 14(1993):181–6.

44. Hajek, P., Jakoubek, B., Radil, T. Gradual increase in cutaneous threshold induced by repeated hypnosis of healthy individuals and patients with atopoic eczema. *Perceptual and Motor Skills* 70(1990):549–50.

45. Ehlers, A., Stangier, U., Gieler, U. Treatment of atopic dermatitis: a comparison of psychological and dermatological approaches to relapse prevention. *Journal of Consulting and Clinical Psychology* 63(1995):624–35.

46. Koldys, K. W., Meyer, R. P. Biofeedback training in the therapy of dyshidrosis. *Cutis* 24(1979):219–21.

47. Schachner, L., Field, T., Hernandez-Rief, M., et al. Atopic dermatitis symptoms decreased in children following massage therapy. *Pediatric Dermatology* 15(1998):390–5.

48. Bjorna, H., Kaada, B. Successful treatment of itching and atopic eczema by transcutaneous nerve stimulation. *Acupuncture and Electrotherapeutics Research* 12(1987):101–12.

49. Spence, D. S. Homeopathic treatment of eczema: a retrospective survey of 130 cases. *British Homeopathic Journal* 80(1991):74–81.

## Chapter 19: Fever

1. Jaber, L., Cohen, I. J., Mor, A. Fever associated with teething. *Archives of Diseases in Childhood* 67(1992):233–4.

2. Inamo, Y., Takeuchi, S., Okuni, M. Host responses and neuroendocrinological changes in pyrexia in childhood. *Acta Paediatrica Japonica* 33(1991):628–32.

3. VanEsch, A., VanSteensel-Moll, H. A., Steyerberg, E. W., et al. Antipyretic efficacy of ibuprofen and acetaminophen in children with febrile seizures. *Archives of Pediatrics and Adolescent Medicine* 149(1995):632–7.

4. Mascolo, N., Sharma, R., Jain, S. C., et al. Ethnopharmacology of *Calotropis procera* flowers. *Journal of Ethnopharmacology* 22(1988):211–21.

5. But, P. P., Tam, Y. K., Lung, L. C. Ethnopharmacology of rhinoceros horn. II. Antipyretic effects of prescriptions containing rhinoceros horn or water buffalo horn. Ibid. 33(1991):45–50.

6. Lanhers, M. C., Fleurentin, J., Dorfman, P., et al. Analgesic, antipyretic and anti-inflammatory properties of *Euphorbia hirta*. *Planta Medica* 57(1991):225–31.

7. Okpanyi, S. N., Schirpke-von-Paczensky, R., Dickson, D. Anti-inflammatory, analgesic and antipyretic effect of various plant extracts and their combinations in an animal model. *Arzneimittel-Forschung* 39(1989):698–703; Sabir, M., Akhter, M. H., Bhide, N. K. Further studies on pharmacology of berberine. *Indian Journal of Physiology and Pharmacology* 22(1978):9–23.

8. Okuyama, E., Nakamura, T., Yamazaki, M. Convulsants from star anise (*Illicium verum* hook. F) *Chemical and Pharmaceutical Bulletin (Tokyo)* 41(1993):1670–1.

9. Sriamarao, P., Nagpal, S., Rao, B. S., et al. Immediate hypersensitivity to *Parthenium hysterophorus*. II. Clinical studies on the preva-

lence of Parthenium rhinitis. *Clinical and Experimental Allergy* 21(1991):55–62.

10. Jacobston, C. S. Effect of a single oral dose of ascorbic acid on body temperature and trace mineral fluxes in healthy men and women. *Journal of the American College of Nutrition* 9(1990):150–4.

11. Mascolo, N., Jain, R., Jain, S. C., et al. Ethnopharmacologic investigation of ginger (*Zingiber officinale*). *Journal of Ethnopharmacology* 27(1987):129–40.

12. Rogers, P. A., Schoen, A. L., Limehouse, J. Acupuncture for immune-mediated disorders. *Problems in Veterinary Medicine* 4(1992): 162–93.

## Chapter 20: Headache

1. Ziegler, D. K., Hur, Y. M., Bouchard, T. J., et al. Migraine in twins raised together and apart. *Headache* 38(1998):417–22.

2. Aromaa, M., Sillanpaa, M., Rautava, P., Helenius, H. Pain experience of children with headaches and their families: a controlled study. *Pediatrics* 106(2000):270–5.

3. Ferrari, M. Migraine. *Lancet* 351(1998):1043–51.

4. Radnitz, C. L. Food-triggered migraine: a critical review. *Annals of Behavioral Medicine* 12(1990):51–65.

5. Moffett, A. L., Swash, M., Scott, D. F. Effect of chocolate in migraine: a double-blind study. *Journal of Neurology, Neurosurgery, and Psychiatry* 37(1974):445–8.

6. Marcus, D. A., Scharff, L., Turk, D., Gourley, L. M. A double-blind provocative study of chocolate as a trigger of headache. *Cephalgia* 17(1997):855–62.

7. Forsythe, W. I., Redmond, A. Two controlled trials of tyramine in children with migraine. *Developmental Medicine and Child Neurology* 16(1974):794–9; Salfield, S. A. W., Wardley, B. L., Houlsby, W. T., et al. Controlled study of exclusion of dietary vasoactive amines in migraine. *Archives of Diseases in Childhood* 62(1987):458–60.

8. Saper, J. R. Daily chronic headache. *Neurologic Clinics* 8(1990):891–901.

9. Jones, H. E., Herning, R. I., Cadet, J. L.,

Griffiths, R. R. Caffeine withdrawal increases cerebral blood flow velocity and alters quantitative electroencephalography (EEG) activity. *Psychopharmacology* 147(2000):371–7.

10. Silverman, K., Evans, S. L., Strain, E. C., et al. Withdrawal syndrome after the double-blind cessation of caffeine consumption. *New England Journal of Medicine* 327(1992):1109–14; Couturier, E. G., Hering, R., Steiner, T. J. Weekend attacks in migraine patients: caused by caffeine withdrawal? *Cephalgia* 12(1992):99–100; Weber, J. G., Ereth, M. H., Danielson, D. R. Perioperative ingestion of caffeine and postoperative headache. *Mayo Clinic Proceedings* 68(1993):842–5.

11. Cooke, L. J., Rose, M. S., Becker, W. J. Chinook winds and migraine headache. *Neurology* 54(2000):302–7.

12. Solomon, G. D. Circadian rhythm and migraine. *Cleveland Clinic Journal of Medicine* 59(1992):326–9.

13. Maytal, J., Bienowski, R. S., Patel, M., Eviatar, L. The value of brain imaging in children with headaches. *Pediatrics* 96(1995):413–6.

14. Lipton, R. B., et al. Efficacy and safety of acetaminophen, aspirin and caffeine in alleviating migraine headache pain: three double-blind, randomized, placebo-controlled trials. *Archives of Neurology* 55(1998):210–17.

15. Holroyd, K. A., Penzien, D. B. Pharmacological versus nonpharmacological prophylaxis of recurrent migraine headache: a meta-analytic review of clinical trials. *Pain* 42(1990):1–13.

16. Schrader, H., Stovner, J., Helde, G., et al. Prophylactic treatment of migraine with angiotensin converting enzyme inhibitor (lisinopril): randomised, placebo-controlled, crossover study. *British Medical Journal* 322(2001):19–22.

17. Couch, J. R., Hassanein, R. S. Amitryptiline in migraine prophylaxis. *Archives of Neurology* 36(1979):695–9.

18. Drummond, P. D. Effectiveness of methysergide in relation to clinical features of migraine. *Headache* 25(1985):145–6.

19. Bille, B., Ludviggson, J., Sanner, G. Prophylaxis of migraine in children. Ibid. 17(1977):61–3.

20. Rompel, H., Bauermeister, P. W. Etiology of

migraines and prevention with carbamazepine (Tegretol): results of a double-blind crossover study. *South African Medical Journal* 44(1970): 75–80.

21. Winner, P., Rothner, D., Saper, J., et al. A randomized, double-blind, placebo-controlled study of sumatriptan nasal spray in the treatment of acute migraine in adolescents. *Pediatrics* 106(2000):989–97.

22. Hansen, P., Henry, P., Mulder, L. J., et al. The effectiveness of combined oral lysine acetylsalicylate and metoclopromide compared with oral sumatriptan for migraine. *Lancet* 346(1995):923–6.

23. Kabbouche, M. A., Vockell, A. L. B., LeCates, S. L., et al. Tolerability and effectiveness of prochlorperazine for intractable migraine in children. *Pediatrics* 107(2000):62.

24. Drazner, D. L., Lacher, M. E., Kulick, R. L. Use of prochlorperazine for treatment of acute migraine headaches in children and adolescents. *Archives of Pediatrics and Adolescent Medicine* 148(1994):67.

25. Maizels, M., Scott, B., Cohen, W., Chen, W. Intranasal lidocain for treatment of migraine. *JAMA.* 276(1996):319–21.

26. Makheja, A. N., Bailey, J. L. The active principle in feverfew. *Lancet* 2(1981):1054; Heptinstall, S., Williamson, L., White, A., et al. Extracts of feverfew inhibit granule secretion in blood platelets and polymorphonuclear leucoclytes. Ibid. 1(1985):1071–4.

27. Johnson, E. S., Kadam, N. P., Hylands, D. L., et al. Efficacy of feverfew as prophylactic treatment of migraine. *British Medical Journal* 291(1985):569–73.

28. Barsby, R. W., Salan, U., Knight, D. W., et al. Feverfew and vascular smooth muscle: extracts from fresh and dried plants show opposing pharmacological profiles, dependent upon sesquiterpene lactone content. *Planta Medica* 59(1993):20–5.

29. Kemper, K. J. Feverfew. www.mcp.edu/herbal/feverfew/feverfew.pdf.

30. Marks, D. R., Rapoport, A., Padla, D., et al. A double-blind, placebo-controlled trial of intranasal capsaicin for cluster headache. *Cephalgia* 13(1993):114–6.

31. Mustafa, T., Srivastava, K. C. Ginger *(Zingiber officinale)* in migraine headache. *Journal of Ethnopharmacology* 29(1990):267–73.

32. Schattner, P., Randerson, D. Tiger Balm as a treatment of tension headache. *Australian Family Physician* 25(1996):216–21.

33. Villegas-Salas, E., Ponce de Leon, R., Juarez-Perez, M. A. Effect of vitamin B6 on the side effects of a low-dose combined oral contraceptive. *Contraception* 55(1997):245–8.

34. Gallai, V., Sarchielli, P., Coata, G., et al. Serum and salivary magnesium levels in migraine. Results in a group of juvenile patients. *Headache* 32(1992):132–5; Mazzotta, G., Sarchielli, P., Alberti, A., Gallai, V. Intracellular Mg concentration and electromyographical ischemic test in juvenile headache. *Cephalgia* 19(1999):802–9.

35. Mishima, K., Takeshima, T., Shimomura, T., Okada, H., et al. Platelet ionized magnesium, cyclic AMP and cyclic GMP levels in migraine and tension-type headache. *Headache* 37(1997):561–4.

36. Aloisi, P., Marrelli, A., Porto, C., et al. Visual evoked potentials and serum magnesium levels in juvenile migraine patients. Ibid. 37(1997):383–5.

37. Facchinetti, F., Sances, G., Borella, P., et al. Magnesium prophylaxis of menstrual migraine: effects on intracellular magnesium. Ibid. 31(1991):298–301.

38. Egger, J., Wilson, J., Carter, C. L., et al. Is migraine food allergy? A double-blind controlled trial of oligoantigenic diet treatment. *Lancet* 2(1983):865–9.

39. Carter, C. M., Egger, J., Soothill, J. F. A dietary management of severe childhood migraine. *Human Nutrition: Applied Nutrition* 39A(1985):294–303.

40. Mansfield, L. E., Vaughan, T. R., Waller, S. F., et al. Food allergy and adult migraine: double-blind and mediator confirmation of an allergic etiology. *Annals of Allergy* 55(1985):126–9.

41. Grant, E. C. Food allergies and migraine. *Lancet* 1(1979):966–8; Monro, J., Brostoff, J., Carini, C., et al. Food allergy in migraine. Ibid. 2(1980):1–4.

42. Atkins, F. M., Ball, B. D., Bock, A. The relation-

ship between the ingestion of specific foods and the development of migraine headaches in children. *Journal of Allergy and Clinical Immunology* 81(1988):185.

43. Guarnieri, P., Radnitz, C. L., Blanchard, E. B. Assessment of dietary risk factors in chronic headache. *Biofeedback and Self-Regulation* 15(1990):15–25.

44. Lockett, D. M., Campbell, J. F. The effects of aerobic exercise on migraine. *Headache* 32(1992):50–4.

45. Landy, S. H. Pressure, heat, and cold help relieve headache pain. *Archives of Family Medicine* 9(2000):792–3.

46. Holden, E. W., Deichmann, M. M., Levy, J. D. Empirically supported treatments in pediatric psychology: recurrent pediatric headache. *Journal of Pediatric Psychology* 24(1999):91–109.

47. Holroyd, K. A., Nash, J. L., Pingel, J. D., et al. A comparison of pharmacological (amitryptiline HCl) and nonpharmacological (cognitive-behavioral) therapies for chronic tension headaches. *Journal of Consulting and Clinical Psychology* 59(1991):387–93.

48. Fentress, D. W., Masek, D. J., Mehegan, J. E., et al. Biofeedback and relaxation-response training in the treatment of pediatric migraine. *Developmental Medicine and Child Neurology* 28(1986):139–46; Engel, J. M. Relaxation training: a self-help approach for children with headaches. *American Journal of Occupational Therapy* 46(1992):591–6.

49. Engel, J. M., Rapoff, M. A., Pressman, A. R. Long-term follow-up of relaxation training for pediatric headache disorders. *Headache* 32(1992):152–6.

50. Primavera, J. P., Kaiser, R. S. Nonpharmacological treatment of headache: is less more? Ibid. 32(1992):393–5.

51. Olness, K., MacDonald, J. T., Uden, D. L. Comparison of self-hypnosis and propranolol in the treatment of juvenile classic migraine. *Pediatrics* 79(1987):593–7.

52. Spinhoven, P., Linssen, A. C., VanDyck, R., et al. Autogenic training and self-hypnosis in the control of tension headache. *General Hospital Psychiatry* 14(1992):408–15; Labbe, E. E. Treatment of childhood migraine with auto-

genic training and skin temperature biofeedback: a component analysis. *Headache* 35(1995):10–3.

53. Bussone, G., Grazzi, L., D'Amico, D., et al. Biofeedback-assisted relaxation training for young adolescents with tension-type headache: a controlled study. *Cephalgia* 18(1998):463–7.

54. Sartory, G., Muller, B., Metsch, J., Pothmann, R. A comparison of psychological and pharmacological treatment of pediatric migraine. *Behaviour Research and Therapy* 36(1998):1155–70.

55. Lisspers, J., Ost, L. G. Long-term follow-up of migraine treatment: do the effects remain up to six years? Ibid. 28(1990):313–22.

56. Powers, S. W., Mitchell, M. J., Byars, K. C., et al. A pilot study of one-session biofeedback training in pediatric headache. *Neurology* 56(2001):133.

57. Budzynski, T. H., Stoyva, J. L., Adler, C. S., et al. EMG biofeedback and tension headache: a controlled outcome study. *Psychosomatic Medicine* 35(1973):484–96; Cox, D. J., Freundlich, A., Meyer, R. G. Differential effectiveness of electromyograph feedback, verbal relaxation instructions and medication placebo with tension headaches. *Journal of Consulting and Clinical Psychology* 43(1975):892–8.

58. Grazzi, L., Leone, M., Frediani, F., et al. A therapeutic alternative for tension headache in children: treatment and one-year follow-up results. *Biofeedback and Self-Regulation* 15(1990):1–6.

59. Nuechterlein, K. H., Holroyd, J. C. Biofeedback in the treatment of tension headache. *Archives of General Psychiatry* 37(1980):866–73.

60. Allen, K. D., McKeen, L. R. Home-based multicomponent treatment of pediatric migraine. *Headache* 31(1991):467–72; Cott, A., Parkinson, W., Fabich, M., et al. Long-term efficacy of combined relaxation: biofeedback treatments for chronic headache. *Pain* 51(1992):49–56.

61. Wylie, K. R., Jackson, C., Crawford P. M. Does psychological testing help to predict response to acupuncture or to massage/relaxation therapy in patients presenting to a general

neurology clinic with headache? *Journal of Traditional Chinese Medicine* 17(1997):130–9.

62. Hernandez-Reif, M., Dieter, J., Field, T., et al. Migraine headaches are reduced by massage therapy. *International Journal of Neuroscience* 96(1998):1–11.

63. Launso, L., Brendstrup, E., Arnberg, S. An exploratory study of reflexological treatment for headache. *Alternative Therapies in Health and Medicine* 5(1999):57–65.

64. Gobel, H., Schmidt, G., Soyka, D. Effect of peppermint and eucalyptus oil preparations on neurophysiological and experimental algesimetric headache parameters. *Cephalgia* 14(1994):228–34.

65. Levoska, S., Keinanen-Kiukaanniemi, S. Active or passive physiotherapy for occupational cervicobrachial disorders? A comparison of two treatment methods with a one-year follow-up. *Archives of Physical Medicine and Rehabilitation* 74(1993):425–30.

66. Tuchin, P. J., Pollard, H., Bonello, R. A randomized, controlled trial of chiropractic spinal manipulative therapy for migraine. *Journal of Manipulative and Physiological Therapeutics* 23(2000):91–5.

67. Bove, G., Nilsson, N. Spinal manipulation in the treatment of episodic tension-type headache: a randomized controlled trial. *JAMA* 280(1998):1576–9.

68. Boivie, J., Brattberg, G. Are there long-lasting effects on migraine headache after one series of acupuncture treatments? *American Journal of Chinese Medicine* 15(1987):69–75; Tavola, T., Gala, C., Conte, G., et al. Traditional Chinese acupuncture in tension-type headache: a controlled study. *Pain* 48(1992):325–9.

69. Dowson, D. I., Lewith, G. T., Machin, D. The effects of acupuncture versus placebo in the treatment of headache. Ibid. 21(1985):35–42; Vincent, C. A. A controlled trial of the treatment of migraine by acupuncture. *Clinical Journal of Pain* 5(1989):305–12.

70. Hu, J. Acupuncture treatment of migraine in Germany. *Journal of Traditional Chinese Medicine* 18(1998):99–101.

71. Jensen, O. K., Nielsen, F. F., Vosmar, L. An open study comparing manual therapy with the use of cold packs in the treatment of post-traumatic headache. *Cephalgia* 10(1990):241–50; Lenhard, L., Waite, P. L. Acupuncture in the prophylactic treatment of migraine headaches: pilot study. *New Zealand Medical Journal* 96(1983):663–6; Baischer, W. Acupuncture and migraine: long-term outcome and predicting factors. *Headache* 35(1995):472–4.

72. Hesse, J., Mogelvang, B., Simonsen, H. Acupuncture versus metoprolol in migraine prophylaxis: a randomized trial of trigger point inactivation. *Journal of Internal Medicine* 235(1994):451–6; Gao, S., Zhao, D., Xie, Y. A comparative study on the treatment of migraine headache with combined distant and local acupuncture points versus conventional drug therapy. *American Journal of Acupuncture* 27(1999):27–30.

73. Pintov, S., Lahat, E., Alstein, M., et al. Acupuncture and the opioid system: implications in the management of migraine. *Pediatric Neurology* 17(1997):129–33.

74. Vincent, C. A. The treatment of tension headache by acupuncture: a controlled single case design with a time series analysis. *Journal of Psychosomatic Research* 34(1990):553–61; Melchart, D., Linde, K., Fischer, P., et al. Acupuncture for recurrent headaches: a systematic review of randomized, controlled trials. *Cephalgia* 19(1999):779–86.

75. Carlsson, J., Fahlcrantz, A., Augustinsson, L. E. Muscle tenderness in tension headache treated with acupuncture or physiotherapy. Ibid. 10(1990):131–41.

76. Hansen, P. E., Hansen, J. H. Acupuncture treatment of chronic tension headache: a controlled, cross-over trial. Ibid. 5(1985):137–42.

77. Keller, E., Bzdek, V. L. Effects of Therapeutic Touch on tension headache pain. *Nursing Research* 35(1986):101–6.

78. Straumshein, P., Borchgrevink, C., Mowinckel, P., et al. Homeopathic treatment of migraine: a double-blind, placebo controlled trial of 68 patients. *The British Homeopathic Journal* 89(2000):4–7.

79. Ernst, E. Homeopathic prophylaxis of headaches and migraine? A systematic review. *Journal of Pain Symptom and Management* 18(1999):353–7.

80. Lipton, R. B., Stewart, W. F., Stone, A. M., Lainez M. J. A., Sawyer J. P. C. Stratified care vs. step care strategies for migraine. *JAMA* 284(2000):2599–605.

## Chapter 21: Hyperactivity (Attention Deficit Hyperactivity Disorder)

1. Zito, J. M., Safer, D. J., dosReis, S., et al. Psychotherapeutic medication patterns for youths with attention deficit hyperactivity disorder. *Archives of Pediatrics and Adolescent Medicine* 153(1999):1257–63.
2. Wasserman, R. C., Kelleher, K. J., Bocian, A., et al. Identification of attentional and hyper-activity problems in primary care: a report from pediatric research in office settings and the ambulatory sentinel practice network. *Pediatrics* 103(1999):E38.
3. Safer, D. J., Malever, M. Stimulant medication in Maryland public schools. Ibid. 106(2000): 533–9.
4. Zito, J. M., Safer, D. J., dosReis, S., et al. Trends in the prescribing of psychotropic medica-tions to preschoolers. *JAMA* 23(2000):1025–30.
5. Committee on Quality Improvement: Subcom-mittee on Attention-Deficit/Hyperactivity Disorder. Clinical Practice Guideline: Diagnosis and evaluation of the child with attention-deficit/hyperactivity disorder. *Pediatrics* 105(2000):1158–70.
6. Fergusson, D. M., Horwood, L. J., Lynskey, M. T. Maternal smoking before and after preg-nancy: effects on behavioral outcomes in middle childhood. Ibid. 92(1993):815–22.
7. Fried, P. A., O'Connell, C. M., Watkinson, B. 60- and 72-month follow-up of children prenatally exposed to marijuana, cigarettes and alcohol: cognitive and language assessment. *Journal of Developmental and Behavioral Pediatrics* 13(1992):383–91.
8. Weitzman, M., Gortmacher, S., Sobol, A. Maternal smoking and behavior problems of children. *Pediatrics* 90(1992):342–9.
9. Byrd, R. S., Roghmann, K. J., Weitzman, M. Predictors of early school failure among chil-dren in the United States. *Archives Journal of Diseases of Children* 147(1993):459.

10. Rydelius, P. A. Children of alcoholic fathers: their social adjustment and health status over twenty years. *Acta Paediatrica Scandinavica* 286(1981)(Suppl):81–85.
11. Roizen, N. J., Blondis, T. A., Irwin, M., et al. Psychiatric and developmental disorders in families of children with attention-deficit hyperactivity disorder. *Archives of Pediatrics and Adolescent Medicine* 150(1996):203–8.
12. Wolraich, M. L., Wilson, D. B., White, J. W. The effect of sugar on behavior or cognition in children. *JAMA* 274(1995):1617–21; Mahan, L. K., Chase, M., Furkawa, C. T., et al. Sugar "allergy" and children's behavior. *Annals of Allergy* 61(1988):453–8.
13. Wender, E. H., Solanto, M. V. Effects of sugar on aggressive and inattentive behavior in chil-dren with attention deficit disorder with hyperactivity and normal children. *Pediatrics* 88(1991):960–6; Gans, D. A., Harper, A. E., Bachorowski, J. A., et al. Sucrose and delin-quency: oral sucrose tolerance test and nutri-tional assessment. Ibid. 86(1990):254–62.
14. Bachoroworski, J. A., Newman, J. P., Nichols, S. L., et al. Sucrose and delinquency: behav-ioral assessment. Ibid. 86(1990):244–53.
15. Behar, D., Rapoport, J. L., Adams, A. J., et al. Sugar challenge testing with children consid-ered behaviorally "sugar reactive." *Nutrion and Behavior* 1(1984):277–88.
16. Blass E. M. and Hoffmeyer, L. B. Sucrose as an analgesic for newborn infants. *Pediatrics* 87(1991):215–8.
17. Saravis, S., Schachar, R., Zlotkin, S., et al. Aspartame: effects on learning, behavior, and mood. Ibid. 86(1990):75–83.
18. Shaywitz, B. A., Sullivan, C. M., Anderson, G. M., et al. Aspartame, behavior, and cognitive func-tion in children with attention deficit disorder. Ibid. 93(1994):70–5.
19. Arbeit, M. L., Nicklas, T. A., Frank, G. C., et al. caffeine intakes of children from a biracial population: the Bogalusa Heart Study. *Journal of the American Dietetic Association* 88(1988): 466–71.
20. Bernstein, G. A., Carroll, M. E., Crosby, R. D., et al. Caffeine effects on learning, performance and anxiety in normal school-age children.

*Journal of the American Academy of Child and Adolescent Psychiatry* 33(1994):407–15.

21. Harley, J., Ray, R., Tomasi, L., et al. Hyperkinesis and food additives: testing the Feingold hypothesis. *Pediatrics* 61(1978):818–28.

22. Conners, C. Goyette, C., Southwick, D., et al. Food additives and hyperkinesis: a double-blind experiment. Ibid. 58(1976):154–66.

23. Salzman, L. Allergy testing, psychological assessment and dietary treatment of the hyperactive child syndrome. *Medical Journal Australia* 2(1976):248–51; Tryphonas, H., Trites, R. Food allergy in children with hyper-sensitivity, learning disabilities and /or mini-mal brain dysfunction. *Annals of Allergy* 42(1979):22–7; Egger, J., Stolla, A. and McEwen, L. M. Controlled trial of hypsensiti-zation in children with food-induced hyperki-netic syndrome. *Lancet* 1(1992):1150–3.

24. Boris, M., Mandel, F. S. Foods and additives are common causes of the attention deficit hyperactive disorder in children. *Annals of Allergy* 72(1994):462–8.

25. Castellanos, F. X. Toward a pathophysiology and attention deficit hyperactivity disorder. *Clinical Pediatrics* (July 1997):381–9; Vandenbergh, D. J. Thompson, M. D., Cook, E. H. Human dopamine transporter gene: coding region conservation among normal, Tourette's disorder, alcohol dependence and attention-deficit hyperactivity disorder popu-lations. *Molecular Psychiatry* 5(2000):283–92.

26. Owens, J. A., Maxim, R., Nobile, C., et al. Parental and self-report of sleep in children with atten-tion deficit hyperactivity disorder. *Archives of Pediatrics and Adolescent Medicine* 154(2000): 549–55.

27. Biederman, J., Faraone, S., Milberger, S., et al. Predictors of persistence and remission of ADHD into adolescence: results from a four-year prospective follow-up study. *Journal of the American Academy of Child Psychiatry* 35(1996):343–51.

28. Barkley, R. A., Murphy, K. R., Kwasnik, D. Motor vehicle competencies and risks in teens and young adults with attention deficit hyper-activity disorder. *Pediatrics* 98(1996):1089–95; Barkley, R. A., Guevremont, D. C., Anastopoulos, A. D., et al. Driving-related risks and outcomes of attention deficit hyperactivity disorder in adolescents and young adults: a 3- to 5-year follow-up survey. Ibid. 92(1993):212–8.

29. Leibson, C. L., Katusic, S. K., Barbaresi, W. J., et al. Use and costs of medical care for children and adolescents with and without attention-deficit/hyperactivty disorder. *JAMA* 285(2001): 60–6; DiScala, C., Lescohier, I., Barthel, M., Li, G. Injuries to children with attention deficit hyperactivity disorder. *Pediatrics* 102(1998):1415–21.

30. Gittelman, R., Mannuzza, S., Shenker, R., et al. Hyperactive boys almost grown up: Psychiatric status. *Archives of General Psychiatry* 42(1985):937–47.

31. Stubberfield, T. G., Wray, J. A., Parry, T. S. Utilization of alternative therapies in attention deficit hyperactivity disorder. *Journal Paediatrics and Child Health* 35(1999):450–3.

32. Safer, D., Krager J. M. Hyperactivity and inat-tentiveness: school assessment of stimulant treatment. *Clinical Pediatrics* 28(1989):216–21; Pelham, W. E., Bender, M. E., Caddell, J., et al. Methylphenidate and children with attention deficit disorder: dose effects on classroom academic and social behavior. *Archives of General Psychiatry* 42(1985):948–52.

33. Committee on Children with Disabilities and Committee on Drugs, American Academy of Pediatrics. Medication for Children with an Attention Deficit Disorder. *Pediatrics* 80(1987):758–60.

34. Rappley, M. D., Mullan, P. B., Alvarez, F. J., et al. Diagnosis of attention-deficit/hyperactivity disorder and use of psychotropic medication in very young children. *Archives of Pediatrics and Adolescent Medicine* 153(1999):1039–45.

35. MTA Cooperative Group. A 14-month random-ized clinical trial of treatment strategies for attention-deficit/hyperactivity disorder. *Archives of General Psychiatry* 56(1999):1073–86.

36. McBride, M. C. An individual double-blind cross-over trial for assessing methylphenidate response in children with attention deficit dis-order. *Journal of Pediatrics* 113(1988):137–45.

37. Kent, M. A., Camfield, C. S., Camfield, P. R. Double-blind methylphenidate trials. *Archives*

*of Pediatrics and Adolescent Medicine* 153(1999): 1292–6.

38. Safer, D. J., Allen, R. P. Absence of tolerance to the behavioral effects of methylphenidate in hyperactive and inattentive children. *Journal of Pediatrics* 115(1989):1003–8.

39. Ahmann, P. A., Waltonen, S. J., Olson, K. A., et al. Placebo-controlled evaluation of Ritalin side effects. *Pediatrics* 91(1993):1101–6.

40. Feldman, H., Crumrine, P., Handen, B. L. Methylphenidate in children with seizures and attention deficit disorder. *Archives Journal of Diseases of Children* 143(1989):1081–6.

41. Kent, J. D., Blader, J. C., Koplewicz, H. S., et al. Effects of late afternoon methylphenidate administration on behavior and sleep in attention-deficit hyperactivity disorder. *Pediatrics* 96(1995):320–5; Stein, M. A., Blondis, T. A., Schnitzler, E. R., et al. Methylphenidate dosing: twice daily versus three times daily. Ibid. 98(1996):748–56.

42. Zametkin, A., Rapoport, J. Neurobiology of attention deficit disorder with hyperactivity: Where have we come in 50 years? *Journal of the American Academy of Child and Adolescent Psychiatry* 26(1987):676–86.

43. Pelham, W. E., Gnagy, E. M., Chronis, A. M., et al. A comparison of morning-only and morning/late afternoon Adderall to morning-only, twice-daily and three times-daily methylphenidate in children with attention-deficit/hyperactivity disorder. *Pediatrics* 104(1999):1300–11.

44. Efron, D., Jarman, F., Barker, M. Side effects of methylphenidate and dexamphetamine in children with attention deficit hyperactivity disorder: a double-blind, crossover trial. Ibid. 100(1997):662–6.

45. White, S., Yadao, C. M. Characterization of methylphenidate exposures reported to a regional poison control center. *Archives of Pediatrics and Adolescent Medicine* 154(2000):1199–1203.

46. Biederman, J., Wilens, T., Mick, E., et al. Pharmacotherapy of attention-deficit/hyperactivity disorder reduces risk for substance abuse disorder. *Pediatrics* 104(1999):20.

47. Spencer, T., Biederman, J., Wilens, T., et al. Effectiveness and tolerability of tomoxetine in adults with attention deficit hyperactivity disorder. *American Journal of Psychiatry* 155(1998):693–5.

48. Rodgers, G. C., Matyunas, N. J., Chenault, B. Clonidine poisoning: an unrecognized complication of attention deficit hyperactivity disorder. *Pediatrics* 102(1998):723.

49. Greenblatt, J. Nutritional supplements in ADHD. *Journal of the American Academy of Child and Adolescent Psychiatry* 38(1999):1209–10, Heimann, S. W. Pycnogenol for ADHD? Ibid. 38(1999):357–8.

50. Firestone, P., Davey, J., Goodman, J. T., et al. The effects of caffeine and methylphenidate on hyperactive children. *Journal of the American Academy of Child Psychiatry* 17(1978):445–56; Huestis, R. D., Arnold, L. E., Smeltzer, D. J. Caffeine versus methylphenidate and d-amphetamine in minimal brain dysfunction: a double-blind comparison. *American Journal of Psychiatry* 132(1975):868–70.

51. Garfinkel, B. D., Webster, C. D., Sloman, L. Responses to methylphenidate and varied doses of caffeine in children with attention deficit disorder. *Canadian Journal of Psychiatry* 26(1981):395–401.

52. Arnold, I. E., Votolato, N. A., Kleykamp, D., et al. Does hair zinc predict amphetamine improvement of ADD/Hyperactivity? *International Journal of Nutrition* 50(1990):103–7; Arnold, L. E., Pinkham, S. M., Votolato, N. Does zinc moderate essential fatty acid and amphetamine treatment of attention-deficit/hyperactivity disorder? *Journal of Child and Adolescent Psychopharmacolgy* 10(2000): 111–7.

53. Baumgaertel, A. Alternative and controversial treatments for attention-deficit/hyperactivity disorder. *Pediatric Clinics of North America* 46(1999):977–92.

54. Chan, E., Gardiner, P., Kemper, K. J. At least it's natural. . . . Herbs and dietary supplements in ADHD. *Contemporary Pediatrics* 17(2000):116–30; Smits, M. G., et al. Melatonin for chronic sleep onset insomnia in children with attention deficit hyperactivity disorder: randomised placebo controlled trial. *Journal of Neurology, Neurosurgery, and Psychiatry* 67(1999):840.

55. Kinsbourne, M. Sugar and the hyperactive child. *New England Journal of Medicine* 330(1994):335–6.

56. Swanson, J. M., Kinsbourne, M. Food dyes impair performance of hyperactive children on a laboratory learning test. *Science* 207(1980):1485–7.

57. Mattes, J. The Feingold diet: a current re-appraisal. *Journal of Learning Disability* 16(1983):319–23; Thorley, G. Pilot study to assess behavioral and cognitive effects of artificial food colours on a group of retarded children. *Developmental Medicine and Child Neurology* 26(1984):56–61.

58. Carter, C. M., Urbanowicz, M., Hemsley, R., et al. Effects of a few food diet in attention deficit disorder. *Archives of Diseases in Childhood* 69(1993):564–8.

59. Loffredo, D. A., Omizo, M., Hammett, V. L. Group relaxation training and parental involvement with hyperactive boys. *Journal of Learning Disabilities* 17(1984):210–3.

60. Klein, P. S. Responses of hyperactive and normal children to variations in tempo of background music. *The Israel Journal of Psychiatry and Related Sciences* 18(1981):157–66.

61. Denkowski, K. M., Denkowski, G. C., Omizo, M. M. The effects of EMG-assisted relaxation training on the academic performance, locus of control and self-esteem of hyperactive boys. *Biofeedback and Self-Regulation* 8(1983):363–75.

62. Potashkin, B. D., Beckles, N. Relative efficacy of Ritalin and biofeedback treatments in the management of hyperactivity. Ibid. 15(1990):305–15.

63. Lee, S. W. Biofeedback as a treatment for childhood hyperactivity: a critical review of the literature. *Psychological Reports* 68(1991): 163–92.

64. Kroll, D. The role of biofeedback in the treatment of attention deficit disorder. *Alternative and Complementary Therapies* Sept(1995): 290–4.

65. Linden, M., Habib, T., Radojevic, V. A controlled study of the effects of EEG biofeedback on cognition and behavior of children with attention deficit disorder and learning disabil-ities. *Biofeedback and Self-Regulation* 21(1996):35; Nash, J. K. Treatment of attention deficit hyperactivity disorder with neurother-apy. *Clinical EEG (Electroencephalography)* 31(2000):30–7.

66. Field, T. M., Quintino, O., Hernandez-Reif, M., Koslovsky, G. Adolescents with attention deficit hyperactivity disorder benefit from massage therapy. *Adolescence* 33(1998):103–8.

67. Smith, M. O. Use of acupressure beads in the treatment of ADHD. *Clinical Acupuncture and Oriental Medicine* 1(1999):31–2.

68. Lamont, J. Homeopathic treatment of Attention Deficit/Hyperactivity Disorder: A controlled study. *British Homeopathic Journal* 86(1997):196–200; Strauss, L. C. The efficacy of a homeopathic preparation in the manage-ment of attention deficit/hyperactivity disor-der. *BT: Biomedical Therapy* 18(2000):197–201.

## Chapter 22: Jaundice

1. Newman, T. B., Klebanoff, M. A. Neonatal hyperbilirubinemia and long-term outcome: another look at the Collaborative Perinatal Project. *Pediatrics* 92(1993):651–7.

2. Stocker, R., Yamamoto, Y., McDonagh, A. F., et al. Bilirubin is an antioxidant of possible phys-iologic importance. *Science* 235(1987):1043–5.

3. Newman, T. B., Easterling, J., Goldman, E. S., et al. Laboratory evaluation of jaundice in newborns. *Archives Journal of Diseases of Children* 144(1990):364–8.

4. Alpay, F., Sarici, S. U., Tosuncuk, D., et al. The value of first-day bilirubin measurement in predicting the development of significant hyperbilirubinemia in healthy term newborns. *Pediatrics* 106(2000):e16.

5. Kemper, K. J., Horwitz, R. I., McCarthy, P. J. Decreased neonatal serum bilirubin with plain agar: a meta-analysis. Ibid. 82(1988):631–8.

6. Yeung, C. Y., Leung, C. S., Chen, Y. Z. An old traditional herbal remedy for neonatal jaun-dice with a newly identified risk. *Journal of Paediatrics and Child Health* 29(1993):292–4; Chan, T. Y. The prevalence, use and harmful potential of some Chinese herbal medicines in

babies and children. *Veterinary and Human Toxicology* 36(1994):238–40.

7. Nicoll, A., Ginsburg, R., Tripp, J. H. Supplementary feeding and jaundice in newborns. *Acta Paediatrica Scandinavica* 71(1982): 759–61; DeCarvalho, M., Hall, M., Harvey, D. Effects of water supplementation of physiologic jaundice in breast-fed babies. *Archives of Diseases in Childhood* 56(1981):568–9.

8. DeCarvalho, M., Klaus, M. H., Merkatz, R. B. Frequency of breast-feeding and serum bilirubin concentration. *Archives Journal of Diseases of Children* 136(1982):737–8.

9. Yamauchi, Y., Yamanouchi, I. Breast-feeding frequency during the first 24 hours after birth in full-term neonates. *Pediatrics* 86(1990):171–5.

10. Elander, G., Lindberg, T. Hospital routines in infants with hyperbilirubinemia influence the duration of breastfeeding. *Acta Paediatrica Scandinavica* 75(1986):708–12.

11. Gourley, G. F., Kreamer, B., Cohnen, M., Kosorok, M. R. Neonatal jaundice and diet. *Archives of Pediatrics and Adolescent Medicine* 153(1999):1002–3.

12. DeAngelis, C., Sargent, J., Chun, M. K. Breast milk jaundice. *Wisconsin Medical Journal* 79(1980):40–2.

13. Provisional Committee for Quality Improvement and Subcommittee on Hyperbilirubinemia. Practice Parameter: Management of hyperbilirubinemia in the healthy term newborn. *Pediatrics* 94(1994):558–65.

14. Kemper, K. J., Forsyth, B. W., McCarthy, P. J. Jaundice, terminating breast-feeding and the vulnerable child. Ibid. 84(1989):773–8.

15. Tan, K. L. Comparison of the efficacy of fiberoptic and conventional phototherapy for neonatal hyperbilirubinemia. *Journal of Pediatrics* 125(1994):607–12; Holtrop, P. C., Ruedisueli, K., Maisels, M. J. Double versus single phototherapy in low birthweight infants. *Pediatrics* 90(1992):674–7.

16. Jackson, J. C. Adverse events associated with exchange transfusion in healthy and ill newborns. Ibid. 99(1997):e7.

17. Braud, W. Distant mental influence of rate of hemolysis of human red blood cells. *Research in Parapsychology* (1989):1–6; Braud, W.,
David, G., Wood, R. Experiments with Matthew Manning. *Journal of Psychical Research* 50(1979):199–223.

18. Krieger, D. *The Therapeutic Touch.* Englewood Cliffs, NJ: Prentice Hall, 1979.

## Chapter 23: Ringworm and Other Fungal Infections

1. Givens, T. G., Murray, M. M., Baker, R. C. Comparison of 1% and 2.5% selenium sulfide in the treatment in tinea capitis. *Archives of Pediatrics and Adolescent Medicine* 149(1995): 808–11.

2. Savin, R., Atton, A. V., Bergstresser, P. R., et al. Efficacy of terbinafine 1% cream in the treatment of moccasin-type tinea pedis: results of placebo-controlled multicenter trials. *Journal of the American Academy of Dermatology* 30(1994): 663–7; Haroon, T. S., Hussain, I., Mahmood, A., et al. An open clinical pilot study of the efficacy and safety of oral terbinafine in dry noninflammatory tinea capitis. *British Journal of Dermatology* 126(1992):47–50.

3. Naftifine Podiatric Study Group. Naftifine cream 1% versus clotrimazole cream 1% in the treatment of tinea pedis. *Journal of the American Podiatric Medical Association* 80(1990):314–8.

4. Chren, M. M., Landefeld, C. S. A cost analysis of topical drug regimens for dermatophyte infections. *JAMA* 272(1994):1922–5.

5. Tong, M. L., Altman, P. L., Barnetson, R. S. Tea tree oil in the treatment of tinea pedis. *Australasian Journal of Dermatology* 33(1992): 145–9.

6. Appleton, J. A., Tansey, M. R. Inhibition of growth of zoopathogenic fungi by garlic extract. *Mycologia* 67(1975):409–13; Yamada, Y., Azuma, K. Evaluation of the in vitro antifungal activity of allicin. *Antimicrobial Agents and Chemotherapy* 11(1977):743–9.

7. Kishore, N., Mishra, A. K., Chansouria, J. P. Fungitoxicity of essential oils against dermatophytes. *Mycoses* 36(1993):211–5; Gundidza, M. Antifungal activity of essential oil from *Artemisia afra* Jacq. *Central African Journal of Medicine* 39(1993):140–2.

8. Daferera, D. J., Ziogas, B. N., Polissiou, M. G. GC-MS analysis of essential oils from some Greek aromatic plants and their fungitoxicity on *Penicillium digitatum*. *Journal of Agricultural and Food Chemistry* 48(2000):2576–81.

9. Garg, A. P., Muller, J. Inhibition of growth of dermatophytes by Indian hair oils. *Mycoses* 35(1992):363–9.

## Chapter 24: Sleep Problems

1. Owens, J. A., Spirito, A., McGuinn, M., et al. Sleep habits and sleep disturbance in elementary and school-age children. *Journal of Developmental and Behavioral Pediatrics* 21(2000):27–36.

2. Meijer, A. M., Habekothe, H. T., Vanden Wittenboer, G. Time in bed, quality of sleep and school functioning of children. *Journal of Sleep Research* 9(2000):145–53.

3. Blader, J. C., Koplewicz, H. S., Abikoff, H., Foley, C. Sleep problems of elementary school children. *Archives of Pediatrics and Adolescent Medicine* 151(1997):473–80.

4. Thunstrom, M. Severe sleep problems among infants: family and infant characteristics. *Ambulatory Child Health* 5(1999):27–41.

5. Stein, M. A., Mendelsohn, J., Obermeyer, W. H., et al. Sleep and behavior problems in school-age children. *Pediatrics* 107(2001):e60.

6. Owens, J. A., Maxim, R., Nobile, C., et al. Parental and self-report of sleep in children with attention-deficit/hyperactivity disorder. *Archives of Pediatrics and Adolescent Medicine* 154(2000):549–55; Gruber, R., Sadeh, A., Raviv, A. Instability of sleep patterns in children with attention-deficit/hyperactivity disorder. *American Academy of Child and Adolescent Psychiatry* 39(2000):495–501.

7. Chang, P. P., Ford, D. E., Mead, L. A., et al. Insomnia in young men and subsequent depression. *American Journal of Epidemiology* 146(1997):105–14.

8. Kahn, A., Mozin, M., Casimir, G., et al. Insomnia and cow's milk allergy in infants *Pediatrics* 76(1985):880–4.

9. Kahn, A., Francois, G., Sottiaux, M., et al. Sleep characteristics in milk-intolerant infants. *Sleep* 11(1988):291–7.

10. Wood, J. M., Bootzin, R. R., Rosenhan, D., et al. Effects of the 1989 San Francisco earthquake on frequency and content of nightmares. *Journal of Abnormal Psychology* 101(1992): 219–24.

11. Owens, J., Maxim, R., McGuinn, M., et al. Television-viewing habits and sleep disturbances in school children. *Pediatrics* 104(1999):27.

12. Gyllenhaal, C., Block, K. I., Peterson, S. D., et al. Herbal remedies: efficacy in controlling sleepiness and promoting sleep. *Nurse Practitioner Forum* 11(2)(2000):87–100.

13. Zuckerman, B., Stevenson, J., Bailey, V. Sleep problems in early childhood: continuities, predictive factors and behavioral correlates. *Pediatrics* 80(1987):664–71.

14. Kaplan, B. J., McNicol, J., Conte, R. A., et al. Sleep disturbances in preschool-aged hyperactive and nonhyperactive children. Ibid. 80(1987):839–44.

15. Pinilla, T., Birch, L. L. Help me make it through the night: behavioral entrainment of breast-fed infants' sleep patterns. Ibid. 91(1993):436–44.

16. Wolfson, A., Lacks, P., Futterman, A. Effects of parent training on infant sleeping patterns, parents' stress, and perceived parental competence. *Journal of Consulting and Clinical Psychology* 60(1992):41–8.

17. Spadafora, A., Hunt, H. T. The multiplicity of dreams: cognitive-affective correlates of lucid, archetypal and nightmare dreaming. *Perceptual and Motor Skills* 71(1990):627–44.

18. Leathwood, P., Chauffard, F., Heck, E., et al. Aqueous extract of valerian root *(Valeriana officianalis L.)* improves sleep quality in man. *Pharmacology, Biochemistry, and Behavior* 17(1982):65–71.

19. Leathwood, P., Chauffard, F. Aqueous extract of valerian reduces latency to fall asleep in man. *Planta Medica* 54(1985):144–8.

20. Lindahl, O., Lindwall, L. Double-blind study of a valerian preparation. *Pharmacology, Biochemistry, and Behavior* 32(1989):1065–6.

21. MacGregor, F. B., Abernethy, V. E., Dahabra, S., et al. Hepatoxicity of herbal remedies. *British Medical Journal.* 299(1989):1156–7.

22. Houghton, P. J. The biological activity of valer-

ian and related plants. *Journal of Ethnopharmacology* 22(1988):121–42.

23. Yogman, M. W. Zeisel, S. H. Diet and sleep patterns in newborn infants. *New England Journal of Medicine* 309(1983):1147–9; Griffiths, W., Lester, B., Coulter, J., et al. Tryptophan and sleep in young adults. *Psychophysiology* 9(1972):345–56.

24. Steinberg, L. A., O'Connell, N. C., Hatch, T. F., et al. Tryptophan intake influences infants' sleep latency. *The Journal of Nutrition* 122(1992):1781–91.

25. Okawa, M., Mishima, K., Nanami, T., et al. Vitamin B12 treatment for sleep-wake rhythm disorders. *Sleep* 13(1990):15–23.

26. Attenburrow, M. E. J., Dowling, B. A., Sharpley, A. L., Cowen, P. J. Case-control study of evening melatonin concentration in primary insomnia. *British Medical Journal* 312(1996):1263–4.

27. Macknin, M. L., Medendorp, S. V., Maier, M. C. Infant sleep and bedtime cereal. *American Journal of Diseases of Children* 143(1989):1066–8.

28. Keane, V., Charney, E., Straus, J., et al. Do solids help baby sleep through the night? Ibid. 142(1988):404–5.

29. King, A. C., Oman, R. F., Brassington, G. S., et al. Moderate-intensity exercise and self-rated quality of sleep. *JAMA* 277(1997):32–7.

30. Youngstedt, S. D., Kripke, D. F., Elliott, J. A. Is sleep disturbed by vigorous late night exercise? *Medicine and Science in Sports and Exercise* 31(1999):864–9.

31. Anderson, J. E. Co-sleeping: can we ever put the issue to rest? *Contemporary Pediatrics* 17(2000):98.

32. Mosko, S., Richard, C., McKenna, J. Infant arousals during mother-infant bed sharing: implications for infant sleep and sudden infant death syndrome research. *Pediatrics* 100(1997):841–9.

33. Latz, S., Wolf, A. W., Lozoff, B. Co-sleeping in context; sleep practices and problems in young children in Japan and the United States. *Archives of Pediatrics and Adolescent Medicine* 153(1999):339–46.

34. Willinger, M., Hoffman, H. J., Wu, K. T., et al. Factors associated with the transition to non-prone sleep positions of infants in the United States. *JAMA* 280(1998):329–35.

35. Brenner, R. A., Simons-Morton, B. G., Bhaskar, B., et al. Prevalence and predictors of the prone sleep position among inner-city infants. Ibid. 280(1998):341–6.

36. Fleming, P. J., Glibert, R., Azaz, Y., et al. Interaction between bedding and sleeping position in the sudden infant death syndrome: a population based case-control study. *British Medical Journal* 301(1990):85–9.

37. Rickert, V. I., Johnson, M. Reducing nocturnal wakening and crying episodes in infants and young children: A comparison between scheduled awakenings and systematic ignoring. *Pediatrics* 90(1992):554–60.

38. Lask, B. Novel and nontoxic treatment for night terrors. *British Medical Journal* 297(1988):502.

39. Adams, L. A, Rickert, V. I. Reducing bedtime tantrums: comparison between positive routines and graduated extinction. *Pediatrics* 84(1989):756–61.

40. NIH Technology Assessment Panel. Integration of behavioral and relaxation approaches into the treatment of chronic pain and insomnia. *JAMA* 276(1996):313–8.

41. Gardner, G. G. and Olness, K. *Hypnosis and hypnotherapy with children.* Orlando, Fla: Grune and Stratton Inc, 1981, p. 113.

42. Neidhardt, E. J., Krakow, B., Kellner, R., et al. The beneficial effects of one treatment session and recording of nightmares on chronic nightmare sufferers. *Sleep* 15(1992):470–3.

43. Kohen, D. P., Mahowald, M. W., Rosen, G. M. Sleep-terror disorder in children: the role of self-hypnosis in management. *American Journal of Clinical Hypnosis* 34(1992):233–44.

44. Kellner, R., Neidbardt, J., Krakow, B., et al. Changes in chronic nightmares after one session of desensitization or rehearsal instructions. *American Journal of Psychiatry* 149(1992):659–63.

45. Palace, E. M., Johnston, C. Treatment of recurrent nightmares by the dream reorganization approach. *Journal of Behavior Therapy and Experimental Psychiatry* 20(1989):219–26.

46. Woolfolk, R. L., Carr-Kaffashan, L., McNulty, T. F. Meditation training as a treatment for insomnia. *Behavior Therapy* 7(1976):359–65.

47. Morin, C. M., Culbert, J. P., Schwartz, S. M. Nonpharmacological interventions for insomnia: a meta-analysis of treatment efficacy. *American Journal of Psychiatry* 151(1994): 1172–80.

48. McMenamy, C., Katz R. C. Brief parent-assisted treatment for children's nighttime fears. *Journal of Developmental and Behavioral Pediatrics* 10(1989):145–8.

49. King, N., Cranstoun, F., Josephs, A. Emotive imagery and children's nighttime fears: a multiple baseline design evaluation. *Journal of Behavior Therapy and Experimental Psychiatry* 20(1989):125–35.

50. Barowsky, E. I., Moskowitz, J., Zweig, J. B. Biofeedback for disorders of initiating and maintaining sleep. *Annals of the New York Academy of Sciences* 602(1990):97–103.

51. Field, T., Morrow, C., Valdeon, C., et al. Massage reduces anxiety in child and adolescent psychiatric patients. *Journal of the American Academy of Child and Adolescent Psychiatry* 31(1992):125–31.

52. Marcus, C. L., Carroll, J. L., Koerner, C. B., et al. Determinants of growth in children with the obstructive sleep apnea syndrome. *Journal of Pediatrics* 125(1994):556–62.

53. Nieto, F. J., Young, T. B., Lind, B. K., et al. Association of sleep-disordered breathing, sleep apnea and hypertension in a large community-based sample. *JAMA* 283(2000):1829–36.

54. Soultan, Z., Wakdowski, S., Rao, M., Kravath, R. E. Effect of treating obstructive sleep apnea by tonsillectomy and /or adenoidectomy on obesity in children. *Archives of Pediatrics and Adolescent Medicine* 153(1999):33–37.

55. Krieger, D., Peper, E., Ancoli, S. The physiological indices of Therapeutic Touch. *American Journal of Nursing* 4(1979):660–5; Heidt, P. Effect of Therapeutic Touch on the anxiety level of hospitalized patients. *Nursing Research* 30(1981):32–7.

56. Heidt, T. R. Helping patients to rest: Clinical studies in Therapeutic Touch. *Holistic Nursing Practice* 5(1991):57–66.

57. Braun, C., Layton, J., Braun, J. Therapeutic Touch improves residents' sleep. *Journal— American Health Care Association* 12(1986): 48–9.

## Chapter 25: Sore Throats

1. Bisno, A. L. Acute pharyngitis: etiology and diagnosis. *Pediatrics* 57(1996):S949–54.

2. Sharland , M., Hodgson, J., Davies, E. G., et al. Enteroviral pharyngitis diagnosed by reverse transcriptase-polymerase chain reaction. *Archives of Diseases in Childhood* 74(1996): 462–3.

3. Pichichero, M. E., Marsocci, S. L., Murphy, M. L., et al. Incidence of streptococcal carriers in private pediatric practice. *Archives of Pediatrics and Adolescent Medicine* 153(1999):624–8.

4. Dajani, A., Taubert, K., Ferrieri, P., et al. Treatment of acute streptococcal pharyngitis and prevention of rheumatic fever: a statement for health professionals. *Pediatrics* 96(1995):758–64.

5. Poses, R. L., Cebul, R. D., Collins, M., Fager, S. S. The accuracy of experienced physicians' probability estimates for patients with sore throats. Implications for decision making. *JAMA* 254(1985):925.

6. Webb, K. H. Does culture confirmation of high-sensitivity rapid streptococcal tests make sense? *Pediatrics* 101(1998):2.

7. Tsevat, J., Kotagal, U. R. Management of sore throats in children: a cost-effectiveness analysis. *Archives of Pediatrics and Adolescent Medicine* 154(2000):93–4.

8. Kaplan, E. L. Recent epidemiology of group A streptococcal infections in North America and Abroad. *Pediatrics* 97(1996):945–8.

9. Bertin, L., Pons, G., D'Athis, P., et al. Randomized, double-blind, multicenter, controlled trial of ibuprofen versus acetaminophen (paracetamol) and placebo for treatment of symptoms of tonsillitis and pharyngitis in children. *Journal of Pediatrics* 119(1991):811–4.

10. Lan, A. J., Colford, J. M. The impact of dosing frequency on the efficacy of 10-day penicillin or amoxicillin therapy for streptococcal tonsillopharyngitis. *Pediatrics* 105(2000):19.

11. Feder, H. L., Gerber, M. A., Randolph, M. F., et al. Once-daily therapy for streptococcal pharyngitis with amoxicillin. Ibid. 103(1999): 47–51.

12. El-Daher, N. T., Hijazi, S. S., Rawashdeh, N. L.,

et al. Immediate vs. delayed treatment of group A beta-hemolytic streptococcal pharyngitis with penicillin, V. *Pediatric Infectious Disease Journal* 10(1991):126–30.

13. Pichichero, M. E., Disney, F. A., Talpey, W. B., et al. Adverse and beneficial effects of immediate treatment of group A beta-hemolytic streptococcal pharyngitis with penicillin. Ibid. 6(1987):635–43.

14. Gerber, M. A., Randolph, M. F., DeMeo, K. K., Kaplan, E. L. Lack of impact of early antibiotic therapy for streptococcal pharyngitis on recurrence rates. *Journal of Pediatrics* 117(1990):853–8.

15. Amir, J., Harel, L., Smetana, Z., Varsano, I. Treatment of herpes simplex gingivostomatitis with acylcovir in children: a randomised double-blind placebo controlled study. *British Medical Journal* 314(1997):1800–3.

16. Partridge, M., Poswillo, D. Topical carbonoxolone sodium in the management of herpes simplex infection. *British Journal of Oromaxillofacial Surgery* 22(1984):138–45; Poswillo, D., Partridge, M. Management of recurrent aphthous ulcers. *British Dental Journal* 157(1984): 55–7.

17. Sun, D., Courtney, H. S., Beachey, E. H. Berberine sulfate blocks adherence of *Streptococcus pyogenese* to epithelial cells, fibronectin, and hexadecane. *Antimicrobial Agents and Chemotherapy* 32(1988):1370–4.

18. Farbman, K. S., Barnett, E. D., Bolduc, G. R., Klein, J. O. Antibacterial activity of garlic and onions: a historical perspective. *Pediatric Infectious Disease Journal* 12(1993):613–4.

19. Paradise, J. L., Bluestone, C. D., Bachman, R. Z., et al. Efficacy of tonsillectomy for recurrent throat infection in severely affected children: results of parallel randomized and nonrandomized clinical trials. *New England Journal of Medicine* 310(1984):674–83.

## Chapter 26: Vomiting and Nausea

1. Chan, T. Y., Tomlinson, B., Critchley, J. A. Aconitine poisoning following the ingestion of Chinese herbal medicines: a report of 8 cases. *Australian and New Zealand Journal of Medicine* 23(1993):268–71; Kao, W. F., Hung, D. Z., Tsai, W. J., et al. Podophyllotoxin intoxication: toxic effect of Bajiaolian in herbal therapeutics. *Human and Experimental Toxicology* 11(1992): 480–7.

2. Venter, C. P., Joubert, P. H. Aspects of poisoning with traditional medicines in Southern Africa. *Biomedical and Environmental Sciences* 1(1988):388–91.

3. Aapro, M. S., Froidevaux, P., Roth, A., et al. Antiemetic efficacy of droperidol or metoclopramide combined with dexamethasone and diphenhydramine. Randomized open parallel study. *Oncology* 48:(1991)116–20; Mori, K., Saito, Y., Tominaga, K. Antiemetic efficacy of alprazolam in the combination of metoclopramide plus methylprednisolone: double-blind randomized crossover study in patients with cisplatin-induced emesis. *American Journal of Clinical Oncology* 16(1993):338–41.

4. Mowrey, D. B., and Clayson, D. E. Motion sickness, ginger and psychophysics. *Lancet* March(1982):655–7; Grontved, A., Brask, T., Kambskard, J., and Hentzer, E. Ginger root against seasickness: a controlled trial on the open sea. *Acta Oto-laryngologica* 105(1988): 45–9; Yamahara, J., Rong, H. Q., Naitoh, Y., et al. Inhibition of cytotoxic drug-induced vomiting in suncus by a ginger constituent. *Journal of Ethnopharmacology* 27(1989):353–5.

5. Bone, M. E., Wilkinson, K. J., Young, J. R., et al. Ginger root—a new antiemetic: the effect of ginger root on postoperative nausea and vomiting after major gynecological surgery. *Anaesthesia* 45(1990):669–71.

6. Weizman, Z., Alkrinawi, S., Goldfarb, D., Bitran, C. Efficacy of herbal tea preparation in infantile colic. *Journal of Pediatrics* 122(1993): 650–2.

7. Sahakian, V., Rouse, D., Sipes, S., et al. Vitamin B6 is effective therapy for nausea and vomiting of pregnancy: a randomized, double-blind placebo-controlled study. *Obstetrics and Gynecology* 78(1991):33–6.

8. McGuinness, B. W., Binns, D. T. "Debendox" in pregnancy sickness. *Journal of the Royal College of General Practitioners* 21(1971):500–3.

9. Mattie, H., Emery, E. W., Hill, I. D., et al.

Treatment of radiation sickness with pyridoxine hydrochloride in outpatients of a radiotherapy unit. *British Medical Journal* 3:(1967): 215–6.

10. Davis, J. M., Burgess, W. A., Slentz, C. A. Effects of ingesting 6% and 12% glucose/electrolyte beverages during prolonged intermittent cycling in the heat. *European Journal of Applied Physiology* 57(1988):563–9.

11. Orenstein, S. R., Magill, H. L., Brooks, P. Thickening of infant feedings for therapy of gastroesophageal reflux. *Journal of Pediatrics* 110(1987):181–6.

12. Iacono, G., Carroccio, A., Cavataio, F., et al. Gastroesophageal reflux and cow's milk allergy in infants: A prospective study. *Journal of Allergy and Clinical Immunology* 97(1996): 822–7.

13. Moses, F. M. The effect of exercise on the gastrointestinal tract. *Sports Medicine* 9(1990): 159–72.

14. Motil, K. J., Ostendorf, J., Bricker, J. T., et al. Exercise-induced gastroesophageal reflux in an athletic child. *Journal of Pediatric Gastroenterology and Nutrition* 6(1987):989–91.

15. Brouns, F., Beckers, E. Is the gut an athletic organ? Digestion, absorption and exercise. *Sports Medicine* 15(1993):242–57.

16. Cheung, B. S., Money, K. E., Jacobs, I. Motion sicknesss susceptibility and aerobic fitness: a longitudinal study. *Aviation, Space, and Environmental Medicine* 61(1990):201–4.

17. Cadranel, J. F., Tarbe de Saint Hardouin, C., Elouaer-Blanc, L., et al. Hypnosis for intractable vomiting. *Lancet* 1(1987):1140.

18. Zeltzer, L. K., Dolgin, M. J., LeBaron, S., et al. A randomized, controlled study of behavioral intervention for chemotherapy distress in children with cancer. *Pediatrics* 88(1991):34–42; Jacknow, D. S., Tschann, J. M., Link, M. P., et al. Hypnosis in the prevention of chemotherapy-related nausea and vomiting in children: a prospective study. *Journal of Developmental and Behavioral Pediatrics* 15(1994):258–64.

19. LaGrone, R. G. Hypnobehavioral therapy to reduce gag and emesis with a 10-year-old pill swallower. *American Journal of Clinical Hypnosis* 36(1993):132–6.

20. Sokel, B. S., Devane, S. P., Bentovim, A., et al. Self hypnotherapeutic treatment of habitual reflex vomiting. *Archives of Disease in Childhood* 65(1990):626–7.

21. Burish, T. G., Jenkins, R. A. Effectiveness of biofeedback and relaxation training in reducing the side effects of cancer chemotherapy. *Health Psychology* 11(1992):17–23; Banks, R. D., Salisbury, D. A., Ceresia, P. J. The Canadian Forces Airsickness Rehabilitation Program, 1981–1991. *Aviation, Space, and Environmental Medicine* 63(1992):1098–101.

22. Dundee, J. W., Chestnutt, W. N., Ghaly, R. G., et al. Traditional Chinese acupuncture: a potentially useful antiemetic? *British Medical Journal* 293(1986):583–4.

23. Barsoum, G., Perry, E. P., Fraser, I. A. Postoperative nausea is relieved by acupressure. *Journal of the Royal Society of Medicine* 83(1990):86–9; Gieron, C., Wieland, B., von der Laage, D., et al. Acupressure in the prevention of postoperative nausea and vomiting. *Anaesthesist* 42(1993):221–6.

24. Ghaly, R. G., Fitzpatrick, K. T., Dundee, J. W. Antiemetic studies with traditional Chinese acupuncture. A comparison of manual needling with electrical stimulation and commonly used antiemetics. Ibid. 42(1987):1108–10.

25. Dundee, J. W. Belfast experience with P6 acupuncture antiemesis. *Ulster Medical Journal* 59(1990):63–70.

26. Dundee, J. W., Sourial, F. B., Ghaly, R. G., et al. P6 acupressure reduces morning sickness. *Journal of the Royal Society of Medicine* 81(1988):456–7.

27. Hyde, E. Acupressure therapy for morning sickness. A controlled clinical trial. *Journal of Nurse-Midwifery* 34(1989):171–8.

28. Dundee, J. W., McMillan, C. M. Clinical uses of P6 acupuncture antiemesis. *Acupuncture and Electrotherapeutics Research* 15(1990):211–5.

29. Dundee, J. W., Yang. J., McMillan, C. Noninvasive stimulation of the P6 (Neiguan) antiemetic acupuncture point in cancer chemotherapy. *Journal of the Royal Society of Medicine* 84(1991):210–2; Lewis, I. H., Pryn, S. J., Reynolds, P. I., et al. Effect of P6 acupres-

sure on postoperative vomiting in children undergoing outpatient strabismus correction. *British Journal of Anaesthesia* 67(1991):73–8; Yentis, S. M., Bissonnette, B. P6 acupuncture and postoperative vomiting after tonsillectomy in children. Ibid. 67(1991):779–80.

30. Dundee, J. W., Ghaly, R. G., Bill, K. M., et al. Effect of stimulation of P6 antiemetic point on postoperative nausea and vomiting. Ibid. 63(1989):612–8.

## Chapter 27: Warts

1. Glass, A. T., Solomon, B. A. Cimetidine therapy for recalcitrant warts in adults. *Archives of Dermatology* 133(1997):530–1.
2. Yilmaz, E., Alpsoy, E., Basaran, E. Cimetidine therapy for warts: a placebo-controlled, double-blind study. *Journal of the American Academy of Dermatology* 34(1996):1005–7.
3. Stern, P., Levine, N. Controlled localized heat therapy in cutaneous warts. *JAMA* 268(1992): 3307.
4. Spanos, N. P., Stenstrom, R. J., Johnston, J. C. Hypnosis, placebo and suggestion in the treatment of warts. *Psychosomatic Medicine* 50(1988):246–60.
5. Noll, R. B. Hypnotherapy for warts in children and adolescents. *Journal of Developmental and Behavioral Pediatrics* 15(1994):170–3.
6. Tasini, M. F., Hackett, T. P. Hypnosis in the treatment of warts in immunodeficient children. *American Journal of Clinical Hypnosis* 19(1977):152–4.
7. Labrecque, M., Audet, D., Latulippe, L. G., et al. Homeopathic treatment of plantar warts. *Canadian Medical Association Journal* 146(1992):1749–53.
8. Smolle, J., Prause, G., Kerl, H. A double-blind, controlled clinical trial of homeopathy and an analysis of lunar phases and postoperative outcome. *Archives of Dermatology* 134(1998): 1368–70.

# INDEX